# www.wadsworth.com

*wadsworth.com* is the World Wide Web site for Wadsworth Publishing Company and is your direct source to dozens of online resources.

At *wadsworth.com* you can find out about supplements, demonstration software, and student resources. You can also send e-mail to many of our authors and preview new publications and exciting new technologies.

**wadsworth.com**
Changing the way the world learns®

# AN INVITATION TO HEALTH

# AN INVITATION TO HEALTH

Brief Third Edition

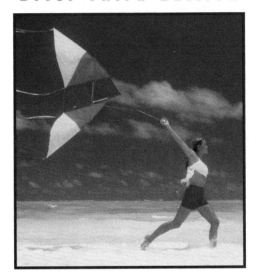

## Dianne Hales

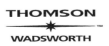

THOMSON

WADSWORTH

Australia · Canada · Mexico · Singapore · Spain · United Kingdom · United States

## THOMSON
*TM*
## WADSWORTH

Acquisitions Editor: April Lemons
Assistant Editor: Andrea Kesterke
Technology Project Manager: Travis Metz
Marketing Manager: Jennifer Somerville
Marketing Assistant: Melanie Wagner
Advertising Project Manager: Shemika Britt
Project Manager, Editorial Production: Sandra Craig
Print/Media Buyer: Karen Hunt
Permissions Editor: Joohee Lee
Production: The Book Company
Text and Cover Designer: Hespenheide Design
Photo Researcher: Myrna Engler
Development Editor: Patricia Brewer
Copy Editor: Lorna Cunkle
Illustrations: Hespenheide Design
Cover Image: Radiance/ImageState
Compositor: Parkwood Composition
Printer: Transcontinental Printing

Printed in Canada
1  2  3  4  5  6  7  07  06  05  04  03

---

For more information about our products, contact us at:
**Thomson Learning Academic Resource Center**
**1-800-423-0563**
For permission to use material from this text, contact us by:
**Phone:** 1-800-730-2214        **Fax:** 1-800-730-2215
**Web:** http://www.thomsonrights.com

---

**Wadsworth/Thomson Learning**
**10 Davis Drive**
**Belmont, CA 94002-3098**
**USA**

**Asia**
Thomson Learning
5 Shenton Way #01-01
UIC Building
Singapore 068808

**Australia/New Zealand**
Thomson Learning
102 Dodds Street
Southbank, Victoria 3006
Australia

**Canada**
Nelson
1120 Birchmount Road
Toronto, Ontario M1K 5G4
Canada

**Europe/Middle East/Africa**
Thomson Learning
High Holborn House
50/51 Bedford Row
London WC1R 4LR
United Kingdom

**Latin America**
Thomson Learning
Seneca, 53
Colonia Polanco
11560 Mexico D.F.
Mexico

**Spain/Portugal**
Paraninfo
Calle/Magallanes, 25
28015 Madrid, Spain

Library of Congress Control Number: 2003104059

ISBN 0-534-59818-8
Instructor's Edition: ISBN 0-534-59819-6

*To my husband, Bob, and my daughter, Julia, who make every day an invitation to joy.*

# Brief Contents

# Contents

# Key Features

✔ Updated statistics on the benefits of exercise.
✔ New section on the possibility of being fat and fit.
✔ New section on the principles of exercise, including a table of FIT guidelines for cardiovascular exercise, strength, and flexibility.
✔ Updated table on exercise heart ranges.
✔ Expanded coverage of sports safety, including temperature considerations.

## Chapter 5   Personal Nutrition

✔ New section on nutrients: macronutrients (protein, carbohydrates, fats) and micronutrients (vitamins and minerals). Includes nutrient data from the new Institute of Medicine report, and tables with key information on vitamins and minerals.
✔ New sections on antioxidants, phytochemicals, and functional foods.
✔ New section on dietary and vitamin supplements.

## Chapter 6   Eating Patterns and Problems

✔ New section on body composition assessment.
✔ Updated table on energy requirements from new Institute of Medicine report.
✔ Updated information on disordered eating in college students, including a table on body weight concerns.
✔ New section on who develops eating disorders.
✔ New information (and figure) on the dangers of obesity.

## Chapter 7   Communication and Sexuality

✔ New discussion on listening.
✔ New section on how sexually active college students are.
✔ New coverage of "sober sex," including a safer sex section.

## Chapter 8   Reproductive Choices

✔ Updated table on contraceptive methods includes effectiveness, level of protection against STDs, and cost.
✔ New sections on the contraceptive ring and the contraceptive patch.
✔ New information from study concerning availability of emergency contraceptives to college students.
✔ Expanded section on infertility now includes information on artificial insemination and infertility treatments.

## Chapter 9   Protecting Yourself from Infectious Diseases

✔ New section on the agents of infection.
✔ Updated statistics on the West Nile virus.
✔ New Strategies for Prevention box on how to protect yourself from insect-borne diseases.
✔ New table on immunization recommendations for adults.
✔ New section on biological warfare.

## Chapter 10   Lowering Your Risk of Major Diseases

✔ Updated information on the best diet for a healthy heart.
✔ New section on metabolic syndrome.
✔ New section helps students understand their lipoprotein profile, and includes methods for reducing cholesterol levels.
✔ Expanded coverage of stroke.
✔ New table on recommended screenings for cancer.
✔ New coverage of studies on breast self-exam and the benefits of mammography.

## Chapter 11   Drug Use, Misuse, and Abuse

✔ New table on common drugs of abuse.
✔ Expanded section on physiological risks of marijuana use.
✔ Expanded section on the club drug ecstasy.

## Chapter 12   Alcohol and Tobacco Use, Misuse, and Abuse

✔ Updated sections on college drinking and binge drinking.
✔ New section on the toll of college drinking.
✔ Expanded section on tobacco use on campus.
✔ New section on smoking and women.
✔ New section on bidis.

## Chapter 13   Consumerism, Complementary and Alternative Medicine, and the Health-Care System

✔ New section on quackery.
✔ New section on doctors and CAM.

## Chapter 14 Staying Safe: Preventing Injury, Violence, and Victimization

✔ New section on individual risk factors for unintentional injury.
✔ Expanded section on road safety including safe driving and safe cycling.
✔ New Strategies for Change box on coping with the threat of violence and terrorism.
✔ New section on hate crimes.

## Chapter 15 A Lifetime of Health (A New Chapter)

In response to instructors and students, this chapter has been added to include coverage of the following important topics:
✔ The aging brain.
✔ Sexuality and aging.
✔ Dealing with death and grief.

## Chapter 16 Working Toward a Healthy Environment

✔ Updated coverage on global warming, including the Kyoto Protocol.
✔ Updated statistics on drinking water.
✔ Updated statistics on chemical risks.

### Features and Pedagogy

**FAQs (Frequently Asked Questions)** are found at the beginning of each chapter to engage students with answers to the most commonly asked health questions, such as "How do you catch an infection?" "Should I take vitamins?" "What can help me relax?" Page references are included after each question, and each corresponding heading is marked with an icon, signaling where the answer can be found.

**The X&Y Files** are boxes found throughout the text that focus on topics related to gender differences in health. Among the topics covered: differences in susceptibility to cancer, differences in stress vulnerabilities, differences in communication styles, differences in vulnerability to alcohol and drug abuse, and more.

**Strategies for Change** boxes appear throughout the text and provide practical, checklist-format behavioral change strategies for achieving better health.

**Strategies for Prevention** boxes appear throughout the text and provide effective, checklist-format strategies for preventing health problems and reducing health risks.

**Student Snapshot** boxes, new to this edition, feature graphs and charts to illustrate data on college populations. Topics include student stress levels, cyber sex on campus, and the social life of college students.

**Savvy Consumer** boxes focus on consumer-related health topics and provide guidelines for being an informed health consumer.

**Making This Chapter Work for You** is a new study feature that reviews important chapter material by asking ten multiple-choice questions. Answers are provided on page 415.

**Sites and Bytes** boxes at the end of every chapter include updated interactive websites and InfoTrac® College Edition activities, encouraging students to use the Internet for additional learning resources.

**Profile Plus®** boxes at the end of every chapter give students a preview of the activities on the CD-ROM that will enhance their study. The Profile Plus CD-ROM is packaged free with every copy of the text.

In addition:

**Learning Objectives** open each chapter and outline the most essential information on which students should focus while reading.

**Key Terms** are boldfaced where they are defined and are listed at the end of each chapter with page references. They are also defined in the Glossary at the end of the book.

**Critical Thinking Questions,** included at the end of each chapter, ask the students to consider some applications of the chapter's coverage or weigh in on health-related controversy.

**CNN Video Discussion Question,** included at the end of each chapter, is designed to work in conjunction with the video of CNN health clips that has been developed for this edition. The CNN health video is complimentary with adoption of this textbook.

**Hales Health Almanac,** bundled free with each copy of this text, is a valuable resource that includes health information on the Internet, advice on what to do in an emergency, a consumer guide to medical tests, tables for counting calories and fat in specific foods, and a health directory.

### Ancillary Package

**Instructor's Manual** The Instructor's Manual provides chapter outlines, learning objectives, key terms, discussion questions, instructor's activities, student handouts, suggestions for additional readings, and video and Internet Resources.

**Test Bank** The test bank contains a variety of questions to assess the students' understanding and comprehension of the text: multiple choice, fill in the blank, matching, and essay questions; and a mid-term exam with questions covering the first eight chapters of the text.

**ExamView** Create, deliver, and customize tests and study guides (both print and online) in minutes with this easy-to-use assessment and tutorial system. ExamView offers both a Quick Test Wizard and an Online Test Wizard that guide you step by step through the process of creating tests, while it allows you to see the test you are creating on the screen exactly as it will print or display online. Using ExamView's complete word-processing capabilities, you can enter an unlimited number of new questions or edit existing ones.

**Multimedia Manager** This dual-platform presentation CD-ROM features illustrations and photographs; a wide array of PowerPoint® slides, featuring art from the text; the Instructor's Manual; and the Test Bank.

**Transparency Acetates** More than 100 transparency acetates of art taken from *An Invitation to Health,* Tenth Edition, plus a correlation guide to help coordinate lectures and reading assignments.

**WebTutor Advantage** WebTutor's text-specific content allows instructors to create and manage a personal website. A course management tool gives instructors the ability to provide virtual office hours, post syllabi, setup threaded discussions, track student progress with quizzing materials, and much more. For students, WebTutor Advantage offers real-time access to a full array of study tools, including chapter outlines, summaries, learning objectives, glossary flashcards (with audio), practice quizzes, web links, InfoTrac College Edition exercises, animations, and videos.

**Study Guide** This excellent aid to students' understanding of the text contains learning objectives, key terms, chapter review questions, and a detailed practice test for each chapter.

**Profile Plus 2004** The most comprehensive software package available with any health textbook, Profile Plus allows students to generate personalized fitness and wellness profiles, conduct self-assessments, analyze their diets, tailor exercise prescriptions to their individual needs, and keep an exercise log. In addition, students have access to a book-specific online study guide complete with practice quizzes, key terms, and much more.

**InfoTrac College Edition Student Guide for Health** This 24-page booklet offers detailed guidance for students on how to use the InfoTrac College Edition database, including log-in help, search tips, and a topic list of key word-search terms for health, fitness, and wellness. Available free when packaged with the text.

**Health, Fitness, and Wellness Internet Explorer** This full-color trifold brochure contains Internet links to more than a dozen of the hottest topics in health, fitness, and wellness.

**Personal Daily Log** The Personal Daily Log contains an exercise pyramid, study and exercise tips, a goal-setting worksheet, a cardiorespiratory exercise record form, a strength training record form, a daily nutrition diary, and helpful Internet links.

**Wellness Worksheets** These detachable self-assessment and wellness worksheets are handy, easy to use, and make a terrific bundle item.

**Careers in Health, Physical Education, and Sport** This comprehensive guide to finding and establishing a career in the field of Health, Physical Education and Sport encourages students to establish personal goals, develop action plans, and research fields of study ranging from entry-level to post-graduate positions. Included are developmental labs at the end of each chapter for students to learn to take a proactive role in the job search process. Helpful hints on topics such as etiquette, ethics, and legal issues as they relate to the career process, make this a tool students will keep long after they graduate.

**Integrative Medicine: The Mind–Body Prescription** Written by Dr. John Janowiak, Appalachian State University, this supplement explains the relationship between Western medical practice and more traditional therapies, and traces the evolution of integrative medicine. Also provided are a detailed list of Internet resources, a comprehensive list of herbs and their interactions and more.

**Diet Analysis 6.0** This unique assessment tool provides students with experience in the estimation and analysis of dietary patterns and practices. Students can track their food intake for up to seven days and create a personal dietary profile based on height, weight, age, gender, and activity level. Diet Analysis Plus calculates dietary reference intakes, goal percentages, and actual percentages of essential nutrients, vitamins, and minerals. Comprehensive dietary data is displayed in attractive, easy-to-read reports that enhance learning. Students can view data as a bar graph, a spreadsheet, in Food Pyramid form, or as a Nutrition Facts panel report. They can identify dietary habits, correct nutritional deficiencies, and truly appreciate the impact of nutrient-dense foods.

**Website** Instructors and students have access to a rich array of teaching and learning resources that cannot be found anywhere else. This outstanding site features student resources, including quizzes, web links, suggested online readings, and discussion forums, and instructor resources, including downloadable supplementary resources and multimedia presentation slides. An online catalog of Wadsworth's health, fitness, wellness, and physical education books and supplements is also available on the website.

**CNN Today: Health and Wellness** Volumes I, II, III These Wadsworth-exclusive videos allow instructors to integrate the news-gathering and programming power of CNN into the classroom to show students the relevance of course topics to their everyday lives. Organized by topics introduced in the text, the clips are presented in two- to five-minute segments. A new video is available each year.

**Relaxation: A Guide to Personal Stress Management** This 30-minute video shows students how to manage their stress. Experts explain relaxation techniques and guide the student through progressive relaxation, guided imagery, breathing, and physical activity.

**Trigger Video Series: Fitness** This 60-minute video focuses on the changing concepts of fitness. Five eight- to ten-minute clips are followed by questions for answer or discussion, and additional material appropriate to the fitness chapter in the text.

**Trigger Video Series: Stress** This 60-minute video focuses on stress. Five eight- to ten-minute clips are followed by questions for answer or discussion, and additional material appropriate to the chapter on stress management.

# Acknowledgments

For the third edition, I was fortunate to work with a terrific team at Wadsworth, with Peter Marshall at its helm. April Lemons, the Health Editor, brought her great expertise and endless enthusiasm to the project. As developmental editor, Pat Brewer contributed the highest levels of skill, creativity, and dedication. Once again, I applaud and admire the production team, headed by Sandra Craig of Wadsworth and Dusty Friedman of The Book Company.

I also am grateful to Hespenheide Design, who has given this edition and the evocative cover the look and feel of a new century; and to Myrna Engler, for her work on photos and permissions. My thanks go to Lorna Cunkle for her meticulous editing of the final manuscript. I also am appreciative of Shemika Britt's work in preparing promotional materials and of Jennifer Somerville's marketing efforts on behalf of the book. Thanks also to editorial assistant Andrea Kesterke.

Finally, I would like to thank the reviewers whose comments have been so valuable:

*Jimmy Anderson,* Macon State College
*Judy B. Backer,* East Carolina University
*Patricia E. Collins-Shotland,* University of North Texas
*Dwalah L. Fisher,* Texas Southern University
*Simone Longpre,* University of British Columbia
*Ann Stine,* Mesa Community College
*Dara M. Vazin,* California State University, Fullerton
*Scott Wolf,* Southwestern Illinois College

For their recent help with the Tenth Edition of the longer book, and for suggestions that influenced the Brief Third Edition as well, I offer my gratitude to:

*Jeremy Barnes,* Southeast Missouri State University
*Carol Biddington,* California University of Pennsylvania
*Richard Capriccioso,* University of Phoenix
*Lori Dewald,* Shippensburg University of Pennsylvania
*Harold Horne,* University of Illinois at Springfield
*Jessica Middlebrooks,* University of Georgia
*Kris Moline,* Lourdes College
*Richard Morris,* Rollins College
*Rosanne Poole,* Tallahassee Community College
*Sadie Sanders,* University of Florida
*Debra Secord,* Coastline College
*Teresa Snow,* Georgia Institute of Technology

# About the Author

Dianne Hales, a contributing editor for *Parade,* has written more than 2,000 articles for national publications. Her trade books include *Just Like a Woman: How Gender Science Is Redefining What Makes Us Female* and the award-winning compendium of mental health information, *Caring for the Mind: The Comprehensive Guide to Mental Health.* Dianne Hales is one of the few journalists to be honored with national awards for excellence in magazine writing by both the American Psychiatric Association and the American Psychological Association. She also has won the EMMA (Exceptional Media Merit Award) for health reporting from the National Women's Political Caucus and Radcliffe College, and numerous writing awards from various organizations, including the Arthritis Foundation, California Psychiatric Society, CHAAD (Children and Adults with Attention-Deficit Disorders), Council for the Advancement of Scientific Education, National Easter Seal Society, and the New York City Public Library.

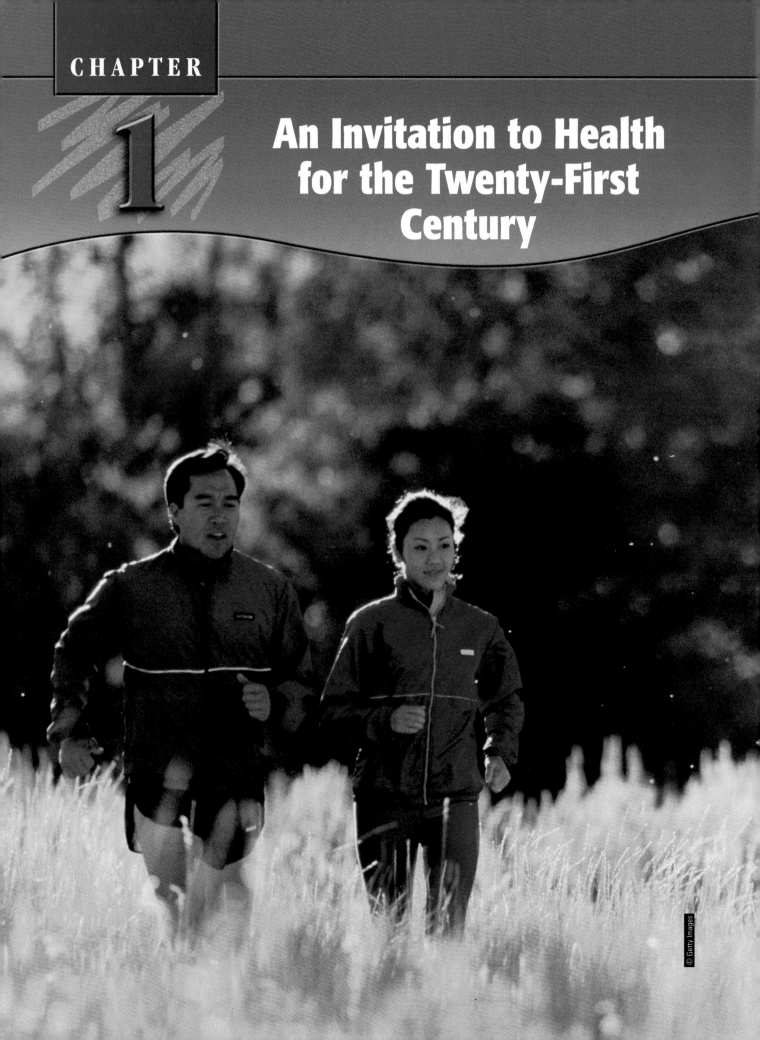

# An Invitation to Health for the Twenty-First Century

**After studying the material in this chapter, you should be able to:**

- **Identify and describe** the components of health and how they relate to total wellness.
- **Describe** how gender, race, and ethnicity can influence health and access to health care.
- **List** the factors that influence the development of health behaviors.
- **Discuss** the principles and goals of prevention, and **differentiate** prevention from protection.
- **Create** a complete plan to change or develop a health behavior.

"How are you?" You may hear that question dozens of times each day.

"Fine," you answer, without thinking. But how often do you ask yourself how you *really* are? How do you feel about yourself and your life? Are you making the most of your life? What do you hope to accomplish before you die?

This book asks these questions and many more. It is a book about you: your mind and your body, your spirit and your social ties, your needs and your wants, your past and your potential. It will help you explore options, discover possibilities, and find new ways to make your life worthwhile.

Health involves more than physical well-being. It is a state of body, mind, and spirit that must be viewed within the context of community, society, and environment. By providing the information and understanding you need to take care of your own health, this brief edition of *An Invitation to Health* can help you live more fully, more happily, and more healthfully. The book's primary themes—prevention of health problems, protection from health threats, and promotion of the health of others—can establish the basis for good health now and in the future.

The invitation to health that we extend to every reader is one offer you literally cannot afford to refuse: The quality of your life depends on it.

 **FREQUENTLY ASKED QUESTIONS**

**FAQ: What is the average life expectancy? p. 7**

**FAQ: Can race affect health? p. 11**

**FAQ: How can I change a bad health habit? p. 17**

# Health and Wellness

By simplest definition, **health** means being sound in body, mind, and spirit. The World Health Organization defines health as "not merely the absence of disease or infirmity," but "a state of complete physical, mental, and social well-being."[1] Health is the process of discovering, using, and protecting all the resources within our bodies, minds, spirits, families, communities, and environment.

Health has many components: physical, psychological, spiritual, social, intellectual, and environmental. This book takes a *holistic* approach, one that looks at health and the individual as a whole, rather than part by part. Your own definition of health may include different elements, but chances are you and your classmates agree that it includes at least some of the following:

✔ A positive, optimistic outlook.
✔ A sense of control over stress and worries; time to relax.
✔ Energy and vitality; freedom from pain or serious illness.
✔ Supportive friends and family, and a nurturing intimate relationship with someone you love.
✔ A personally satisfying job.
✔ A clean environment.

**Wellness** can be defined as purposeful, enjoyable living or, more specifically, a deliberate lifestyle choice characterized by personal responsibility and optimal enhancement of physical, mental, and spiritual health. Wellness means more than not being sick; it means taking steps to prevent illness and to lead a richer, more balanced, and more satisfying life.

Although physical well-being is essential to health, the term *wellness*, as used by health professionals, has a broader meaning. To understand how the concepts of wellness and health fit together, think of an automobile transmission: Having a disease (illness) is like being in reverse; absence of disease (health) puts you in neutral; positive health changes (wellness) push you into forward motion. When

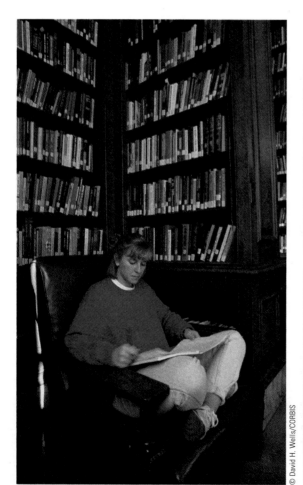

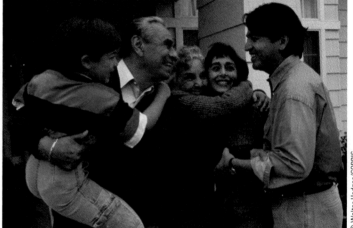

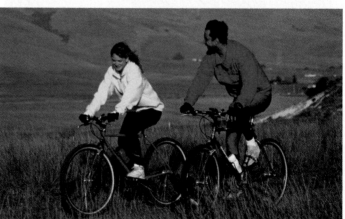

▲ Health is the process of discovering, using, and protecting all the resources within our bodies, minds, spirits, families, communities, and environment.

your entire lifestyle is based on health-enhancing behaviors, you're in high gear and going at top speed—and you've achieved total wellness.

John Travis, M.D., compares the various levels of wellness to an iceberg (see Figure 1-1). Only about one-tenth of the mass of an iceberg is visible—the rest is submerged. Your current state of health is like the tip of the iceberg, the part that shows.

"To understand all that creates and supports your current state of health," says Travis, "you have to look 'underwater.'" The first hidden level—the "lifestyle/behavioral" level—consists of what you eat, how active you are, how you manage stress, and how you protect yourself from hazards. Below this level is the "cultural/psychological/motivational" level, the often invisible influences that lead us to choose a certain lifestyle. The foundation of the iceberg is the "spiritual/being/meaning" realm, which encompasses issues such as your reason for being, the meaning of your life, and your place in the universe. "Ultimately," says Travis, "this realm determines whether the tip of the iceberg, representing your state of health, is one of disease or wellness."[2]

In wellness, health, and sickness, there is considerable overlap of the functions of the mind, body, and spirit. As scientists have shown again and again in recent decades, psychological factors play a major role in enhancing physical well-being and preventing illness, but they can also trigger, worsen, or prolong physical symptoms.

"The mind clearly can have a profound effect on every aspect of physiologic functioning," says James Gordon, M.D., Director of the Center for Mind–Body Studies in Washington, DC. "Individuals who are chronically pessimistic, angry, anxious or depressed are clearly more susceptible to stress and illness, including heart disease and cancer."[3] Similarly, almost every medical illness affects people psychologically as well as physically.

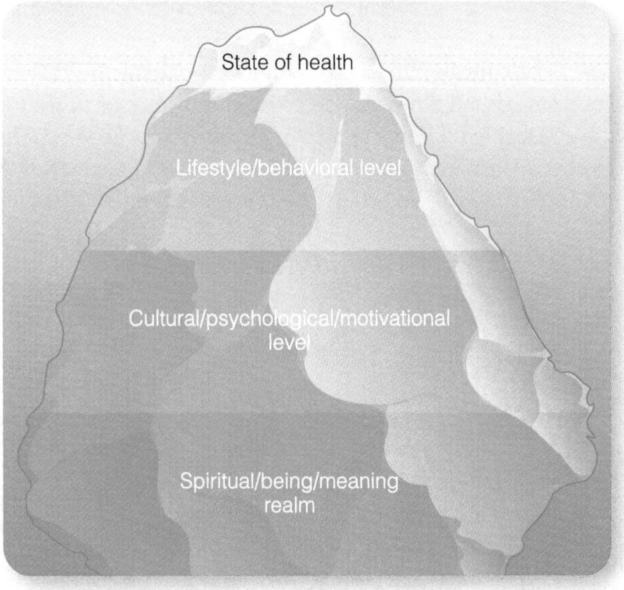

## Physical Health

The various states of good and ill physical health can be viewed as points on a continuum (see Figure 1-2). At one end is early and needless death; at the other is optimal wellness, in which you feel and perform at your very best. In the middle, individuals are neither sick enough to need medical attention nor well enough to live each day with zest and vigor. For the sake of optimal physical health, we must take positive steps away from illness and toward well-being. We must feed our bodies nutritiously, exercise them regularly, avoid harmful behaviors and substances, watch out for early signs of sickness, and protect ourselves from accidents.

## Psychological Health

Like physical well-being, psychological health is more than the absence of problems or illness. Psychological health refers to both our emotional and mental states—that is, to our feelings and our thoughts. It involves awareness and acceptance of a wide range of feelings in oneself and others, the ability to express emotions, to function independently, and to cope with the challenges of daily stressors. (Chapter 3 provides more information on psychological health.)

## Spiritual Health

Spiritually healthy individuals identify their own basic purpose in life; learn how to experience love, joy, peace, and fulfillment; and help themselves and others achieve their full potential. As they devote themselves to others' needs more than their own, their spiritual development produces a sense of greater meaning in their lives.

Americans tend to be both spiritual and religious. According to the most recent in a series of national Gallup polls conducted over the last 60-plus years, 95 percent of Americans believe in God—an all-time high. Most Americans also say that prayer is an important part of their lives, that they believe miracles are performed by a divine

State of health

Lifestyle/behavioral level

Cultural/psychological/motivational level

Spiritual/being/meaning realm

▲ **Figure 1-1** Iceberg Model of Wellness
Like an iceberg, only a small part of your total wellness is visible: your current state of health. Just as important are hidden dimensions, including lifestyle habits, cultural and psychological factors, and the realm of spiritual meaning and being.

Source: Reprinted with permission, Wellness Workbook, Travis & Ryan, Ten Speed Press, Berkeley, CA. © 1981, 1988 by John W. Travis, MD <www.thewellspring.com>

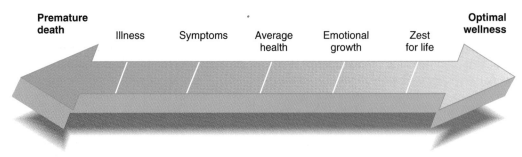

▲ **Figure 1-2** Wellness-Illness Continuum

power, and that they are sometimes conscious of the presence of God.[4] Faced with physical or psychological difficulties, most Americans turn to prayer, reading the Bible, or meditation as a way of coping.[5]

Prayer is the most commonly used form of complementary/alternative medicine. Being prayed for also may have some benefits. In a controlled study of 40 adults with moderately severe rheumatoid arthritis, those who were the recipients of intense praying aloud and "laying on of hands," followed by educational sessions on spirituality and healing, showed improvements in joint swelling and other symptoms. However, blood tests showed no changes in inflammatory markers, a finding suggesting that prayer changed perceptions of illness rather than the illness itself.[6]

The data on the effects of spirituality on health have mounted steadily in recent years. Using data from 126,000 people, scientists at the National Institute for Healthcare Research found that those with some religious involvement, such as attending worship services, were almost 30 percent more likely to live longer than less involved men and women.[7] Open-heart surgery patients who reported drawing strength and comfort from religion had only one-third the risk of dying within six months of the surgery as those who didn't. Believers recovered from depression earlier,[8] and believers became pregnant sooner than other patients at a fertility clinic.[9] Frequent churchgoers also have lower blood pressure and more rigorous immune systems, and they report fewer physical symptoms.[10]

Are religious people simply healthier to begin with? At the very least, they're well enough to get to church. By avoiding sin, they may stay away from harmful habits, such as excessive drinking, taking drugs, smoking, or risky sexual practices.[11] In addition, belonging to a religious congregation may broaden and cement social bonds that buffer the harmful effects of stress, anxiety, and depression. Prayer itself may have a therapeutic effect, inducing the relaxation responses by producing a tranquil state of mind. Faith also may help people understand and interpret negative life situations so they cope better with unexpected upsets.[12]

In one survey of family practitioners, 99 percent said they believe that religious beliefs can heal; 75 percent believe that others' prayers can promote healing. However, more than half felt uncertain about questioning or discussing spirituality with a patient.[13] About half of America's medical schools now offer courses on spirituality and healing. And a growing number of doctors, while not endorsing or prescribing any one approach to religion, are encouraging patients to cultivate a spiritual commitment—for the sake of their mortal bodies as well as their immortal souls.[14]

Some health professionals have long recognized the power and potential of spirituality. For 30 years, Herbert Benson, M.D., head of the Mind/Body Medical Institute at Harvard Medical School, has conducted rigorous experiments to document the influence of the spirit on health. His conclusion: The combination of relaxation and behavioral methods, such as prayer and meditation, with standard surgical and medical treatments can help relieve a host of medical problems, including chronic pain, arthritis, insomnia, and premenstrual symptoms. Improving spiritual health may not cure an illness, but it may help patients feel better, prevent certain illnesses, and cope with disease or death.[15]

"Deeply religious people of all faiths appear to benefit in five major areas," reports Dale Matthews of Georgetown School of Medicine, who reviewed more than 300 studies

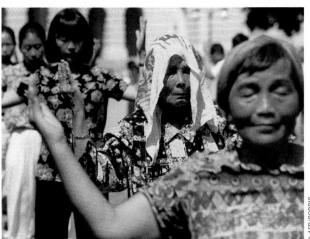

▲ In every culture, religious rituals play an important role in the lives and health of individuals.

on healing and religion.[16] The benefits are: less substance abuse; lower rates of depression and anxiety, especially among women; enhanced quality of life; quicker recovery from injury or illness; and longer life expectancy.

Skeptics point out that none of the research has pinpointed religion rather than another alternative as the direct cause of health benefits. As they note, meditation, exercise, healthful habits, and a strong social network may provide similar benefits.

## Social Health

Social health refers to the ability to interact effectively with other people and the social environment, to develop satisfying interpersonal relationships, and to fulfill social roles. It involves participating in and contributing to your community, living in harmony with fellow human beings, developing positive interdependent relationships with others (discussed in Chapter 7), and practicing healthy sexual behaviors.

For Americans, the terrorist attacks of September 11, 2001, dramatically demonstrated the importance of social connections. As the routines of everyday life stopped, people checked on the safety of loved ones and gathered together in churches, synagogues, university centers, living rooms, parks, and plazas. In times of crisis, social connections provide comfort and support. "Ultimately, community helps us heal from trauma," says psychiatrist Robert Ursano, M.D., author of *The Psychiatric Aspects of Terrorism*.[17]

Even in tranquil times, social isolation increases the risk of sickness and mortality. In a landmark study of 4,725 men and women in Alameda County, California, death rates were

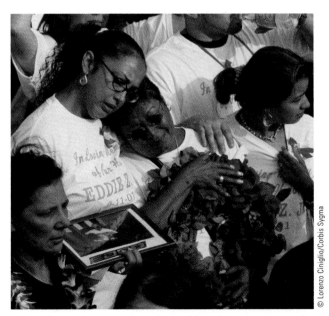

© Lorenzo Ciniglio/Corbis Sygma

▲ Mourners gather together at the World Trade Center memorial service at Ground Zero in New York City.

twice as high for loners as for those with strong social ties. In other studies, social isolation greatly increased the risk of dying of a heart attack. Heart attack patients have a better chance of long-term survival if they believe they have adequate help in performing daily tasks from family and friends. People with spouses, friends, and a rich social network may outlive isolated loners by as much as 30 years.[18]

Health educators are placing greater emphasis on social health in its broadest sense as they expand the traditional individualistic concept of health to include the complex interrelationships between one person's health and the health of the community and environment. This change in perspective has given rise to a new emphasis on **health promotion,** which enhances health by building knowledge and skills among individuals and modifying their environment to foster healthier lifestyles.

## Intellectual Health

Your brain is the only one of your organs capable of self-awareness. Every day you use your mind to gather, process, and act on information; to think through your values; to make decisions, set goals, and figure out how to handle a problem or challenge. Intellectual health refers to your ability to think and learn from life experience, your openness to new ideas, and your capacity to question and evaluate information. Throughout your life, you'll use your critical thinking skills, including your ability to evaluate health information, to safeguard your well-being.

## Environmental Health

You live in a physical and social setting that can affect every aspect of your health. Environmental health refers to the impact your world has on your well-being. It means protecting yourself from dangers in the air, water, and soil, and in products you use—and also working to preserve the environment itself. (Chapter 16 offers a thorough discussion of environmental health.)

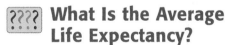

## Health in a New Millennium

### ???? What Is the Average Life Expectancy?

In 1900, the average American woman could expect to live to an age of 50.9 years, compared with 47.9 years for a man. Infectious diseases, such as smallpox and tuberculosis, claimed tens of thousands of lives, particularly among the young and the poor. A high percentage of women died during childbirth or shortly afterward.

At the beginning of the twenty-first century, life expectancy reached a record high of 76.9 years. Both gender and race affect how long we live. (See Figure 1-3 and The X & Y Files: "Do Sex and Gender Matter?") A white girl born in the year 2000 can expect to live to 79.5 years; a black girl, to 75 years. A white baby boy's life expectancy is 74.8 years; a black baby boy's, 68.3 years.[19] While life expectancy has increased by about three years since 1980, African Americans still lag six years behind—regardless of sex or age.[20]

Gains in life expectancy are slowing, primarily because adding decades, or even years, to the lives of people who have already lived for 70 years is much more difficult than adding decades to the lives of children who might otherwise die of infectious diseases. According to current predictions, the practical upper limit for life expectancy is 88 years for women and 82 for men. The French may reach this limit in the year 2033; the Japanese, in 2035; Americans, not until 2182.[21]

## U.S. Health

It may surprise you, but U.S. health is not the best in the world. See Figure 1-4, which ranks the healthiest countries in the world. Why does American health come in 12th in a

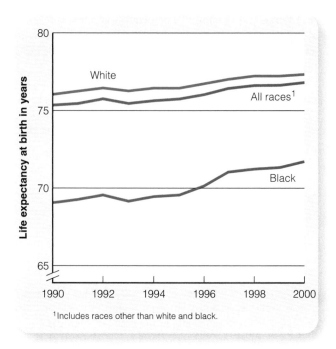

▲ **Figure 1-3** Increases in Life Expectancy in the United States: 1990–2000

Source: *National Vital Statistics Report,* Vol. 49, No. 12, October 9, 2001.

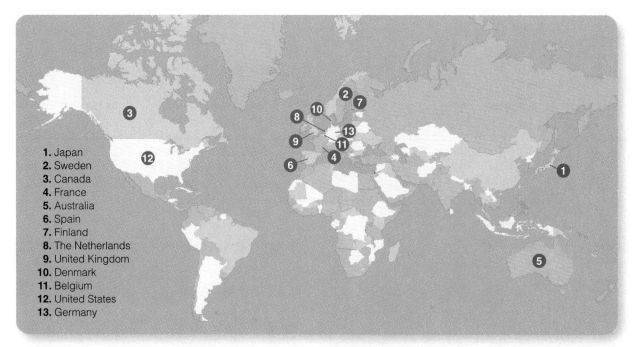

1. Japan
2. Sweden
3. Canada
4. France
5. Australia
6. Spain
7. Finland
8. The Netherlands
9. United Kingdom
10. Denmark
11. Belgium
12. United States
13. Germany

▲ **Figure 1-4** What Are the Healthiest Countries in the World?
Although the United States ranks 7th for life expectancy at age 65, the nation ranks 13th for percentage of low birthweight babies, mortality at birth and during infancy, and years of potential life lost (excluding intentional and nonintentional injury).

Source: Starfield, Barbara. "Is U.S. Health Really the Best in the World?" *Journal of the American Medical Association,* Vol. 284, No. 4, July 26, 2000.

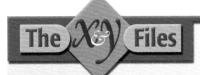

## Do Sex and Gender Matter?

"Sex does matter. It matters in ways that we did not expect. Undoubtedly, it also matters in ways that we have not begun to imagine." This was the conclusion of the Institute of Medicine Committee on Understanding the Biology of Sex and Gender Differences in the first significant review of the status of sex and gender differences in biomedical research.

*Sex,* the committee stated, is "a classification, generally as male or female, according to the reproductive organs and functions that derive from the chromosomal complement." *Gender* refers to "a person's self-representation as male or female, or how that person is responded to by social institutions on the basis of the individual's gender presentation." Rooted in biology, gender is shaped by environment and experience.

In animals other than humans, sex alone influences the prevalence and severity of a broad range of diseases, disorders, and conditions. In human beings, gender also matters. The experience of being male or female in a particular culture and society can and does have an effect on physical and psychological well-being. In fact, sex and gender may have a greater impact than any other variable on how our bodies function, how long we live, and the symptoms, course, and treatment of the diseases that strike us.

This realization is both new and revolutionary. For centuries, scientists based biological theories solely on a male model and viewed women as shorter, smaller, and rounder versions of men. Even modern medicine is based on the assumption that, except for their reproductive organs, both sexes are biologically interchangeable. We now know that this simply isn't so. Sex begins in the womb, but sex and gender differences affect behavior, perception, and health throughout life.

The X & Y Files throughout this book show that virtually every part and organ system of the body differ in men and women (see Figure 1-5). A man's core body temperature runs lower than a woman's; his heart beats at a slower rate. A woman takes 9 breaths a minute; a man averages 12. Her blood carries higher levels of protective immunoglobulin; his has more oxygen-rich hemoglobin. Her ears are more sensitive to sound; his eyes are more sensitive to light. Male brains are 10 percent larger, but certain areas in female brains contain more neurons.

Gender differences persist in sickness as well as in health. Before age 50, men are more prone to lethal diseases, including heart attacks, cancer, and liver failure. Women show greater vulnerability to chronic but non–life-threatening problems such as arthritis and autoimmune disorders. Women are twice as likely to suffer depression; men have a fivefold greater rate of alcoholism. Women outlive men by more than six years, yet they're more prone to age-related problems, such as osteoporosis and Alzheimer's disease. Health behaviors—patterns of drinking, smoking, or using seat belts—also are different in men and women.

More than half of men between ages 18 and 29 do not have a regular physician, compared with a third of women. Seven in ten of those who have not visited a doctor in more than five years are men. Men have fewer dental as well as medical checkups. They're less likely to seek psychiatric services, to have their cholesterol levels and blood pressure checked regularly, and to undergo some form of screening for colon cancer. More women than men are overweight, and fewer women are physically active. Although college men are among those at highest risk of testicular cancer, three out of four do not know how to perform a self-examination. Male undergraduates are much less likely to examine their testicles than female students are to examine their breasts. College-age men also are significantly more likely to engage in risky and physically dangerous behaviors, and to suffer more injuries, including fatal ones, as a result.

Recognition of these gender differences is transforming medical research and practice. A new science called *gender-specific medicine* is replacing one-size-fits-all health care with new definitions of what is normal in both men and women, more complex concepts of disease, more precise diagnostic tests, and more effective treatments.

Sources: Committee on Understanding the Biology of Sex and Gender Differences. *Exploring the Biological Contributions to Human Health: Does Sex Matter?* Washington, DC: Institute of Medicine, National Academy of Sciences, 2001. Hales, Dianne. *Just Like a Woman.* New York: Bantam, 2001. "Biology Shows Women and Men Are Different." *Mayo Clinic Women's Healthsource.* Vol. 6, No. 9, September 2002, p. 1.

---

comparison of 13 countries? Some point to the fact that more than 40 million people have no health insurance. Others observe that among those who can afford health care, 20 to 30 percent receive treatments that may be more harmful than beneficial.[22]

Are health behaviors to blame? Not necessarily. The proportion of men and women who smoke is higher in many other nations. The United States ranks fifth lowest in alcohol consumption. Americans also have relatively low consumption of animal fats. However, our nation has the dubious distinction of outranking all others in deaths due to motor vehicle accidents and violence.

Americans are living healthier lifestyles than they did 25 years ago. Fewer smoke. More have lowered their blood

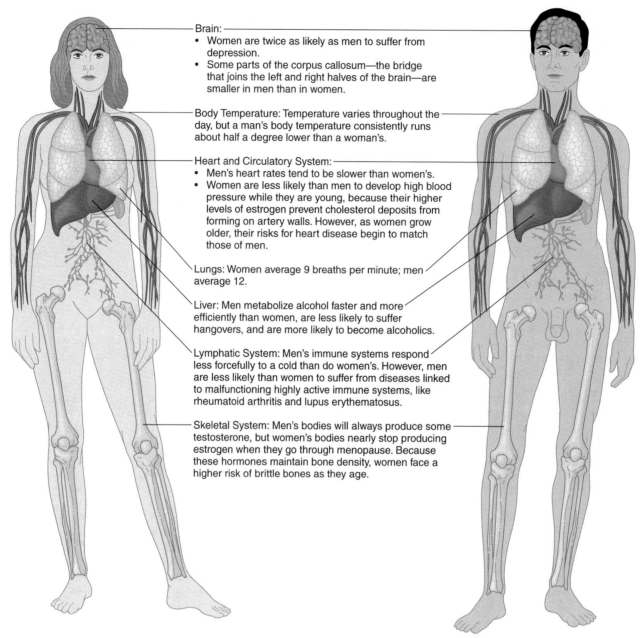

**Brain:**
- Women are twice as likely as men to suffer from depression.
- Some parts of the corpus callosum—the bridge that joins the left and right halves of the brain—are smaller in men than in women.

**Body Temperature:** Temperature varies throughout the day, but a man's body temperature consistently runs about half a degree lower than a woman's.

**Heart and Circulatory System:**
- Men's heart rates tend to be slower than women's.
- Women are less likely than men to develop high blood pressure while they are young, because their higher levels of estrogen prevent cholesterol deposits from forming on artery walls. However, as women grow older, their risks for heart disease begin to match those of men.

**Lungs:** Women average 9 breaths per minute; men average 12.

**Liver:** Men metabolize alcohol faster and more efficiently than women, are less likely to suffer hangovers, and are more likely to become alcoholics.

**Lymphatic System:** Men's immune systems respond less forcefully to a cold than do women's. However, men are less likely than women to suffer from diseases linked to malfunctioning highly active immune systems, like rheumatoid arthritis and lupus erythematosus.

**Skeletal System:** Men's bodies will always produce some testosterone, but women's bodies nearly stop producing estrogen when they go through menopause. Because these hormones maintain bone density, women face a higher risk of brittle bones as they age.

▲ **Figure 1-5** Sex Differences in Health

pressure and cholesterol levels. But Americans in small towns and rural areas lag behind others. They tend to smoke more, lose more teeth as they age, exercise less, and die sooner than residents of suburbs and big cities.[23]

Chronic diseases, such as heart disease, cancer, and diabetes, currently account for 75 percent of deaths in the United States.[24] However, fewer people are dying of heart disease and cancer, according to the Centers for Disease Control and Prevention (CDC). Death rates from murder, suicide, accidents, stroke, diabetes, chronic respiratory disease, chronic liver disease, and AIDS also have fallen.[25]

Homicide and suicide have declined as causes of death for the total population, but among young persons 15 to 24 years of age, they remain, respectively, the second and third leading causes of death. Accidents are the number-one cause of death in this age group.

## Healthy People 2010

Americans entered the twenty-first century in fairly good shape but with a way to go to attain optimal wellness and fitness. *Healthy People 2000,* a federal initiative for health promotion and disease prevention, announced that Americans had achieved or "nearly met" about 60 percent of their health goals. On 18 percent of the objectives, however, the nation did worse rather than better. For example, the number of overweight people increased in the last decade, and physical activity levels decreased.

*Healthy People 2010* has more than 450 health objectives organized into 28 areas and two overarching goals: to increase years of healthy life and to eliminate racial and ethnic health disparities.[26] Among the specific goals related to wellness and fitness in *Healthy People 2010* are the following:

- ✔ Increase the number of adolescents engaging in vigorous physical activity three or more days per week for 20 or more minutes per occasion.
- ✔ Encourage adults to engage in moderate physical activity for at least 30 minutes on a regular basis, if not daily.
- ✔ Reduce the proportion of obese adults from 23 percent of the population to 15 percent.
- ✔ Reduce the proportion of obese children and adolescents from 11 percent to 5 percent.
- ✔ Reduce the number of adolescents and adults using illegal substances.
- ✔ Reduce the number of adults engaging in binge drinking.
- ✔ Reduce the percentage of teens and adults who report having smoked cigarettes in the past month.[27]

## Diversity and Health

We live in the most diverse nation on Earth, and in one that is becoming increasingly diverse. During the 1990s, the Hispanic and Asian populations of the United States surged, growing by 35 and 40 percent, respectively. The number of African Americans grew by almost 13 percent.

For society, this variety can be both enriching and divisive. Tolerance and acceptance of others have always been part of the American creed. By working together, Americans have created a country that remains, to those outside our borders, a symbol of opportunity. Yet members of different ethnic groups still have to struggle against discrimination. Today, in this country's third century, all Americans still aren't equal in their access to health care. Poverty remains a major barrier to quality health care for minorities. Without adequate insurance or the ability to pay, many cannot afford the tests and treatments that could prevent illness or overcome it at the earliest possible stages.

As public health experts explore the links between race, culture, and health, they are moving beyond any narrow definition of *minority* to the broader concept of *underserved,* a group made up of many cultures that also includes the homeless, rural Americans, and women. Special problems also exist for illegal immigrants, who often live in extreme poverty; perform difficult, haz-

ardous jobs; and have little or no access to health services. Even when they desperately need medical care, they may be so fearful of deportation that they do not seek help.[28]

Diversity poses special challenges in health care. Racial and ethnic minority communities have a disproportionately high burden of disability from inadequately treated mental health problems and illnesses.[29] In some cultures, physicians are seen as less effective than other healers, who are believed to cure illness caused by bad karma or evil spirits. American physicians, trained to believe that high-tech medicine is best, may not understand or appreciate traditional healing practices. In many communities, innovative programs have begun to educate patients from other cultures about the American health-care system, as well as to educate American health-care providers about the beliefs and health practices of their diverse patients.

## Can Race Affect Health?

Different racial and ethnic groups often face different health risks. Consider the following statistics:

- ✔ The infant mortality rate for African-American babies remains higher than for white babies.[30]
- ✔ Life expectancy for African Americans, though increasing, is six years lower than for whites.[31]
- ✔ African Americans have higher rates of high blood pressure (hypertension), develop this problem earlier in life, suffer more severe hypertension, and have higher rates of strokes and hypertension-related deaths than whites. Cardiovascular risk is higher in minority than white youth.
- ✔ African Americans have higher rates of glaucoma, systemic lupus erythematosus, liver disease, and kidney failure than whites.
- ✔ The death rate for heart disease among middle-aged black women is 150 percent higher than among white women the same age. Among those with diabetes, the death rate is 134 percent higher than for white female diabetics.
- ✔ Of all black women diagnosed with breast cancer, 37 percent are younger than 50—compared with 22 percent of white women.
- ✔ Caucasians are prone to osteoporosis (progressive weakening of bone tissue); cystic fibrosis; skin cancer; and phenylketonuria (PKU), a metabolic disorder that can lead to mental retardation.
- ✔ Women with Chinese or Hispanic backgrounds face a significantly greater risk of developing diabetes during pregnancy than African Americans or whites.
- ✔ Asians and Asian Americans metabolize some medications faster than whites and thus require much smaller doses.

✔ Hispanics have higher rates of death from diabetes and infectious and parasitic diseases than African Americans or whites.

✔ Native Americans have the highest rate of diabetes in the world. Among the Pima Indians, half of all adults have diabetes.

✔ Native Hawaiian women have a higher rate of breast cancer than women from other racial and ethnic groups.

✔ Native Americans, including those indigenous to Alaska, are more likely to die young than the population as a whole, primarily as a result of accidental injuries, cirrhosis of the liver, homicide, pneumonia, and the complications of diabetes.[32]

✔ The suicide rate among American Indians and Alaska natives is 50 percent higher than the national rate. The rates of co-occurring mental illness and substance abuse (especially alcohol) are also higher among Native American youth and adults.[33]

✔ Disproportionate numbers of African Americans are among the groups most vulnerable to mental illness: the homeless, the incarcerated, those in the child welfare system, and the victims of trauma.

Are these increased susceptibilities the result of genetics, the stress of living with discrimination, an unhealthy lifestyle, lack of access to health services, or poverty? It is hard to say precisely. Certainly, poverty presents a major barrier to seeking preventive care and getting timely and effective treatment.

In some cases, both genetic and environmental factors may play a role. Take, for example, the high rates of diabetes among the Pima Indians. Until 50 years ago, these Native Americans were not notably obese or prone to diabetes. After World War II, the tribe started trading handmade baskets for lard and flour. Their lifestyle became more sedentary, and their diet, higher in fats. In addition, researchers have discovered that many Pima Indians have an inherited resistance to insulin that increases their susceptibility to diabetes. The combination of a hereditary predisposition and environmental factors may explain why the Pimas now have epidemic levels of diabetes.

Health-care providers often fail to recognize racial health risks, in part because the discussion of ethnicity in health is politically controversial. Yet recognition of different health needs and risks is the first step toward overcoming the health problems of many Americans.

## Closing the Minority Health Gap

In the words of a National Institutes of Health (NIH) report, minorities have carried "an unequal burden with respect to disease and disability, resulting in a lower life expectancy." Each year minorities in the United States—African Americans, Hispanics, Asian Americans, Pacific Islanders, Native Americans, and other groups—experience as many as 75,000 more deaths than they would if they lived under the same health conditions as the white population.

But race itself isn't the primary reason for the health problems faced by minorities in the United States. Poverty is. One in three Hispanics under age 65 has no health insurance.[34] According to public health experts, low income may account for one-third of the racial differences in death rates for middle-aged African-American adults. High blood pressure, high cholesterol, obesity, diabetes, and smoking are responsible for another third. The final third has been blamed on "unexplained factors," which may well include poor access to health care and the stress of living in a society in which skin color remains a major barrier to equality.

When African Americans receive the same cancer treatments as whites, they are equally likely to survive. In a study of nearly 3,400 colon cancer patients, white and black patients treated with surgery and chemotherapy had virtually the same five-year survival rates. In past studies, African Americans were less likely to survive for five years than whites.[35] When blacks and whites have equal access to quality health care, perhaps some of the racial-based differences in overall health will also be reduced.

NIH has established an Office of Research on Minority Health (ORMH) with the goal of "closing the gap that currently exists between the health of minorities and the majority population." Funds have been provided for research and prevention efforts aimed at improving minority health. Some researchers focus on prenatal care to improve survival rates. Others are educating minority youths about HIV infection and AIDS.

## The Health of College Students

As one of the nation's 14.5 million full- or part-time college students, you belong to one of the most diverse groups in America. A quarter of all 18- to 24-year-olds in the United States are enrolled at one of the nation's 3,800 colleges and universities.[36] Some of you are reentry students, back on campus for the second time; half of all college dropouts return to school within 15 years.

College students often engage in behaviors that put them at risk for serious health problems. College-age men are more likely than women to engage in risk-taking behaviors—to use drugs and alcohol; to engage in risky sexual behaviors, such as having multiple partners and having sex while under the influence of alcohol; and to drive dangerously. Men also are more likely to be hospitalized for injuries and to commit suicide. Three-fourths of the deaths in the 15- to 24-year age range are men.[37]

College itself can seem hazardous to health. Dormitories have proven to be breeding grounds for serious infectious diseases, such as meningitis (discussed in Chapter 9). Secondhand smoke can present a long-term threat to smokers' roommates. Binge drinking imperils not only the drinkers but those in their immediate environment, including anyone on the road if an intoxicated student gets behind the wheel of a car.[38]

Undergraduates also face risks to their psychological health. In a Canadian survey, college students reported more distress than the general Canadian population and than same-age peers not enrolled in college.[39] Nearly a third of more than 7,500 undergraduates surveyed had significantly elevated psychological distress—women more than men, younger students more than upperclassmen.

Freshman year seems to take the greatest toll. A survey of 3,680 students, interviewed at the beginning and end of their freshman year, found significant drops in physical and emotional well-being. As entering freshmen, 51 percent rated their physical health as "above average"; at the end of the year, only 41 percent did. The percentage of students reporting above-average emotional health dropped from 52 percent to 45 percent.[40] In 1985, 60 percent ranked themselves as above average in emotional health.[41] (See Student Snapshot, "How Freshmen Rate Their Health.")

Chapter 2 will discuss the sources of stress on campus: academic pressures, financial worries, adjustment to new people and expectations, anxieties about the future. One often-overlooked stressor is unpleasant interaction with others. In a recent study of students, hostile or upsetting exchanges with friends, ex-friends, loved ones, and even strangers—in person, by phone, or online—strongly correlated with both emotional and physical well-being.[42] Students who endure harassment or abuse of any sort are more likely to report health-related symptoms. Those most at risk include minority students as well as gay, lesbian, and bisexual undergraduates.[43]

Colleges and universities can take varied steps to protect students' well-being. These range from offering vaccination against meningitis to banning alcohol at athletic and social events.[44] Reliable health-related information also can make a difference. Although the majority of college students report receiving some health information, only 6 percent in one recent survey had information on a comprehensive range of health topics. Full-time, single students between ages 18 and 25 are most likely to receive health information. Students who are black, Hispanic, or belong to another racial or ethnic group are more likely than white students to have received information from campus sources.[45]

According to a survey of 1,200 Americans between the ages of 15 and 24, school is their number-one source for health information, followed by parents and doctors. Three out of four young people who have ever gone online have used the Internet at least once to find health information. Half looked up information on a specific disease, such as cancer or diabetes, while 40 percent sought information about pregnancy, birth control, HIV-AIDS, or other sexually transmitted diseases.[46] (See Figure 1-6.)

Despite potential health risks, the great majority of students not only survive college but, simply by acquiring more years of schooling, increase their chances of a long and healthful life. Many risk factors for disease—including high blood pressure, elevated cholesterol, and cigarette smoking—decline steadily as education increases, regardless of how much money people make. Education may be good for the body as well as the mind by influencing lifestyle behaviors, problem-solving abilities, and values. People who earn college degrees gain positive attitudes

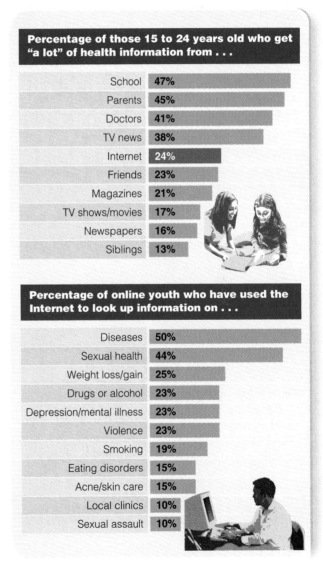

▲ **Figure 1-6** Where Young People Get Health Information

Note: A total of 75 percent of online youth have looked for information on one or more of these topics.

Source: Rideout, Victoria. *Generation Rx.com: How Young People Use the Internet for Health Information.* Menlo Park, CA Kaiser Family Foundation, December 2001. Used with permission.

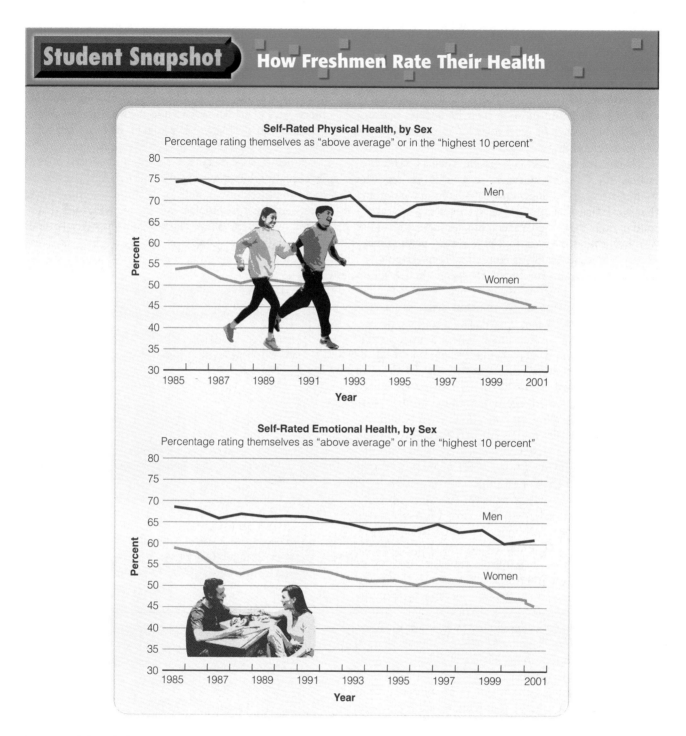

**Student Snapshot** How Freshmen Rate Their Health

**Self-Rated Physical Health, by Sex**
Percentage rating themselves as "above average" or in the "highest 10 percent"

Men

Women

**Self-Rated Emotional Health, by Sex**
Percentage rating themselves as "above average" or in the "highest 10 percent"

Men

Women

Source: Sax, Linda, et al. *The American Freshman: National Norms for Fall 2001*. Los Angeles: Higher Education Research Institute, UCLA, 2001.

about the benefits of healthy living, learn how to gain access to preventive health services, join peer groups that promote healthy behavior, and develop higher self-esteem and greater control over their lives.

Do healthy behaviors have an effect on academic performance? In a study of 200 students living in on-campus residence halls at a large private university, researchers weighed the impact of various health-related variables on first-year students' grade point averages (GPAs). Variables associated with higher grades included female gender, age, studying spiritually oriented material, eating breakfast, and using a planner to organize time. Students with lower GPAs were more likely to stay up and wake up later on weekdays and weekends, sleep more on weekend nights, and work longer hours.[47]

In its National College Health Assessment, the American College Health Association found the conditions that most affect a student's grade or class attendance are stress, depression, sleep problems, family concerns, and time spent on the Internet.[48] The academic performance of African Americans has improved, with most students getting average grades and some excelling. However, Caucasian students typically get better grades. One reason may be higher stress levels for minority students at predominantly white universities.[49] (See Chapter 2 for a discussion of minority stress.) Caucasian students also report feeling more parental pressure to get good grades.[50]

## Becoming All You Can Be

Your choices and behaviors affect how long and how well you live. Nearly half of all deaths in the United States are linked to behaviors such as tobacco use, improper diet, abuse of alcohol and other drugs, use of firearms, motor vehicle accidents, risky sexual practices, and lack of exercise. Yet doctors rarely counsel patients about behavior changes.[51] Among young Americans ages 10 to 24, motor vehicle accidents, homicides, and suicides are responsible for 73 percent of deaths.[52]

What aspects of your life could use some attention and improvement? As Savvy Consumer:"Too Good to Be True?" points out, there are no easy answers or quick solutions. Use this course as an opportunity to zero in on at least one less-than-healthful behavior and improve it. The following sections discuss some of the processes you'll have to go through to make a successful change for the better.

## Understanding Health Behavior

Behaviors that affect your health include exercising regularly, eating a balanced, nutritious diet, seeking care for symptoms, and taking the necessary steps to overcome illness and restore well-being. If you would like to improve one health behavior, you have to realize that change isn't easy. Between 40 and 80 percent of those who try to kick bad health habits lapse back into their unhealthy ways within six weeks. To make lasting beneficial changes, you have to understand the three types of influences that shape behavior: predisposing, enabling, and reinforcing factors (Figure 1-7).

### Predisposing Factors

Predisposing factors include knowledge, attitudes, beliefs, values, and perceptions. Unfortunately, knowledge isn't enough to cause most people to change their behavior; for

## Savvy Consumer

### Too Good to Be True?

Almost every week you're likely to come across a commercial or an ad for a new health product that promises better sleep, more energy, clearer skin, firmer muscles, lower weight, brighter moods, longer life—or all of these combined. As the Savvy Consumer throughout this book points out, you can't believe every promise you read or hear. Keep these general guidelines in mind the next time you come across a health claim:

- If it sounds too good to be true, it probably is. If a magic pill could really trim off excess pounds or banish wrinkles, the world would be filled with thin people with unlined skin. Look around and you'll realize that's not the case.

- Look for objective evaluations. If you're watching an infomercial for a treatment or technique, you can be

sure that the enthusiastic endorsements have been skillfully scripted and rehearsed. Even ads that claim to be presenting the science behind a new breakthrough are really sales pitches in disguise.

- Consider the sources. Research findings from carefully controlled scientific studies are reviewed by leading experts in the field and published in scholarly journals. Just because someone has conducted a study doesn't mean it was a valid scientific investigation.

- Check credentials. Anyone can claim to be a scientist or a health expert. Find out if advocates of any type of therapy have legitimate degrees from recognized institutions and are fully licensed in their fields.

- Do your own research. Check with your doctor or with the student health center. Go to the library or do some online research to gather as much information as you can.

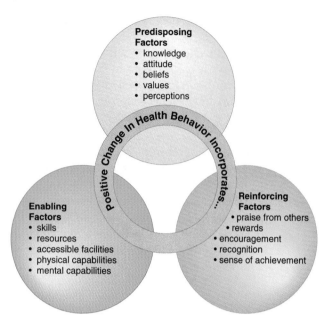

**Predisposing Factors**
- knowledge
- attitude
- beliefs
- values
- perceptions

**Positive Change In Health Behavior Incorporates...**

**Enabling Factors**
- skills
- resources
- accessible facilities
- physical capabilities
- mental capabilities

**Reinforcing Factors**
- praise from others
- rewards
- encouragement
- recognition
- sense of achievement

▲ **Figure 1-7** Factors That Shape Positive Behavior

example, people fully aware of the grim consequences of smoking often continue to puff away. Nor is attitude—one's likes and dislikes—sufficient; an individual may dislike the smell and taste of cigarettes but continue to smoke regardless.

Beliefs are more powerful than knowledge and attitudes, and researchers report that people are most likely to change health behavior if they hold three beliefs:

✔ **Susceptibility.** They acknowledge that they are at risk for the negative consequences of their behavior.
✔ **Severity.** They believe that they may pay a very high price if they don't make a change.
✔ **Benefits.** They believe that the proposed change will be advantageous to their health.

There can be a gap between stated and actual beliefs, however. Young adults may say they recognize the very real dangers of casual, careless sex in this day and age. Yet, rather than act in accordance with these statements, they may impulsively engage in unprotected sex with individuals whose health status and histories they do not know. The reason: Like young people everywhere and in every time, they feel invulnerable, that nothing bad can or will happen to them, that if there were a real danger, they would somehow know it. Often it's not until something happens—a former lover may admit to having a sexually transmitted disease (STD)—that their behaviors become consistent with their stated beliefs.

Young people, especially young men, are the greatest risk takers, a fact reflected in their high rates of auto accidents, binge drinking, drug use, and pathological gambling.[53] The death rates for injuries related to swimming,

boating, driving, cycling, and even crossing the street are higher in college-age men than women.[54]

The value or importance we give to health also plays a major role in changing behavior. Many people aren't concerned about their health just for the sake of being healthy. Usually they want to look or feel better, be more productive or competitive, or behave more independently. They're more likely to change, and to stick with a change, if they can see that the health benefits also enhance other important aspects of their lives.

Perceptions are the way we see things from our unique perspective; they vary greatly with age. As a student, you may not think that living a few hours longer is a significant gain; as you grow older, however, you may prize every additional second.

## Enabling Factors

Enabling factors include skills, resources, accessible facilities, and physical and mental capacities. Before you initiate a change, assess the means available to reach your goal. No matter how motivated you are, you'll become frustrated if you keep encountering obstacles. That's why breaking a task or goal down into step-by-step strategies is so important in behavioral change.

## Reinforcing Factors

Reinforcing factors may be praise from family and friends, rewards from teachers or parents, or encouragement and recognition for meeting a goal. Although these help a great deal in the short run, lasting change depends not on external rewards, but on an internal commitment and sense of achievement. To make a difference, reinforcement must come from within.

A decision to change a health behavior should stem from a permanent, personal goal, not from a desire to please or impress someone else. If you lose weight for the homecoming dance, you're almost sure to regain pounds afterward. But if you shed extra pounds because you want to feel better about yourself or get into shape, you're far more likely to keep off the weight.

## Making Decisions

Every day you make decisions that have immediate and long-term effects on your health. You decide what to eat, whether to drink or smoke, when to exercise, and how to cope with a sudden crisis. Beyond these daily matters, you decide when to see a doctor, what kind of doctor, and with what sense of urgency. You decide what to tell your doctor and whether to follow the advice given, whether to keep up your immunizations, whether to have a prescription filled and comply with the medication instructions, and whether to seek further help or a second opinion. The entire process of maintaining or restoring health depends on your decisions; it cannot start or continue without them.

The small decisions of everyday life—what to eat, where to go, when to study—are straightforward choices. Larger decisions—which major to choose, what to do about a dead-end relationship, how to handle an awkward work situation—are more challenging. However, if you think of decision making as a process, you can break down even the most difficult choices into manageable steps:

✔ **Set priorities.** Rather than getting bogged down in details, step back and look at the big picture. What matters most to you? What would you like to accomplish in the next week, month, year? Look at the decision you're about to make in the context of your values and goals.

✔ **Inform yourself.** The more you know—about a person, a position, a place, a project—the better you'll be able to evaluate it. Gathering information may involve formal research, such as an online or library search for relevant data, or informal conversations with teachers, counselors, family members, or friends.

✔ **Consider all your options.** Most complex decisions don't involve simple either-or alternatives. List as many options you can think of, along with the advantages and disadvantages of each.

✔ **Tune in to your gut feelings.** After you've gotten the facts and analyzed them, listen to your intuition. While it's not infallible, your sixth sense can provide valuable feedback. If something just doesn't feel right, try to figure out why. Are there any fears you haven't dealt with? Do you have doubts about taking a certain path?

✔ **Consider a worst-case scenario.** When you've come close to a final decision, imagine what will happen if everything goes wrong—the workload becomes overwhelming, your partner betrays your trust, your expectations turn out to be unrealistic. If you can live with the worst consequences of a decision, you're probably making the right choice.

### ???? How Can I Change a Bad Health Habit?

Change is never easy—even if it's done for the best possible reasons. When you decide to change a behavior, you have to give up something familiar and easy for something new and challenging. Change always involves risk—and the prospect of rewards.

Researchers have identified various approaches that people use to make beneficial changes. In the moral model, you take responsibility for a problem (such as smoking) and its solution; success depends on adequate motivation, while failure is seen as a sign of character weakness. In the enlightenment model, you submit to strict discipline to correct a problem; this is the approach used in Alcoholics Anonymous. The behavioral model involves rewarding yourself when you make positive changes. The medical model sees the behavior as caused by forces beyond your control (a genetic predisposition to being overweight, for example) and employs an expert to provide advice or treatment. For many people, the most effective approach is the compensatory model, which doesn't assign blame but puts responsibility on individuals to acquire whatever skills or power they need to overcome their problems.

Before they reach the stage where they can and do take action to change, most people go through a process comparable to religious conversion. First they reach a level of accumulated unhappiness that makes them ready for change. Then they have a moment of truth that makes them want to change. One pregnant woman, for instance, felt her unborn baby quiver when she drank a beer and swore never to drink again. As people change their behavior, they change their lifestyles and identities as well. Ex-smokers, for instance, may start an aggressive exercise program, make new friends at the track or gym, and participate in new types of activities, like racquetball games or fun runs.

## STRATEGIES FOR PREVENTION

### Setting Realistic Goals

Here's a framework for setting goals and objectives, the crucial preliminary step for prevention:

▲ Determine your goal or objective. Define it in words and on paper. Then test your definition against your own value system. Can you attain your goal and still be the person you want to be?

▲ Think in terms of evolution, not revolution. Revolutionary changes only inspire counterrevolutions. If you want to change the way you eat, start by changing just one meal a week.

▲ Identify your resources. Do you have the knowledge, skills, finances, time—whatever it takes? Find out from others who know. Be sure you're ready for the next step.

▲ Systematically analyze barriers. How can missing resources be acquired? Identify and select alternative plans. List solutions for any obstacles you foresee.

▲ Choose a plan. Think it through, step by step, trying to anticipate what might go wrong and why.

## ▶ STRATEGIES FOR CHANGE ▶

### How to Make a Change

▲ Get support from friends, but don't expect them to supply all the reinforcement you need. You may join a group of overweight individuals and rely on their encouragement to stick to your diet. That's a great way to get going; but in the long run, your own commitment to losing weight has got to be strong enough to help you keep eating right and light.

▲ Focus on the immediate rewards of your new behavior. You may stop smoking so that you'll live longer, but take note of every other benefit it brings you—more stamina, less coughing, more spending money, no more stale tobacco taste in your mouth.

▲ Remind yourself of past successes you've had in making changes. Give yourself pep talks, commending yourself on how well you've done so far and how well you'll continue to do. This will boost your self-confidence.

▲ Reward yourself regularly. Plan a pleasant reward as an incentive for every week you stick to your new behavior—sleeping in on a Saturday morning, going out with some friends, or spending a sunny afternoon outdoors. Small, regular rewards are more effective in keeping up motivation than one big reward that won't come for many months.

▲ Expect and accept some relapses. The greatest rate of relapse occurs in the first few weeks after making a behavior change. During this critical time, get as much support as you can. In addition, work hard on self-motivation, reminding yourself daily of what you have to gain by sticking with your new health habit.

Social and cultural **norms**—behaviors that are expected, accepted, or supported by a group—can make change much harder if they're constantly working against a person's best intentions. You may resolve to eat less, for instance, yet your mother may keep offering you homemade fudge and brownies because your family's norm is to show love by making and offering delicious treats. Or you might decide to drink less, yet your friends' norm may be to equate drinking with having a good time.

If you're aware of the norms that influence your behavior, you can devise strategies either to change them (by encouraging your friends to dance more and drink less at parties, for example) or adapt to them (having just a bite of your mother's sweets). Another option is to develop relationships with people who share your goals and whose norms can reinforce your behavior.

## Stages of Change

According to the transtheoretical model of change, developed by psychologist James Prochaska, individuals progress through a sequence of stages as they make a change. Certain activities and experiences, called *change processes,* can help individuals progress through these stages.[55] (See Figure 1-8.)

1. **Precontemplation**
   Whether or not they're aware of a problem behavior, people in this stage have no intention of making a change in the next six months. Busy college students in good health, for instance, might never think about getting more exercise.

2. **Contemplation**
   Individuals in this stage are aware they have a problem behavior and are considering changing it within the next six months. However, they may be torn between the positives of the new behavior and the amount of energy, time, and other resources required to change. Students in a health course, for instance, may start thinking about exercising but struggle to balance potential benefits with the effort of getting up early to jog or go to the gym.

3. **Preparation**
   People in this stage intend to change a problem behavior within the next month. Some focus on a master plan. For instance, they might look into fitness classes, gyms, or other options for working out. Others might start by making small changes, such as walking to classes rather than taking a campus shuttle bus.

4. **Action**
   People in this stage are modifying their behavior according to their plan. For instance, they might be jogging or working out at the gym three times a week.

5. **Maintenance**
   In this stage, individuals have continued to work at changing their behavior and have avoided relapse for at least six months. New exercisers are likely to stop during the first three to six months. One reason that researchers have identified: the "temptation to not exercise."[56]

6. **Termination**
   While it may take two to five years, a behavior becomes so deeply ingrained that a person can't imagine abandoning it. As discussed in Chapter 4, more than eight in

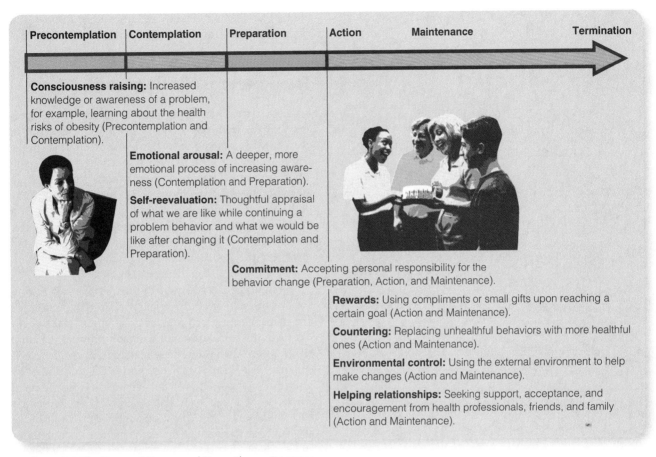

| Precontemplation | Contemplation | Preparation | Action | Maintenance | Termination |

**Consciousness raising:** Increased knowledge or awareness of a problem, for example, learning about the health risks of obesity (Precontemplation and Contemplation).

**Emotional arousal:** A deeper, more emotional process of increasing awareness (Contemplation and Preparation).

**Self-reevaluation:** Thoughtful appraisal of what we are like while continuing a problem behavior and what we would be like after changing it (Contemplation and Preparation).

**Commitment:** Accepting personal responsibility for the behavior change (Preparation, Action, and Maintenance).

**Rewards:** Using compliments or small gifts upon reaching a certain goal (Action and Maintenance).

**Countering:** Replacing unhealthful behaviors with more healthful ones (Action and Maintenance).

**Environmental control:** Using the external environment to help make changes (Action and Maintenance).

**Helping relationships:** Seeking support, acceptance, and encouragement from health professionals, friends, and family (Action and Maintenance).

▲ **Figure 1-8** The Stages of Change and Some Change Processes
These change processes can help you progress through the stages of change. Each can be used through more than one stage.

Source: Petrocelli, John. "Processes and Stages of Change: Counseling with the Transtheoretical Model of Change. *Journal of Counseling and Development,* Vol. 8, No. 1, Winter 2002, p. 22.

ten college seniors who exercised regularly remain as active, or even more active, after graduation.[57]

## Successful Change

"The process of changing from what you are to what you would like to become can be either arduous and frustrating or easy and rewarding," observes Stan Goldberg, Ph.D., who has spent 25 years researching how people change. Because change can be frightening, he encourages individuals to examine the consequences of both sticking with the status quo and switching to the desired behavior.[58]

Some people find it helpful to sign a contract, a written agreement in which they make a commitment to change, with their partner, parent, or health educator. Spelling out what they intend to do, and why, underscores the seriousness of what they're trying to accomplish (see Figure 1-9).

Above all else, change depends on the belief that you can and will succeed. In his research on **self-efficacy,** psychologist Albert Bandura of Stanford University found that the individuals most likely to reach a goal are those who believe they can. The more strongly they feel that they can and will change their behavior, the more energy and per-sistence they put into making the change. Other researchers have linked positive health change with optimism. Individuals who see themselves as optimists may underestimate their susceptibility to problems, such as hypertension, because they always expect things to turn out well. Individuals who perceive themselves as susceptible—that is, who anticipate potentially negative consequences—may be more cautious.

Another crucial factor is **locus of control.** If you believe that your actions will make a difference in your health, your locus of control is internal. If you believe that external forces or factors play a greater role, your locus of control is external. Individuals with an external locus of control for health are less likely to seek preventive health care, are less optimistic about early treatment, rate their own health as poorer, and spend more time in bed because of illness than those with an internal locus of control.

**Reinforcements**—either positive (a reward) or negative (a punishment)—also can play a role. If you decide to set up a regular exercise program, for instance, you might reward yourself with a new sweat suit if you stick to it for three months or you might punish yourself for skipping a day by doing an extra ten minutes of exercises the following day.

## My Contract For Change

Date: _____

Personal Goal: _____

_____

Motivating Factors: _____

_____

Change(s) I Promise to Make to Reach This Goal: ___

_____

Plan for Making This Change: _____

_____

_____

Start Date: _____

Assessment Plan: _____

_____

_____

_____

If I Need Help: _____

_____

_____

Target Date for Reaching Goal: _____

Reward for Achieving Goal: _____

Penalty for Failing to Achieve Goal: _____

Signed: _____

Witnessed By: _____

▲ **Figure 1-9** Sample Health-Change Contract

Your **self-talk**—the messages you send yourself—also can play a role. In recent decades, mental health professionals have recognized the conscious use of positive self-talk as a powerful force for changing the way individuals think, feel, and behave. "We have a choice about how we think," explains psychologist Martin Seligman, Ph.D., author of *Learned Optimism.* As he notes, by learning to challenge automatic negative thoughts that enter our brains and asserting our own statements of self-worth, we can transform ourselves into optimists who see what's right rather than pessimists forever focusing on what's wrong. "Optimism is a learned set of skills," Seligman contends. "Once learned, these skills persist because they feel so good to use. And reality is usually on our side."[59]

## A New Era in Health Education

In the past, health education focused on individual change. Today many educators are using a new framework in which behavior change occurs within the context of the entire environment of a person's life. Its primary themes—prevention

of health problems and protection from health threats—can establish the basis for good health now and in the future.

## The Power of Prevention

No medical treatment, however successful or sophisticated, can compare with the power of **prevention.** Two out of every three deaths and one in three hospitalizations in the United States could be prevented by changes in six main risk factors: tobacco use, alcohol abuse, accidents, high blood pressure, obesity, and gaps in screening and primary health care. Preventive efforts have already proved helpful in increasing physical activity, quitting smoking, reducing dietary fat, preventing sexually transmitted diseases and unwanted pregnancy, reducing intolerance and violence, and avoiding alcohol and drug abuse.

Prevention can take many forms. Primary or before-the-fact prevention efforts might seek to reduce stressors and increase support to prevent problems in healthy people. Consumer education, for instance, provides guidance about how to change our lifestyle to prevent problems and enhance well-being. Other preventive programs identify people at risk and empower them with information and support so they can avoid potential problems. Prevention efforts may target an entire community and try to educate all of its members about the dangers of alcohol abuse or environmental hazards, or they may zero in on a particular group (for instance, seminars on safer sex practices offered to teens) or an individual (one-on-one counseling about substance abuse).

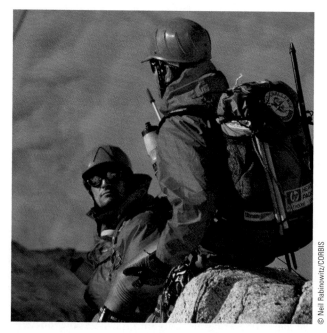

▲ Wearing a helmet is a health choice that diminishes your risk of serious injury.

In the past, physicians did not routinely incorporate prevention into their professional practices. Instead, consumers played the role of Humpty-Dumpty: As long as they sat quietly on the wall, they were ignored. When they fell, the medical equivalents of all the king's horses and all the king's men came running to put them back together again. Often, however, even the best these professionals could provide was still too little, too late.

But times have changed. Medical schools are providing more training in preventive care. A growing number of studies have demonstrated that prevention saves not only money but also productivity, health, and lives. As many as 50 to 80 percent of the deaths caused by cardiovascular disease, strokes, and cancer could be avoided or delayed by preventive measures. Eliminating smoking could prevent more than 300,000 deaths each year, for instance, while changes in diet could prevent 35 percent of unnecessary deaths from heart disease.

## The Potential of Protection

There is a great deal of overlap between prevention and **protection.** Some people might think of immunizations (discussed in Chapter 9) as a way of preventing illness; others see them as a form of protection against dangerous diseases. In many ways, protection picks up where prevention leaves off. You can prevent STDs or unwanted pregnancy by abstaining from sex. But if you decide to engage in potentially risky sexual activities, you can protect yourself with condoms and spermicides (discussed in Chapter 8). Similarly, you can prevent many automobile accidents by not driving when road conditions are hazardous. But if you do have to drive, you can protect yourself by wearing a seat belt and using defensive driving techniques (discussed in Chapter 14).

The very concept of protection implies some degree of risk—immediate and direct (for instance, the risk of intentional injury from an assailant or unintentional harm from a fire) or long-term and indirect (such as the risk of heart disease and cancer as a result of smoking). To know how best to protect yourself, you have to be able to realistically assess risks.

## Assessing Risks

Young people face a host of risks, from the danger of being the victim of violence to the hazards of self-destructive behaviors like drinking and using illegal drugs. At any age, the greatest health threats stem from high-risk behaviors—smoking, excessive drinking, not getting enough exercise, eating too many high-fat foods, and not getting regular medical checkups, to name just a few. That's why changing unhealthy habits is the best way to reduce risks and prevent health problems.

Environmental health risks are the subject of newspaper headlines. Every year brings calls of alarm about a new hazard to health: electromagnetic radiation, fluoride in drinking water, hair dyes, silicone implants, radon, lead. Often the public response is panic. Consumers picket and protest. Individuals arrange for elaborate testing. Yet how do we know whether or not alleged health risks are acceptable? Some key factors to consider:

- ✔ **Are there possible benefits?** Advantages—such as the high salary paid for working with toxic chemicals or radioactive materials—may make some risks seem worth taking.
- ✔ **Is the risk voluntary?** All of us tend to accept risks that we freely choose to take, such as playing a sport that could lead to injuries, as opposed to risks imposed on us, such as threats of terrorism.
- ✔ **Is the risk fair?** The risk of skin cancer affects us all. We may worry about it and take action to protect ourselves and our planet, but we don't resent it the way we resent living with the risk of violence because the only housing we can afford is in a high-crime area.
- ✔ **Are there alternatives?** As consumers, we may become upset about cancer-causing pesticides or food additives when we learn about safer chemicals or methods of preservation.
- ✔ **Are lives saved or lost?** Our thinking about risks often depends on how they're presented. For instance, if we're told that a new drug may kill 1 out of every 100 people, we react differently than if we're told that it may save the lives of 99 percent of those who use it.

## The Future of Medicine

Medical science is moving ahead at astounding speed. Every week seems to bring a new discovery or breakthrough. In their quest for new cures for deadly or disabling diseases, scientists have ventured into uncharted and highly controversial territory. The ethics of cloning, whether of animals or of human embryos, and the use of embryonic stem cells (which have the potential to grow into any type of cell, such as muscle, bone, or skin) have stirred passionate debate among legislators, scientists, religious leaders, and patient advocacy groups. Gene therapy, which replaces defective genes with normal ones, also has come under attack after the death of a volunteer in an experimental program. The federal government has restricted funding for certain types of research and has set up a panel of doctors, lawyers, and ethicists to advise the president on stem cells, cloning, and other challenging research issues.

One of the most exciting scientific frontiers has been genetic research. The completion of the mapping of the human genome sequence in 2001 was a milestone in biological science. Two teams of scientists have positively identified 26,588 human genes, with another 12,731 possibilities. The total—probably somewhere between 30,000 and 40,000 genes—is far less than the estimated 100,000 genes that scientists had predicted.[60] When all human genes are identified, scientists will have the tools to study the details of human development and disease.[61]

Each individual carries about 20 abnormal genes, including six that are potentially deadly.[62] Most are hidden, but in combination with other genes or in certain environmental conditions, they can become dangerous. According to the American Society of Human Genetics, about 5 percent of adults under age 25 have a genetically linked disease; 60 percent of adults older than 25 develop a genetically influenced disorder. In addition to rare genetic syndromes, hereditary diseases include common problems such as certain types of cataracts, glaucoma, gallbladder disease, hypertension, nearsightedness, ulcers, and dyslexia.

 Why is taking the stairs a healthier alternative than riding an elevator?

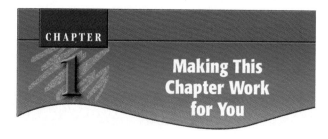

**CHAPTER**
**1**

**Making This Chapter Work for You**

1. The components of health include all of the following except
   a. supportive friends and family.
   b. a well-paying job.
   c. energy and vitality.
   d. a clean environment.

2. Wellness is defined as
   a. purposeful, enjoyable living, characterized by personal responsibility and enhancement of physical, mental, and spiritual health.
   b. a state of complete physical, mental, and social well-being.
   c. attitudes and beliefs that contribute to a healthy state of mind.
   d. the absence of physical or mental illness.

3. Which of the following statements about the dimensions of health are true?
   a. Spirituality provides solace and comfort for those who are severely ill, but it has no health benefits.

   b. The people who reflect the highest levels of social health are usually among the most popular individuals in a group and are often thought of as the life of the party.
   c. Intellectual health refers to one's academic abilities.
   d. Optimal physical health requires a nutritious diet, regular exercise, avoidance of harmful behaviors and substances, and self-protection from accidents.

4. The goals of the *Healthy People 2010* initiative include all of the following except
   a. reduce the proportion of obese adults and children in the population.
   b. decrease the number of teens using illegal substances.
   c. increase the number of adults engaging in daily vigorous physical activity for 30 minutes per occasion.
   d. reduce the percentage of teens and adults who report smoking cigarettes in the past month.

5. Health risks faced by different ethnic and racial groups include all of the following except:
   a. Whites have higher rates of hypertension, lupus, liver disease, and kidney failure than African Americans.
   b. Native Hawaiian women have a higher rate of breast cancer than women from other racial and ethnic groups.
   c. Infant mortality is higher for African-American babies than for white babies.
   d. Chinese and Hispanic women are at greater risk of developing diabetes during pregnancy than African-American and white women.

6. Which of the following health hazards faced by college students can be avoided?
   a. binge drinking
   b. unprotected sex
   c. smoking
   d. all of the above

7. The development of health behaviors is influenced by all of the following except
   a. reinforcing factors, which involve external recognition for achieving a goal.
   b. preexisting health factors, which take into account the individual's current position on the wellness continuum.
   c. predisposing factors, which include knowledge, attitudes, and beliefs.
   d. enabling factors, which are related to an individual's skills and capabilities to make behavior changes.

8. If you want to change unhealthy behavior, which of the following strategies is least likely to promote success?

a. Believe that you can make the change.

b. Reward yourself regularly.

c. During self-talks, remind yourself about all your faults.

d. Accept that you are in control of your health.

9. According to the stages of change in the transtheoretical model of change, which statement is incorrect?

a. In the maintenance stage, individuals have avoided relapse for six months.

b. In the contemplation stage, individuals are considering changing a problem behavior in the next six months.

c. In the action stage, individuals are actually modifying their behavior according to their plan.

d. In the preparation stage, individuals intend to change a problem behavior in the next six months.

10. Which of the following statements is incorrect?

a. Prevention involves specific actions that an individual can take when participating in risky behavior to prevent health threats.

b. You can prevent health problems by educating yourself about them and then avoiding the risky behavior that may cause them.

c. An example of a preventive measure is to avoid driving in icy, snowy conditions, and an example of a protective measure is to put chains on your tires.

d. In assessing risks, two questions to ask are: Is the risk voluntary? Are there alternatives?

Answers to these questions can be found on page 415.

## Critical Thinking

1. What is the definition of health according to the text? Does your personal definition differ from this? If so, in what ways? How would you have defined health before reading this chapter?

2. Talk to classmates from different racial or ethnic backgrounds than yours about their culture's health attitudes. Ask them what is considered healthy behavior in their culture. For example, is having a good appetite a sign of health? What kinds of self-care practices did their parents and grandparents use to treat colds, fevers, rashes, and other health problems? What are their attitudes about the health-care system?

3. Where are you on the wellness–illness continuum? What variables might affect your place on the scale? What do you consider your optimum state of health to be?

4. In what ways would you like to change your present lifestyle? What steps could you take to make those changes?

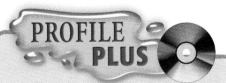

## PROFILE PLUS

Get on the road to wellness by participating in the following activities on your Profile Plus CD-ROM:

Wellness Inventory * Life Expectancy and Physiological Age Prediction Questionnaire * Self-Evaluation and Behavioral Objectives for the Future * Behavior Change Plan.

# SITES & BYTES

### Healthy People 2010
**http://web.health.gov/healthypeople**

*Healthy People 2010* is a statement of national health objectives designed to identify the most significant preventable causes of acute and chronic illnesses and accidents, and to establish national goals to reduce these threats to health.

### LiveWell Health Risk Appraisal
**http://wellness.uwsp.edu/Health_Service/services/livewell**

This comprehensive site sponsored by the National Wellness Institute features a series of self-assessment surveys composed of questions in a variety of wellness dimensions, including physical fitness, nutrition, self-care, drugs, emotional health, and spiritual wellness.

### Selfgrowth.com
**www.selfgrowth.com**

This site is an online guide to self-help, self-improvement, and personal growth, featuring information on psychology, dieting, recovery, relationships, health and fitness, natural medicine, and spiritual development. An online IQ test, daily and weekly newsletters, and links to more than 4,000 websites are included.

Please note that links are subject to change. If you find a broken link, use a search engine such as www.yahoo.com and search for the website by typing in keywords.

### InfoTrac College Edition Activity
David E. Nelson, Shayne Bland, Eve Powell-Griner, Richard Klein, Henry E. Wells, Gary Hogelin, and James S. Marks. "State Trends in Health Risk Factors and Receipt of Clinical Preventive Services Among U.S. Adults During the 1990s." *Journal of the American Medical Association,* Vol. 287, No. 20, May 22, 2002 p. 2659 (9).

1. During the decade of the 1990s, what measured behavior has shown the greatest improvement in most states?
2. According to strong scientific consensus, name five health risk factors that have been shown to increase mortality risk.
3. What have been the trends in cigarette smoking, obesity, and binge alcohol use during the 1990s?

You can find additional readings relating to personal health with InfoTrac College Edition, an online library of more than 900 journals and publications. Follow the instructions for accessing InfoTrac that were packaged with your textbook; then search for articles using a keyword search.

For additional links, resources, and suggested readings on InfoTrac, visit our Health & Wellness Resource Center at http://health.wadsworth.com.

## Key Terms

The terms listed here are used within the chapter on the page indicated. Definitions of terms are in the Glossary at the end of the book.

| | | | |
|---|---|---|---|
| **health** 4 | **norms** 18 | **reinforcement** 19 | **wellness** 4 |
| **health promotion** 7 | **prevention** 20 | **self-efficacy** 19 | |
| **locus of control** 19 | **protection** 21 | **self-talk** 20 | |

## References

1. "Constitution of the World Health Organization." *Chronicle of the World Health Organization.* Geneva, Switzerland: WHO, 1947.
2. Travis, John. Personal interview.
3. Gordon, James. Personal interview.
4. Amandarajah, Gowri, and Ellen Hight. "Spirituality and Medical Practice." *American Family Physician,* Vol. 63, No. 1, January 1, 2001.
5. Ferraro, Kenneth, et al. "Religious Consolation Among Men and Women: Do Health Problems Spur Seeking?" *Journal for the Scientific Study of Religion,* Vol. 39, No. 2, June 2000, p. 220.
6. "Can Your Prayer Heal Others?" *Spirituality & Health,* Fall 2001, p. 15.
7. "Spiritual Matters, Earthly Benefits." *Tufts University Health & Nutrition Letter,* Vol. 19, No. 6, August 2001, p. 1.
8. Schnittker, Jason. "When Is Faith Enough?" *Journal for the Scientific Study of Religion,* Vol. 40, No. 3, September 2001, p. 393.
9. Nagourney, Eric. "A Study Links Prayer and Pregnancy." *New York Times,* October 2, 2001.
10. Garfield, A. M., et al. "Religion/Spirituality, Education and Physical Health in Mid-Life Adults." *Gerontologist,* October 15, 2001, p. 160.

11. Strawbridge, William, et al. "Frequent Religious Attendance May Encourage Better Health Behaviors." *Annals of Behavioral Medicine,* February 2001.

12. Van Ness, Peter, and Jeff Levin. *God, Faith, and Health: Exploring the Spirituality–Healing Connection.* Chicago: University of Chicago Press, 2002.

13. Larrimore, Walter. "Providing Basic Spiritual Care for Patients: Should It Be the Exclusive Domain of Pastoral Professionals?" *American Family Physician,* Vol. 63, No. 1, January 1, 2001.

14. Sloan, Richard, and Emilia Bagiella. "Spirituality and Medical Practice: A Look at the Evidence." *American Family Physician,* Vol. 63, No. 1, January 1, 2001.

15. Benson, Herbert. "Spirituality and Health." *American Family Physician,* Vol. 63, No. 1, January 1, 2001.

16. Matthews, Dale. Personal interview.

17. Ursano, Robert. Personal interview.

18. Roizen, Michael. *RealAge: Are You As Young As You Can Be?* New York: HarperCollins, 2000.

19. Minino, Arialdi, et al. "Deaths: Preliminary Data for 2000." *National Vital Statistics Reports,* Vol. 49, No. 12, October 9, 2001.

20. Kiefe, Catarina. "Race/Ethnicity and Cancer Survival: The Elusive Target of Biological Differences." *Journal of the American Medical Association,* Vol. 287, No. 16, April 24, 2002, p. 2106.

21. Olshanky, S. Jay, et al. "Life Expectancy." *Science,* Vol. 291, No. 5508, February 23, 2001.

22. *Crossing the Quality Chasm: A New Health System for the 21st Century.* Washington, DC: Institute of Medicine, 2001.

23. www.cdc.gov/nchs.

24. Gorin, Stephen. "Inequality and Health: Implications for Social Work." *Health and Social Work,* Vol. 25, No. 4, November 2000.

25. Minino, et al., "Deaths: Preliminary Data for 2000."

26. *Healthy People 2010 Fact Sheet:* "Healthy People in Healthy Communities." *Healthy People 2010* is available on the Internet at http://web.health.gov/healthypeople.

27. Ibid.

28. Swanbrow, Diane. "Black–White Health Gap Is As Large As It Was in 1950." University of Michigan News Service, February 24, 2000.

29. *Mental Health: Culture, Race, and Ethnicity.* Washington, DC: Office of the Surgeon General, August 2001. www.surgeongeneral.gov/library/mentalhealth/cre/

30. Scanlan, James. "Race and Mortality." *Society,* Vol. 37, No. 2, January 2000.

31. Guyer, Bernard, et al. "Annual Summary of Vital Statistics: Trends in the Health of Americans During the 20th Century." *Pediatrics,* Vol. 106, No. 6, December 2000.

32. McCollum, David, et al. "Outcomes and Toxicity in African-American and Caucasian Patients in a Randomized Adjuvant Chemotherapy Trial for Colon Cancer." *Journal of the National Cancer Institute,* Vol. 94, August 7, 2002, p. 1160.

33. United States Department of Health and Human Services.

34. *Mental Health: Culture, Race, and Ethnicity.*

35. Vitucci, Jeff. "The State of Hispanic Health." *Hispanic Business,* Vol. 21, No. 6, June 1999.

36. National Center for Education Statistics. Office of Educational Improvement. U.S. Department of Statistics. http://nces.ed.gov.

37. Davies, Jon, et al. "Identifying Male College Students' Perceived Health Needs, Barriers to Seeking Help, and Recommendations to Help Men Adopt Healthier Lifestyles." *Journal of American College Health,* Vol. 48, No. 5, May 2000.

38. Keeling, Richard. "Is College Dangerous?" *Journal of American College Health,* Vol. 50, No. 2, September 2001, p. 53.

39. Adlaf, Edward, et al. "The Prevalence of Elevated Psychological Distress Among Canadian Undergraduates: Findings from the 1998 Canadian Campus Survey." *Journal of American College Health,* Vol. 50, No. 2, September 2001, p. 67.

40. Bartlett, Thomas. "Freshman Pay, Mentally and Physically, As They Adjust to Life in College." *Chronicle of Higher Education,* February 1, 2002.

41. Bartlett, Thomas. "Evaluating Student Attitudes Is More Difficult This Year." *Chronicle of Higher Education,* February 1, 2002.

42. Edwards, Kevi, et al. "Stress, Negative Social Exchange, and Health Symptoms in University Students." *Journal of American College Health,* Vol. 50, No. 2, September 2001, p. 75.

43. Bowen, Anne, and Martin Bourgeois. "Attitudes Toward Lesbian, Gay, and Bisexual College Students." *Journal of American College Health,* Vol. 50, No. 2, September 2001, p. 91.

44. Bormann, Carol, and Michael Stone. "The Effects of Eliminating Alcohol in a College Stadium: The Folsom Field Beer Ban." *Journal of American College Health,* Vol. 50, No. 2, September 2001, p. 81.

45. Brener, Nancy, and Vani Gowda. "U.S. College Students' Reports of Receiving Health Information on College Campuses." *Journal of American College Health,* Vol. 49, No. 5, March 2001, p. 223.

46. Rideout, Victoria. *Generation Rx.com: How Young People Use the Internet for Health Information.* Menlo Park, CA: Kaiser Family Foundation, December 2001.

47. Trockel, Mickey, et al. "Health-Related Variables and Academic Performance Among First-Year College Students: Implications for Sleep and Other Behaviors." *Journal of American College Health,* Vol. 49, No. 3, November 2000.

48. Swinford, Paula. "Advancing the Health of Students: A Rationale for College Health Programs." *Journal of American College Health,* Vol. 50, No. 6, May 2002, p. 261.

49. Jackson, Pamela Braboy, and Montenique Finney. "Negative Life Events and Psychological Distress Among Young Adults." *Social Psychology Quarterly,* Vol. 65, No. 2, p. 186.

50. Walker, Katrina, and Tammy Satterwhite. "Academic Performance Among African American and Caucasian College Students: Is the Family Still Important?" *College Student Journal,* Vol. 36, No. 1, March 2002, p. 113.

51. Gruman, Jessie. "Integration of Health Behavior Counseling in Routine Medical Care." Washington, DC: Center for the Advancement of Health, 2001. This report is also available at www.cfah.org.

52. "Social and Emotional Competence: Healthy Behaviors for Youth." *Facts of Life: Issue Briefing for Health Reporters,* Vol. 6, No. 4, May 2001, p. 1.

53. Zuckerman, Marvin. "Are You a Risk Taker?" *Psychology Today,* November–December 2000.

54. Courtenay, Will. "Behavioral Factors Associated with Disease, Injury and Death Among Men: Evidence and Implications for Prevention." *Journal of Men's Studies,* Vol. 9, No. 1, Fall 2000.

55. Petrocelli, John. "Processes and Stages of Change: Counseling with the Transtheoretical Model of Change." *Journal of Counseling and Development,* Vol. 80, No. 1, Winter 2002, p. 22.

56. Dannecker, Erin, et al. "The Missing Piece of the Transtheoretical Model: Development and Validation of the Exercise Temptation Scale." *Research Quarterly for Exercise and Sport,* Vol. 71, No. 1, March 2000, p. A-87.

57. Sparling, Phillip, and Teresa Snow. "Physical Activity Patterns in Recent College Alumni," *Research Quarterly for Exercise and Sport,* Vol. 73, No. 2, June 2002, p. 200.

58. Goldberg, Stan. "The 10 Rules of Change." *Psychology Today,* Vol. 35, No. 5, September–October 2002, p. 38.

59. Martin Seligman, personal interview.

60. Venter, J. Craig, et al. "The Sequence of the Human Genome." *Science,* Vol. 291, No. 5507, February 15, 2001.

61. Peltonen, Leena, and Victor A. McKusick. "Genomics and Medicine: Dissecting Human Disease in the Postgenomic Era." *Science,* Vol. 291, No. 5507, February 16, 2001.

62. Friedrich, M. J. "Preserving Privacy, Preventing Discrimination Become the Province of Genetics Experts." *Journal of the American Medical Association,* Vol. 288, No. 7, August 21, 2002, p. 2106.

# Personal Stress Management

**After studying the material in this chapter, you should be able to:**

- **Define** stress and stressors and **describe** how the body responds to stress according to the general adaptation syndrome theory.
- **List** the physical changes associated with frequent or severe stress and discuss how stress can affect the cardiovascular, immune, and digestive systems.
- **Explain** how stressful events can affect psychological health, including posttraumatic stress disorder.
- **Describe** some personal causes of stress, especially those experienced by students, and **discuss** how their effects can be prevented or minimized.
- **Discuss** the major social issues that can cause stress.
- **Identify** ways of managing time more efficiently.
- **Describe** some techniques to help manage stress.

Y ou know about stress. You live with it every day: the stress of passing exams, preparing for a career, meeting people, facing new experiences. Everyone, regardless of age, gender, race, or income, has to deal with stress—as an individual and as a member of society.

As researchers have demonstrated, stress has profound effects, both immediate and long-term, on our bodies and minds. While stress alone doesn't cause disease, it triggers molecular changes throughout the body that make us more susceptible to many illnesses. Its impact on the mind is no less significant. The burden of chronic stress can undermine the ability to cope with day-to-day hassles and can exacerbate psychological problems like depression and anxiety disorders.

Yet stress in itself isn't necessarily bad. What matters most is not the stressful situation, but an individual's response to it. By learning to anticipate stressful events, to manage day-to-day hassles, and to prevent stress overload, you can find alternatives to running endlessly on a treadmill of alarm, panic, and exhaustion. As you organize your schedule, find ways to release tension, and build up coping skills, you will begin to experience the sense of control and the confidence that make stress a challenge rather than an ordeal.

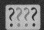

## What Is Stress?

People use the word *stress* in different ways: as an external force that causes a person to become tense or upset, as the internal state of arousal, and as the physical response of the body to various demands. Dr. Hans Selye, a pioneer in studying physiological responses to challenge, defined **stress** as "the nonspecific response of the body to any demand made upon it." In other words, the body reacts to **stressors**—the things that upset or excite us—in the same way, regardless of whether they are positive or negative.

Stress can be acute, episodic, or chronic, depending on the nature of the stressors or external events that cause the stress response. Acute or short-term stressors, which can range from a pop quiz to a bomb threat in a crowded stadium, trigger a brief but intense response to a specific incident. Episodic stressors like monthly bills or quarterly exams cause regular but intermittent elevations in stress levels. Chronic stressors include everything from rush-hour traffic to a learning disability to living with an alcoholic parent or spouse.

Not all stressors are negative. Some of life's happiest moments—births, reunions, weddings—are enormously stressful. We weep with the stress of frustration or loss; we weep, too, with the stress of love and joy. Selye coined the term **eustress** for positive stress in our lives (*eu* is a Greek prefix meaning "good"). Eustress challenges us to grow, adapt, and find creative solutions in our lives. **Distress** refers to the negative effects of stress that can deplete or even destroy life energy. Ideally, the level of stress in our lives should be just high enough to motivate us to satisfy our needs and not so high that it interferes with our ability to reach our fullest potential.

## What Causes Stress?

Of the many biological theories of stress, the best known may be the **general adaptation syndrome (GAS),** developed by Hans Selye. He postulated that our bodies constantly strive to maintain a stable and consistent physiological state, called **homeostasis.** Stressors, whether in the form of physical illness or a demanding job, disturb this state and trigger a nonspecific physiological response. The body attempts to restore homeostasis by means of an **adaptive response.**

Selye's general adaptation syndrome, which describes the body's response to a stressor—whether threatening or exhilarating—consists of three distinct stages:

1. *Alarm.* When a stressor first occurs, the body responds with changes that temporarily lower resistance. Levels of certain hormones may rise; blood pressure may increase (see Figure 2-1). The body quickly makes internal adjustments to cope with the stressor and return to normal activity.
2. *Resistance.* If the stressor continues, the body mobilizes its internal resources to try to sustain homeostasis. For example, if a loved one is seriously hurt in an accident, we initially respond intensely and feel great anxiety. During the subsequent stressful period of recuperation, we struggle to carry on as normally as possible, but this requires considerable effort.
3. *Exhaustion.* If the stress continues long enough, we cannot keep up our normal functioning. Even a small amount of additional stress at this point can cause a breakdown.

Among the nonbiological theories is the cognitive-transactional model of stress, developed by Richard

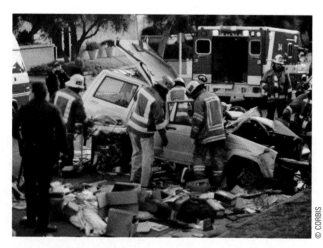

▲ An automobile accident is an example of an acute stressor. Getting married is an example of a positive stressor.

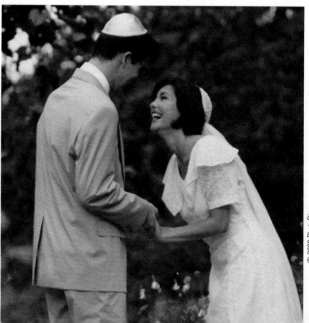

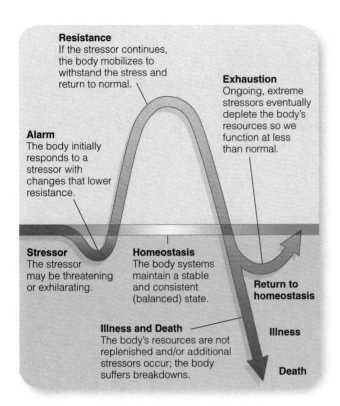

**▲ Figure 2-1** General Adaptation Syndrome (GAS)
The three stages of Hans Selye's GAS are alarm, resistance, exhaustion.

Lazarus, which looks at the relation between stress and health. As he sees it, stress can have a powerful impact on health. Conversely, health can affect a person's resistance or coping ability. Stress, according to Lazarus, is "neither an environmental stimulus, a characteristic of the person, nor a response, but a relationship between demands and the power to deal with them without unreasonable or destructive costs."[1] Thus, an event may be stressful for one person but not for another, or it may seem stressful on one occasion but not on another. For instance, one student may think of speaking in front of the class as extremely stressful, while another relishes the chance to do so—except on days when he's not well-prepared.

At any age, some of us are more vulnerable to life changes and crises than others. The stress of growing up in families troubled by alcoholism, drug dependence, or physical, sexual, or psychological abuse may have a lifelong impact—particularly if these problems are not recognized and dealt with. Other early experiences, positive and negative, also can affect our attitude toward stress—and our resilience to it. Our general outlook on life, whether we're optimistic or pessimistic, can determine whether we expect the worst and feel stressed or anticipate a challenge and feel confident. The number and frequency of changes in our lives, along with the time and setting in which they occur, have a great impact on how we'll respond.

## Is Stress Hazardous to Physical Health?

These days we've grown accustomed to warning labels advising us of the health risks of substances like alcohol and cigarettes. Medical researchers speculate that another component of twenty-first–century living also warrants a warning: stress.[2] In recent years, an ever-growing number of studies has implicated stress as a culprit in a range of medical problems. Mental stress, according to recent investigations, may even kill. In individuals with heart disease, severe mental stress, which increases oxygen demand by causing elevations in blood pressure and heart rate, can trigger a lack of blood flow to the heart and increase the risk of dying.[3]

Stress triggers complex changes in the body's endocrine, or hormone-secreting, system. When you confront a stressor, your body responds by producing stress hormones that speed up heart rate and blood pressure and prepare the body to deal with the threat. This fight-or-flight response prepares you for quick action: Your heart works harder to pump more blood to your legs and arms. Your muscles tense, your breathing quickens, and your brain becomes extra alert. And because they're nonessential in a crisis, your digestive and immune systems practically shut down.

Cortisol, one of the stress hormones, speeds the conversion of proteins and fats into carbohydrates, the body's basic fuel, so we have the energy to fight or flee from a threat. However, stress increases the amount of time required to clear triglycerides, a type of fat linked to heart disease, from the bloodstream.[4] Thus, cortisol can cause excessive central or abdominal fat, which heightens the risk of diseases such as diabetes, high blood pressure, and stroke.[5] Even slender, premenopausal women faced with increased stress and lacking good coping skills are more likely to accumulate excess weight around their waists, thereby increasing their risk of heart disease and other health problems.[6]

Figure 2-2 illustrates how persistent or repeated increases in the stress hormones can be hazardous throughout the body. In the brain, stress hormones linked to powerful emotions may help create long-lasting memories of events such as the collapse of the World Trade Center towers. But very prolonged or severe stress can damage the brain's ability to remember and can actually cause brain cells, or neurons, to atrophy and die.

Hundreds of studies over the last 20 years have shown that stress contributes to approximately 80 percent of all major illnesses: cardiovascular disease, cancer, endocrine and metabolic disease, skin rashes, ulcers, ulcerative colitis, emotional disorders, musculoskeletal disease, infectious ailments, premenstrual syndrome (PMS), uterine fibroid cysts, and breast cysts. As many as 75 to 90 percent of visits to physicians are related to stress.

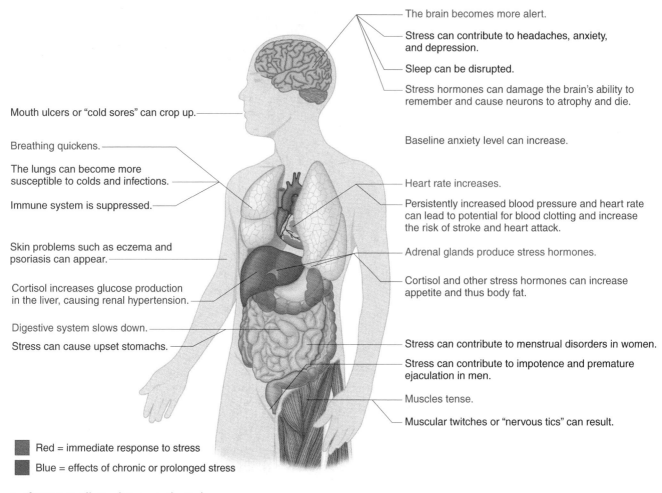

The brain becomes more alert.

Stress can contribute to headaches, anxiety, and depression.

Sleep can be disrupted.

Stress hormones can damage the brain's ability to remember and cause neurons to atrophy and die.

Baseline anxiety level can increase.

Heart rate increases.

Persistently increased blood pressure and heart rate can lead to potential for blood clotting and increase the risk of stroke and heart attack.

Adrenal glands produce stress hormones.

Cortisol and other stress hormones can increase appetite and thus body fat.

Stress can contribute to menstrual disorders in women.

Stress can contribute to impotence and premature ejaculation in men.

Muscles tense.

Muscular twitches or "nervous tics" can result.

Mouth ulcers or "cold sores" can crop up.

Breathing quickens.

The lungs can become more susceptible to colds and infections.

Immune system is suppressed.

Skin problems such as eczema and psoriasis can appear.

Cortisol increases glucose production in the liver, causing renal hypertension.

Digestive system slows down.

Stress can cause upset stomachs.

Red = immediate response to stress

Blue = effects of chronic or prolonged stress

▲ **Figure 2-2** Effects of Stress on the Body

## Stress and the Heart

In the 1970s, cardiologists Meyer Friedman, M.D., and Ray Rosenman, M.D., suggested that excess stress could be the most important factor in the development of heart disease. They compared their patients to individuals of the same age with healthy hearts and developed two general categories: Type A and Type B.

Hardworking, aggressive, and competitive, Type A's never have time for all they want to accomplish, even though they usually try to do several tasks at once. Type B's are more relaxed, though not necessarily less ambitious or successful. The degree of danger associated with Type-A behavior remains controversial. Of all the personality traits linked with Type-A behavior, the one that has emerged as most sinister is chronic hostility or cynicism. People who are always mistrustful, angry, and suspicious are twice as likely to suffer blockages of their coronary arteries.

## Stress and the Immune System

The powerful chemicals triggered by stress dampen or suppress the immune system—the network of organs, tissues, and white blood cells that defend against disease. Impaired immunity makes the body more susceptible to many diseases, including infections (from the common cold to tuberculosis) and disorders of the immune system itself. Research has shown that traumatic stress, such as losing a loved one through death or divorce, can impair immunity for as long as a year.

 Even minor hassles take a toll. Under exam stress, students experience a dip in immune function and a higher rate of infections. In a study of medical students during exam periods, Ohio State University researchers found a significant drop in the immune cells that normally ward off infection and cancer.[7] Studies of university students and staff in the

United States and in Spain have implicated stress and a generally negative outlook as increasing susceptibility to the common cold, even in individuals taking vitamin C and zinc to ward off infection.[8]

 Certain uplifts, including humor and volunteerism, may buffer the harmful effects of stress. In studies of college students, watching videotapes of comedians bolstered immune function. Students who provided services to others showed a temporary boost in immunity.

## Stress and the Digestive System

Do you ever get butterflies in your stomach before giving a speech in class or before a big game? The digestive system is, as one psychologist quips, "an important stop on the tension trail." To avoid problems, pay attention to how you eat: Eating on the run, gulping food, or overeating results in poorly chewed foods, an overworked stomach, and increased abdominal pressure.

Some simple strategies can help you avoid stress-related stomachaches. Many people experience dry mouth or sweat more under stress. By drinking plenty of water, you replenish lost fluids and prevent dehydration. Fiber-rich foods counteract common stress-related problems, such as cramps and constipation. Do not skip meals. If you do, you're more likely to feel fatigued and irritable.

Be wary of overeating under stress. Some people eat more because they scarf down meals too quickly. Others reach for snacks to calm their nerves or comfort themselves. Watch out for caffeine. Coffee, tea, and cola drinks can make your strained nerves jangle even more. Also avoid sugary snacks. They'll send your blood sugar levels on a roller-coaster ride—up one minute, down the next.

ing depression, anxiety, and panic attacks (discussed in Chapter 3).

In the past, **posttraumatic stress disorder (PTSD)** was viewed as a psychological response to out-of-the-ordinary stressors, such as captivity or combat. However, other experiences can also forever change the way people view themselves and their world. Thousands of individuals experience or witness traumatic events, such as fires or floods. Children, in particular, are likely to develop PTSD symptoms when they live through a traumatic event or witness a loved one or friend being assaulted. Those with preexisting psychological problems may be the most vulnerable. Following the terrorist attacks of September 11, 2001, one in three people in psychotherapy in the New York City region developed significant symptoms.[9] Sometimes an entire community, such as the residents of a town hit by a devastating hurricane or a terrorist attack, develops symptoms.

According to recent research, almost half of car-accident victims may develop PTSD. Those who were seriously injured are especially vulnerable.[10] A history of childhood sexual abuse can greatly increase the likelihood of developing PTSD.[11] In PTSD, individuals re-experience their terror and helplessness again and again in their dreams or intrusive thoughts.

The sooner trauma survivors receive psychological help, the better they are likely to fare. Often talking about what happened with an empathic person or someone who's shared the experience—preferably before going to sleep on the day of the event—can help an individual begin to deal with what has occurred. Group sessions, ideally beginning soon after the trauma, allow individuals to share views and experiences. Behavioral, cognitive, and psychodynamic therapy (described in Chapter 3) can help individuals suffering PTSD.

## Is Stress Hazardous to Psychological Health?

Traumatic events (such as a robbery, assault, or death of a loved one) always take a toll on an individual, and it's normal to feel sad, tense, overwhelmed, angry, or incapable of coping with the ordinary demands of daily living. Usually such feelings and behaviors subside with time. The stressful event fades into the past, and those whose lives it has touched adapt to its lasting impact. But sometimes individuals remain extremely distressed and unable to function as they once did. While the majority of individuals who survive a trauma recover, at least a quarter of such individuals later develop serious psychological symptoms, includ-

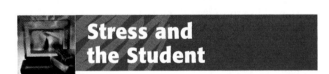

## Stress and the Student

You've probably heard that these are the best years of your life, but being a student—full-time or part-time, in your late teens, early twenties, or later in life—can be extremely stressful. You may feel pressure to perform well to qualify for a good job or graduate school. To meet steep tuition payments, you may have to juggle part-time work and coursework. You may feel stressed about choosing a major, getting along with a difficult roommate, passing a particularly hard course, or living up to your parents' and teachers' expectations. If you're an older student, you may have children, housework, and homework to balance. Your days may seem so busy and your life so full that you worry about coming apart at the seams. One thing is for certain: You're not alone. Stress levels among college students have risen, especially among women. (See the X & Y Files: "Men, Women, and Stress.")

 According to surveys of students at colleges and universities around the country and the world, stress levels are consistently high and stressors are remarkably similar.[12] Among the most common are:

- Test pressures.
- Financial problems.
- Frustrations, such as delays in reaching goals.
- Problems in friendships and dating relationships.

- Daily hassles.
- Academic failure.
- Pressures as a result of competition, deadlines, and the like.
- Changes, which may be unpleasant, disruptive, or too frequent.
- Losses, whether caused by the breakup of a relationship or the death of a loved one.

Nontraditional students face increased stress simply by being different. About 97 percent of entering freshmen are age 19 or younger; 99.6 percent are single. Three in four (76 percent) live on campus, most in dormitories, while 17 percent live with parents or relatives.[13] Students who are older, living off campus, or married may feel like outsiders who do

---

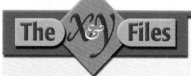 **Men, Women, and Stress**

Women, who make up 56 percent of today's college students, also shoulder the majority of the stress load. In a nationwide survey of students in the class of 2005, freshmen women were twice as likely to be anxious as men. More women (36.6 percent) described themselves as "overwhelmed by all I have to do," compared with just 17.4 percent of men. More women than men reported feeling depressed, insecure about their physical and mental health, and worried about paying for college. More men—60.4 percent, compared with 47.7 percent of women—considered themselves above average or in the top 10 percent of people their age in terms of emotional health.

Gender differences in lifestyle may help explain why women feel so stressed. College men, the survey revealed, spend significantly more time doing things that are fun and relaxing: exercising, partying, watching TV, and playing video games. Women, on the other hand, tend to study more, do more volunteer work, and handle more household and child-care chores.

The stress gender gap, which appeared in the mid-1980s, is "one of the ironies of the women's movement," says Alexander Astin of UCLA, founder of the annual American Freshman Survey, which has tracked shifting student attitudes for 35 years. By adding more commitments and responsibilities on top of all the other things they have to cope with, he believes that college women are experiencing an early version of the stress that "super-moms" feel later in life when they pursue a career, care for children, and maintain a household.

Where can stressed-out college women turn for support? The best source, according to University of

California research, is other women. In general, the social support women offer their friends and relatives seems more effective in reducing the blood-pressure response to stress than that provided by men.

At all ages, women and men tend to respond to stress differently. While males (human and those of other species) react with the classic fight-or-flight response, females under attack try to protect their children and seek help from other females—a strategy dubbed *tend-and-befriend*. When exposed to experimental stress (such as a loud, harsh noise), women show more affection for friends and relatives; men show less. When working mothers studied by psychologists had a bad day, they coped by concentrating on their children when they got home. Stressed-out fathers were more likely to withdraw.

The gender difference in stress responses may be the result of hormones and evolution. While both men and women release stress hormones, men also secrete testosterone, which tends to increase hostility and aggression. For prehistoric women, who were usually pregnant, nursing, or caring for small children, neither fight nor flight were a wise strategy. Smaller and weaker than males, women may long ago have reached out to other women to form a social support system that helped ensure their safety and that of their children.

Sources: Sax, Linda, et al. *The American Freshman: National Norms for Fall 2001.* Los Angeles: Higher Education Research Institute, UCLA, 2001. "How Women Handle Stress: Is There a Difference?" *Harvard Mental Health Letter,* Vol. 17, No. 10, April 2001. "Women's Response to Stress," *Harvard Women's Health Watch,* Vol. 9, No. 9, May 2002.

not fit in as well as more typical undergraduates. Simply commuting from off-campus housing or working part-time means fewer hours for study and school activities.

Many students bring complex psychological problems with them to campus, including learning disabilities and mood disorders like depression and anxiety. "Students arrive with the underpinnings of problems that are brought out by the stress of campus life," says one counselor. Some have grown up in broken homes and bear the scars of family troubles. Others fall into the same patterns of alcohol abuse that they observed for years in their families or suffer lingering emotional scars from childhood physical or sexual abuse.

 For many students, the first year at college is the most challenging. Almost a third of freshmen feel overwhelmed by all they have to do at the beginning of the academic year; by the year's end, 44 percent feel overwhelmed.[14] (See Student Snapshot: "Freshman Stress.") In a recent study of students at three universities, underclassmen were most vulnerable to negative life events, perhaps because they lacked experience in coping with stressful situations. Freshmen had the highest levels of depression; sophomores had the most anger and hostility. Seniors may handle life's challenges better because they have developed better coping mechanisms. In the study, more seniors reported that they faced problems squarely and took action to resolve them, while younger students were more likely to respond passively, for instance, by trying not to let things bother them.[15]

First-generation college students—those whose parents never experienced at least one full year of college—encounter more difficulties with social adjustment than freshmen whose parents attended college. Second-generation students may have several advantages: more knowledge of college life, greater social support, more preparation for college in high school, a greater focus on college activities, and more financial resources.[16]

In college students, excessive levels of stress have been linked to increased headaches, sleep disturbances, and colds.[17] Students say they react to stress in various ways: physiologically (by sweating, stuttering, trembling, or developing physical symptoms); emotionally (by becoming anxious, fearful, angry, guilty, or depressed); behaviorally (by crying, eating, smoking, being irritable or abusive); or cognitively (by thinking about and analyzing stressful situations and strategies that might be useful in dealing with them).

Social support makes a difference. Students with a truly supportive network of friends and family available to them report greater satisfaction and less psychological distress.[18] Effective time management, discussed later in this chapter, helps buffer academic stress.[19] Higher levels of positive experiences, such as forming close friendships, also

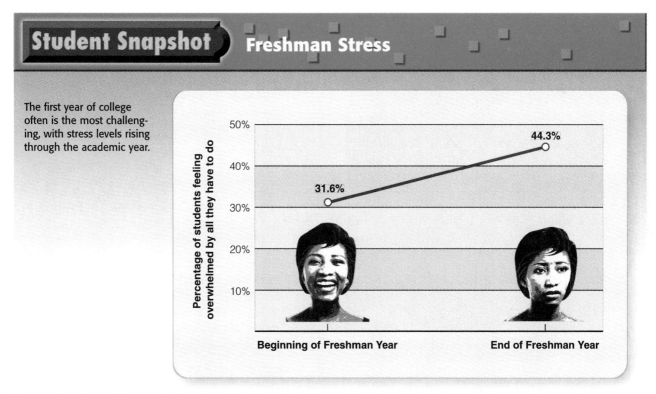

**Student Snapshot** **Freshman Stress**

The first year of college often is the most challenging, with stress levels rising through the academic year.

Percentage of students feeling overwhelmed by all they have to do

44.3%

31.6%

Beginning of Freshman Year    End of Freshman Year

Source: Bartlett, Thomas. "Freshmen Pay, Mentally and Physically, As They Adjust to Life in College." *Chronicle of Higher Education,* February 1, 2002.

reduce stress and compensate for the depressive effects of negative experiences, such as failing a test.[20]

Campuses are providing more frontline services than they have in the past, including career-guidance workshops, telephone hot lines, and special social programs for lonely, homesick freshmen. In one study of 128 undergraduates, those who learned relaxation and stress-reduction techniques in a six-week program reported less stress, anxiety, and psychological distress than a control group of students. The participants—who had described themselves as "extremely stressed" before the intervention—also began to increase health-promoting behaviors.[21]

## Test Stress

For many students, midterms and final exams are the most stressful times of the year. Studies at various colleges and universities found that the incidence of colds and flu soared during finals. Some students feel the impact of test stress in other ways—headaches, upset stomachs, skin flare-ups, or insomnia.

Test stress affects people in different ways. Sometimes students become so preoccupied with the possibility of failing that they can't concentrate on studying. Others, including many of the best and brightest students, freeze up during tests and can't comprehend multiple-choice questions or write essay answers, even if they know the material.

The students most susceptible to exam stress are those who believe they'll do poorly and who see tests as extremely threatening. Unfortunately, such negative thoughts often become a self-fulfilling prophecy. As they study, these students keep wondering, "What good will studying do? I never do well on tests." As their fear increases, they try harder, pulling all-nighters. Fueled by caffeine, munching on sugary snacks, they become edgy and find it harder and harder to concentrate. By the time of the test, they're nervous wrecks, scarcely able to sit still and focus on the exam.

Can you do anything to reduce test stress and feel more in control? Absolutely. One way is to defuse stress through relaxation. In a study by researchers Janice Kiecolt-Glaser and Ron

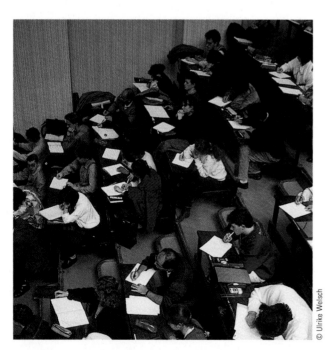

▲ Test stress can affect your immune system, cause digestive problems, and even cause you to freeze during the exam. But you can take control of your stress responses by practicing relaxation techniques, avoiding cramming, and being positive about your performance on the test.

© Ulrike Welsch

## STRATEGIES FOR PREVENTION

### Defusing Test Stress

▲ Plan ahead. A month before finals, map out a study schedule for each course. Set aside a small amount of time every day or every other day to review the course materials.

▲ Be positive. Picture yourself taking your final exam. Imagine yourself walking into the exam room feeling confident, opening up the test booklet, and seeing questions for which you know the answers.

▲ Take regular breaks. Get up from your desk, breathe deeply, stretch, and visualize a pleasant scene. You'll feel more refreshed than you would if you chugged another cup of coffee.

▲ Practice. Some teachers are willing to give practice finals to prepare students for test situations, or you and your friends can test each other.

▲ Talk to other students. Chances are that many of them share your fears about test taking and may have discovered some helpful techniques of their own. Sometimes talking to your adviser or a counselor can also help.

▲ Be satisfied with doing your best. You can't expect to ace every test; all you can and should expect is your best effort. Once you've completed the exam, allow yourself the sweet pleasure of relief that it's over.

Glaser of Ohio State University, a month before finals one group of students was taught relaxation techniques—such as controlled breathing, meditation, progressive relaxation, and guided imagery (visualization). The more the students used these stress busters, the higher were their levels of immune cells during the exam period. The extra payoff was that they felt calmer and in better control during their tests.[22]

## Minorities and Stress

Regardless of your race or ethnic background, college may bring culture shock. You may never have encountered such a degree of diversity in one setting. You probably will meet students with different values, unfamiliar customs, entirely new ways of looking at the world—experiences you may find both stimulating and stressful.

Mental health professionals have long assumed that minority students may feel a double burden of stress. Racism has indeed been shown to be a source of stress that can affect health and well-being.[23] In the past, some African-American students have described predominately white campuses as hostile, alienating, and socially isolating; they have reported greater estrangement from the campus community and heightened estrangement in interactions with faculty and peers.[24] However, the generalization that all minority students are more stressed may not be valid.

A recent study conducted at a racially diverse university in a large metropolitan area in the Northeast evaluated 595 freshmen. The study group was made up of both genders and students of various racial and ethnic backgrounds, including Asians, African Americans, and Hispanics.[25] Less than 15 percent of these students—whether Asian, African American, Hispanic, white, or another ethnic minority—reported clinically significant levels of anger, anxiety, and depression, and there was no correlation between these stress-linked symptoms and ethnicity or race.

"Diversity, in and of itself, is unlikely to be related to higher levels of reported psychological symptoms on campus," the researchers concluded, theorizing that minority students "may have developed strengths while growing up within their particular cultures, subcommunities, and families that have often gone unrecognized or unnoted."[26] And some coping mechanisms, especially spirituality, can buffer the negative effects of racism.[27]

All minority students do share some common stressors. In one study of minority freshmen entering a large, competitive university, Asian, Hispanic, Filipino, African-American, and Native-American students all felt more sensitive and vulnerable to the college social climate, to interpersonal tensions between themselves and nonminority students and faculty, to experiences of actual or perceived racism, and to racist attitudes and discrimination (discussed later in this chapter, under Societal Stressors). Despite scoring above the national average on the SAT, the minority students in this study did not feel accepted as legitimate students and sensed that others viewed them as unworthy beneficiaries of affirmative action initiatives. While most said that overt racism was rare and relatively easy to deal with, they reported subtle pressures that undermined their academic confidence and their ability to bond with the university. Balancing these stressors, however, was a strong sense of ethnic identity, which helped buffer some stressful effects.

Hispanic students have identified three major types of stressors in their college experiences: academic (related to exam preparation and faculty interaction), social (related to ethnicity and interpersonal competence), and financial (related to their economic situation). Some Asian students who recently immigrated to the United States report feeling ostracized by students of similar ancestry who are second- or third-generation Americans. While they take pride in being truly bicultural and bilingual, the newcomers feel ambivalent about mainstream American culture. "My parents stress the importance of traditions; my friends tell me to get with it and act like an American," says one Asian-born student who has spent five years in the United States. "I feel trapped between cultures."

## Other Personal Stressors

### Job Stress

More so than ever, many people find that they are working more—up to 55 or 60 hours per week—and enjoying it less. This exhausting cycle of overwork causes stress, which makes work harder, which leads to more stress. Even the workplace itself can contribute to stress. A noisy, open-office environment can increase levels of stress without workers even realizing it.

Yet work in itself is not hazardous to health. Attitudes about work and habits related to how we work are the true threats. In fact, a job—stressful or not, enjoyable or not—can be therapeutic.

### Illness and Disability

Just as the mind can have profound effects on the body, the body can have an enormous impact on our emotions. Whenever we come down with the flu or pull a muscle, we feel under par. When the problem is more serious or persistent—a chronic disease like diabetes, for instance, or a lifelong hearing impairment—the emotional stress of constantly coping with it is even greater.

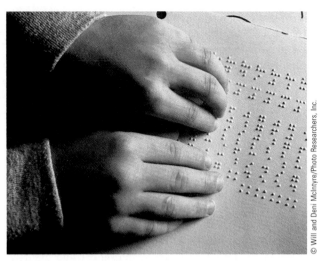

© Will and Deni McIntyre/Photo Researchers, Inc.

▲ The blind college student has unique challenges and stressors that sighted students do not.

A common source of stress for college students is a learning disability, which may affect one of every ten Americans. Most learning-disabled have average or above-average intelligence, but they rarely live up to their ability in school. Some have only one area of difficulty, such as reading or math. Others have problems with attention, writing, communicating, reasoning, coordination, social competence, and emotional maturity—all of which may make it difficult, if not impossible, for them to find and keep jobs. Special training and a better understanding of what's wrong can make an enormous difference.

Learning disorders can be hard to recognize in adults, who often become adept at covering up or compensating for their difficulties. However, someone with a learning disability may exhibit the following traits:

✔ Unable to engage in a focused activity such as reading.
✔ Extremely distractible, forgetful, or absentminded.
✔ Easily frustrated by waiting, delays, or traffic.
✔ Disorganized, unable to manage time efficiently and complete tasks on time.
✔ Hot tempered, explosive, constantly irritated.
✔ Impulsive, making decisions with little reflection or information.
✔ Easily overwhelmed by ordinary hassles.
✔ Clumsy, with a poor body image and poor sense of direction.
✔ Emotionally immature.
✔ Physically restless.

Individuals with several of these characteristics should undergo diagnostic tests to evaluate their skills and abilities and to determine whether remedial training, available through state offices of vocational rehabilitation, can help.

Not all students with learning disabilities may experience greater stress. In one in-depth study comparing 34 undergraduates with and without learning disabilities, the learning-disabled (LD) students reported significantly fewer college stressors and demonstrated a higher need for achievement. The LD students also scored significantly higher in resiliency and initiative in solving problems and working toward goals.[28]

## Societal Stressors

Not all stressors are personal. Centuries ago the poet John Donne observed that no man is an island. Today, on an increasingly crowded and troubled planet, these words seem truer than ever. Problems such as discrimination and terrorism can no longer be viewed only as economic or political issues. Directly or indirectly, they affect the well-being of all who inhabit the Earth—now and in the future. Even more mundane stressors, such as traffic, can lead to outbursts of anger that have come to be known as *road rage*.[29]

### Discrimination

Discrimination can take many forms—some as subtle as not being included in a conversation or joke, some as blatant as threats scrawled on a wall, some as violent as brutal beatings and other hate crimes. Because it can be hard to deal with individually, discrimination is a particularly sinister form of stress. By banding together, however, those who experience discrimination can take action to protect themselves, challenge the ignorance and hateful assumptions that fuel bigotry, and promote a healthier environment for all.

In the last decade, there have been reports of increased intolerance among young people and a greater tolerance for overt expressions and acts of hatred on college campuses. To counteract this trend, many schools have set up programs and classes to educate students about each other's backgrounds and to acknowledge and celebrate the richness diversity brings to campus life. Educators have called on universities to make campuses less alienating and more culturally and emotionally accessible, with programs and policies targeted not only at minority students but also at the university population as a whole.

### Violence and Terrorism

The deliberate use of physical force to abuse or injure is a leading killer of young people in the United States—and a potential source of stress in all our lives. Chances are that

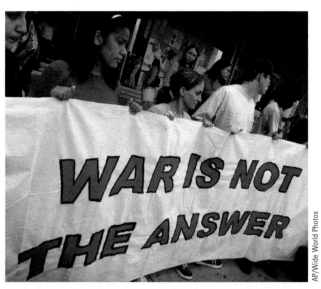

▲ Protest marches are one way in which college students have often responded to national and international crises, including global conflicts.

you or someone you know has been the victim of a violent crime, and awareness of our own vulnerability adds to the stress of daily living.

In the weeks after the September 11, 2001, terrorist attacks in New York and Washington, many Americans reported one or more significant symptoms of psychological distress. The residents of New York City suffered the greatest impact. According to an epidemiologic survey conducted in the second month after the attacks, more than half a million people in the metropolitan area were likely to develop posttraumatic stress disorder (PTSD).[30]

## Stress Survival

Sometimes we respond to stress or challenge with self-destructive behaviors, such as drinking or using drugs. These responses can lead to psychological problems, such as anxiety or depression, and physical problems, including psychosomatic illnesses.

**Defense mechanisms,** such as those described in Table 2-1, are another response to stress. These psychological devices are mental processes that help us cope with personal problems. Such responses are also not the answer to stress—and learning to recognize them in yourself will enable you to deal with your stress in a healthier way.

The key to coping with stress is realizing that your *perception* of and *response* to a stressor are crucial. Changing the way you interpret events or situations—a skill called *reframing*—makes all the difference. An event, such as a move to a new city, is not stressful in itself. A move becomes stressful if you see it as a traumatic upheaval rather than an exciting beginning of a new chapter in your life.

In times of stress, the following simple exercises can stop the stress buildup inside your body and help you regain a sense of calm and control.

✔ **Breathing.** Deep breathing relaxes the body and quiets the mind. Draw air deeply into your lungs, allowing your chest to fill with air and your belly to rise and fall. You will feel the muscle tension and stress begin to melt away. When you're feeling extremely stressed, try this calming breath: Sit or lie with your back straight and place the tip of your tongue on the roof of your mouth behind your teeth. Exhale completely through the mouth, then inhale through the nose for 4 seconds.

| ▼ Table 2-1  Common Defense Mechanisms Used to Alleviate Anxiety and Eliminate Conflict | |
|---|---|
| **Defense Mechanism** | **Example** |
| **Denial:** the refusal to accept a painful reality. | You don't accept as true the news that a loved one is seriously ill. |
| **Displacement:** the redirection of feelings from their true object to a more acceptable or safer substitute. | Instead of lashing out at a coach or a teacher, you snap at your best friend. |
| **Projection:** the attribution of unacceptable feelings or impulses to someone else. | When you want to end a relationship, you project your unhappiness onto your partner. |
| **Rationalization:** the substitution of "good," acceptable reasons for the real motivations for our behavior. | You report a classmate who has been mean to you for cheating on an exam and explain that cheating is unfair to other students. |
| **Reaction formation:** adopting attitudes and behaviors that are the opposite of what you feel. | You lavishly compliment an acquaintance whom you really despise. |
| **Repression:** the way we keep threatening impulses, fantasies, memories, feelings, or wishes from becoming conscious. | You don't "hear" the alarm after a late night, or you "forget" to take out the trash. |

## STRATEGIES FOR PREVENTION

### Recognize the Warning Signals of Stress Overload

▲ Experiencing physical symptoms, including chronic fatigue, headaches, indigestion, diarrhea, and sleep problems.

▲ Having frequent illness or worrying about illness.

▲ Self-medicating, including nonprescription drugs.

▲ Having problems concentrating on studies or work.

▲ Feeling irritable, anxious, or apathetic.

▲ Working or studying longer and harder than usual.

▲ Exaggerating, to yourself and others, the importance of what you do.

▲ Becoming accident-prone.

▲ Breaking rules, whether it's a curfew at home or a speed limit on the highway.

▲ Going to extremes, such as drinking too much, overspending, or gambling.

Hold the breath for 7 seconds, then exhale audibly through the mouth for 8 seconds. Repeat four times.

✔ **Refocusing.** Thinking about a situation you can't change or control only increases the stress you feel. Force your mind to focus on other subjects. If you're stuck in a long line, distract yourself. Check out what other people are buying or imagine what they do for a living. In a traffic jam, turn on the car radio to a music station you like. Imagine that you're in a hot shower and a wave of relaxation is washing your stress down the drain.

✔ **Serenity breaks.** Build moments of tranquility into your day. For instance, while waiting for your computer to warm up or a file to download, look at a photograph of someone you love or a poster of a tropical island. If none is available, close your eyes and visualize a soothing scene, such as walking in a meadow or along a beach.

✔ **Stress signals.** Learn to recognize the first signs that your stress load is getting out of hand: Is your back bothering you? Do you have a headache? Do you find yourself speeding or misplacing things? Whenever you spot these early warnings, force yourself to stop and say, "I'm under stress. I need to do something about it."

✔ **Reality checks.** To put things into proper perspective, ask yourself: Will I remember what's made me so upset a month from now? If I had to rank this problem on a scale of 1 to 10, with worldwide catastrophe as 10, where would it rate?

✔ **Stress inoculation.** Rehearse everyday situations that you find stressful, such as speaking in class. Think of

## Savvy Consumer

### Can Stress-Relief Products Help?

You're stressed out, and you see an ad for a product—an oil, candle, cream, herbal tea, pill, or potion—that promises to make all your cares disappear. Should you soak in an aromatic bath, have a massage, try kava, squeeze foam balls? In most cases, you're probably not doing yourself much harm, but you aren't necessarily doing yourself much good either. Keep these considerations in mind:

• Be wary of instant cures. Regardless of the promises on the label, it's unrealistic to expect any magic ingredient or product to make all your problems disappear.

• Focus on stress-reducing behavior, rather than a product. An aromatic candle may not bring instant serenity, but if you light a candle and meditate, you may indeed feel more at peace. A scented pillow may

not be a cure for a stress, but if it helps you get a good night's sleep, you'll cope better the next day.

• Exercise is one of the best ways to lower your stress levels. Try walking, running, swimming, cycling, kickboxing—anything physical that helps you release tension.

• Don't make matters worse by smoking (the chemicals in cigarettes increase heart rate, blood pressure, and stress hormone), consuming too much caffeine (it speeds up your system for hours), eating snacks high in sugar (it produces a quick high followed by a sudden slump), or turning to drugs or alcohol (they can only add to your stress when their effects wear off).

• Remember that stress is a matter of attitude. Remind yourself of some basic words of wisdom: Don't sweat the small stuff—and it's all small stuff.

how you might make the situation less tense, for instance, by breathing deeply before you talk or jotting down notes beforehand. Think of these small doses of stress as the psychological equivalent of allergy shots: They immunize you so you feel less stressed when bigger challenges come along.[31]

✓ **Laughter.** Humor counters stress by focusing on comic aspects of difficult situations and may, as various studies have shown, lessen harmful effects on the immune system and overall health.

 Humor may have different effects on stress in men and women. In a study of 131 undergraduates, humor buffered stress-related physical symptoms in men and women. However, it reduced stress-linked anxiety only in men. The researchers theorized that men may prefer humor as a more appropriate way of expressing emotions such as anxiety, whereas women are more likely to use self-disclosure, that is, to confide in friends.[32]

✓ **Spiritual coping.** Saying a prayer under stress is one of the oldest and most effective ways of calming yourself. Other forms of spiritual coping, such as putting trust in God and helping others (for instance, by volunteering at a shelter for battered women) also can provide a different perspective on daily hassles and stresses.

✓ **Sublimation.** This term refers to the redirection of any drives considered unacceptable into socially acceptable channels. Outdoor activity is one of the best ways to reduce stress through sublimation. For instance, if you're furious with a friend who betrayed your trust or frustrated because your boss rejects all of your proposals, you might go for a long run or hike to sublimate your anger.

✓ **Journaling.** One of the simplest, yet most effective, ways to work through stress is by putting your feelings into words that only you will read. The more honest and open you are as you write, the better. According to the research of psychologist James Pennebaker of the University of Texas, Austin, college students who wrote in their journals about traumatic events felt much better afterward than those who wrote about superficial topics.[33]

## ???? What Can Help Me Relax?

Relaxation is the physical and mental state opposite that of stress. Rather than gearing up for fight or flight, our bodies and minds grow calmer and work more smoothly. We're less likely to become frazzled and more capable of staying in control. The most effective relaxation techniques include progressive relaxation, visualization, meditation, mindfulness, and biofeedback.

**Progressive relaxation** works by intentionally increasing and then decreasing tension in the muscles. While sitting or lying down in a quiet, comfortable setting,

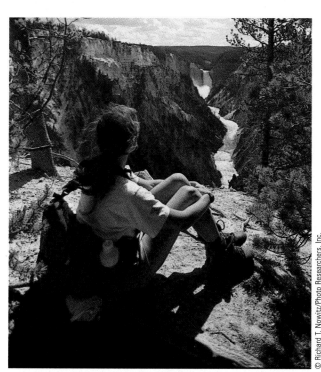

▲ Spending time outdoors is a great way to leave behind daily tensions and gain a new perspective.

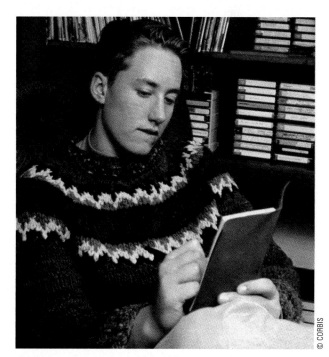

▲ Writing in your journal about feelings and difficulties is a simple and very effective way to help control your stress.

you tense and release various muscles, beginning with those of the hand, for instance, and then proceeding to the arms, shoulders, neck, face, scalp, chest, stomach, buttocks, genitals, and so on, down each leg to the toes. Relaxing the muscles can quiet the mind and restore internal balance.

**Visualization,** or **guided imagery,** involves creating mental pictures that calm you down and focus your mind. Some people use this technique to promote healing when they are ill. Visualization skills require practice and, in some cases, instruction by qualified health professionals.

**Meditation** has been practiced in many forms over the ages, from the yogic techniques of the Far East to the Quaker silence of more modern times. Brain scans have shown that meditation activates the sections of the brain in charge of the autonomic nervous system, which governs bodily functions, such as digestion and blood pressure, that we cannot consciously control.[34] Although many studies have documented the benefits of meditation for overall health, it may be particularly helpful for people dealing with stress-related medical conditions such as high blood pressure.

 In a study of African Americans with arteriosclerosis, or hardening of the arteries, those who meditated showed a marked decrease in the thickness of their artery walls, while the nonmeditators showed an increase. This benefit is particularly important because African Americans are twice as likely to die from cardiovascular disease as are whites.[35]

Meditation helps a person reach a state of relaxation, but with the goal of achieving inner peace and harmony. There is no one right way to meditate, and many people have discovered how to meditate on their own, without even knowing what it is they are doing. Among college students, meditation has proven especially effective in increasing relaxation. Most forms of meditation have common elements: sitting quietly for 15 to 20 minutes once or twice a day, concentrating on a word or image, and breathing slowly and rhythmically. If you wish to try meditation, it often helps to have someone guide you through your first sessions.

**Mindfulness** is a modern form of an ancient Asian technique that involves maintaining awareness in the present moment. You tune in to each part of your body, scanning from head to toe, noting the slightest sensation. You allow whatever you experience—an itch, an ache, a feeling of warmth—to enter your awareness. Then you open yourself to focus on all the thoughts, sensations, sounds, and feelings that enter your awareness. Mindfulness keeps you in the here and now, thinking about what *is* rather than about *what if* or *if only.*

**Biofeedback** is a method of obtaining feedback, or information, about some physiological activity occurring in the body. An electronic monitoring device attached to the body detects a change in an internal function and communicates it back to the person through a tone, light, or meter. By paying attention to this feedback, most people can gain some control over functions previously thought to be beyond conscious control, such as body temperature, heart rate, muscle tension, and brain waves. The goal of biofeedback for stress reduction is a state of tranquility, usually associated with the brain's production of alpha waves, which are slower and more regular than normal waking waves.

## Time Management

We live in what some sociologists call hyperculture, a society that moves at warp speed. Information constantly bombards us. The rate of change seems to accelerate every year. Our time-saving devices—pagers, cell phones, modems, faxes, palm-sized organizers, laptop computers—have simply extended the boundaries of where and how we work.

As a result, more and more people are suffering from time sickness, a nerve-racking feeling that life has become little more than an endless to-do list. The best antidote is time management, and hundreds of books, seminars, and experts offer training in making the most of the hours in the day. Yet these well-intentioned methods often fail, and sooner or later most of us find ourselves caught in a time trap.

###  How Can I Better Manage My Time?

Time management involves skills that anyone can learn, but they require commitment and practice to make a difference in your life. It may help to know the techniques that other students have found most useful:

- ✔ **Schedule your time.** Use a calendar or planner. Beginning the first week of class, mark down deadlines for each assignment, paper, project, and test scheduled that semester. Develop a daily schedule, listing very specifically what you will do the next day, along with the times. Block out times for working out, eating dinner, calling home, and talking with friends as well as for studying.
- ✔ **Develop a game plan.** Allow at least two nights to study for any major exam. Set aside more time for researching and writing papers. Make sure to allow time to type and print out a paper—and to deal with emergencies like a computer breakdown. Set daily and weekly goals for every class. When working on a big project, don't neglect your other courses. Whenever possible, try to work ahead in all your classes.

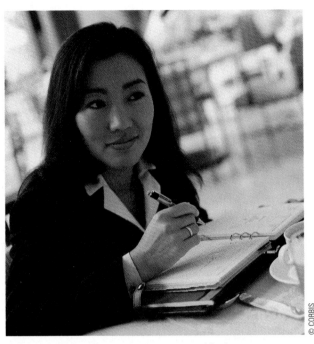

▲ A calendar or planner is an important tool in time management. You can use it to keep track of assignment due dates, class meetings, and other "to do's."

✔ **Identify time robbers.** For several days keep a log of what you do and how much time you spend doing it. You may discover that disorganization is eating away at your time or that you have a problem getting started. (See the following section on Overcoming Procrastination.)

✔ **Make the most of classes.** Read the assignments before class rather than waiting until just before you have a test. By reading ahead of time, you'll make it easier to understand the lectures. Go to class yourself. Your own notes will be more helpful than a friend's or those from a note-taking service. Read your lecture notes at the end of each day or at least at the end of each week.

✔ **Develop an efficient study style.** Some experts recommend studying for 50 minutes, then breaking for 10 minutes. Small incentives, such as allowing yourself to call or visit a friend during these 10 minutes, can provide the motivation to keep you at the books longer. When you're reading, don't just highlight passages. Instead, write notes or questions to yourself in the margins, which will help you retain more information. Even if you're racing to start a paper, take a few extra minutes to prepare a workable outline. It will be easier to structure your paper when you start writing.

✔ **Focus on the task at hand.** Rather than worrying about how you did on yesterday's test or how you'll ever finish next week's project, focus intently on whatever you're doing at any given moment. If your mind starts to wander, use any distraction—the sound of the phone ringing or a noise from the hall—as a reminder to stay in the moment.

✔ **Turn elephants into hors d'oeuvres.** Cut a huge task into smaller chunks so it seems less enormous. For instance, break down your term paper into a series of steps, such as selecting a topic, identifying sources of research information, taking notes, developing an outline, and so on.

✔ **Keep your workspace in order.** Even if the rest of your room is a shambles, try to keep your desk clear. Piles of papers are distracting, and you can end up wasting lots of time looking for notes you misplaced or an article you have to read by morning. Try to spend the last ten minutes of the day cleaning up your desk so you will have a fresh start on the new day.

## Overcoming Procrastination

 Putting off until tomorrow what should be done today is a habit that creates a great deal of stress for many students. It also takes a surprising toll. In a study of students taking a health psychology course, researchers found that although procrastinating provided short-term benefits, including periods of low stress, the tendency to dawdle had long-term costs, including poorer health and lower grades. Early in the semester, the procrastinators reported less stress and fewer health problems than students who scored low on procrastination. However, by the end of the semester, procrastinators reported more health-related symptoms, more stress, and more visits to health-care professionals than nonprocrastinators.[36] Students who procrastinate also get poorer grades in courses with many deadlines.[37]

The three most common types of procrastination are: putting off unpleasant things, putting off difficult tasks, and putting off tough decisions. Procrastinators are most likely to delay by wishing they didn't have to do what they must or by telling themselves they "just can't get started," which means they never do.

To get out of the procrastination trap, keep track of the tasks you're most likely to put off, and try to figure out why you don't want to tackle them. Think of alternative ways to complete these tasks. If you put off library readings, for instance, is the problem getting to the library or the reading itself? If it's the trip to the library, arrange to walk over with a friend whose company you enjoy.

Develop daily time-management techniques, such as a to-do list. Rank items according to priorities (A, B, C), and schedule your days to make sure the A's get accomplished. Try not to fixate on half-completed projects. Divide large tasks, such as a term paper, into smaller ones, and reward yourself when you complete a part.

Do what you like least first. Once you have it out of the way, you can concentrate on the tasks you enjoy. Learn to live according to a three-word motto: Just do it!

© CORBIS

What is the difference between short-term and long-term stress? How does stress affect your health?

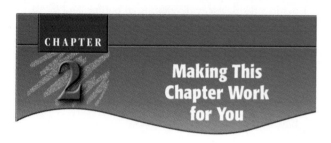

CHAPTER 2

**Making This Chapter Work for You**

1. Stress can be defined as
   a. a negative emotional state related to fatigue and similar to depression.
   b. the physiological and psychological response to any event or situation that either upsets or excites us.
   c. the end result of the general adaptation syndrome.
   d. a motivational strategy for making life changes.

2. According to the general adaptation syndrome theory, how does the body typically respond to an acute stressor?
   a. The heart rate slows, blood pressure declines, and eye movement increases.
   b. The body enters a physical state called eustress and then moves into the physical state referred to as distress.
   c. If the stressor is viewed as a positive event, there are no physical changes.
   d. The body demonstrates three stages of change: alarm, resistance, and exhaustion.

3. Over time, increased levels of stress hormones have been shown to increase a person's risk for which of the following conditions?
   a. diabetes, high blood pressure, memory loss, and skin disorders
   b. stress fractures, male pattern baldness, and hypothyroidism
   c. hemophilia, AIDS, and hay fever
   d. none of the above

4. A person suffering from posttraumatic stress disorder may experience which of the following symptoms?
   a. procrastination
   b. constant thirst
   c. drowsiness
   d. terror-filled dreams

5. Stress levels in college students
   a. may be high due to stressors such as academic pressures, financial concerns, learning disabilities, and relationship problems.

   b. are usually low because students feel empowered, living independently of their parents.
   c. are typically highest in seniors because their self-esteem diminishes during the college years.
   d. are lower in minority students because they are used to stressors such as a hostile social climate and actual or perceived discrimination.

6. Which of the following situations is representative of a societal stressor?
   a. Peter has been told that his transfer application has been denied because his transcripts were not sent in by the deadline.
   b. Nia and Kwame find an unsigned note pinned to the door of their new home, ordering them to move out or face the consequences.
   c. Kelli's boyfriend drives her car after he had been drinking and has an accident.
   d. Joshua, who is the leading basketball player on his college varsity team, has just been diagnosed with diabetes.

7. Which of the following illustrates the defense mechanism of displacement?
   a. You have a beer in the evening after a tough day.
   b. You act as if nothing has happened after you have been laid off from your job.
   c. You start an argument with your sister after being laid off from your job.
   d. You argue with your boss after he lays you off from your job.

8. If you are stuck in a traffic jam, which of the following actions will help reduce your stress level?
   a. deep slow breathing
   b. honking your horn
   c. berating yourself for not taking a different route
   d. getting on your cell phone to reschedule appointments

9. A relaxed peaceful state of being can be achieved with which of the following activities?
   a. an aerobic exercise class
   b. playing a computer game
   c. meditating for 15 minutes
   d. attending a rap concert

10. To effectively manage your time, which of these techniques should you try?
    a. Use a calendar or planner.
    b. Keep a log of your activities for a week.
    c. Tackle a large task by breaking it down into a series of smaller tasks.
    d. All of the above.

Answers to these questions can be found on page 415.

## Critical Thinking

1. Stress levels among college students have reached record highs. What reasons can you think of to account for this? Consider possible social, cultural, and economic factors that may play a role.

2. Identify three stressful situations in your life and determine whether they are examples of eustress or distress. Describe both the positive and negative aspects of each situation.

3. Can you think of any ways in which your behavior or attitudes might create stress for others? What changes could you make to avoid doing so?

4. What advice might you give an incoming freshman at your school about managing stress in college? What techniques have been most helpful for you in dealing with stress? Suppose that this student is from a different ethnic group than you? What additional suggestions would you have for this student?

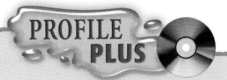

## PROFILE PLUS

How is stress affecting you? Discover how you respond to stressful situations by participating in the following activities on your Profile Plus CD-ROM:

Life Experiences Survey * Type A Behavior * The Stress Test * Stress Vulnerability Questionnaire * Hostile Personality Assessment

## SITES & BYTES

### Stress Assess
**http://wellness.uwsp.edu/Health_Service/Services/stress.htm**

This site features a comprehensive educational tool to help assess your current stress sources, distress symptoms, and lifestyle behaviors. It is not a clinical or diagnostic tool. Based on your personalized assessment, you can learn healthy and effective strategies to balance the stress in your life. (Be careful when you key in this case-sensitive address.)

### National Center for PTSD
**www.ncptsd.org**

This site features comprehensive information and publications on posttraumatic stress disorder, including causes, frequently asked questions, treatment, and research.

### Stress Inc.
**stress.irn.columbia.edu**

This interactive website from Columbia University features a variety of stress management resources, includ-

ing tension breakers and a stress quiz to test your knowledge.

Please note that links are subject to change. If you find a broken link, use a search engine such as http://www.yahoo.com and search for the website by typing in keywords.

### InfoTrac College Edition Activity

Gerd Karin Natvig, Grethe Albrektsen, and Ulla Qvarnstrom. "School-Related Stress Experience As a Risk Factor for Bullying Behavior." *Journal of Youth and Adolescence,* Vol. 30, No. 5, October 2001, p. 561.

1. What are some personality characteristics of bullying behavior?
2. Describe some of the various ways of coping with stressful environments.
3. According to the authors, what personal resource may prevent the negative consequences of stress resulting from bullying behaviors?

Kevin J. Edwards, Paul J. Hershberger, Richard K. Russell, and Ronald J. Markert. "Stress, Negative Social Exchange, and Health Symptoms in University Students." *Journal of American College Health,* Vol. 50, No. 2, September 2001, p. 75.

1. Based on this study, what is the relationship between negative social interaction and physical symptoms?
2. How did the investigators measure chronic life stress in the college students at Ohio State University?
3. What did this study reveal about the relationship between physical health and the negative social support due to abusive relationships?

You can find additional readings relating to stress management with InfoTrac College Edition, an online library of more than 900 journals and publications. Follow the instructions for accessing InfoTrac that were packaged with your textbook; then search for articles using a keyword search.

For additional links, resources, and suggested readings on InfoTrac, visit our Health & Wellness Resource Center at http://health.wadsworth.com.

## Key Terms

The terms listed here are used within the chapter on the page indicated. Definitions of the terms are in the Glossary at the end of the book.

**adaptive response** 28
**biofeedback** 40
**defense mechanism** 37
**distress** 28
**eustress** 28

**general adaptation syndrome (GAS)** 28
**guided imagery** 40
**homeostasis** 28
**meditation** 40

**mindfulness** 40
**posttraumatic stress disorder (PTSD)** 31
**progressive relaxation** 39
**stress** 28

**stressor** 28
**visualization** 40

## References

1. Lazarus, R., and R. Launier. "Stress-Related Transactions Between Person and Environment" in *Perspectives in Interactional Psychology.* New York: Plenum, 1978.
2. Senior, Kathryn. "Should Stress Carry a Health Warning?" *Lancet,* Vol. 357, No. 9250, January 13, 2001, p. 126.
3. Sheps, David, et al. "Mental Stress–Induced Ischemia and All-Cause Mortality in Patients with Coronary Artery Disease: Results from the Psychophysiological Investigations of Myocardial Ischemia Study." *Circulation,* Vol. 105, March 26, 2002, p. 1780.
4. "Stress Increases Fat's Staying Power." *American Medical News,* Vol. 45, No. 9, March 4, 2002, p. 38.
5. Davis, Mary, et al. "Body Fat Distribution and Hemodynamic Stress Responses in Premenopausal Obese Women: A Preliminary Study." *Health Psychology,* Vol. 18, No. 6, November 1999, p. 625.
6. Epel, Elissa. "Can Stress Shape Your Body? Stress and Cortisol Reactivity Among Women with Central Body Fat Distribution." *Yale University, U.S. Dissertation Abstracts International, Section B: The Sciences & Engineering,* Vol. 60, No. 5-B, December 1999, p. 2403.
7. Glaser, Ronald, and Janice Kiecolt-Glaser. *Handbook of Human Stress and Immunity.* San Diego: Academic Press, 1994.
8. Takkouche, Bahi, et al. "Stress and Susceptibility to the Common Cold." *Epidemiology,* Vol. 11, April 2001, p. 345.
9. Baker, Lori. "9/11 Toll on Mentally Ill." *Psychology Today,* March–April 2002, p. 15.
10. Schnyder, Ulrich, et al. "Incidence and Prediction of Posttraumatic Stress Disorder Symptoms in Severely Injured Accident Victims." *American Journal of Psychiatry,* Vol. 158, No. 4, April 2001, p. 594.
11. Wijma, Klaas, et al. "Prevalence of Post-Traumatic Stress Disorder Among Gynecological Patients with a History of Sexual and Physical Abuse." *Journal of Interpersonal Violence,* Vol. 15, No. 9, September 2000, p. 944.
12. "Stressed Out on Campus." *Techniques,* Vol. 75, No. 3, March 2000.
13. Sax, Linda, et al. *The American Freshman: National Norms for Fall 2001.* Los Angeles: Higher Education Research Institute, UCLA, 2001.
14. Bartlett, Thomas. "Freshmen Pay, Mentally and Physically, As They Adjust to Life in College." *Chronicle of Higher Education,* February 1, 2002.
15. Jackson, Pamela Braboy, and Montenique Finney. "Negative Life Events and Psychological Distress Among Young Adults." *Social Psychology Quarterly,* Vol. 65, No. 2, p. 186.
16. Hertel, James. "College Students Generational Status: Similarities, Differences, and Factors in College Adjustment." *The Psychological Record,* Vol. 52, No. 1, Winter 2002, p. 3.
17. Deckro, Gloria, et al. "The Evaluation of a Mind/Body Intervention to Reduce Psychological Distress and Perceived Stress in College Students." *Journal of American College Health,* Vol. 50, No. 6, May 2002, p. 281.
18. Hertel, "College Students Generational Status."

19. Misra, Ranjita, and Michelle McKean. "College Students, Academic Stress and Its Relation to Their Anxiety, Time Management and Leisure Satisfaction." *American Journal of Health Studies,* Vol. 16, No. 1, Winter 2000.

20. Dixon, Wayne, and Jon Reid. "Positive Life Events As a Moderator of Stress-Related Depressive Symptoms." *Journal of Counseling and Development,* Vol. 78, No. 3, Summer 2000.

21. Deckro, et al. "The Evaluation of a Mind/Body Intervention."

22. Glaser and Kiecolt-Glaser, *Handbook of Human Stress and Immunity.* Hornig-Rohan, Mary. "Stress, Immune-Mediators, and Immune-Mediated Disease." *Advances: The Journal of Mind-Body Health,* Vol. 11, No. 2, Spring 1995.

23. Harrell, Shelly. "A Multidimensional Conceptualization of Racism-Related Stress: Implications for the Well-Being of People of Color." *American Journal of Orthopsychiatry,* Vol. 70, No. 1, January 2000.

24. Launier, Raymond. "Stress Balance and Emotional Life Complexes in Students in a Historically African American College." *Journal of Psychology,* Vol. 131, No. 2, March 1997.

25. Rosenthal, Beth Spenciner, and Arleen Cedeno Schreiner. "Prevalence of Psychological Symptoms Among Undergraduate Students in an Ethnically Diverse Urban Public College." *Journal of American College Health,* Vol. 49, No. 1, July 2000.

26. Ibid.

27. Bowen-Reid, Terra, and Jules Harrell. "Racist Experiences and Health Outcomes: An Examination of Spirituality As a Buffer." *Journal of Black Psychology,* Vol. 28, No. 1, February 2002, p. 18.

28. Hall, Cathy, et al. "Motivational and Attitudinal Factors in College Students With and Without Learning Disabilities." *Learning Disability Quarterly,* Vol. 25, No. 1, Spring 2002, p. 79.

29. "Driving-Induced Stress in Urban College Students." *Perceptual and Motor Skills,* Vol. 90, No. 2, April 2000.

30. Schlenger, William, et al. "Psychological Reactions to Terrorist Attacks: Findings from the National Study of Americans' Reactions to September 11." *Journal of the American Medical Association,* Vol. 288, No. 5, August 7, 2002, p. 581.

31. Saunders, Teri, et al. "The Effect of Stress Inoculation Training on Anxiety and Performance." *Journal of Occupational Health Psychology,* Vol. 1, No. 2, pp. 170–186.

32. Abel, Millicent. "Interaction of Humor and Gender in Moderating Relationships Between Stress and Outcomes." *Journal of Psychology,* Vol. 132, No. 3, May 1998.

33. Pennebaker, James. "Putting Stress into Words: Health, Linguistic and Therapeutic Implications." *Behavioral Research,* Vol. 31, No. 6, 1993.

34. Barbar, Cary. "The Science of Meditation." *Psychology Today,* May–June 2001, p. 54.

35. "Is Meditation Good Medicine?" *Harvard Women's Health Watch,* Vol. 8, No. 5, January 2001, p. 1.

36. "Procrastinators Always Finish Last, Even in Health," *American Psychological Monitor,* Vol. 20, No. 1, January 1998.

37. Tuchman, Bruce. "Procrastinators." Presentation, American Psychological Association, Chicago, August 22, 2002.

# Psychological Health

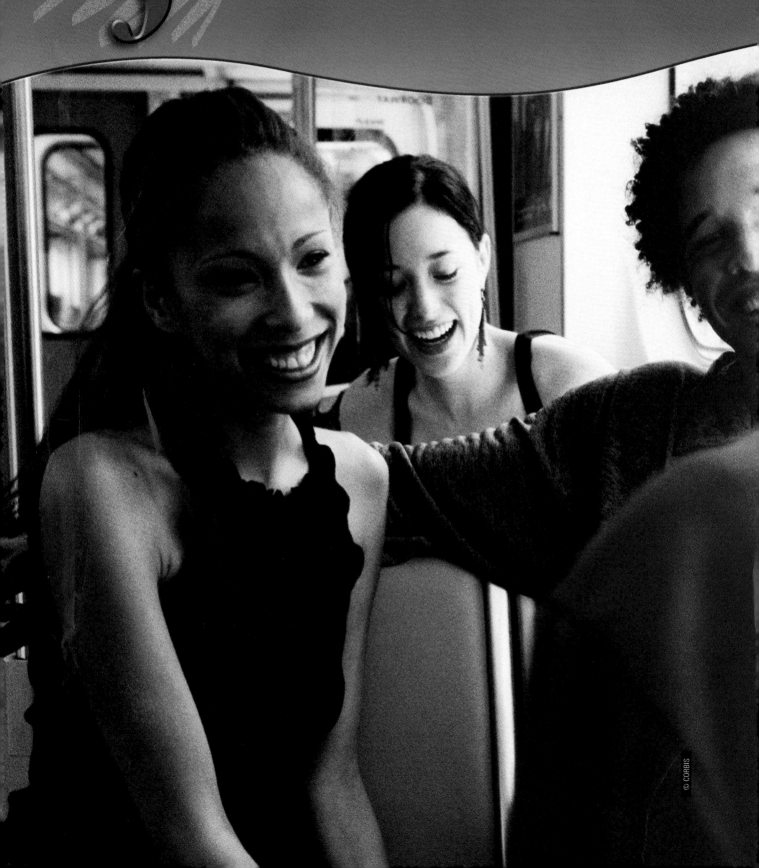

## After studying the material in this chapter, you should be able to:

- **Identify** the characteristics of emotional, mental, and spiritual health.
- **Discuss** the concepts of emotional and spiritual intelligence.
- **Describe** the relationship of needs, values, self-esteem, a sense of control, and relationships to psychological health.
- **Explain** the differences between mental health and mental illness, and **list** some effects of mental illness on physical health.
- **Describe** the major mental illnesses—anxiety disorders, depressive disorders, attention disorders, and schizophrenia—and the characteristic symptoms of each type.
- **Discuss** some of the factors that may lead to suicide as well as strategies for prevention.
- **Describe** the treatment options available for those with psychological problems.

outh can seem a golden time, when body and mind glow with potential. However, the process of becoming an adult is challenging in every culture and country. Psychological health can make the difference between facing this challenge with optimism and confidence or feeling overwhelmed by expectations and responsibilities.

Unlike physical health, psychological well-being cannot be measured, tested, X-rayed, or dissected. Yet psychologically healthy men and women generally share certain characteristics: They value themselves and strive toward happiness and fulfillment. They establish and maintain close relationships with others. They accept the limitations as well as the possibilities that life has to offer. And they feel a sense of meaning and purpose that makes the gestures of living worth the effort required. Feeling good does not depend on money, success, recognition, or status.

At some point in life, one of every three people develops an emotional disorder. Young adulthood—the years from the late teens to the mid-twenties—is a time when many serious disorders, including bipolar illness (manic depression) and schizophrenia, often develop.

The saddest fact is not that so many feel so bad, but that so few realize they can feel better. Only one of every five men and women who could use treatment ever seeks help. Yet 80 to 90 percent of those treated for psychological problems recover, most within a few months.[1]

By learning about psychological disorders, you may be able to recognize early warning

 **FREQUENTLY ASKED QUESTIONS**

**FAQ: How can I lead a fulfilling life? p. 50**

**FAQ: What is a mental disorder? p. 55**

**FAQ: Why are so many young people depressed? p. 59**

**FAQ: What leads to suicide? p. 62**

**FAQ: Where can I turn for help? p. 65**

signals in yourself or your loved ones so you can deal with potential difficulties or seek professional help for more serious problems.

## What Is Psychological Health?

"A sound mind in a sound body is a short but full description of a happy state in this world," the philosopher John Locke wrote in 1693. More than 300 years later his statement still rings true. Both physical and psychological well-being are essential to total wellness. However, modern theorists have gone beyond these general requirements to analyze other components of well-being, including coping styles, goals, and adaptation to stress and change.[2]

Psychological health encompasses both our emotional and mental states—that is, our feelings and our thoughts. **Emotional health** generally refers to feelings and moods, both of which are discussed later in this chapter. Characteristics of emotionally healthy persons, identified in an analysis of major studies of emotional wellness, include the following:

- Determination and effort to be healthy.
- Flexibility and adaptability to a variety of circumstances.
- Development of a sense of meaning of and affirmation for life.
- An understanding that the self is not the center of the universe.
- Compassion for others.
- The ability to be unselfish in serving or relating to others.
- Increased depth and satisfaction in intimate relationships.
- A sense of control over the mind and body that leads to health-enhancing choices and decisions.[3]

**Mental health** describes our ability to perceive reality as it is, to respond to its challenges, and to develop rational strategies for living. The mentally healthy person doesn't try to avoid conflicts and distress, but copes with life's transitions, traumas, and losses in a way that allows for emotional stability and growth. The characteristics of mental health include:

- The ability to function and carry out responsibilities.
- The ability to form relationships.
- Realistic perceptions of the motivations of others.
- Rational, logical thought processes.

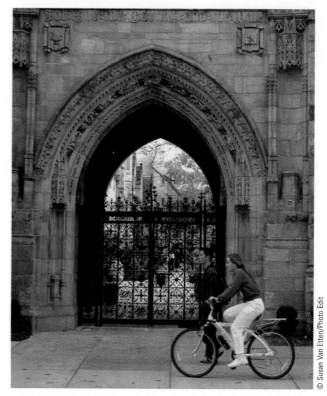

▲ Psychologically healthy people can adapt to a variety of circumstances, have the ability to form relationships, and strive to achieve their full potential.

- The ability to adapt to change and to cope with adversity.[4]

There is considerable overlap between psychological health and **spiritual health,** which involves our ability to identify our basic purpose in life and to experience the fulfillment of achieving our full potential. However, many people consider the two separate. "We like to think that emotional problems have to do with the family, childhood, and trauma—with personal life but not with spirituality," observes Thomas Moore, author of *Care of the Soul,* "Yet it is obvious that the soul, seat of the deepest emotions, can benefit greatly from the gifts of a vivid spiritual life and can suffer when it is deprived of them."[5]

In addition, **culture** helps to define psychological health. In one culture, men and women may express feelings with great intensity, shouting with joy or wailing in grief, while in another culture such behavior might be considered abnormal or unhealthy. In our diverse society, many cultural influences affect Americans' sense of who they are, where they came from, and what they believe. Cultural rituals help bring people together, strengthen their bonds, reinforce the values and beliefs they share, and provide a sense of belonging, meaning, and purpose.

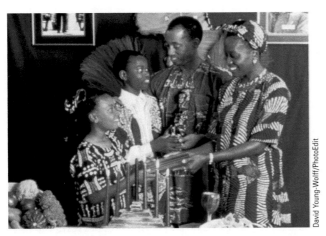

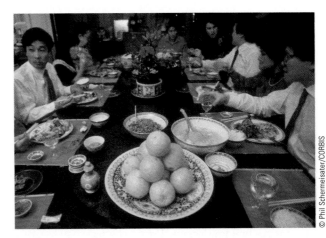

▲ Special holidays, such as Kwanza and Chinese New Year, bring people together in cultural celebration.

## Emotional Intelligence

A person's IQ—intelligence quotient—was once considered the leading determinant of achievement. However, psychologists have determined that another way of knowing, dubbed **emotional intelligence,** may make an even greater difference in a person's personal and professional success. In his international best-seller on what some call EQ (for emotional quotient), psychologist Daniel Goleman identifies five components of emotional intelligence: self-awareness, altruism, personal motivation, empathy, and the ability to love and be loved by friends, partners, and family members. People who possess high emotional intelligence are the people who truly succeed in work as well as play, building flourishing careers and lasting, meaningful relationships.[6]

 Men and women, who vary more in the intensity of their emotional experiences than in the nature of their emotions, are equally capable of cultivating greater emotional intelligence. Emotional intelligence isn't fixed at birth, nor is it the same as intuition. The emotional competencies that most benefit students are focusing on clear, manageable goals, and identifying and understanding emotions rather than relying on gut feelings.[7]

## Spiritual Intelligence

Spiritual approaches to knowledge and well-being are the focus of much scholarly interest and research. As noted in Chapter 1, a growing number of research studies are assessing the impact of spirituality on health, and nearly 30 medical schools include courses on religion, spirituality, and health in their curricula.[8]

Mental health professionals also are recognizing the power of **spiritual intelligence,** which some define as the capacity to sense, understand, and tap into the highest parts of ourselves, others, and the world around us. Unlike spirituality, spiritual intelligence does not center on the worship of a God above, but on the discovery of a wisdom within. All of us are born with the potential to develop spiritual intelligence, but relatively few do. Yet its dividends are many. As one minister put it, this way of knowing provides solutions—often surprising and unexpected—to problems that had seemed insolvable.[9]

Here are some guidelines for tapping into your own spiritual intelligence:

- Build silence and solitude into your daily life. Even a few stolen moments in the early morning or evening hours can help quiet the hum of constant distractions. "There is an inner wisdom," says cardiologist Dean Ornish, "but it speaks very, very softly." He suggests ending each session with a question like "What am I not paying attention to that's important?"[10]
- Spend time in nature. A walk on the beach, a stroll through a park, or simply looking up at the night sky has value—perhaps because nature helps put our mostly man-made problems into perspective.
- Keep company with the wise, either in person or through their words. Inspirational people and their writings provide factual knowledge and insight that enable us to examine serious issues.
- Reflect on the nature of life and death. You don't need a doctorate in philosophy for this task because the basic principles are simple: Life is precious. Life is short. Death is certain. While life involves difficulties, these can be transcended rather than avoided.
- Practice spiritual values. Spiritual intelligence is not a spectator sport. Rather than just contemplating kindness and honesty, we have to live them as best we can. One of the best places to learn and practice forgiveness is on the highway.

# ?????How Can I Lead a Fulfilling Life?

What's life all about? We all ask this question sooner or later. Whether dreams come true or fade away, whether we achieve our goals or not, we find ourselves confronting profound questions about the purpose of our time on Earth. No recipe can guarantee a life worth living. Each of us must create life satisfaction on our own.

Psychology, a field that traditionally concentrated on what goes wrong in our lives and in our minds, has shifted its focus to the study of what goes right. *Positive psychology* emphasizes building personal strengths rather than treating weaknesses. One of its key beliefs is that young people who learn to be **optimistic** and resilient are less likely to suffer from mental disorders and more likely to lead happy, productive lives.

Positive attitudes may even prolong life. In a study that has followed 678 Catholic nuns into old age, those who expressed more positive emotions (such as joy, love, hope, and happiness) in autobiographies written in their twenties lived as much as ten years longer than those expressing fewer positive emotions.[11]

## Knowing Your Needs

Newborns are unable to survive on their own. They depend on others for the satisfaction of their physical needs for food, shelter, warmth, and protection, as well as their less tangible emotional needs. In growing to maturity, children take on more responsibility and become more independent. No one, however, becomes totally self-sufficient. As adults, we easily recognize our basic physical needs, but we often fail to acknowledge our emotional needs. Yet they, too, must be met if we are to be as fulfilled as possible.

The humanist theorist Abraham Maslow believed that human needs are the motivating factors in personality development. First we must satisfy basic physiological needs, such as those for food, shelter, and sleep. Only then can we pursue fulfillment of our higher needs—for safety and security, love and affection, and self-esteem. Few individuals reach the state of **self-actualization,** in which one functions at the highest possible level and derives the greatest possible satisfaction from life. (See Figure 3-1.)

## Clarifying Your Values

Your **values**—the criteria by which you evaluate things, people, events, and yourself—represent what's most important to you. In a world of almost dizzying complexity, values can provide guidelines for making decisions that are right for you. If understood and applied, they help give life meaning and structure.

Social psychologist Milton Rokeach distinguished between two types of values. *Instrumental values* represent ways of thinking and acting that we hold important, such as being loving or loyal. *Terminal values* represent goals, achievements, or ideal states that we strive toward, such as happiness. Instrumental and terminal values form the basis for your attitudes and your behavior.

There can be a large discrepancy between what people say they value and what their actions indicate about their values. That's why it's important to clarify your own values, making sure you understand what you believe so you can live in accordance with your beliefs. To do so, follow these steps:

1. Carefully consider the consequences of each choice.
2. Choose freely from among all the options.

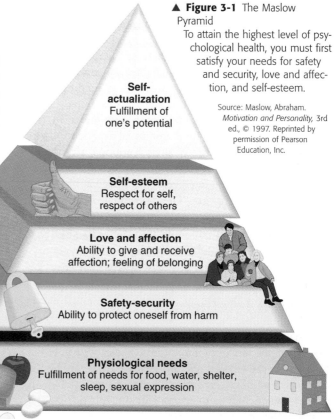

▲ **Figure 3-1** The Maslow Pyramid
To attain the highest level of psychological health, you must first satisfy your needs for safety and security, love and affection, and self-esteem.

Source: Maslow, Abraham. *Motivation and Personality,* 3rd ed., © 1997. Reprinted by permission of Pearson Education, Inc.

**Self-actualization**
Fulfillment of one's potential

**Self-esteem**
Respect for self, respect of others

**Love and affection**
Ability to give and receive affection; feeling of belonging

**Safety-security**
Ability to protect oneself from harm

**Physiological needs**
Fulfillment of needs for food, water, shelter, sleep, sexual expression

3. Publicly affirm your values by sharing them with others.
4. Act out your values.

Values clarification is not a once-in-a-lifetime task, but an ongoing process of sorting out what matters most to you. If you believe in protecting the environment, do you shut off lights and walk rather than drive to conserve energy? Do you vote for political candidates who support environmental protection? Do you recycle newspapers, bottles, and cans? Values are more than ideals we'd like to attain; they should be reflected in the way we live day by day.

## Boosting Self-Esteem

Each of us wants and needs to feel significant as a human being with unique talents, abilities, and roles in life. A sense of **self-esteem,** of belief or pride in ourselves, gives us the confidence to achieve at school or work and to reach out to others to form friendships and close relationships. Self-esteem is the little voice that whispers, "You're worth it. You can do it. You're okay."

Self-esteem is not based on external factors like wealth or beauty, but on what you believe about yourself. It's not something you're born with; self-esteem develops over time. It's also not something anyone else can give you, although those around you can either help boost or diminish your self-esteem.

The seeds of self-esteem are planted in childhood when parents provide the assurance and appreciation youngsters need to push themselves toward new accomplishments: crawling, walking, forming words and sentences, learning control over their bladder and bowels.

Adults, too, must consider themselves worthy of love, friendship, and success if they are to be loved, to make friends, and to achieve their goals. Low self-esteem is more common in people who have been abused as children and in those with psychiatric disorders, including depression, anxiety, alcoholism, and drug dependence. Feeling neglected as a child can also lead to poor self-esteem. Adults with poor self-esteem may unconsciously enter into relationships that reinforce their negative self-perceptions, and may prefer and even seek out people who think poorly of them.

One of the most useful techniques for bolstering self-esteem and achieving your goals is developing the habit of positive thinking and talking. Negative observations, such as constant criticism or reminders of the most minor of faults, can undermine self-image, while positive affirmations—compliments, kudos, encouragements—have proven effective in enhancing self-esteem and psychological well-being. Individuals who fight off negative thoughts fare bet-

ter psychologically than those who collapse when a setback occurs or who rely on others to make them feel better.

Self-esteem has proven to be one of the best predictors of college adjustment. Students with high self-esteem report better personal, emotional, social, and academic adjustment.[12] However, true self-esteem requires an honest sense of your own worth. In a study of college students, psychology professors followed self-enhancers who began their freshman year with an inflated sense of their own academic ability. These students expected to get much higher college grades than might be expected based on their high school grades and test scores. While they felt confident and happy for a while, they did no better academically and were no more likely to graduate than their realistic or self-deprecating peers. In fact, the short-term benefits of their self-illusions took a toll over the long term: Their self-esteem and interest in school declined with each passing year.[13]

## Managing Your Moods

Feelings come and go within minutes. A **mood** is a more sustained emotional state that colors our view of the world for hours or days. According to surveys by University of Michigan psychologist Randy Larsen, bad moods descend upon us an average of three out of every ten days. "A few people—about 2 percent—are happy just about every day," he says. "About 5 percent report bad moods four out of every five days."[14] Some personality types are prone to longer bad moods, which can lead to health problems.[15]

There are gender differences in mood management: Men typically try to distract themselves (a partially successful strategy) or use alcohol or drugs (an ineffective tactic). Women are more likely to talk to someone (which can help) or to ruminate on why they feel bad (which doesn't help).[16] Learning effective mood-boosting, mood-regulating strategies can help both men and women pull themselves up and out of an emotional slump.

The most effective way to banish sadness or a bad mood is by changing what caused it in the first place—if you can figure out what made you upset and why. "Most bad moods are caused by loss or failure in work or intimate relationships," says Larsen. "The questions to ask are: What can I do to fix the failure? What can I do to remedy the loss? Is there anything under my control that I can change? If there is, take action and solve it." Rewrite the report. Ask to take a make-up exam. Apologize to the friend whose feelings you hurt. Tell your parents you feel bad about the argument you had.

If there's nothing you can do, accept what happened and focus on doing things differently next time. "In our studies, resolving to try harder actually was as effective in improving mood as taking action in the present," says Larsen. You also can try to think about what happened in a different way and put a positive spin on it. This technique, known as *cognitive reappraisal* or *reframing,* helps you look at a setback in a new light: What lessons did it teach you? What would you have done differently? Could there be a silver lining or hidden benefit?

If you can't identify or resolve the problem responsible for your emotional funk, the next-best solution is to concentrate on altering your negative feelings. For example, try setting a quick, achievable goal that can boost your spirits with a small success. Clean out a closet; sort through the piles of paper on your desk; write the letter to your aunt you've been putting off for weeks.

Another good option is to get moving. In studies of mood regulation, exercise consistently ranks as the single most effective strategy for banishing bad feelings. Numerous studies have confirmed that aerobic workouts, such as walking or jogging, significantly improve mood. Even nonaerobic exercise, such as weight lifting, can boost spirits; improve sleep and appetite; reduce anxiety, irritability, and anger; and produce feelings of mastery and accomplishment.

Although it's tempting to pull away from others when you're in a slump, it's better not to withdraw. "It's never a good idea to sulk by yourself when you're feeling down," says Larsen. "Pretend to be extroverted if you have to, but do spend time with other people." As he notes, friends often can help improve your mood by giving you good feedback. But be wary of seeking out companions solely for a gripe-and-groan session. You might end up feeling worse rather than better.

Taking your mind off your troubles, rather than mulling over what's wrong, is one of the most often used mood boosters, but it's only partly successful. Simple distractions—watching television, for instance, or reading—work only temporarily. Activities that engage the imagination, on the other hand, seem to have more lasting effects. Listening to music, for instance, is one of the most popular and effective ways of distracting people from their troubles and changing their bad moods.

## Doing Good

**Altruism**—helping or giving to others—enhances self-esteem, relieves physical and mental stress, and protects psychological well-being. Hans Selye, the father of stress research, described cooperation with others for the self's sake as *altruistic egotism,* whereby we satisfy our own needs while helping others satisfy theirs. This concept is essentially an updated version of the golden rule: Do unto others as you would have them do unto you. The important difference is that you earn your neighbor's love and help by offering them love and help.

Volunteerism helps those who give as well as those who receive. People involved in community organizations, for instance, consistently report a surge of well-being, called *helper's high,* which they describe as a unique sense  of calmness, warmth, and enhanced self-worth. College students who provided community service as part of a semester-long course reported changes in attitude (including a decreased tendency to blame people for their misfortunes), self-esteem (primarily a belief that they can make a difference), and behavior (a greater commitment to do more volunteer work).

The options for volunteerism and giving of yourself are limitless: Volunteer to serve a meal at a homeless shelter. Collect donations for a charity auction. Teach reading in an illiteracy program. Perform the simplest act of charity: Pray for others.

## Feeling in Control

Although no one has absolute control over destiny, we can do a great deal to control how we think, feel, and behave. By realistically assessing our life situations, we can live in a way that allows us to make the most of our circumstances. By doing so, we gain a sense of mastery. In nationwide surveys, Americans who feel in control of their lives report greater psychological well-being than those who do not, as well as "extraordinarily positive feelings of happiness."[17]

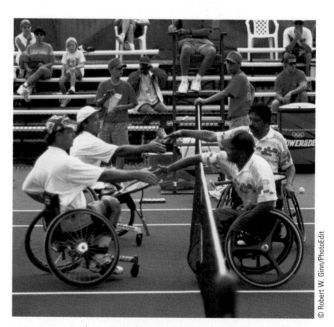

▲ You may not have complete control over your destiny, but you can control how you respond to challenges. Even under the most difficult of circumstances, it is usually not impossible to gain a sense of mastery.

## Developing Autonomy

One goal that many people strive for is **autonomy,** or independence. Both family and society influence our ability to grow toward independence. Autonomous individuals are true to themselves. As they weigh the pros and cons of any decision, whether it's using or refusing drugs or choosing a major or career, they base their judgment on their own values, not those of others. Their ability to draw on internal resources and cope with challenges has a positive impact on both their psychological well-being and their physical health, including recovery from illness. Those who've achieved autonomy may seek the opinions of others, but they do not allow their decisions to be dictated by external influences. For autonomous individuals, their **locus of control**—that is, where they view control as originating—is *internal* (from within themselves) rather than *external* (from others).

## Asserting Yourself

Being **assertive** means recognizing your feelings and making your needs and desires clear to others. Unlike aggression, a far less healthy means of expression, assertiveness usually works. You can change a situation you don't like by communicating your feelings and thoughts in nonprovoca-

tive words, by focusing on specifics, and by making sure you're talking with the person who is directly responsible.

Becoming assertive isn't always easy. Many people have learned to cope by being passive and not communicating their feelings or opinions. Sooner or later they become so irritated, frustrated, or overwhelmed that they explode in an outburst—which they think of as being assertive. However, such behavior is so distasteful to them that they'd rather be passive. Assertiveness doesn't mean screaming or telling someone off. You can communicate your wishes calmly and clearly. Assertiveness is a behavior that respects your rights and the rights of other people, even when you disagree.

Even at its mildest, assertiveness can make you feel better about yourself and your life. The reason: When you speak up or take action, you're in the pilot's seat. And that's always much less stressful than taking a backseat and trying to hang on for dear life.

## STRATEGIES FOR CHANGE

### Asserting Yourself

▲ Use I statements to explain your feelings. This allows you to take ownership of your opinions and feelings without putting down others for how they feel and think.

▲ Listen to and acknowledge what the other person says. After you speak, find out if the other person understands your position. Ask how he or she feels about what you've said.

▲ Be direct and specific. Describe the problem as you see it, using neutral language rather than assigning blame. Also suggest a specific solution, but make clear that you'd like the lines of communication and negotiation to remain open.

▲ Don't think you have to be obnoxious in order to be assertive. It's most effective to state your needs and preferences without any sarcasm or hostility.

## Connecting with Others

At every age, people who feel connected to others tend to be healthier physically and psychologically.[18] College students are no exception: Those who have a supportive, readily available network of relationships are less psychologically distressed and more satisfied with life. (See Chapter 7 for a comprehensive discussion of communication, friendship, and intimacy.)

The opposite of *connectedness* is **social isolation,** a major risk factor for illness and early death. Individuals with few social contacts face two to four times the mortality rate of others. The reason may be that their social isolation weakens the body's ability to ward off disease. Medical students with higher-than-average scores on a loneliness scale had lower levels of protective immune cells.[19] The end of a long-term relationship—through separation, divorce, or death—also dampens immunity.

It is part of our nature as mammals and as human beings to crave relationships. But we invariably end up alone at times. Solitude is not without its own quiet joys—time for introspection, self-assessment, learning from the past, and looking toward the future. Each of us can cultivate the joy of our company, of being alone without becoming lonely.

## Overcoming Loneliness

More so than many other countries, we are a nation of loners. Recent trends—longer work hours, busy family schedules, frequent moves, high divorce rates—have created even more lonely people. Only 23 percent of Americans say they're never lonely. Loneliest of all are those who are divorced, separated, or widowed, and those who live alone or solely with children. Among single adults who have never been married, 42 percent feel lonely at least sometimes. However, loneliness is most likely to cause emotional distress when it is a chronic rather than an episodic condition.[20]

To combat loneliness, people may join groups, fling themselves into projects and activities, or surround themselves with superficial acquaintances. Others avoid the effort of trying to connect, sometimes limiting most of their personal interactions to chat groups on the Internet. The Internet may actually make people feel lonelier. In the first study of the social and psychological effects of Internet use at home, researchers at Carnegie Mellon University found that people who spend even a few hours a week online have higher levels of depression and loneliness than those who use the Internet less frequently.[21]

The true keys to overcoming loneliness are developing resources to fulfill our own potential and learning to reach out to others. In this way, loneliness can become a means to personal growth and discovery.

Race and gender affect the experience of loneliness. In a study of 100 African-American undergraduates, having a best friend was the most important factor in low levels of emotional loneliness in men and high levels of feeling in control in women.[22] Some studies have found that men are lonelier than women. Others find no gender differences in loneliness, but researchers note that men, particularly those who score high on measures of masculinity, are more hesitant than women to admit that they're lonely.[23]

Loneliness affects positive health practices among college students. Those who do not have a network of supportive relationships report feeling a sense of utter aloneness, of living in a barren environment, of feeling empty and hollow, and of frequently experiencing boredom and aimlessness. These students also feel least motivated to take the best possible care of their minds and bodies.

## Facing Social Anxieties

Many people are uncomfortable meeting strangers or speaking or performing in public. In some surveys, as many as 40 percent of people describe themselves as shy or socially anxious. Some shy people—an estimated 10 to 15 percent of children—are born with a predisposition to shyness. Others become shy because they don't learn proper social responses or because they experience rejection or shame.

Social anxieties often become a problem in late adolescence. Students may develop symptoms when they go to a party or are called on in class. Some experience symptoms when they try to perform any sort of action in the

presence of others, even such everyday activities as eating in public, using a public restroom, or writing a check. About 7 percent of the population could be diagnosed with **social phobia,** a severe form of social anxiety in which individuals typically fear and avoid various social situations.[24] Adolescents and young adults with severe social anxiety are at increased risk of major depression.[25] Phobias are discussed later in this chapter. The key difference between these problems and normal shyness and self-consciousness is the degree of distress and impairment that individuals experience.

If you're shy, you can overcome much of your social apprehensiveness on your own, the same way you might set out to stop smoking or lose weight. For example, you can improve your social skills by pushing yourself to talk with a stranger at a party or to chat about the food selections with the person next to you in a cafeteria line. Gradually you'll acquire a sense of social timing and a verbal ease that will take the worry out of close encounters with others.

Those with more disabling social anxiety may do best with professional guidance, which has proven highly effective. One common technique used by experts is role playing, in which individuals act out situations that normally produce butterflies in the stomach, such as returning a defective product to a store or calling for a date. With practice and time, most people are able to emerge from the

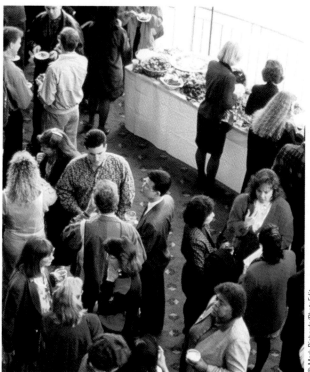

▲ Social situations can be extremely uncomfortable if you suffer from social anxieties. But over time you can overcome shyness by forcing yourself to interact with others.

walls that shyness has built around them and take pleasure in interacting with others.

## Understanding Mental Health

Mentally healthy individuals value themselves, perceive reality as it is, accept their limitations and possibilities, carry out their responsibilities, establish and maintain close relationships, pursue work that suits their talent and training, and feel a sense of fulfillment that makes the efforts of daily living worthwhile (see Figure 3-2).

According to research conducted by the World Health Organization (WHO), mental disorders affect 400 million people around the world, and these numbers will surge even higher in the coming decades.[26] In its first-ever official report on mental health, the U.S. Surgeon General called for increased efforts to recognize, treat, and prevent mental disorders.[27]

### ???? What Is a Mental Disorder?

While lay people may speak of nervous breakdowns or insanity, these are not scientific terms. The U.S. government's official definition describes a serious mental illness as "a diagnosable mental, behavioral, or emotional disorder that interferes with one or more major activities in life, like dressing, eating, or working." According to the U.S. Surgeon General, one in five Americans experiences a mental disorder in the course of a year.[28]

The mental health profession's standard for diagnosing a mental disorder is the pattern of symptoms, or diagnostic criteria, spelled out for the almost 300 disorders in the American Psychiatric Association's *Diagnostic and Statistical Manual,* 4th edition (DSM-IV). It defines a **mental disorder** as "a clinically significant behavioral or psychological syndrome or pattern that occurs in an individual and that is associated with present distress (a painful symptom) or disability (impairment in one or more important areas of functioning) or with a significantly increased risk of suffering death, pain, disability, or an important loss of freedom."[29]

## Does Mental Health Affect Physical Health?

Mental disorders affect not just the mind but also the body. **Anxiety** can lead to intensified asthmatic reactions, skin conditions, and digestive disorders. Stress can play a role in hypertension, heart attacks, sudden cardiac death, and immune disorders.

**Depression** has increasingly been recognized as a serious risk factor for physical illness. According to a recent review of large-scale studies on depression of more than 36,000 men and women, depressed individuals were 1.5 to 4 times more likely to develop heart problems.[30] In still-unknown ways, depression may increase risk factors for heart disease, such as high blood pressure.[31] Together, depression and heart disease worsen a patient's prognosis more than either condition alone. One in five heart-attack survivors suffers major depression.[32] They are two to five times more likely to die in the first 6 to 12 months following a heart attack.[33] Since depression can and often does recur, physicians now view it as a chronic illness with lifelong implications for mental and physical health.[34]

By some estimates, as many as 60 percent of those who seek help from physicians suffer primarily from a psychological problem. Treating mental health problems leads not only to improved health but also to lower health-care costs. Psychiatric treatment reduces hospitalizations, cuts medical expenses, and reduces work disability.

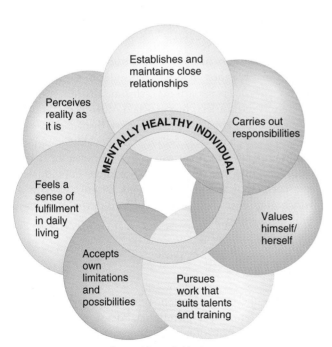

▲ **Figure 3-2** Mentally Healthy Individual
Mental well-being is a combination of many factors.

## Diversity and Mental Health on Campus

 College students have traditionally been viewed as psychologically troubled. Studies in the 1970s and 1980s concluded that half to three-quarters of students might have

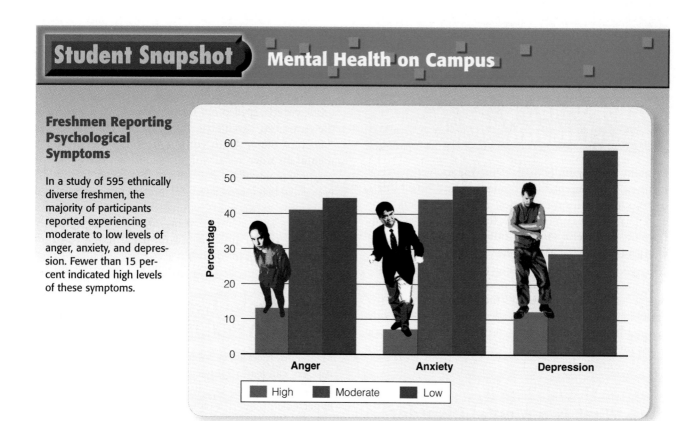

**Student Snapshot** — **Mental Health on Campus**

**Freshmen Reporting Psychological Symptoms**

In a study of 595 ethnically diverse freshmen, the majority of participants reported experiencing moderate to low levels of anger, anxiety, and depression. Fewer than 15 percent indicated high levels of these symptoms.

*(Bar chart: Percentage (y-axis, 0 to 60) vs. Anger, Anxiety, Depression (x-axis). Legend: High, Moderate, Low)*

Source: Rosenthal, Beth, et al. "Prevalence of Psychological Symptoms Among Undergraduate Students in an Ethnically Diverse Urban Public College." *Journal of American College Health,* Vol. 49, No. 1, July 2000.

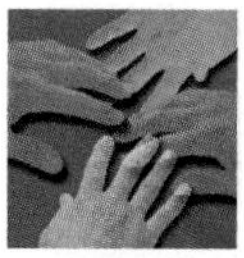

significant emotional difficulties, while a smaller number—estimated from 10 to 40 percent—suffered more serious psychological impairment. Many predicted that as campuses became more diverse in ethnicity and gender, rates of mental disorders would rise.

More recent studies of ethnic and gender differences challenged this assumption. The few researchers who have looked into ethnic variations yielded conflicting or inconclusive results: Some found no differences; others suggested higher rates of depression among Korean and south Asian students. Studies comparing male and female students have also been inconclusive. Some reported higher rates of depression and anxiety in women; others showed no difference.

A study of 595 freshmen at an ethnically diverse urban public college found that less than 15 percent reported high levels of anger, anxiety, and depression. (See Student Snapshot: "Mental Health on Campus.") There were no statistically significant differences among Asian, African-American, Hispanic, and white students on any of the three psychological symptoms. Although women reported higher levels of anger, anxiety, and depression, the differences compared with men were small.[35] (See the X & Y Files: "Are Men's and Women's Brains Different?")

## Anxiety Disorders

**Anxiety disorders** may involve inordinate fears of certain objects or situations (phobias), episodes of sudden, inexplicable terror (panic attacks), chronic distress (generalized anxiety disorder), or persistent, disturbing thoughts and behaviors (obsessive-compulsive disorder). Over a lifetime, according to the National Comorbidity Survey, as many as one in four Americans may experience an anxiety disorder. Only one of every four of these individuals is ever correctly diagnosed and treated. Yet most who do get treatment, even for severe and disabling problems, improve dramatically.

### Phobias

**Phobias**—the most prevalent type of anxiety disorder—are out-of-the-ordinary, irrational, intense, persistent fears of certain objects or situations. About 2 million Americans develop such acute terror that they go to extremes to avoid whatever they fear, even though they realize these feelings are excessive or unreasonable.[36] The most common pho-

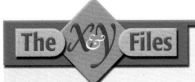

## Are Men's and Women's Brains Different?

"The brain is not an organ of sex," the pioneering feminist and economist Charlotte Perkins Gilman declared in 1898. "[We might] as well speak of the female liver." These days, gender scientists do indeed speak of the female liver, describing it as one of the most gender-distinctive organs. What then of the brain? Consider these recent findings:

- **Men's brains are bigger; women use more neurons.** A woman's brain, like her body, is 10 to 15 percent smaller than a man's, yet the regions dedicated to higher cognitive functions such as language are more densely packed with neurons—and women use more of them. When a male puts his mind to work, neurons turn on in highly specific areas. When females set their minds on similar tasks, cells light up all over the brain.
- **Male and female brains perceive light and sound differently.** A man's eyes are more sensitive to bright light and retain their ability to see well at long distances later in life. A woman hears a much broader range of sounds and her hearing remains sharper longer.
- **The female brain responds more intensely to emotion.** According to neuro-imaging studies, the genders respond differently to emotions, especially sadness, which activates neurons in an area eight times larger in women than men.
- **Male and female brains age in different ways.** The male brain loses tissue at almost three times the rate of the female brain. Because of this gender difference, the all-important frontal lobes, which are larger in men in youth and early adulthood, reach approximately the same size in men and women by the time they reach their forties. Other parts of men's brains—including the corpus callosum and the left hemisphere—also atrophy more rapidly.
- **Neither gender's brain is better.** Intelligence appears equal in men and women. The greatest gender differences appear at the top and at the bottom of the intelligence scale. Men outnumber women as both geniuses and morons.

Nevertheless, more than half the time, regardless of the type of test, most women and men perform more or less equally—even though they may take different routes to arrive at the same answers. Cognitive skills show greater variability among women and among men than between the genders. The best evaluation of all may have come from the essayist Samuel Johnson. When asked whether women or men are more intelligent, he responded, "Which man? Which woman?"

---

bias involve animals, particularly dogs, snakes, insects, and mice; the sight of blood; closed spaces *(claustrophobia);* heights *(acrophobia);* air travel; and being in places or situations from which they perceive it would be difficult or embarrassing to escape *(agoraphobia).*

Although various medications have been tried, none is effective by itself in relieving phobias. The best approach is behavior therapy, which consists of gradual, systematic exposure to the feared object (a process called *systematic desensitization).* Numerous studies have proven that exposure—especially in-vivo exposure, in which individuals are exposed to the actual source of their fear rather than simply imagining it—is highly effective. *Medical hypnosis,* the use of induction of an altered state of consciousness, also can help.

The characteristic symptoms of a phobia include:

- ✔ Excessive or unreasonable fear of a specific object or situation.
- ✔ Immediate, invariable anxiety when exposed to the object or situation.
- ✔ Recognition that the fear is excessive or unreasonable.
- ✔ Avoidance of the feared object or situation, or enduring it only with intense anxiety or distress.
- ✔ Inability to function as usual at school or work or in social relationships because of the phobia.

## Panic Attacks and Panic Disorder

Individuals who have had **panic attacks** describe them as the most frightening experiences of their lives. Without reason or warning, their hearts race wildly. They may become light-headed or dizzy. Because they can't catch their breath, they may start breathing rapidly and hyperventilate. Parts of their bodies, such as their fingers or toes, may tingle or feel numb. Worst of all is the terrible sense that something horrible is about to happen: that they will die, lose their minds, or have a heart attack. Most attacks reach peak intensity within ten minutes. Afterward, individuals live in dread of another one. In the course of a lifetime, your risk of having a single panic attack is 7.2 percent.

**Panic disorder** develops when attacks recur or apprehension about them becomes so intense that individuals cannot function normally. Full-blown panic disorder occurs in about 1.6 percent of all adults in the course of a lifetime and usually develops before age 30. The lifetime risk of panic disorder is about 2.5 times greater in women than men.[37] Parents, siblings, and children of individuals with panic disorders also are more likely to develop them than are others.[38]

The two primary treatments for panic disorder are: (1) *cognitive-behavioral therapy,* which teaches specific strategies for coping with symptoms like rapid breathing, and (2) *medication.* Treatment helps as many as 90 percent of those with panic disorder improve significantly or recover completely, usually within six to eight weeks. Individuals who receive cognitive-behavior therapy as well as medication are less likely to suffer relapses than those taking medication alone, and often can learn to control their symptoms without drugs.[39]

## Generalized Anxiety Disorder

About 10 million adults in the United States suffer from a **generalized anxiety disorder (GAD),** excessive or unrealistic apprehension that causes physical symptoms and lasts for six months or longer. It usually starts when people are in their twenties.[40] Unlike fear, which helps us recognize and avoid real danger, GAD is an exaggerated, irrational, or unwarranted response to harmless objects or situations. The most common symptoms are faster heart rate, sweating, increased blood pressure, muscle aches, intestinal pains, irritability, sleep problems, and difficulty concentrating.

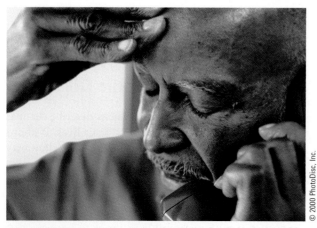

© 2000 PhotoDisc, Inc.

▲ Worry is a normal part of daily life, but individuals with generalized anxiety disorder worry constantly about everything and anything that might go wrong.

Chronically anxious individuals worry—not just some of the time, and not just about the stresses and strains of ordinary life. They worry constantly, about almost everything: their health, families, finances, marriages, potential dangers. Treatment for GAD may consist of a combination of psychotherapy, behavioral therapy, and antianxiety drugs.

## Obsessive-Compulsive Disorder

As many as 1 in 40 Americans has a type of anxiety called **obsessive-compulsive disorder (OCD).** Some of these individuals suffer only from an *obsession,* a recurring idea, thought, or image that they realize, at least initially, is senseless. The most common obsessions are repetitive thoughts of violence (for example, killing a child), contamination (becoming infected by shaking hands), and doubt (wondering whether one has performed some act, such as having hurt someone in a traffic accident). Most people with OCD also suffer from a *compulsion,* repetitive behavior performed according to certain rules or in a stereotyped fashion. The most common compulsions involve handwashing, cleaning, hoarding useless items, counting, or checking (for example, making sure dozens of times that a door is locked).[41]

Individuals with OCD realize that their thoughts or behaviors are bizarre, but they cannot resist or control them. Eventually, the obsessions or compulsions consume a great deal of time and significantly interfere with normal routine, job functioning, social activities, and relationships with others. A young woman who must follow a very rigid dressing routine may always be late for class, for example; a student who must count each letter of the alphabet as he types may not be able to complete a term paper.

OCD is believed to have biological roots. It may be a result of gene abnormalities, head injury, or even an autoimmune reaction after childhood infection with the strep bacteria. Treatment may consist of cognitive therapy to correct irrational assumptions, behavioral techniques such as progressively limiting the amount of time someone obsessed with cleanliness can spend washing and scrubbing, and medication. About 70 to 80 percent of those with OCD improve with treatment.

## Depressive Disorders

Depression, the world's most common mental ailment, affects the brain, the mind, and the body in complex ways. According to a survey of 2,000 adults, more than 20 percent of Americans feel unhappy or depressed. About 12 percent suffer from clinical depression and require psychiatric treatment.[42] Stress-related events may trigger half of all

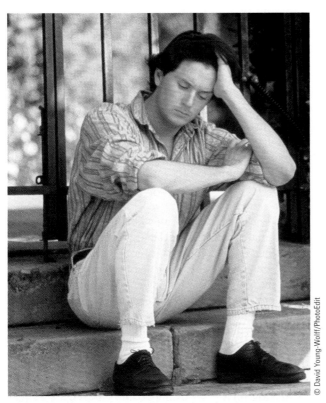

© David Young-Wolff/PhotoEdit

▲ A number of factors can contribute to the development of depression during your college years, including stressful events, poor academic performance, loneliness, and relationship problems.

depressive episodes; great trauma in childhood can increase vulnerability to depression later in life.[43] An estimated 15 to 40 percent of college-age men and women (18- to 24-year-olds) may develop depression.[44]

Depression has become so widespread that the U.S. Preventive Services Task Force is encouraging physicians to screen all their adult patients for this disorder.[45] Public attitudes also have changed. According to the National Mental Health Association, 55 percent of Americans recognize depression as an illness—up from 38 percent in 1991. Almost half of all Americans have a family member, close friend, or both who has been diagnosed with depression.[46]

Comparing everyday blues to a **depressive disorder** is like comparing a cold to pneumonia. Major depression can destroy a person's joy for living. Food, friends, sex, or any form of pleasure no longer appeals. It is impossible to concentrate on work and responsibilities. Unable to escape a sense of utter hopelessness, depressed individuals may fight back tears throughout the day and toss and turn through long, empty nights. Thoughts of death or suicide may push into their minds.

But there is good news: Depression is a treatable disease. Psychotherapy is remarkably effective for mild depression. In more serious cases, **antidepressant** medica-

tion can lead to dramatic improvement in 40 to 80 percent of depressed patients.

Exercise also is a good way to both prevent and treat psychological problems. Several studies have shown that exercise effectively lifts mild to moderate depression; for some patients with major depression, exercise may be more effective than drug treatment.[47] In a study of 150 individuals diagnosed with major depression, one group was assigned to four months of walking, jogging, or cycling; another took antidepressant medication; and a third both exercised and took medication. At the end of four months, all had improved significantly. Six months later, the exercisers were in better shape physically and mentally—and much less likely to have suffered a relapse. At ten months, the chance of a patient still being depressed was reduced by 50 percent for every 50 minutes of current weekly exercise.[48] In older adults, low-intensity exercise that included weight training improved overall mood more than just aerobic exercise.[49]

## ???? Why Are So Many Young People Depressed?

Once young people were considered immune to sadness. Now mental health professionals know better. An estimated 5 to 10 percent of American teenagers suffer from a serious depressive disorder; girls are twice as susceptible as boys. Prior to puberty, girls and boys are equally likely to develop depression. Even preschoolers can develop symptoms of depression, such as irritability, sadness, and withdrawal.[50]

The risks of depression in the young are high. Four in ten depressed adolescents think about killing themselves; two in ten actually try to do so. Every year an estimated 11 to 13 of every 100,000 teens take their own lives, twice as many as the number who die from all natural causes combined.

"Depression is the most common emotional problem in adolescence and the single greatest risk factor for teen suicide," says child psychiatrist Peter Jensen, M.D., director of the Center for the Advancement of Children's Mental Health at Columbia University. He also notes that depression rates have been rising over the last half century: "Teens born in the 1980s are more likely to develop depression than those who were born in the 1970s, whose rate of depression is higher than for those born in the 1960s."[51]

No one knows the reason for this steady surge in sadness, but experts point to the breakdown of families, the pressures of the information age, and increased isolation. "Social environment doesn't cause depression," explains psychiatrist John March, M.D., of Duke University, who is heading a nationwide study of therapies for teen depression. "But environmental stress can bring out depression in people who are susceptible. Depression is more than teenage angst. It is an illness of the central nervous system that is common, impairing, and lethal."[52]

A family history of depression greatly increases a young person's vulnerability. In one recent study of high school students diagnosed with depression, family members of depressed adolescents had much higher rates of major depression.[53] However, the strongest predictor of depression is cigarette smoking. Depressed teens may smoke because they think smoking will make them feel better, but nicotine alters brain chemistry and actually worsens symptoms of depression.[54]

Depression can be hard to recognize in the young. Many depressed teens don't look or act sad. Rather than crying, they may snap grouchily at parents or burst into angry tirades. Some turn to alcohol or drugs in hopes of feeling better; others become depressed after they start abusing these substances. As they drop out of activities and pull away from friends, depressed teens spend more time alone. Their schoolwork suffers, and many are labeled as underachievers. Those whose anger explodes in public are branded as troublemakers

Only in the last decade have mental health researchers studied specific treatments for teen depression. They now know that 60 to 75 percent of teenagers—the same percentage as adults—respond to treatment with the medications called SSRIs (a group of antidepressants that includes Prozac and Paxil). The use of these antidepressants in children and teenagers has increased three- to fivefold in recent years.[55] Older antidepressants called tricyclics, once the mainstay of treatment for adults, are not effective in adolescents. Some therapies are as effective as the SSRIs—particularly cognitive behavior therapy, which focuses on teaching new ways to deal with stress and sadness, such as changing unrealistic or highly negative ways of thinking.

## Major Depression

The simplest definition of **major depression** is sadness that does not end. The incidence of major depression has soared over the last two decades, especially among young adults. The National Comorbidity Survey found that major depression affects 10.3 percent of Americans in any given year.

The characteristic symptoms of major depression include:

- Feeling depressed, sad, empty, discouraged, tearful.
- Loss of interest or pleasure in once-enjoyable activities.
- Eating more or less than usual and either gaining or losing weight.
- Having trouble sleeping or sleeping much more than usual.
- Feeling slowed down, or feeling restless and unable to sit still.
- Lack of energy.
- Feeling helpless, hopeless, worthless, inadequate.
- Difficulty concentrating, forgetfulness.
- Difficulty thinking clearly or making decisions.
- Persistent thoughts of death or suicide.
- Withdrawal from others, lack of interest in sex.
- Physical symptoms (headaches, digestive problems, aches and pains).

Neuroscience, the study of the brain, has revealed that major depression is as physical as diabetes or heart disease. Dozens of brain-imaging studies have revealed abnormalities in the front part of the brain, which is involved in regulating emotions, and the shrinking of certain brain regions during depressive episodes.[56]

Most cases of major depression can be treated successfully, usually with psychotherapy, medication, or both. Psychotherapy alone works in more than half of mild-to-moderate episodes of major depression. Psychotherapy helps individuals pinpoint the life problems that contribute to their depression, identify negative or distorted thinking patterns, explore behaviors that contribute to depression, and regain a sense of control and pleasure in life. Two specific psychotherapies—cognitive-behavioral therapy and interpersonal therapy (described later in this chapter)—have proven as helpful as antidepressant drugs in treating mild cases of depression, although they take longer than medication to achieve results.

Three of four patients treated for depression take antidepressant medications.[57] (See the section on psychiatric drug therapy later in this chapter.) These prescription drugs generally take three or four weeks to produce significant benefits and may not have their full impact for up to eight weeks.

Newer antidepressants that boost levels of the neurotransmitter serotonin have proven equally effective as older medications, but their side effects are different. Patients report higher rates of diarrhea, nausea, insomnia, and headache.[58] The older drugs are more likely to adversely affect the heart and blood pressure and to cause dry mouth, constipation, dizziness, blurred vision, and tremors.

Modest exercise—30 minutes on a treadmill or stationary bicycle three times a week—also has proven effective.[59]

Eighty percent of people who have one episode of depression are likely to have another. Because of this high risk of recurrence, many psychiatrists now view depression as a chronic disease and advise ongoing treatment with antidepressants. However, little is known about the long-term effects of these medications.[60]

For individuals who cannot take antidepressant medications because of medical problems, or who do not improve with psychotherapy or drugs, *electroconvulsive therapy* (ECT)—the administration of a controlled electrical current through electrodes attached to the scalp—remains the safest and most effective treatment. About 50 percent of depressed individuals who do not get better with antidepressant medication and psychotherapy improve after ECT.

# Bipolar Disorder (Manic Depression)

**Bipolar disorder,** or manic depression, consists of mood swings that may take individuals from *manic* states of feeling euphoric and energetic to *depressive* states of utter despair. In episodes of full mania, they may become so impulsive and out of touch with reality that they endanger their careers, relationships, health, or even survival. One percent of the population—about 2 million American adults—suffers from this serious but treatable disorder, which affects both genders and all races equally.

The characteristic symptoms of bipolar disorder include:

✔ Mood swings (from happy to miserable, optimistic to despairing, and so on).

✔ Changes in thinking (thoughts speeding through one's mind, unrealistic self-confidence, difficulty concentrating, delusions, hallucinations).

✔ Changes in behavior (sudden immersion in plans and projects, talking very rapidly and much more than usual, excessive spending, impaired judgment, impulsive sexual involvement).

✔ Changes in physical condition (less need for sleep, increased energy, fewer health complaints than usual).

During manic periods, individuals may make grandiose plans or take dangerous risks. But they often plunge from this highest of highs to a horrible low depressive episode, during which they may feel sad, hopeless, and helpless, and develop other symptoms of major depression. The risk of suicide is very real.

Professional therapy is essential in treating bipolar disorders. Mood-stabilizing medications are the keystone of treatment, although psychotherapy plays a critical role in helping individuals understand their illness and rebuild their lives. Most individuals continue taking medication indefinitely after remission of their symptoms because the risk of recurrence is high.

## Suicide

Suicide is not in itself a psychiatric disorder, but it can be the tragic consequence of emotional and psychological problems. Every 18 minutes an American dies by suicide; 80 lives are lost every day.[61] An estimated 752,000 Americans attempt to take their own lives every year; there may be 4.5 million suicide survivors in the U.S.[62]

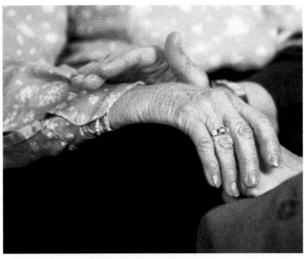

Paul Avis/Getty Image

▲ Depression and suicidal thoughts are closely linked. If you know someone who is severely depressed, be willing to offer help and comfort during difficult times.

Depressed teens are more likely than adults to attempt suicide—and to die. "In psychological interviews after a teen suicide, we see that the warning signs were there," notes child psychiatrist Madelyn Gould, M.D., of Columbia University, "but no one realized the underlying problem was depression."[63] Stressors that may contribute to the soaring suicide rate among the young are psychological problems, mental disorders, drug abuse, school pressures, social difficulties, concern and confusion about sexual orientation, and family problems.

After tripling between 1955 and 1985, the suicide rate among Americans between ages 15 and 19 has dropped 27 percent. One reason may be increased diagnoses of depression and treatment with antidepressant medications. The total number of annual youth suicides has dropped below 30,000 for the first time since 1985.[64]

At all ages, men commit suicide three times more frequently than women, but women attempt suicide much more often than men. Elderly men are ten times more likely to take their own lives than older women. Native Americans have a suicide rate five times higher than that of the general population.

 Suicide is the third leading cause of death among children and adolescents 10 to 19 years old in the United States. The age-adjusted death rate for suicide has decreased in recent years, but the death rate for suicide among children 10 to 14 years old has doubled. Although black youths have historically had lower suicide rates than whites, the gap between suicide rates for black and white youths has narrowed.[65] Among all young people under age 25, firearms-related deaths account for 67 percent of suicides.

Among the factors that increase the likelihood of teen suicide are a previous suicide attempt, violence (either as

## STRATEGIES FOR PREVENTION

### If You Start Thinking About Suicide

At some point, the thought of ending it all—the disappointments, problems, and bad feelings—may cross your mind. This experience isn't unusual. But if the idea of taking your life persists or intensifies, you should respond as you would to other warnings of potential threats to your health—by getting the help you need:

▲ *Talk to a mental health professional.* If you have a therapist, call immediately. If not, call a suicide hot line.

▲ *Find someone you trust and can talk with honestly about what you're feeling.* If you suffer from depression or another mental disorder, educate trusted friends or relatives about your condition so they are prepared if called upon to help.

▲ *Write down your more uplifting thoughts.* Even if you are despondent, you can help yourself by taking the time to retrieve some more positive thoughts or memories. A simple record of your hopes for the future and the people you value in your life can remind you of why your own life is worth continuing.

▲ *Avoid drugs and alcohol.* Most suicides are the result of sudden, uncontrolled impulses, and drugs and alcohol can make it harder to resist these destructive urges.

▲ *Go to the hospital.* Hospitalization can sometimes be the best way to protect your health and safety.

victim or perpetrator), and use of alcohol or marijuana. For girls, medical symptoms, having a friend attempt or complete suicide, illicit drug use, and a history of mental health problems also increase the risk. Among boys, risk factors include carrying a weapon at school, same-sex romantic attraction, a family history of suicide or suicide attempts, easy household access to guns, cutting school, and being held back or skipping a grade.

Researchers also have identified factors that protect young people from suicide. Number one for both boys and girls was feeling connected to their parents and family. For girls, emotional well-being was also protective. A high grade point average was an additional protective factor for boys. High parental expectations for their child's school achievement, more people living in the household, and religiosity were protective for some of the boys, but not for the girls. Availability of counseling services at school and parental presence at key times during the day were protective for some of the girls, but not for the boys.

Suicide is the third leading cause of death among college-aged Americans.[66] Males in this age group have a suicide rate six times greater than that of females.[67] Participation in sports seems to have a protective effect and decreases the odds of suicide among male and female college students.[68]

Suicide is not inevitable. Appropriate treatment can help as many as 70 to 80 percent of those at risk for suicide. Among young people, early recognition and treatment for depressive disorders and alcohol and drug abuse could save thousands of lives each year.

## ???? What Leads to Suicide?

Researchers have looked for explanations for suicide by studying everything from phases of the moon to seasons (suicides peak in the spring and early summer) to birth order in the family.[69] They have found no conclusive answers. A constellation of influences—mental disorders, personality traits, biologic and genetic vulnerability, medical illness, and psychosocial stressors—may combine in ways that lower an individual's threshold of vulnerability. The risk of suicide is higher in people who live in cities, are single, have a low income, or are unemployed.[70] No one factor in itself may ever explain fully why a person chooses death.[71]

### Mental Disorders

More than 95 percent of those who commit suicide have a mental disorder. Two in particular—depression and alcoholism—account for two-thirds of all suicides. Suicide also is a risk for those with schizophrenia and other personality disorders.

Psychiatrists have revised the estimated risk of suicide among their patients, which had been set on the basis of theoretical calculations at 15 percent—or 30 times the lifetime rate in the general population. Suicide risk calculated from data on actual fatalities is lower: 2 percent for depressed patients outside of hospitals, 4 percent for depressed patients in hospitals, and 6 percent for hospitalized patients are diagnosed as suicidal. These figures are 5 or 6 (rather than 30) times the rate in the general population.[72]

### Substance Abuse

Many of those who commit suicide drink beforehand, and their use of alcohol may lower their inhibitions. Since alcohol itself is a depressant, it can intensify the despondency suicidal individuals are already feeling. Alcoholics who attempt suicide often have other risk factors, including major depression, poor social support, serious medical illness, and unemployment. Drugs of abuse also can alter thinking and lower inhibitions against suicide.

## Hopelessness

The sense of utter hopelessness and helplessness may be the most common contributing factor in suicide. When hope dies, individuals view every experience in negative terms and come to expect the worst possible outcomes for their problems. Given this way of thinking, suicide often seems a reasonable response to a life seen as not worth living.

## Family History

One of every four people who attempt suicide has a family member who also tried to commit suicide. While a family history of suicide is not in itself considered a predictor of suicide, two mental disorders that can lead to suicide—depression and bipolar disorder (manic depression)—do run in families.

## Physical Illness

People who commit suicide are likely to be ill or to believe that they are. About 5 percent actually have a serious physical disorder, such as AIDS or cancer. While suicide may seem to be a decision rationally arrived at in those with serious or fatal illnesses, this may not be the case. Depression, not uncommon in such instances, can warp judgment. When the depression is treated, the person may no longer have suicidal intentions.

More than 80 percent of those who commit suicide have seen a physician about a medical complaint within the six months preceding suicide. To help general physicians identify people at risk of suicide, researchers at Johns Hopkins University developed a set of four crucial questions:

- ✔ Have you ever had a period of two weeks or more when you had trouble falling asleep, staying asleep, waking up too early, or sleeping too much?
- ✔ Have you ever had two weeks or more during which you felt sad, blue, or depressed, or when you lost interest and pleasure in things you usually cared about or enjoyed?
- ✔ Has there ever been a period of two weeks or more when you felt worthless, sinful, or guilty?
- ✔ Has there ever been a period of time when you felt that life was hopeless?

Anyone who answers yes to these questions should be referred immediately to a mental health professional.

## Brain Chemistry

Investigators have found abnormalities in the brain chemistry of those who complete suicide, especially low levels of a metabolite of the neurotransmitter serotonin. There are indications that individuals with a deficiency of this substance may have as much as a ten times greater risk of committing suicide than those with higher levels.

## Access to Guns

For individuals already facing a combination of predisposing factors, access to a means of committing suicide, particularly to guns, can add to the risk. Unlike other methods of suicide, guns almost always work. States with strict gun-control laws have much lower rates of suicides than states with more lenient laws. Health professionals are urging parents whose children undergo psychological treatment or assessment to remove all weapons from their homes and to make sure their youngsters do not have access to alcohol or potentially lethal medications.

## Other Factors

Individuals who kill themselves often have gone through more major life crises—job changes, births, financial reversals, divorce, retirement—in the previous six months, compared with others. Long-standing, intense conflict with family members or other important people may add to the danger. In some cases, suicide may be an act of revenge that offers the person a sense of control, however temporary or illusory. For example, a husband whose wife has had an affair may rationalize that he can get back at her, and have the final word, by killing himself. Others may feel that by rejecting life they are rejecting a partner or parent who abandoned or betrayed them.

## Suicide Prevention

If someone you know has talked about suicide, behaved unpredictably, or suddenly emerged from a severe depression into a calm, settled state of mind, don't rule out the possibility that he or she may attempt suicide.

- ✔ Encourage your friend to talk. Ask concerned questions. Listen attentively. Show that you take the person's feelings seriously and truly care.
- ✔ Don't offer trite reassurances. List reasons to go on living, try to analyze the person's motives, or try to shock or challenge him or her.
- ✔ Suggest alternative solutions to problems. Make plans. Encourage positive action, such as getting away for a while to gain a better perspective on a problem.
- ✔ Don't be afraid to ask whether your friend has considered suicide. The opportunity to talk about thoughts

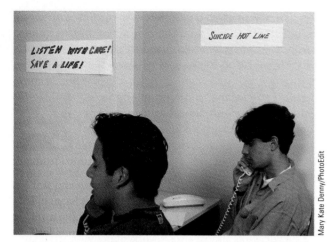

▲ About 20 percent of teenagers seriously consider suicide; a much smaller number actually attempts to take their own lives. Talking to a counselor at a suicide hot line may help depressed teens deal with their feelings of despondency.

of suicide may be an enormous relief, and—contrary to a long-standing myth—will not fix the idea of suicide more firmly in a person's mind.

✔ Don't think that people who talk about killing themselves never carry out their threat. Most individuals who commit suicide give definite indications of their intent to die.

## Attention Disorders

Approximately 10 percent of boys and 2 percent of girls in the United States have **attention deficit/hyperactivity disorder (ADHD),** the most common psychiatric diagnosis of childhood.[73] Its causes are complex and include genetic and biological factors, including differences within the brain. Research has shown that children with ADHD often have smaller overall brain volumes than others, particularly in the right frontal region, an area of the brain associated with the processes of paying attention and focusing concentration.[74]

Between 40 and 70 percent of youngsters with ADHD do not outgrow their restless, reckless ways at puberty. In all, 1 to 2 percent of adult men and women—at least 5 million Americans—have problems sustaining attention or controlling their movements and impulses.[75]

Adults with ADHD have one or more of three primary symptoms: hyperactivity, impulsivity, and distractibility. Rather than scooting around a room, they may tap their fingers or jiggle their feet. Some appear calm and organized but cannot concentrate long enough to finish reading a paragraph or follow a list of directions. Others, on a whim, go on buying sprees or take wild dares.

An estimated 1 percent of college students have an attention disorder that can have a significant impact on their academic performance. At one midwestern university,

for instance, the counseling service estimates that students with attention disorders have an average GPA of 2.4, compared to a university average mean of 3.1.

## Schizophrenia

**Schizophrenia,** one of the most debilitating mental disorders, profoundly impairs an individual's sense of reality. As the National Institute of Mental Health (NIMH) puts it, schizophrenia, which is characterized by abnormalities in brain structure and chemistry, destroys "the inner unity of the mind" and weakens "the will and drive that constitute our essential character." It affects every aspect of psychological functioning, including the ways people think, feel, view themselves, and relate to others.

The symptoms of schizophrenia include:

✔ Hallucinations.
✔ Delusions.
✔ Inability to think in a logical manner.
✔ Talking in rambling or incoherent ways.
✔ Making odd or purposeless movements or not moving at all.
✔ Repeating others' words or mimicking their gestures.
✔ Showing few, if any, feelings; responding with inappropriate emotions.
✔ Lacking will or motivation to complete a task or accomplish something.
✔ Functioning at a much lower level than in the past at work, in interpersonal relations, or in taking care of themselves.

Individuals with schizophrenia may hear, see, or feel things that do not exist—a voice telling them to jump from a bridge, a statue crying tears of blood, a spaceship beaming a light upon them. Frightened and vulnerable, they may devote all their energy to warding off the demons within. Unable to take care of themselves, they may look messy and disheveled. They often move in unusual ways, such as rocking or pacing, and they tend to repeat certain gestures again and again. They may believe that someone or something, such as the devil, is putting thoughts into their heads or controlling their actions. Some think they are reincarnations of Christ or Napoleon. About a third attempt to take their own lives, often in response to a command they hear inside their heads. Researchers have identified early markers of schizophrenia, including impaired social skills, intellectual ability, and capacity for organization.[76]

Schizophrenia is most likely to occur between the ages of 17 and 30 in men and between 20 and 40 in women.[77] Although symptoms do not occur until then, they are almost certainly the result of a failure in brain development that occurs very early in life. The underlying defect is probably present before birth. Schizophrenia has a strong genetic basis and is not the result of upbringing, social conditions, or traumatic experiences.[78]

According to NIMH's epidemiological data, the total lifetime prevalence for schizophrenia in the United States ranges from 1 to 1.9 percent. This means that between 2.5 million and 4.75 million Americans may have schizophrenia at any one time. For the vast majority of individuals with schizophrenia, antipsychotic drugs are the foundation of treatment.

Some individuals with schizophrenia recover completely. However, many thousands—perhaps as many as 200,000—live on the street or in homeless shelters.

## Overcoming Problems of the Mind

Mental illness costs our society an estimated $150 billion a year in lost work time and productivity, employee turnover, disability payments, and death. Yet many Americans do not have access to mental health services, nor do they have insurance for such services. Despite the fact that treatments for mental disorders have a higher success rate than those for many other diseases, employers often restrict mental health benefits. HMOs and health insurance plans are much

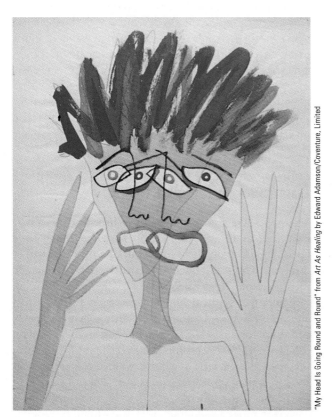

▲ "My Head Is Going Round and Round," a drawing by a patient suffering from schizophrenia, expresses the anxiety and agitation that may occur with this brain abnormality.

*"My Head Is Going Round and Round" from Art As Healing by Edward Adamson/Coventure, Limited*

more likely to limit psychotherapy visits and psychiatric hospitalizations than treatments for medical illnesses.

Even when cost is not a barrier, many people do not seek treatment because they see psychological problems as a sign of weakness rather than illness. They also may not realize that scientifically proven therapies can bring relief, often in a matter of weeks or months.

 Because an individual's perception of a problem is culture-specific—that is, influenced by cultural, social, and religious beliefs—immigrants to the United States may treat symptoms of psychological distress in different ways. For instance, Asian-American college students tend to seek medical care for physical symptoms, such as aches, pains, or sleep problems, but forgo counseling for a mental disorder, because it is more appropriate in their native cultures to do so.

## ???? Where Can I Turn for Help?

As a student, your best contact for identifying local services may be your school's health department. Health instructors can tell you about general and mental health counseling available on campus, school-based support groups, community-based programs, and special emergency services. On campus, you can also turn to the student health services or the office of the dean of student services or student affairs.

Within the community, you may find help through the city or county health department, neighborhood health centers, and local hospitals. Most communities have local branches of national service organizations, such as United Way, Alcoholics Anonymous, other 12-step programs, and various support groups. You can call the psychiatric or psychological association in your city or state for the names of licensed professionals. Your primary physician may also be able to help.

The telephone directory is another good resource. Special programs are often listed—by the nature of the service, by the name of the neighborhood or city, or by the name of the sponsoring group. In some places, the city's name may precede a listing: the New York City Suicide Hot Line, for instance. In addition to suicide-prevention programs, other listings usually include crisis intervention, violence prevention, and child-abuse prevention programs; drug-treatment information; shelters for battered women; senior citizen centers; and self-help and counseling services. Many services have special hot lines for coping with emergencies. Others provide information as well as counseling over the phone.

## Types of Therapists

Only professionally trained individuals who have met state licensing requirements are certified as psychiatrists, psychologists, social workers, psychiatric nurses, and marriage and family therapists. Before selecting any of these mental health professionals, be sure to check the person's background and credentials.

**Psychiatrists** are licensed medical doctors (M.D.) who have training in various forms of psychotherapy, psychopharmacology and both outpatient and inpatient treatment of mental disorders. They can prescribe medications and make medical decisions.

**Psychologists** complete a graduate program (including clinical training and internships) in human psychology but do not study medicine and cannot prescribe medication.

**Certified social workers** or **licensed clinical social workers (LCSWs)** usually complete a two-year graduate program and have specialized training in helping people with mental problems in addition to conventional social work.

**Psychiatric nurses** have nursing degrees and have passed a state examination. They usually have special training and experience in mental health care, although no specialty licensing or certification is required.

**Marriage and family therapists,** licensed in some but not all states, usually have a graduate degree, often in psychology, and at least two years of supervised clinical training in dealing with relationship problems.

Other therapists include pastoral counselors, members of the clergy who offer psychological counseling; hypnotherapists, stress-management counselors, and alcohol and drug counselors. Anyone can use these terms to describe themselves professionally, and there are no licensing requirements.

## Options for Treatment

The term **psychotherapy** refers to any type of counseling based on the exchange of words in the context of the unique relationship that develops between a mental health professional and a person seeking help. The process of talking and listening can lead to new insight, relief from distressing psychological symptoms, changes in unhealthy or maladaptive behaviors, and more effective ways of dealing with the world.

Most mental health professionals today are trained in a variety of psychotherapeutic techniques and tailor their approach to the problem, personality, and needs of each person seeking their help. Because skilled therapists may combine different techniques in the course of therapy, the lines between the various approaches often blur.

Because insurance companies and health-care plans often limit the duration of psychotherapy, many mental health professionals are adopting a *time-limited format* in order to make the most of every session, regardless of the length of treatment. Brief or short-term psychotherapy typically focuses on a central theme, problem, or topic and may continue for several weeks to several months. The individuals most likely to benefit are those interested in solving immediate problems rather than changing their

characters, those who can think in psychological terms, and those who are motivated to change.

## Psychodynamic Psychotherapy

For the most part, today's mental health professionals base their assessment of individuals on a **psychodynamic** understanding that takes into account the role of early experiences and unconscious influences in *actively* shaping behavior. (This is the *dynamic* in psychodynamic.) Psychodynamic treatments work toward the goal of providing greater insight into problems and bringing about behavioral change. Therapy may be brief, consisting of 12 to 25 sessions, or may continue for several years. According to current thinking, psychotherapy can actually rewire the network of neurons within the brain in ways that ease distress and improve functioning in many areas of daily life.

## Interpersonal Therapy

**Interpersonal therapy (IPT),** originally developed for research into the treatment of major depression, focuses on relationships in order to help individuals deal with unrecognized feelings and needs and improve their communication skills. IPT does not deal with the psychological origins of symptoms but rather concentrates on the current problems of getting along with others. The supportive, empathic relationship that is developed with the therapist, who takes an even more active role than in psychodynamic psychotherapy, is the most crucial component of this therapy. The emphasis is on the here and now and on interpersonal—rather than intrapsychic—issues. Individuals with major depression, chronic difficulties developing relationships, chronic mild depression, or bulimia (see Chapter 6 on eating disorders) are most likely to benefit. IPT usually consists of 12 to 16 sessions.

## Cognitive-Behavioral Therapy

This approach, also called cognitive-behavior therapy or CBT, focuses on inappropriate or inaccurate thoughts or beliefs to help individuals break out of a distorted way of thinking. The techniques of **cognitive therapy** include identification of an individual's beliefs and attitudes, recognition of negative thought patterns, and education in alternative ways of thinking. Individuals with major depression or anxiety disorders are most likely to benefit, usually in 15 to 25 sessions. In a recent study, cognitive therapy proved at least as effective as medication for long-term treatment of severe depression.[79] However, many of the positive messages used in cognitive therapy can help anyone improve a bad mood or negative outlook.

**Behavior therapy** strives to substitute healthier ways of behaving for maladaptive patterns used in the past. Its

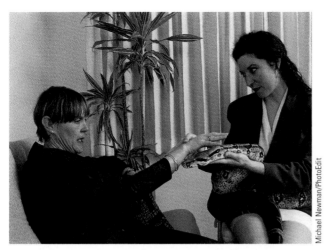

▲ Systematic desensitization is one of the behavior therapies used to treat phobias.

premise is that distressing psychological symptoms, like all behaviors, are learned responses that can be modified or unlearned. Some therapists believe that changing behavior also changes how people think and feel. As they put it, "Change the behavior, and the feelings will follow." Behavior therapies work best for disorders characterized by specific, abnormal patterns of acting—such as alcohol and drug abuse, anxiety disorders, and phobias—and for individuals who want to change bad habits.

## Psychiatric Drug Therapy

Medications that alter brain chemistry and relieve psychiatric symptoms have brought great hope and help to millions of people. Thanks to the recent development of a new generation of more precise and effective **psychiatric drugs,** success rates for treating many common and disabling disorders—depression, panic disorder, schizophrenia, and others—have soared. Often used in conjunction with psychotherapy, sometimes used as the primary treatment, these medications have revolutionized mental health care.[80]

At some point in their lives, about half of all Americans will take a psychiatric drug. The reason may be depression, anxiety, a sleep difficulty, an eating disorder, alcohol or drug dependence, impaired memory, or another disorder that disrupts the intricate chemistry of the brain. (See Savvy Consumer: "What You Need to Know About Mind–Mood Medications.")

Psychiatric drugs are now among the most widely prescribed drugs in the United States. Three of the top ten prescription drugs sold in this country are serotonin-boosting antidepressants—best known by their trade names Prozac, Paxil, and Zoloft—that are used to treat a variety of problems, including obsessive-compulsive disorder, premenstrual syndrome, and attention deficits, as well as depression.[81]

Psychiatric medications affect every aspect of a person's physical, mental, and emotional functioning. Some take effect immediately; others take several weeks to relieve symptoms. A few continue to exert their effects even after an individual discontinues their use. When taken appropriately, psychiatric agents can alleviate tremendous suffering and reduce the financial and personal costs of mental illness by lessening the need for hospitalization and by restoring an individual's ability to function normally, to work, and to contribute to society. But they do have side effects and must be used with care.

## Alternative Mind–Mood Medicine

Increasingly consumers are trying natural products, such as herbs and enzymes that claim to have psychological

## Savvy Consumer

### What You Need to Know About Mind–Mood Medications

Before taking any *psychoactive* drug (one that affects the brain), talk to a qualified health professional. Here are some points to raise:

- What can this medication do for me? What specific symptoms will it relieve? Are there other possible benefits?
- Are there any risks? What about side effects? Do I have to take it before or after eating? Will it affect my ability to study, work, drive, or operate machinery?
- When will I notice a difference? How long does it take for the medicine to have an effect?
- How will I be able to tell if the medication is working? What are the odds that it will help me?
- How long will I have to take medication? Is there any danger that I'll become addicted?
- What if it doesn't help?
- Is there an herbal or natural alternative? If so, has it been studied? What do you know about its possible risks and side effects?

effects. Because they are not classified as drugs, they have not undergone the rigorous scientific testing required of psychiatric medications, and little is known about their safety or efficacy. "Natural" doesn't mean risk-free. Opium and cocaine are natural substances that have dramatic and potentially deadly effects on the mind.[82]

St. John's wort (named after St. John the Baptist because the yellow flowers of the *Hypericum perforatum* plant bloom in June, the anniversary month of his execution) has been used to treat anxiety and depression in Europe for many years. Although more than 24 clinical trials have investigated St. John's wort, many researchers feel that most had significant flaws in design. In recent scientifically rigorous studies, St. John's wort has proved no more effective than a placebo, or inactive substance, in treating major depression.[83] Side effects include dizziness, abdominal pain and bloating, constipation, nausea, fatigue, and dry mouth. St. John's wort should not be taken in combination with other prescription antidepressants.[84]

 What is known about biofeedback in the treatment of attention deficit disorder?

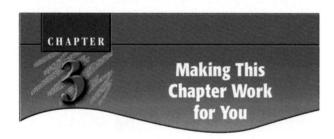

**CHAPTER 3**

**Making This Chapter Work for You**

1. Psychological health is influenced by all of the following *except*
   a. spiritual health.
   b. physical agility.
   c. culture.
   d. a firm grasp on reality.

2. Emotional intelligence encompasses which of the following components?
   a. creativity, sense of humor, scholastic achievement
   b. integrity, honesty, and perseverance
   c. piety, tolerance, and self-esteem
   d. empathy, self-awareness, and altruism

3. Which of the following activities can contribute to a lasting sense of personal fulfillment?
   a. becoming a Big Sister or Big Brother to a child from an inner city single-parent home
   b. volunteering at a local soup kitchen on Thanksgiving
   c. being a regular participant in an Internet chat room

   d. going on a shopping spree

4. Individuals who have developed a sense of mastery over their lives are
   a. skilled at controlling the actions of others.
   b. usually passive and silent when faced with a situation they don't like.
   c. aware that their locus of control is internal, not external.
   d. aware that their locus of control is external, not internal.

5. A mental disorder can be described as
   a. a condition associated with migraine headaches and narcolepsy.
   b. a condition that is usually caused by severe trauma to the brain.
   c. a behavioral or psychological disorder that impairs an individual's ability to conduct one or more important activities of daily life.
   d. a psychological disorder that is easily controlled with medication and a change in diet.

6. Which of the following statements about psychological health is *incorrect*?
   a. Individuals with social phobia typically fear and avoid various social situations.
   b. Mentally healthy individuals value themselves, accept their limitations, and carry out their responsibilities.
   c. In one study, less than 15 percent of college students reported high levels of anger, anxiety, and depression.
   d. Depressed individuals are less likely to develop heart problems.

7. Which of the following statements about anxiety disorders is true?
   a. Anxiety disorders are the least prevalent type of mental illness.
   b. An individual suffering from a panic attack may mistake her symptoms for a heart attack.
   c. The primary symptom of obsessive-compulsive disorder is irrational, intense, and persistent fear of a specific object or situation.
   d. Generalized anxiety disorders respond to systematic desensitization behavior therapy.

8. Some characteristic symptoms of major depression are
   a. difficulty concentrating, lack of energy, and eating more than usual.
   b. exaggerated sense of euphoria and energy.
   c. palpitations, sweating, numbness, and tingling sensations.
   d. talking in rambling ways, inability to think in a logical manner, and delusions.

9. A person may be at higher risk of committing suicide if
   a. he is taking antidepressant medication.

b. he lives in a rural environment and is married.

c. he has been diagnosed with hyperactivity disorder.

d. he has lost his job because of alcoholism.

10. Which of the following statements is true?

a. Individuals with schizophrenia are most likely to benefit from psychodynamic therapy in combination with nutritional supplements.

b. The antidepressants Prozac, Paxil, and Zoloft can also be used to treat premenstrual syndrome and attention deficit disorder.

c. Psychologists are usually trained in a variety of psychotherapeutic techniques and are licensed to prescribe psychiatric medications.

d. Interpersonal therapy focuses on the role of early experiences and unconscious influences in shaping patterns of behavior, such as repeated failed relationships.

Answers to these questions can be found on page 415.

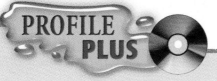

## Critical Thinking

1. Would you say that you view life positively or negatively? Would your friends and family agree with your assessment? Ask two of your closest friends for feedback about what they perceive are your typical responses to a problematic situation. Are these indicative of positive attitudes? If not, what could you do to become more psychologically positive?

2. Paula went to a therapist when she was feeling depressed and was given a prescription for an antidepressant called fluoxetine (trade name Prozac). Her therapist recommended the drug because it causes fewer side effects than other medications. However, Paula later read in a news magazine that some patients, claiming that Prozac had made them violent or suicidal, had sued the drug's manufacturers. Their

suits didn't win in court, but Paula was less certain about taking the prescribed medication. What do you think she should do? How would you weigh the risks and benefits of taking a psychiatric drug?

3. Research has indicated that many homeless men and women are in need of outpatient psychiatric care, often because they suffer from chronic mental illnesses or alcoholism. Yet government funding for the mentally ill is inadequate, and homelessness itself can make it difficult, if not impossible, for people to gain access to the care they need. How do you feel when you pass homeless individuals who seem disoriented or out of touch with reality? Who should take responsibility for their welfare? Should they be forced to undergo treatment at psychiatric institutions?

## PROFILE PLUS

Take stock of your emotional and mental state with these activities on your Profile Plus CD-ROM:

Well Being Scale * Is Something Wrong?

## SITES & BYTES

### American Psychological Association
**www.apa.org**
This site features a help center for general advice and access to psychological services. In addition, the site regularly updates current events on mental health topics as well as information for the public, mental health professionals, and researchers.

### Wellplace
**www.wellplace.com**
This site is sponsored by Pioneer Behavioral Health and features fact sheets on a variety of mental health topics,

including depression, stress, posttraumatic stress disorder, and personality disorders. In addition, the site has several self-assessment tools, wellness articles, chat forums, advice from experts, and a list of online resources for self-help recovery groups and national hotlines.

### National Mental Health Information Center
**www.mentalhealth.org**
Sponsored by the National Mental Health Information Center of the U.S. Department of Health and Human Services, this site features current mental health topics, including posttraumatic stress disorder, children's mental

health, substance abuse prevention, suicide prevention, and a comprehensive list of online mental health resources.

### 🔍 InfoTrac College Edition Activity

David M. Fergusson and Lianne J. Woodward. "Mental Health, Educational, and Social Role Outcomes of Adolescents with Depression." *Archives of General Psychiatry,* Vol. 59, No. 3, March 2002, p. 225(7).

1. Depression occurring during early adolescence is associated with an increased risk of developing which other adverse psychosocial life events?
2. What are the pathways that may link adolescent depression to later outcomes?

3. Based on the results of the research, what gender differences were found to exist between the onset of adolescent depression and later life outcomes?

You can find additional readings related to psychological health with InfoTrac College Edition, an online library of more than 900 journals and publications. Follow the instructions for accessing InfoTrac that were packaged with your textbook; then search for articles using a key-word search.

For additional links, resources, and suggested readings on InfoTrac, visit our Health & Wellness Resource Center at http://health.wadsworth.com.

## Key Terms

The terms listed here are used within the chapter on the page indicated. Definitions of the terms are in the Glossary at the end of the book.

altruism 52
antidepressant 59
anxiety 55
anxiety disorders 56
assertive 53
attention deficit/
  hyperactivity disorder
  (ADHD) 64
autonomy 53
behavior therapy 66
bipolar disorder 61
certified social worker 66
cognitive therapy 66

culture 48
depression 55
depressive disorders 59
emotional health 48
emotional intelligence 49
generalized anxiety disorder
  (GAD) 58
interpersonal therapy
  (IPT) 66
licensed clinical social
  worker (LCSW) 66
locus of control 53
major depression 60

marriage and family
  therapist 66
mental disorder 55
mental health 48
mood 51
obsessive-compulsive
  disorder (OCD) 58
optimistic 50
panic attack 57
panic disorder 58
phobia 56
psychiatric drugs 67
psychiatric nurse 66

psychodynamic 66
psychologists 66
psychotherapy 66
schizophrenia 64
self-actualization 50
self-esteem 51
social isolation 53
social phobia 54
spiritual health 48
spiritual intelligence 49
values 50

## References

1. Satcher, David. "Executive Summary: A Report of the Surgeon General on Mental Health." *Public Health Reports,* Vol. 115, No. 1, January 2000.
2. Diener, Ed, et al. "Subjective Well-Being: Three Decades of Progress." *Psychological Bulletin,* Vol. 125, No. 2, March 1999.
3. Shapiro, Deane, and Roger Walsh. *Beyond Health and Normalcy.* New York: Van Nostrand Reinhold, 1983.
4. Satcher, "Executive Summary: A Report of the Surgeon General on Mental Health."
5. Moore, Thomas. *Care of the Soul.* New York: Harper Perennial, 1994.
6. Goleman, Daniel. *Emotional Intelligence.* New York: Bantam Books, 1997.
7. Chatterjee, Camille. "Emotional Ignorance." *Psychology Today,* Vol. 33, No. 6, November 2000, p. 12.
8. Sloan, R. P., et al. "Religion, Spirituality, and Medicine." *Lancet,* Vol. 353, No. 9153, February 20, 1999.
9. Harris, T. George. "Spiritual Intelligence." Symposium at American Psychological Association, Annual Meeting, San Francisco, August 1998.
10. Ornish, Dean. Personal interview.
11. Danner, Deborah, et al. "Positive Emotions in Early Life and Longevity: Findings from the Nun Study." *Journal of Personality & Social Psychology,* Vol. 80, No. 5, May 2001, p. 804.
12. Hertel, James. "College Students Generational Status: Similarities,

Differences, and Factors in College Adjustment." *The Psychological Record,* Vol. 52, No. 1, Winter 2002, p. 3.
13. Robins, Richard, and Jennifer Beer. "Positive Illusions about the Self: Short-Term Benefits and Long-Term Costs." *Journal of Personality & Social Psychology,* Vol. 80, No. 2, February 2001, p. 340.
14. Larsen, Randy. Personal interview.
15. "Persistent Bad Mood Leads to Poor Health." *Health & Medicine Week,* June 3, 2002, p. 4.
16. Larsen, Randy. Personal interview.
17. Ibid.
18. "What Is the Psychiatric Significance of Loneliness?" *Harvard Mental Health Letter,* Vol. 16, No. 10, April 2000.
19. Schwartz, Richard. "Loneliness." *Harvard Review of Psychiatry,* Vol. 5, No. 2, July–August 1997.
20. "What Is the Psychiatric Significance of Loneliness?"
21. Preboth, Monica, and Shyla Wright. "Does the Internet Make People Unhappy?" *American Family Physician,* Vol. 59, No. 6, March 15, 1999.
22. Clinton, Monique, and Lynn Anderson. "Social and Emotional Loneliness: Gender Differences and Relationships with Self-Monitoring and Perceived Control." *Journal of Black Psychology,* Vol. 25, No. 1, February 1999.
23. Cramer, Kenneth, and Kimberley Neyedley. "Sex Differences in Loneliness: The Role of Masculinity and Femininity." *Sex Roles: A Journal of Research,* Vol. 38, Nos. 7–8, April 1998.

24. Stein, Murray, et al. "Social Phobia Symptoms, Subtypes, and Severity." *Archives of General Psychiatry,* Vol. 57, No. 11, November 2000.

25. Lang, Ariel, and Murray Stein. "Social Phobia: Prevalence and Diagnostic Threshold." *Journal of Clinical Psychiatry,* Vol. 62, Suppl. 1, 2001, pp. 5–10.

26. "This Year's International Mental Health Agenda: Erasing the Stigma of Mental Illness." *WHO Reports,* May 2001, p. 24.

27. Satcher, David. "Heads Up." *Psychology Today,* May–June 2001, p. 13.

28. Ibid.

29. American Psychiatric Association. *Diagnostic and Statistical Manual of Mental Disorders.* 4th ed. Washington, DC: American Psychiatric Association, 1994.

30. "Mounting Evidence Indicates Heart Disease Link." *Medical Letter on the CDC & FDA,* July 21, 2002, p. 14.

31. "Depression Doubles Risk of Later Hypertension." *Family Practice News,* Vol. 32, No. 9, May 1, 2002, p. 13.

32. Parmet, Sharon. "Depression and Heart Disease." *Journal of the American Medical Association,* Vol. 288, No. 6, August 14, 2002, p. 792.

33. "Depression and Heart Disease." *Harvard Heart Letter,* Vol. 11, No. 8, April 2001.

34. Andrews, Gavin. "Should Depression Be Managed As a Chronic Disease?" *British Medical Journal,* Vol. 322, No. 7283, February 17, 2001, p. 419.

35. Rosenthal, Beth, et al. "Prevalence of Psychological Symptoms Among Undergraduate Students in an Ethnically Diverse Urban Public College," *Journal of American College Health,* Vol. 49, No. 1, July 2000.

36. Stein, "Social Phobia Symptoms, Subtypes, and Severity."

37. Rabatin, Joseph, and Lynn Buckvar. "Generalized Anxiety and Panic Disorder." *Western Journal of Medicine,* Vol. 176, No. 3, May 2002, p. 164.

38. "What Are the Current Treatments for Panic Disorder?" *Harvard Mental Health Letter,* Vol. 16, No. 11, May 2000.

39. "CBT May Help Patients Control Panic Disorder." *Mental Health Weekly,* Vol. 12, No. 7, February 18, 2002, p. 7.

40. "What You Should Know About Generalized Anxiety Disorders." *American Family Physician,* Vol. 62, No. 7, October 1, 2000.

41. "Obsessive-Compulsive Disorder: What It Is and How to Treat It." *American Family Physician,* Vol. 61, No. 5, March 1, 2000.

42. "Depressing." Short Takes, *UCSF Today,* November 9, 2000.

43. Pullen, Lisa, et al. "Adolescent Depression: Important Facts That Matter." *Journal of Child and Adolescent Psychiatric Nursing,* Vol. 13, No. 2, April 2000.

44. Walling, Anne. "Depression in Young Adults." *American Family Physician,* Vol. 62, No. 1, July 1, 2000.

45. Torrey, Brian. "USPSTF Depression Screening Recommendations." *American Family Physician,* Vol. 66, No. 12, July 15, 2002, p. 335.

46. "Depression Survey Reveals Dramatic Change in Public Opinion." *Healthcare Review,* Vol. 15, No. 4, April 22, 2002, p. 8.

47. "Exercise Against Depression." *Harvard Mental Health Letter,* Vol. 17, No. 19, March 2001.

48. Babyak, Michael, et al. "Exercise Treatment for Major Depression: Maintenance of Therapeutic Benefit at 10 Months." *Psychosomatic Medicine,* Vol. 62, No. 5, September–October 2000, pp. 633–638.

49. LeTourneau, Melanie. "Pump Up to Cheer Up." *Psychology Today,* May–June 2001, p. 27.

50. Dubin, Julie Weingarden. "More Than a Mood." *Psychology Today,* May–June 2001, p. 26.

51. Jensen, Peter. Personal interview.

52. March, John. Personal interview.

53. "Teenage Depression Shows Family Ties." *Science News,* Vol. 159, No. 1, February 3, 2001, p. 72.

54. Hughes, Alice, et al. "Depressive Symptoms and Cigarette Smoking Among Teens." *Journal of the American Medical Association,* Vol. 284, No. 23, December 20, 2000, p. 2980.

55. Zito, Julia. "Antidepressant Use in Youth." Presentation, American Psychiatric Association Annual Meeting, New Orleans, May 2001.

56. Vastag, Brian. "Decade of Work Shows Depression Is Physical." *Journal of the American Medical Association,* Vol. 287, No. 14, April 10, 2002, p. 1787.

57. Olfson, Mark, et al. "National Trends in the Outpatient Treatment of Depression." *Journal of the American Academy of Child and Adolescent Psychiatry,* Vol. 41, No. 7, July 2002, p. 837.

58. Straton, Joseph, and Peter Cronholm. "Are Paroxetine, Fluoxetine, and Sertraline Equally Effective for Depression?" *Journal of Family Practice,* Vol. 51, No. 3, March 2002, p. 285.

59. Babyak, "Exercise Treatment for Major Depression."

60. Hales, Robert E., and Dianne Hales. The *Mind–Mood Pill Book.* New York: Bantam, 2001.

61. "Drop in Suicide Rates Related to Wider Use of Antidepressants." *Pain & Central Nervous System Week,* July 8, 2002, p. 12.

62. Wetzstein, Cheryl. "Preventing Suicide." *Insight on the News,* Vol. 16, No. 16, May 1, 2000.

63. Gould, Madelyn. Personal interview.

64. "Drop in Suicide Rates Related to Wider Use of Antidepressants."

65. Borowsky, Iris, et al. "Adolescent Suicide Attempts: Risks and Protectors." *Pediatrics,* Vol. 107, No. 3, March 2001, p. 485.

66. Barrios, Lisa, et al. "Suicide Ideation Among U.S. College Students." *Journal of American College Health,* Vol. 48, No. 5, March 2000.

67. "Suicide and Suicide Attempts in Adolescents." *Pediatrics,* Vol. 105, No. 4, April 2000.

68. Brown, David, and Curtis Blanton. "Physical Activity, Sports Participation, and Suicidal Behavior Among College Students." *Science in Sports and Exercise,* Vol. 34, No. 7, July 2002, p. 1087.

69. "The Seasons of Suicide." *Harvard Mental Health Letter,* Vol. 16, No. 11, May 2000.

70. Walling, Anne. "Which Patients Are at Greatest Risk of Committing Suicide?" *American Family Physician,* Vol. 61, No. 8, April 15, 2000, p. 2487.

71. "Analysis of Suicide Risk Factors and Suicidal Self-Injury and Concurrent Health Risk Behaviors Among Adolescents." *Research Quarterly for Exercise and Sport,* Vol. 71, March 2000.

72. Bostwick, J. M., et al. "Affective Disorders and Suicide Risk: A Re-examination." *American Journal of Psychiatry,* Vol. 157, No. 12, December 2000, p. 1925.

73. Popper, Charles, and Scott West. "Disorders Usually Diagnosed in Infancy, Childhood or Adolescence." *American Psychiatric Press Textbook of Psychiatry,* 3rd ed. Washington, DC: American Psychiatric Press, 1999.

74. Mostofsky, Stewart. "Brain Abnormalities in Children with ADHD." American Academy of Neurology, Annual Meeting, Toronto, April 1999.

75. Young, Joel. "ADHD in Adults: Contemporary Approaches." *Behavioral Health Management,* Vol. 22, No. 3, May–June, 2002, p. 21.

76. "Harbingers of Schizophrenia." *Harvard Mental Health Letter,* Vol. 17, No. 5, November 2000.

77. Walling, Anne. "Update on Schizophrenia." *American Family Physician,* Vol. 61, No. 12, June 15, 2000.

78. "How Schizophrenia Develops: New Evidence and New Ideas." *Harvard Mental Health Letter,* Vol. 17, No. 8, February 2001.

79. "Cognitive Therapy Tops Medication." *Pain & Central Nervous System Week,* June 17, 2002, p. 6.

80. Hart, Valerie. "The Balance of Psychotherapy and Pharmacotherapy." *Perspectives in Psychiatric Care,* Vol. 36, No. 2, April–June 2000.

81. Hales and Hales, *The Mind–Mood Pill Book.*

82. Ibid.

83. Davidson, Jonathan. "Effect of Hypericum Perforatum (St. John's Wort) in Major Depressive Disorder: A Randomized Controlled Trial." *Journal of the American Medical Association,* Vol. 287, No. 14, April 10, 2002, p. 1807.

84. Dickstein, Leah. "Nature's Pharmacy Is Full of Surprises." *Psychology Today,* March–April 1999.

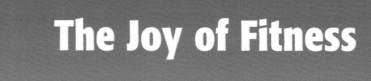

# The Joy of Fitness

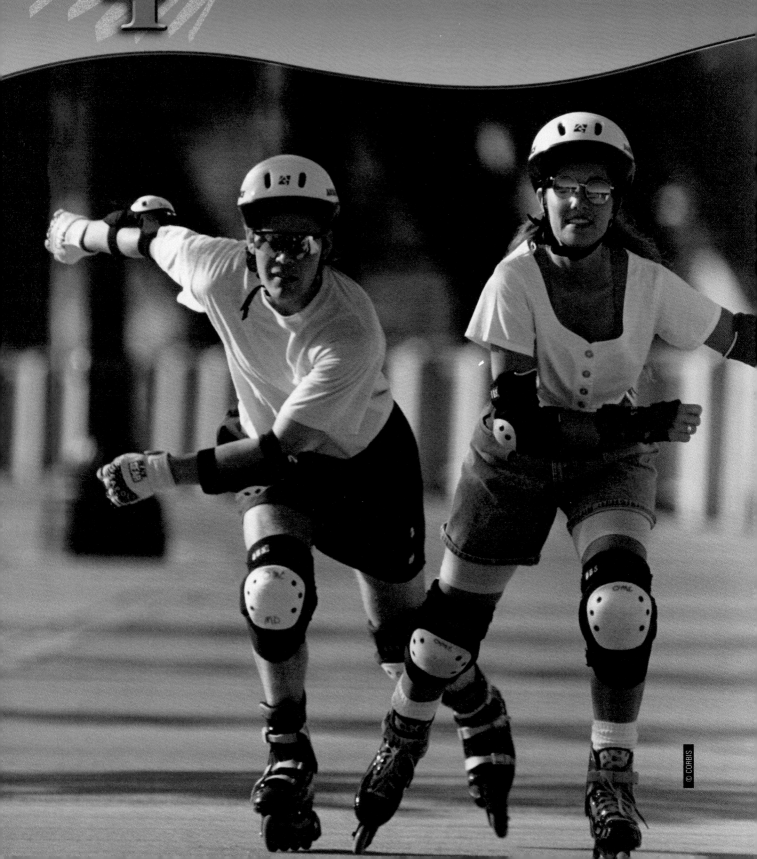

© CORBIS

**After studying the material in this chapter, you should be able to:**

- **Describe** the components of physical fitness.
- **Describe** the health benefits of regular physical activity.
- **List** the different forms of cardiorespiratory activities and **describe** their potential health benefits and risks.
- **Explain** the benefits of a muscle training program and **describe** how to design a workout.
- **Define** flexibility and **describe** the different types of stretching exercises.
- **List** safety strategies for physically active individuals.

You are designed to move. In ways far more complex than the fastest airplane or sleekest car, your body runs, stretches, bends, swims, climbs, glides, and strides—day after day, year after year, decade after decade. While mere machines break down from constant wear and tear, your body thrives on physical activity. The more you use your body, the stronger and healthier you can become.

Often the college years represent a turning point in physical fitness. In the bustle of campus life, students typically log more hours in classes and in front of computers, and spend less time walking, jogging, swimming, cycling, or working  out. In one recent survey at a Southern university in a large metropolitan area, 43 percent of college seniors were regular exercisers who worked out three days a week or more, and 17 percent didn't exercise at all. About 85 percent of the regularly active seniors remained as or even more active in the years after graduation. Most of the nonexercisers reported being as or less active than in their college days.[1] (See Student Snapshot: "Exercising During College—and After.")

As you'll see in this chapter, exercise yields immediate rewards: It boosts energy, improves mood, soothes stress, improves sleep, and makes you look and feel better. In the long term, physical activity slows many of the changes associated with chronological aging, such as loss of calcium and bone density, lowers the risk of serious chronic illnesses, and extends the lifespan.

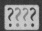

To get these benefits, you don't have to turn into a jock or fitness fanatic. But you do have to get moving. This chapter can help. It presents the latest activity recommendations, documents the benefits of exercise, describes types of exercise, and provides guidelines for getting into shape and exercising safely.

## What Is Physical Fitness?

The simplest, most practical definition of **physical fitness** is the ability to respond to routine physical demands with enough reserve energy to cope with a sudden challenge. Consider yourself fit if you meet your daily energy needs, can handle unexpected extra demands, have a realistic but positive self-image, and are protecting yourself against potential health problems, such as heart disease.

Fitness is important—for health and for athletic performance. The health-related components of physical fit-

ness, which this chapter emphasizes, include aerobic or cardiorespiratory endurance, muscular strength and endurance, body composition (the ratio of fat to lean body tissue), and flexibility. Athletic performance depends on additional skills, such as agility, coordination, balance, and speed, which vary with specific sports. While many amateur and professional athletes are in superb overall condition, you do not need athletic skills to keep your body operating at maximum capacity throughout life.

**Cardiorespiratory fitness** refers to the ability of the body to sustain prolonged rhythmic activity. It is achieved through **aerobic exercise**—any activity, such as brisk walking or swimming, in which the amount of oxygen taken into the body is slightly more than, or equal to, the amount of oxygen used by the body. In other words, aerobic exercise involves working out strenuously without pushing to the point of breathlessness.

**Muscular fitness** has two components: strength and endurance. **Strength** refers to the force within muscles; it is measured by the absolute maximum weight that a person can lift, push, or press in one effort. **Endurance** is the ability to perform repeated muscular effort; it is measured by counting how many times a person can lift, push, or press

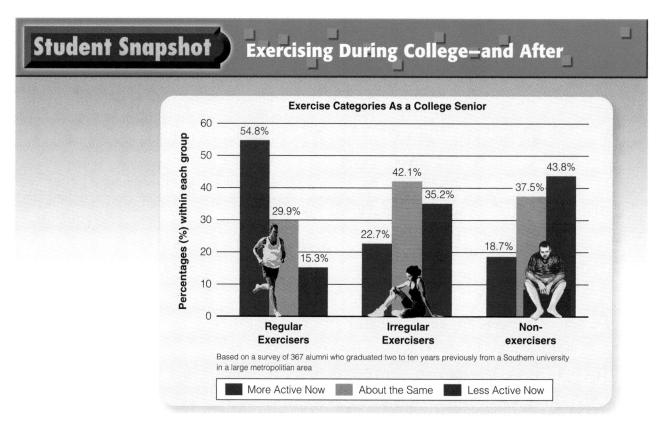

**Student Snapshot** — **Exercising During College—and After**

**Exercise Categories As a College Senior**

*Regular Exercisers:* More Active Now 54.8%, About the Same 29.9%, Less Active Now 15.3%

*Irregular Exercisers:* More Active Now 22.7%, About the Same 42.1%, Less Active Now 35.2%

*Non-exercisers:* More Active Now 18.7%, About the Same 37.5%, Less Active Now 43.8%

Percentages (%) within each group

Based on a survey of 367 alumni who graduated two to ten years previously from a Southern university in a large metropolitan area

■ More Active Now   ■ About the Same   ■ Less Active Now

Adapted with permission from Phillip Sparling and Teresa Snow. "Physical Activity Patterns in Recent College Alumni," *Research Quarterly for Exercise and Sport*, Vol. 73, No. 2, June 2002, p. 200.

a given weight. Both are equally important. It's not enough to be able to hoist a shovelful of snow; you've got to be able to keep shoveling until the entire driveway is clear.

**Body composition** refers to the relative amounts of fat and of lean tissue (bone, muscle, organs, water) in the body. A high proportion of body fat has serious health implications, including increased incidence of heart disease, high blood pressure, diabetes, stroke, gallbladder problems, back and joint problems, and some forms of  cancer. College-age men average 15 percent body fat; college-age women, 23 percent. On average, women have 11 percent more body fat and 8 percent less muscle mass than men.[2] (See The X&Y Files: "Gender Differences and Physical Fitness.")

A combination of regular exercise and good nutrition is the best way to maintain a healthy body composition. Aerobic exercise helps by burning calories and increasing metabolic rate (the rate at which the body uses calories) for several hours after a workout. Strength training increases the proportion of lean body tissue by building muscle mass, which also increases the metabolic rate.

**Flexibility** is the range of motion around specific joints—for example, the stretching you do to touch your toes or twist your torso. Flexibility depends on many factors: your age, gender, and posture; bone spurs; and how fat or muscular you are. As children develop, their flexibility increases until adolescence. Then a gradual loss of joint mobility begins and continues throughout adult life. Both muscles and connective tissue, such as tendons and

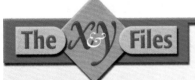

## Gender Differences and Physical Fitness

Men and women benefit equally from physical activity and exercise. Nevertheless, the components of physical fitness do have gender differences. Many are related to size. On average, men are 10 to 15 percent bigger than women, with roughly twice the percentage of muscle mass and half the percentage of body fat. Overall, men are about 30 percent stronger, particularly above the waist. They have more sweat glands and a greater maximum oxygen uptake. A man's bigger heart pumps more blood with each beat. His larger lungs take in 10 to 20 percent more oxygen. His longer legs cover more distance with each stride. If a man jogs along at 50 percent of his capacity, a woman has to push to 73 percent of hers to keep up.

Women have a higher percentage of body fat than men, and more is distributed around the hips and thighs; men carry more body fat around the waist and stomach. The average woman has a smaller heart, a lower percentage of slow twitch muscle fibers, and a smaller blood volume than a man. Because women have a lower concentration of red blood cells, their bodies are less effective at transporting oxygen to their working muscles during exercise.

Even though training produces the same relative increases for both genders, a woman's maximum oxygen intake remains about 25 to 30 percent lower than that of an equally well-conditioned man. In elite athletes, the gender difference is smaller: 8 to 12 percent. Because the angle of the upper leg bone (femur) to the pelvis is greater in a woman, her legs are less efficient at running.

In some endurance events, such as ultramarathon running and long-distance swimming, female anatomy and physiology may have some aerobic advantages. The longer a race—on land, water, or ice—the better women perform. In an analysis of world-record times in running, swimming, and speed skating, researchers at Northeastern University observed that in all three sports the superiority of men's performances diminished with increasing distance.

|  | Female | Male |
|---|---|---|
| Percent fat | 27% | 15% |
| Lean body mass | 107.8 pounds | 134.2 pounds |
| Blood volume | 4.5–5 liters | 5–6 liters |
| Maximum oxygen consumption | 3–3.5 liters per minute | 5.5–9 liters per minute |

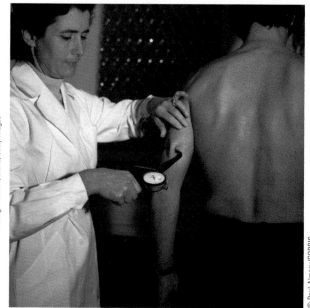

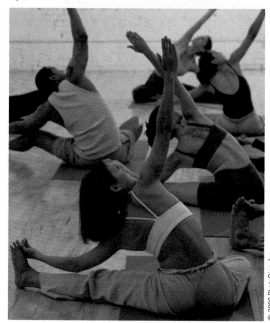

Body composition

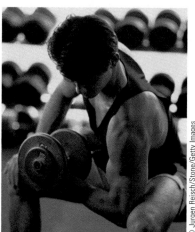

Muscular strength and endurance

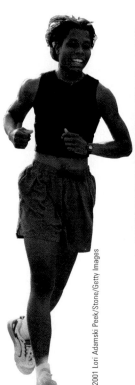

Cardiorespiratory fitness

▲ Four components of physical fitness.

ligaments, shorten and become tighter if not used at all or not used through their full range of motion.

Physical **conditioning** (or training) refers to the gradual building up of the body to enhance cardiorespiratory or aerobic fitness, muscular strength and endurance, and flexibility.

## 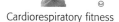 Why Should I Exercise?

If exercise could be packed into a pill, it would be the single most widely prescribed and beneficial medicine in the nation. Why? Because nothing can do more to help your body function at its best (Figure 4-1). With regular activity, your heart muscles become stronger and pump blood more efficiently. Your heart rate and resting pulse slow down. Your blood pressure may drop slightly from its normal level.

Regular physical activity thickens the bones and can slow the loss of calcium that normally occurs with age. Exercise increases flexibility in the joints and improves digestion and elimination. It speeds up metabolism, so the body burns up more calories and body fat decreases. It heightens sensitivity to insulin (a great benefit for diabetics) and may lower the risk of developing diabetes. In addition, exercise enhances clot-dissolving substances in the

Flexibility

blood, helping to prevent strokes, heart attacks, and pulmonary embolisms (clots in the lungs). Regular, vigorous exercise can actually extend the lifespan.

 These are not the benefits most college students mention. Unlike middle-aged and older individuals, traditional-age college students cite improved fitness as the number-one advantage that exercise offers, followed by improved appearance and muscle tone. But undergraduates who recognize any benefits from exercise are more likely to be physically active than those who focus on barriers to working out.[3] (See Table 4-1.)

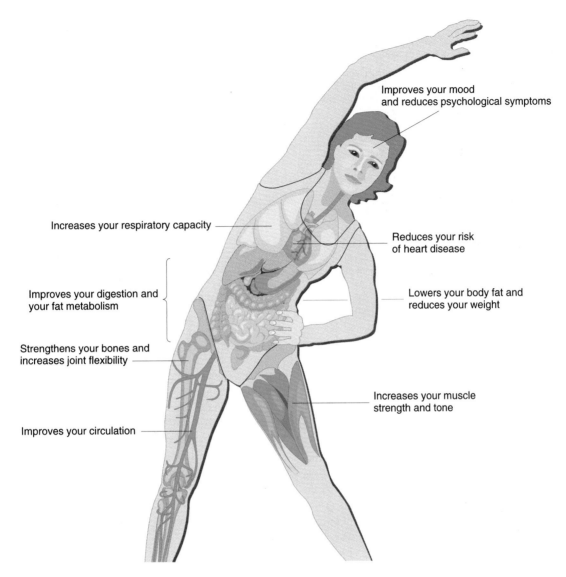

Improves your mood
and reduces psychological symptoms

Increases your respiratory capacity

Reduces your risk
of heart disease

Improves your digestion and
your fat metabolism

Lowers your body fat and
reduces your weight

Strengthens your bones and
increases joint flexibility

Improves your circulation

Increases your muscle
strength and tone

▲ **Figure 4-1** Benefits of Exercise
Regular physical activity enhances your overall health and helps prevent disease.

Here is a summary of the benefits of getting in shape:

## Longer Life

An estimated 2 million people around the globe die every year because they are not physically active, according to the World Health Organization.[4] In the United States, poor cardiorespiratory fitness accounts for 12 percent of deaths.[5] Inactivity increases all causes of mortality, doubles the risk of cardiovascular diseases, diabetes, and obesity, and increases the risk of colon cancer, high blood pressure, osteoporosis, depression, and anxiety.[6]

Capacity for exercise has proven a better predictor of whether a man would die in the next few years than other risk factors, such as high blood pressure, high total cholesterol, or smoking.[7] Formerly sedentary people, even the elderly, who begin to exercise live longer, on average, than those who remain inactive.[8]

## Protection Against Heart Disease and Certain Cancers

Sedentary people are about twice as likely to die of a heart attack as people who are physically active. (See Chapter 10 for a discussion of heart disease.) In addition to its effects on the heart, exercise makes the lungs more efficient. They take in more oxygen, and their vital capacity (ability to take in and expel air) is increased, providing more energy for

### ▼ Table 4-1 Why College Students Exercise—or Don't

In a sample of 147 graduates, the regular exercisers—92 percent of the men and 63.8 percent of the women—perceived more benefits than those who didn't exercise.

**Top Exercise Benefits**

1. Exercise increases my level of physical fitness.
2. Exercise improves the way my body looks.
3. My muscle tone is improved with exercise.
4. Exercise gives me a sense of personal accomplishment.
5. Exercise increases my muscle strength.

**Top Exercise Barriers**

1. Exercise tires me.
2. Exercise is hard work for me.
3. I am fatigued by exercise.
4. Exercising takes too much of my time.
5. My family members do not encourage me to exercise.

Source: Grubbs, Laurie and Jason Carter. "The Relationship of Perceived Benefits and Barriers to Reported Exercise Behaviors in College Undergraduates." *Family and Community Health,* Vol. 25, No. 2, July 2002, p. 76.

you to use. As demonstrated in a 20-year study of almost 4,000 men, regular physical activity also makes blood less likely to clot and cause a stroke or heart attack.[9]

Recent studies have shown that exercise reduces the risk of colon and rectal cancers, possibly by enhancing digestion and elimination. Fitter men are less likely to die of prostate and colon cancer than others.[10] Regular moderate exercise lowers blood levels of estrogen in postmenopausal women, which may lower their risk of breast cancer.[11]

## Better Bones

Weak and brittle bones are common among people who don't exercise. **Osteoporosis,** a condition in which bones lose their mineral density and become increasingly susceptible to injury, affects a great many older people. Women, in particular, are more vulnerable because their bones are less dense to begin with. Researchers estimate that a minimum of two 45-minute exercise sessions per week may protect the bones of postmenopausal women.[12]

## Enhanced Immunity

Moderate exercise correlates with a reduced number of sick days. Researchers speculate that exercise may enhance immune function by reducing stress hormones like cortisol that can dampen resistance to disease. In recent studies, women who walked briskly for 35 to 45 minutes five days a week experienced half the number of sick days with cold symptoms as inactive women. While moderate exercise seems to bolster a person's immune system, heavy training may increase the risk of upper respiratory tract infections for endurance athletes.[13]

## Brighter Mood

Exercise makes people feel good from the inside out. Exercise boosts mood, increases energy, reduces anxiety, improves concentration and alertness, and increases the ability to handle stress. During long workouts, some people experience what is called *runner's high,* which may be the result of increased levels of mood-elevating brain chemicals called **endorphins.**

## Better Mental Health

Exercise is an effective—but underused—treatment for mild to moderate depression and may help in treating other mental disorders.[14] Regular, moderate exercise, such as walking, running, or lifting weights, three times a week, has proven helpful for depression and anxiety disorders, including panic attacks.[15] It also eases certain symptoms, such as agitation and hallucinations, in schizophrenic patients.[16] In a recent study of people with major depression, exercise proved as effective as medication in improving mood and also helped prevent relapse.[17]

## Lower Weight

Aerobic exercise burns off calories during your workout. As your body responds to the increased demand from your muscles for nutrients, your metabolic rate rises. Moreover, this surge persists for as long as 12 hours after exercise, so you continue to use up more calories than usual even after you've stopped sweating. In addition, aerobic exercise suppresses appetite, so you aren't as tempted to eat. It also helps dieters lose fat rather than lean muscle tissue when they cut back on calories. (See Chapter 6 for information on exercise and weight control.)

## A More Active Old Age

Exercise slows the changes that are associated with advancing age: loss of lean muscle tissue, increase in body fat, and decrease in work capacity. In addition to lowering the risk of heart disease and stroke, exercise also helps older men and women retain the strength and mobility needed to live independently. Even in old age, exercise boosts strength and stamina, lessens time in wheelchairs, and improves outlook and the sense of being in control.[18]

# Physical Activity and Health

Alarmed by Americans' sedentary ways, health officials have shifted their emphasis from promoting regular and rigorous exercise to urging people to become more active in any way possible. As they point out, all forms of physical activity—any bodily movement that requires energy and is carried out by the muscles—can produce some health benefits. Studies have confirmed that lifestyle activities, such as walking, housecleaning, and gardening, are as effective as a structured exercise program in improving heart function, lowering blood pressure, and maintaining or losing weight.[19]

While lifestyle activity can improve health, exercise—the structured movement of the body for the purpose of improving or maintaining physical fitness—offers more benefits. Light exercise, activities that increase oxygen consumption no more than three times the level burned by the body at rest, can produce cardiorespiratory benefits.[20] Though light activity is good, moderate is better.

▲ **Figure 4-2** Activity Pyramid
Use the pyramid to create a physical activity plan for your life.

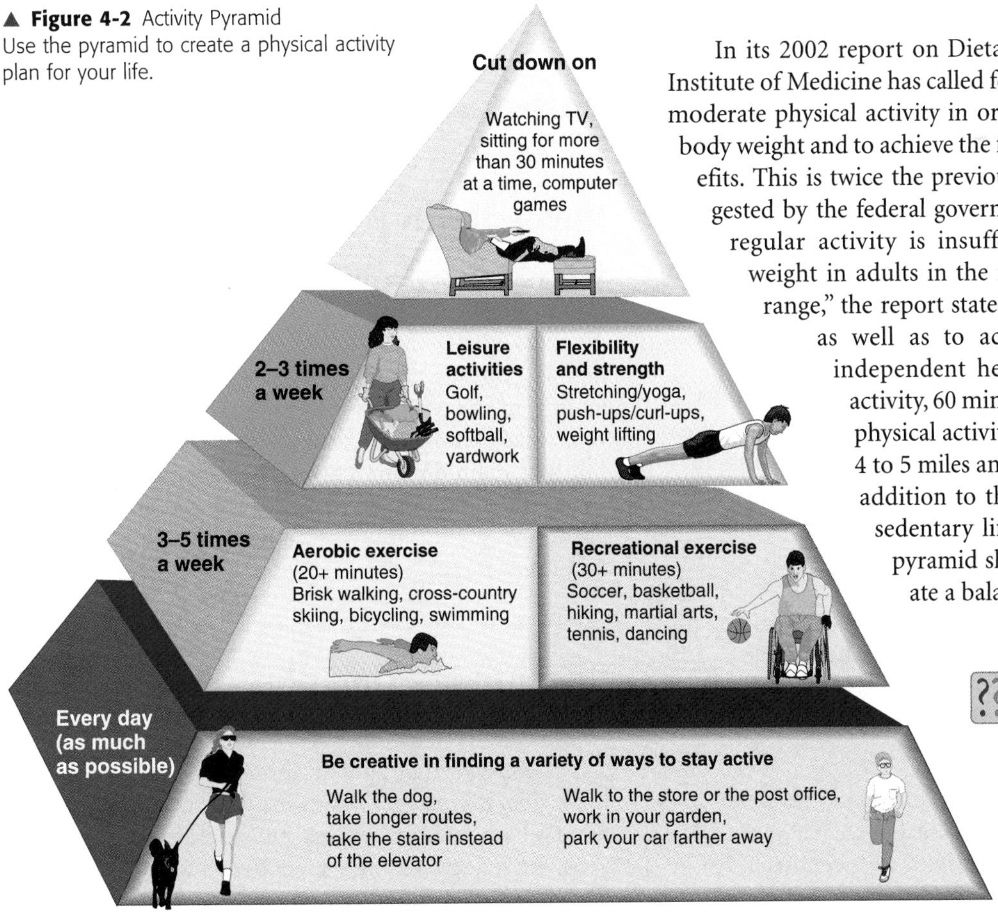

## STRATEGIES FOR CHANGE

### Activating Your Lifestyle

Here are some little ways to add short spurts of activity to your day:

▲ Add a physical component to passive activities. Stand while talking on the phone. Stretch during television commercials.

▲ Actively use waiting time. If you have to wait for a delayed appointment, take a quick walk down the hall or up the stairs.

▲ Put extra oomph into your chores. Use wide, sweeping motions when you mop the floor. Turn on the radio and dance as you fold laundry or dust.

▲ Create opportunities for getting physical. Go dancing instead of to the movies. Shoot hoops with friends instead of sipping coffee. When unloading groceries, carry them into the house one bag at a time.

**Cut down on**

Watching TV, sitting for more than 30 minutes at a time, computer games

**2–3 times a week**

**Leisure activities**
Golf, bowling, softball, yardwork

**Flexibility and strength**
Stretching/yoga, push-ups/curl-ups, weight lifting

**3–5 times a week**

**Aerobic exercise**
(20+ minutes)
Brisk walking, cross-country skiing, bicycling, swimming

**Recreational exercise**
(30+ minutes)
Soccer, basketball, hiking, martial arts, tennis, dancing

**Every day (as much as possible)**

**Be creative in finding a variety of ways to stay active**

Walk the dog, take longer routes, take the stairs instead of the elevator

Walk to the store or the post office, work in your garden, park your car farther away

In its 2002 report on Dietary Reference Intakes, the Institute of Medicine has called for at least an hour of daily, moderate physical activity in order to maintain a healthy body weight and to achieve the fullest possible health benefits. This is twice the previous half-hour amount suggested by the federal government. "Thirty minutes of regular activity is insufficient to maintain body weight in adults in the recommended body mass range," the report states. "To prevent weight gain as well as to accrue additional weight-independent health benefits of physical activity, 60 minutes of moderate intensity physical activity (e.g., walking/jogging at 4 to 5 miles an hour) is recommended in addition to the activities required by a sedentary lifestyle."[21] Use the activity pyramid shown in Figure 4-2 to create a balanced exercise "diet."

## ???? Can a Person Be Fat and Fit?

Most people assume that fitness comes in only one size: small.

That's not necessarily so. As discussed in Chapter 6, there is considerable controversy over how to define a healthy weight. But individuals of every size can improve their physical fitness.

In ten years of research on 25,000 men and 8,000 women, scientists led by Steven Blair, director of research at the Cooper Institute for Aerobics Research in Dallas, have found that heavier individuals can be just as healthy and physically fit as their leaner counterparts. In their studies, obese people who exercised moderately (30 minutes of daily walking at three or four miles per hour) had half the death rate of those who were slimmer but more sedentary. Low cardiorespiratory fitness, regardless of an individual's weight, is as great a risk factor for dying of heart disease or other causes such as diabetes, high blood pressure, and other well-recognized threats.[22]

## The Principles of Exercise

Why does exercise work? As you begin working toward fitness, keep these three principles of exercise in mind: the overload principle, the reversibility principle, and the specificity principle.

## Overload Principle

The **overload principle** requires a person exercising to provide a greater stress or demand on the body than it's usually accustomed to handling. For any muscle, including the heart, to get stronger, it must work against a greater-than-normal resistance or challenge. To continue to improve, you need further increases in the demands—but not too much too quickly. **Progressive overloading**—gradually increasing physical challenges—provides the benefits of exercise without the risk of injuries.

Although slow and gentle activity can enhance basic health, you need to work harder—that is, at a greater intensity—to improve fitness. Whatever exercise you do, there is a level, or threshold, at which fitness begins to improve; a target zone, where you can achieve maximum benefits; and an upper level, at which potential risks outweigh any further benefits. The acronym FIT sums up the three dimensions of progressive overload: *frequency* (how often you exercise) *intensity* (how hard), and *time* (how long).

### Frequency

To attain and maintain physical fitness, you need to exercise regularly, but the recommended frequency varies with different types of exercise and with an individual's fitness goals. The minimum frequency recommended by federal health officials is three to five days of cardiovascular or aerobic exercise a week and two to three days of resistance and flexibility training a week.

### Intensity

Exercise intensity varies with the type of exercise and with personal goals. To improve cardiovascular fitness, you need to increase your heart rate to a target zone (the level that produces benefits). To develop muscular strength and endurance, you need to increase the amount of weight you lift or the resistance you work against and/or the number of repetitions. For enhanced flexibility, you need to stretch muscles beyond their normal length.

### Time (Duration)

The amount of time, or duration, of your workouts is also important, particularly for cardiovascular exercise. In general, experts have found similar health benefits from a single 30-minute session of moderate exercise as from several shorter sessions throughout the day. Duration and intensity are interlinked. If you're exercising at high intensity (biking or running at a brisk pace, for instance), you don't need to exercise as long as when you're working at lower intensity (walking or swimming at a moderate pace). For muscular strength and endurance and for flexibility, duration is defined by the number of sets or repetitions rather than total time.

## Reversibility Principle

The **principle of reversibility** is the opposite of the overload principle. Just as the body adapts to greater physical demands, it also adjusts to lower levels. If you stop exercising, you can lose as much as 50 percent of your fitness improvements within two months. If you have to curtail your usual exercise routine because of a busy schedule, you can best maintain your fitness by keeping the intensity constant and reducing frequency or duration. The principle of reversibility is aptly summed up by the phrase, "Use it or lose it."

## Specificity Principle

The **specificity principle** refers to the body's adaptation to a paticular type of activity or amount of stress placed upon it. Jogging, for instance, trains the heart and lungs to work more efficiently and strengthens certain leg muscles. However, it does not build upper body strength or enhance flexibility.

▼ **Table 4-2 Guidelines for Physical Fitness**

| | Cardiorespiratory | Strength | Flexibility |
|---|---|---|---|
| | © 2001 PhotoDisc | © David Hanover | © David Hanover |
| **Type of Activity** | Aerobic activity that uses large-muscle groups and can be maintained continuously | Resistance activity that is performed at a controlled speed and through a full range of motion | Stretching activity that uses the major muscle groups |
| **Frequency** | A minimum of 3 to 5 days per week | 2 to 3 days per week | A minimum of 2 to 3 days per week |
| **Intensity** | 55 to 90% of maximum heart rate | Enough to enhance muscle strength and improve body composition | Enough to develop and maintain a full range of motion |
| **Time (Duration)** | 20 to 60 minutes | 8 to 12 repetitions of 8 to 10 different exercises (minimum) | 4 repetitions of 10 to 30 seconds per muscle group (minimum) |

Source: Adapted from American College of Sports Medicine, "Position Stand: The Recommended Quantity and Quality of Exercise for Developing and Maintaining Cardiorespiratory and Muscular Fitness, and Flexibility in Healthy Adults." *Medicine and Science in Sports and Exercise,* Vol. 30, 1998, pp. 975–991.

In other words, the overload principle is specific to each body part and to each component of fitness. Leg exercises develop only the lower limbs; arm exercises, only the upper limbs. This is why you need a comprehensive fitness plan that includes a variety of exercises to develop all parts of the body.

## ???? How Much Exercise Is Enough?

If you're not active at all, any physical exercise will produce some benefits. In the beginning, don't worry about frequency or intensity. You're better off starting slow and small, with just a 10-minute walk or bike ride a few days a week, than pushing to do too much and giving up because of injury or discomfort.[23] Although exercising just once or twice a week is not enough to improve cardiorespiratory or aerobic fitness, it does produce benefits: In a study of 45 healthy office workers, even those who exercised just once a week had lower body weights and lower body fat than those who didn't work out at all.[24] Simply walking one hour a week reduced the risk of heart disease for sedentary middle-aged women, even those who were overweight, smoked, or had high cholesterol.[25]

While some exercise is better than none, more is better. Federal health guidelines call for at least 30 minutes of brisk walking on most days of the week. The American College of Sports Medicine recommends the following weekly minimums (see Table 4-2):

✔ Three to five days of aerobic workouts of 20- to 60-minute duration, either in a single session or in several 10-minute sessions.
✔ Two to three strength training sessions that involve at least one set of eight to twelve repetitions of eight to ten exercises that work all major muscle groups.
✔ Two to three flexibility workouts that stretch the major muscles throughout the body.

## Cardiorespiratory or Aerobic Fitness

Since physical activity requires more energy, the heart, lungs, and blood vessels have to work harder to deliver more oxygen to the cells. A person with good cardiorespiratory endurance can engage in a physical activity for a long time without becoming fatigued. The heart of a person who isn't in good condition has to pump more often; as a result, it becomes fatigued more easily.

Unlike muscular endurance, which is specific to individual muscles, cardiorespiratory endurance involves the entire body. The exercises that improve cardiorespiratory endurance are referred to as aerobic because the body uses as much, or slightly more, oxygen than it takes in. Aerobic exercise can take many forms, as noted later in this chapter, but all involve working strenuously without pushing to the point of breathlessness.

In **anaerobic exercise,** the amount of oxygen taken in by the body cannot meet the demands of the activity. This quickly creates an oxygen deficit that must be made up later. Anaerobic activities are high in intensity but short in duration, usually lasting only about ten seconds to two minutes. An example is sprinting the quarter-mile, which leaves even the best-trained athletes gasping for air.

In nonaerobic exercise, such as bowling, softball, or doubles tennis, there is frequent rest between activities. Because the body can take in all the oxygen it needs, the heart and lungs really don't get much of a workout.

## Your Target Heart Rate

To be sure you're working hard enough to condition your heart and lungs, but not overdoing it, use your pulse, or heart rate, as a guide. One of the easiest places to feel your pulse is in the carotid artery in your neck. Slightly tilt your head back and to one side. Use your middle finger or forefinger, or both, to feel for your pulse. (Do not use your thumb; it has a beat of its own.) To determine your heart rate, count the number of pulses you feel for 10 seconds and multiply that number by six, or count for 30 seconds and multiply that number by two. Learn to recognize the pulsing of your heart when you're sitting or lying down. This is your **resting heart rate.**

Start taking your pulse during, or immediately after, exercise, when it's much more pronounced than when you're at rest. Three minutes after heavy exercise, take your pulse again. The closer that reading is to your resting heart rate, the better your condition. If it takes a long time for your pulse to recover and return to its resting level, your body's ability to handle physical stress is poor. As you continue working out, however, your pulse will return to normal much more quickly.

You don't want to push yourself to your maximum heart rate, yet you must exercise at about 60 to 85 percent of that maximum to get cardiovascular benefits from your training. This range is called your **target heart rate.** If you don't exercise intensely enough to raise your heart rate at least this high, your heart and lungs won't benefit from the workout. If you push too hard, and exercise at or near your absolute maximum heart rate, you run the risk of placing too great a burden on your heart. Table 4-3 lists target heart rates for various ages. The following formula can also be used to calculate your maximum and target heart rates (in beats per minute):

1.  Estimate your maximum heart rate. Take 220 − age = ___ (this is your maximum)

| ▼ Table 4-3  Target Heart Ranges Based on Age | | | |
|---|---|---|---|
| **Age** | **Average Maximum Heart Rate (100%)** | **Target Heart Rate (60–90%)** | |
| 20 | 200 | 120 | 180 |
| 25 | 195 | 117 | 175 |
| 30 | 190 | 114 | 171 |
| 35 | 185 | 111 | 166 |
| 40 | 180 | 108 | 162 |
| 45 | 175 | 105 | 157 |
| 50 | 170 | 102 | 153 |
| 55 | 165 | 99 | 148 |
| 60 | 160 | 96 | 144 |
| 65 | 155 | 93 | 139 |
| 70 | 150 | 90 | 135 |

2.  Determine your lower-limit target heart rate by multiplying your maximum heart rate by 0.6 = ___
3.  Determine your upper-limit target heart rate by multiplying your maximum heart rate by 0.9 = ___

Your target heart rate range is between your lower and upper limits.

According to the American College of Sports Medicine, for most people exercising at the lower end of the target heart rate range for a long time is more beneficial than exercising at the higher end of the range for a short time.[26] If your goal is losing weight, exercise at 60 to 70 percent of your maximum heart rate in order to burn fat calories. To improve aerobic endurance and strengthen your heart, work at 70 to 80 percent of your maximum heart rate. Competitive athletes may train at 80 to 100 percent of their maximum heart rate.[27] (See Table 4-4.)

## How Do I Design an Aerobic Workout?

Whatever activity you choose, your aerobic workout should consist of several stages, including a warm-up and a cool-down.

### Warm-Up

Just as you don't get in your car and immediately gun your engine to 60 miles per hour, you shouldn't do the same with your body. You need to prepare your cardiorespiratory system for a workout, speed up the blood flow to your lungs, and increase the temperature and elasticity of your muscles and connective tissue to avoid injury.

▼ **Table 4-4  Target Heart Rates Based on Type of Activity**

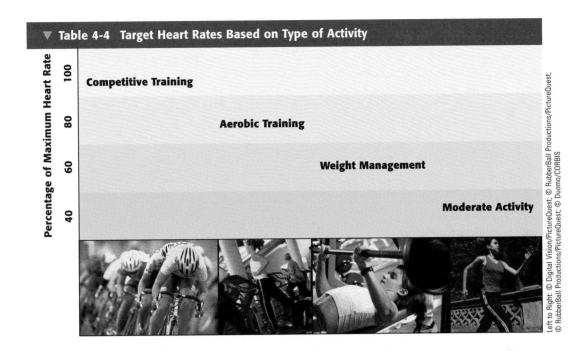

Start by walking briskly for about 5 minutes. This helps your body make the transition from inactivity to exertion. Follow this general warm-up with about 5 minutes of simple stretches of the muscles you'll be exercising most. Before a jog, for instance, you can stretch the muscles in your ankle and the back of your leg by leaning against a wall, with one leg bent and tilted forward and the other straight. Lean forward until you feel the stretch and hold.

## Aerobic Activity

The two key components of this part of your workout are intensity and duration. As described in the previous section, you can use your target heart rate range to make sure you are working at the proper intensity. The current recommendation is to keep moving for at least 60 minutes, either in one session or several briefer sessions, each lasting at least 10 minutes.

## Cool-Down

After you've pushed your heart rate up to its target level and kept it there for a while, the worst thing you can do is slam on the brakes. If you come to a sudden stop, you put your heart at risk. When you stand or sit immediately after vigorous exercise, blood can pool in your legs. You need to keep moving at a slower pace to ensure an adequate supply of blood to your heart. Ideally, you should walk for 5 to 10 minutes at a comfortable pace before you end your workout session.

## Your Long-Term Plan

One of the most common mistakes people make is to push too hard too fast. Often they end up injured or discouraged and quit entirely. If you are just starting an aerobic program, think of it as a series of phases: beginning, progression, and maintenance:

✔ **Beginning (4–6 weeks).** Start slow and low (in intensity). If you're walking, monitor your heart rate and aim for 55 percent of your maximum heart rate. Another good rule of thumb to make sure you're moving at the right pace: If you can sing as you walk, you're going too slow; if you can't talk, you're going too fast.
✔ **Progression (16–20 weeks).** Gradually increase the duration and/or intensity of your workouts. For instance, you might add 5 minutes every two weeks to your walking time. You also can gradually pick up your pace, using your target heart rate as your guide. Keep a log of your workouts so you can chart your progress until you reach your goal.
✔ **Maintenance (lifelong).** Once you've reached the stage of exercising for an hour every day, you may want to develop a repertoire of aerobic activities you enjoy. Combine or alternate activities to avoid monotony and keep up your enthusiasm. This is called *cross-training*.

## Walking

More men and women are taking to their feet. Some are casualties of high-intensity sports and can no longer withstand the wear and tear of rigorous workouts. Others want to shape up, slim down, or ward off heart disease and other health problems. The good news for all is that walking may well be the perfect exercise. Walking at least 30 minutes a day at a moderate pace is as effective as more vigorous exercise in reducing the risk of heart disease, according to the Women's Health Initiative Observational study of more than 70,000 postmenopausal women.[28]

Recent research has demonstrated the health benefits of walking for both men and women and for both healthy individuals and those with heart disease. One major study of women, the Nurses' Health Study, found that women who walk briskly three hours a week are as well protected from heart disease as women who spend an hour and a half a week in more vigorous activities, such as aerobics or running. Women engaged in either form of exercise had a rate of heart attacks 30 to 40 percent lower than that of sedentary women. The Women's Health Study, a randomized, controlled trial of aspirin and heart disease, found that even walking one hour per week can lower heart disease risk among relatively sedentary women.[29] Walking also protects men's hearts, whether they're healthy or have had heart problems. In a recent British study of 772 men, those who regularly engaged in light exercise, including walking, had a risk of death that was 58 percent lower than that of their sedentary counterparts.[30]

Walking is good for the brain as well as the body. In a study that followed almost 6,000 women age 65 or older for up to eight years, those who walked regularly were less likely to experience memory loss and other age-related declines in mental function.[31] Another bonus is stress reduction. Since you can do it during a break or at lunchtime, walking builds relaxation into your day.

Treadmills are a good alternative to outdoor walks—and not just in bad weather. They keep you moving at a certain pace, they're easier on the knees, and they allow you to exercise in a climate-controlled, pollution-free environment—a definite plus for many city dwellers. Holding onto the handrails while walking on a treadmill reduces both heart rate and oxygen consumption, so you burn fewer calories. Experts advise slowing the pace if necessary so you can let go of the handrails while working out.[32]

Here are some guidelines for putting your best foot forward:

✔ Walk very slowly for 5 minutes, and then do some simple stretches.

✔ Maintain good posture. Focus your eyes ahead of you, stand erect, and pull in your stomach.

✔ Use the heel-to-toe method of walking. The heel of your leading foot should touch the ground before the ball or toes of that foot do. When you push off with your trailing foot, bend your knee as you raise your heel. You should be able to feel the action in your calf muscles.

✔ Pump your arms back and forth to burn 5 to 10 percent more calories and get an upper-body workout as well.

✔ End your walk the way you started it—let your pace become more leisurely for the last 5 minutes.

## Jogging and Running

The difference between jogging and running is speed. You should be able to carry on a conversation with someone on a long jog or run; if you're too breathless to talk, you're pushing too hard.

If your goal is to enhance aerobic fitness, long, slow, distance running is best. If you want to improve your speed, try *interval training,* which consists of repeated hard runs over a certain distance, with intervals of relaxed jogging in between. Depending on what suits you and what your training goals are, you can vary the distance, duration, and number of fast runs, as well as the time and activity between them. Interval training is usually done on a track and should not be attempted unless you're in top shape.

If you have been sedentary, it's best to launch a walking program before attempting to jog or run. Start by walking for 15 to 20 minutes three times a week at a comfortable pace. Continue at this same level until you no longer feel sore or unduly fatigued the day after exercising. Then increase your walking time to 20 to 25 minutes, speeding up your pace as well.

When you can handle a brisk 25-minute walk, alternate fast walking with slow jogging. Begin each session walking, and gradually increase the amount of time you spend jogging. If you feel breathless while jogging, slow down and walk. Continue to alternate in this manner until you can jog for 10 minutes without stopping. If you gradually increase your jogging time by 1 or 2 minutes with each workout, you'll slowly build up to 20 or 25 minutes per session. For optimal fitness, you should jog at least three times a week.

Here's how to be sure you're running right:

✔ Always take time to warm up and to stretch. Warm up with jumping jacks or running in place for 3 to 5 minutes. Spend at least one-fourth of the time that you plan to run on stretching exercises.[33]

✔ As you run, keep your back straight and your head up. Run tall, with your buttocks tucked in. Look straight ahead. Hold your arms slightly away from your body. Your elbows should be bent slightly so that your forearms are almost parallel to the ground. Move your arms rhythmically to propel yourself along.

## Savvy Consumer

### How to Buy Athletic Shoes

For many aerobic activities, good shoes are the most important purchase you'll make. Take the time to choose well. Here are some basic guidelines:

- Shop for shoes in the late afternoon, when your feet are most likely to be somewhat swollen—just as they will be after a workout.

- For walking shoes, look for a shoe that's lightweight, flexible, and roomy enough for your toes to wiggle, with a well-cushioned, curved sole; good support at the heel; and an upper made of a material that breathes (allows air in and out).

- For running shoes (see the figure), look for good cushioning, support, and stability. You should be able to wiggle your toes easily, but the front of your foot shouldn't slide from side to side, which could cause blisters. Your toes should not touch the end of the shoe because your feet will swell with activity. Allow about half an inch from the longest toe to the tip of the shoe.

- For tennis shoes, look for reinforcement at the toe. The sole at the ball of the foot should be well padded, because that's where most pressure is exerted. The sides of the shoe should be sturdy, for stability during continuous lateral movements. The toe box should allow ample room and some cushioning at the tips. A long throat ensures greater control by the laces.

Don't wear wet shoes for training. Let wet shoes airdry, because a heater will cause them to stiffen or shrink. Use powder in your shoes to absorb moisture, lessen friction, and prevent fungal infections. Break in new shoes for several days before wearing them for a long-distance run or during competition.

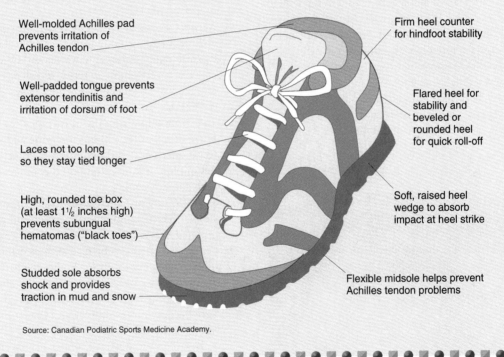

Well-molded Achilles pad prevents irritation of Achilles tendon

Well-padded tongue prevents extensor tendinitis and irritation of dorsum of foot

Laces not too long so they stay tied longer

High, rounded toe box (at least 1½ inches high) prevents subungual hematomas ("black toes")

Studded sole absorbs shock and provides traction in mud and snow

Firm heel counter for hindfoot stability

Flared heel for stability and beveled or rounded heel for quick roll-off

Soft, raised heel wedge to absorb impact at heel strike

Flexible midsole helps prevent Achilles tendon problems

Source: Canadian Podiatric Sports Medicine Academy.

✔ Have your heels hit the ground first. Land on your heel, rock forward, and push off the ball of your foot. If this is difficult, try a more flat-footed style.

✔ Avoid running on the balls of your feet; this produces soreness in the calves because the muscles must contract for a longer time. To avoid shin splints (a dull ache in the lower shins), stretch regularly to strengthen the shin muscles and to develop greater flexibility in your ankles.

✔ Avoid running on hard surfaces and making sudden stops or turns.

## Other Aerobic Activities

Because variety is the spice of an active life, many people prefer different forms of aerobic exercise. All can provide many health benefits. Among the popular options:

✔ **Swimming.** For aerobic conditioning, you have to swim laps using the freestyle, butterfly, breaststroke, or backstroke. (The sidestroke is too easy.) You must also be a good enough swimmer to keep churning through the water for at least 20 minutes. Your heart will beat more slowly in water than on land, so your heart rate while swimming is not an accurate guide to exercise intensity. You should try to keep up a steady pace that's fast enough to make you feel pleasantly tired, but not completely exhausted, by the time you get out of the pool.

✔ **Cycling.** Bicycling, indoors and out, can be an excellent cardiovascular conditioner, as well as an effective way to control weight—provided you aren't just along for the ride. If you coast down too many hills, you'll have to ride longer up hills or on level ground to get a good workout. Half of all bikes now sold in the United States are mountain bikes, sturdy cycles with knobby tires that allow bikers to climb up and zoom down dirt trails and explore places traditional racing bikes couldn't go. An 18-speed bike can make pedaling too easy, however, unless you choose gears carefully. To gain aerobic benefits, mountain bikers have to work hard enough to raise their heart rates to their target zone and keep up that intensity for at least 20 minutes.

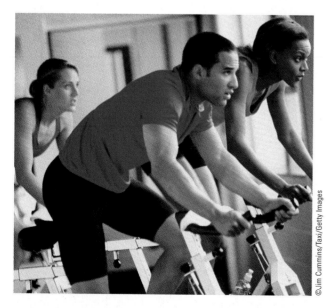

Spinning has become a popular option for aerobic exercise because people of different ages, skills, and fitness levels can participate in the same class.

✔ **Spinning.**™ Spinning is a cardiovascular workout for the whole body that utilizes a special stationary bicycle. Led by an instructor, a group of bikers listens to music, and modifies their individual bike's resistance and their own pace according to the rhythm. An average spinning class lasts 45 minutes and has between 20 and 40 participants.

Unlike an ordinary stationary bike, a spinning bike has a larger saddle area and a heavier flywheel to create greater resistance; the rider, rather than a built-in computer, monitors performance. Introduced in 1987, this indoor cycling program has grown in appeal because it is time efficient and nonimpact, and because people of all ages, skills, and fitness levels can participate in the same class.

✔ **Skipping rope.** Essentially a form of stationary jogging with some extra arm action thrown in, skipping rope is excellent as both a heart conditioner and a way of losing weight. Always warm up before starting and cool down afterward. To alleviate boredom, try skipping to music and vary the steps: both feet together, alternating left and right feet, or jumping up and down on one leg.

✔ **Aerobic dancing.** This activity combines music with kicking, bending, and jumping. A typical class (you can also dance at home to a video or TV program) consists of stretching exercises and sit-ups, followed by aerobic dances and cool-down exercises. A particular benefit of aerobic dance is that people get enjoyment and stimulation from the music; they're also able to move their bodies without worrying about skill and technique. "Soft," or low-impact, aerobic dancing doesn't put as much strain on the joints as "hard," or high-impact, routines.

✔ **Step training or bench aerobics.** "Stepping" combines step, or bench, climbing with music and choreographed movements. Basic equipment consists of a bench 4 to 12 inches high. The fitter you are, the higher the bench—but the higher the bench, the greater the risk of knee injury. Injuries have skyrocketed in recent years as movements and choreography have become more complex and the pace of the music has picked up.[34]

Tugging on supersized rubber stretch cords, which has the same effect as weight training, can increase the benefits of a step workout. In a controlled study, exercisers who added resistance exercises with stretch cords to their step routines showed improvements in aerobic capacity as well as muscle strength and size.[35] A 40-minute step workout is equivalent to running seven miles an hour in terms of oxygen uptake and calories burned.

✔ **Stair-climbing.** An estimated 4 million Americans are stepping up to fitness, according to the American Sports Data Institute. You could run up the stairs in an office building or dormitory, but most people use stair-climbing machines available in home models and at gyms and health clubs. On most versions of these machines, exercisers push a pair of pedals up and down, which is much easier on the feet and legs than many other activities.

✔ **Inline skating.** Inline skating can increase aerobic endurance and muscular strength, and is less stressful on joints and bones than running or high-impact aerobics. Skaters can adjust the intensity of their workout by varying the terrain. (Obviously, they'll have to work harder while going up hills, and less so on the slide down.) They can also buy special training wheels and weights to increase resistance and make muscles work harder. One caution: Protective gear, including a helmet, knee and elbow pads, and wrist guards, is essential.

✔ **Tennis.** As with other sports, tennis can be an aerobic activity—depending on the number of players and their skill level. In general, a singles match requires more continuous exertion than playing doubles. Intermediate to advanced players, who engage in prolonged volleys, experience a more challenging workout than beginners, who spend less time in motion.

## Muscular Strength and Endurance

Although aerobic workouts condition your insides (heart, blood vessels, and lungs), they don't exercise many of the muscles that shape your outsides and provide power when you need it. Strength workouts are important because they enable muscles to work more efficiently and reliably. Conditioned muscles function more smoothly, and contract somewhat more vigorously and with less effort. With exercise, muscle tissue becomes firmer and can withstand much more strain—the result of toughening the sheath protecting the muscle and developing more connective tissue within it (see Figure 4-3).

Muscular strength and endurance are critical for handling everyday burdens, such as cramming a 20-pound suitcase into an overhead luggage bin or hauling a trunk down from the attic. Prolonged exercise prepares the muscles for sustained work by improving the circulation of blood in the tissue. The number of tiny blood vessels, called capillaries, increases by as much as 50 percent in regularly exercised muscles, and existing capillaries open wider so that the total circulation increases by as much as 400 percent, thus providing the muscles with a much greater supply of nutrients. This increase occurs after about 8 to 12 weeks in young persons, but takes longer in older individuals. Inactivity reverses the process, gradually shutting down the extra capillaries that have developed.

The latest research on fat-burning shows that the best way to reduce your body fat is to add muscle-strengthening exercise to your workouts. Muscle tissue is your very best calorie-burning tissue, and the more you have, the more calories you burn, even when you are resting. You don't have to become a serious body builder. Using handheld weights (also called *free weights*) two or three times a week is enough. Just be sure you learn how to use them properly because you can tear or strain muscles if you don't practice the proper weight-lifting techniques. As more people have begun to lift weights, injuries have soared.[36]

A balanced workout regimen of muscle building and aerobic exercise does more for you than just burn fat. It gives you more endurance by promoting better distribution of oxygen to your tissues and increasing the blood flow to your heart.

## Exercise and Muscles

Your muscles never stay the same. If you don't use them, they atrophy, weaken, or break down. If you use them rigorously and regularly, they grow stronger. The only way to develop muscles is by demanding more of them than you usually do. This is called **overloading.** (Remember the overload principle?) As you train, you have to gradually increase the number of repetitions or the amount of resistance and work the muscle to temporary fatigue. That's why it's important not to quit when your muscles start to tire. Some exercise enthusiasts believe that the experience of pain—the *burn*—signals that exercise is paying off; others contend that it means you're pushing too hard and risking injury.

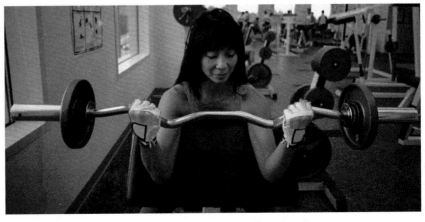

© 2000 PhotoDisc, Inc.

▲ Build up muscular strength and endurance through weight training.

## Strength workouts increase circulation

The heart's right half pumps oxygen-poor blood to capillary beds in lungs. There, $O_2$ diffuses into blood and $CO_2$ diffuses out. The oxygenated blood flows into the heart's left half, where it is then pumped to capillary beds throughout the body

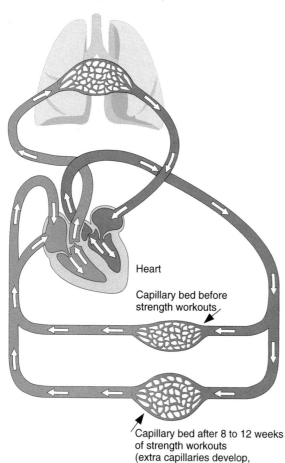

Heart

Capillary bed before strength workouts

Capillary bed after 8 to 12 weeks of strength workouts (extra capillaries develop, circulation increases)

## Strength workouts build muscles

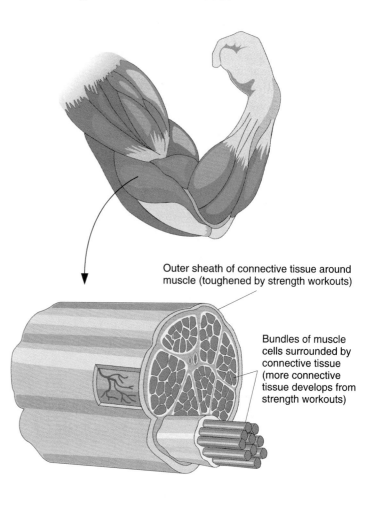

Outer sheath of connective tissue around muscle (toughened by strength workouts)

Bundles of muscle cells surrounded by connective tissue (more connective tissue develops from strength workouts)

▲ **Figure 4-3** Benefits of Strength Training on the Body
Strength training in combination with aerobic exercise increases blood circulation and oxygen supply to body tissues and develops muscles.

You need to exercise differently for strength than for endurance. *To develop strength,* do a few repetitions with heavy loads. As you increase the weight your muscles must move, you increase your strength. *To increase endurance,* you do many more repetitions with lighter loads. If your muscles are weak and you need to gain strength in your upper body, you may have to work for weeks to do a half-dozen regular push-ups. Then you can start building endurance by doing as many push-ups as you can before collapsing in exhaustion.

Muscles can do only two things: contract or relax. As they do so, skeletal muscles either pull on bones or stop pulling on bones. All exercise involves muscles pulling on bones across a joint. The movement that takes place depends on the structure of the joint and the position of the muscle attachments involved.

In an **isometric** contraction, the muscle applies force while maintaining an equal length. The muscle contracts and tries to shorten but cannot overcome the resistance. An example is pushing against an immovable object, like a wall, or tightening an abdominal muscle while sitting. The muscle contracts but there is no movement. Push or pull against the immovable object, with each muscle contraction held for 5 to 8 seconds; repeat five to ten times daily.

An **isotonic** contraction involves movement, but the muscle tension remains the same. In an isotonic exercise, the muscle moves a moderate load several times, as in weight lifting or calisthenics. The best isotonic exercise for producing muscular strength involves high resistance and a low number of repetitions. On the other hand, you can develop the greatest flexibility, coordination, and endurance with isotonic exercises that incorporate lower resistance and frequent repetitions.

True **isokinetic** contraction is a constant speed contraction. Isokinetic exercises require special machines that provide resistance to overload muscles throughout the entire range of motion.

## ???? How Do I Design a Muscle Workout?

A workout with weights should exercise your body's primary muscle groups: the *deltoids* (shoulders), *pectorals* (chest), *triceps* and *biceps* (back and front of upper arms), *quadriceps* and *hamstrings* (front and back of thighs), *gluteus maximus* (buttocks), *trapezius* and *rhomboids* (back), and *abdomen* (see Figure 4-4). Various machines and free-weight routines focus on each muscle group, but the principle is always the same: Muscles contract as you raise and lower a weight, and you repeat the lift-and-lower routine until the muscle group is tired.

A weight training program is made up of *reps* (the single performance, or *repetition,* of an exercise, such as lifting 50 pounds one time) and *sets* (a *set* number of repetitions of the same movement, such as a set of 20 push-ups). You should allow your breath to return to normal before moving on to each new set. Pushing yourself to the limit builds strength.

Maintaining proper breathing during weight training is crucial. To breathe correctly, inhale when muscles are relaxed, and exhale when you push or lift. Don't ever hold your breath because oxygen flow helps prevent muscle fatigue and injury.

No one type of equipment— free weight or machine—has a clear advantage in terms of building fat-free body mass, enhancing strength and endurance, or improving a sport-specific skill. Each type offers benefits but also has drawbacks.

Free weights offer great versatility for strength training. With dumbbells, for example, you can perform a variety of exercises to work specific muscle groups, such as the chest and shoulders. Machines, in contrast, are much more limited; most allow only one exercise.

Strength-training machines have several advantages. They ensure correct movement for a lift, which helps protect against injury and prevent cheating when fatigue sets in. They isolate specific muscles, which is good for rehabilitating an injury or strengthening a specific body part. Because they offer high-tech options like varying resistance during the lifting motion, they can tax muscles in ways that a traditional barbell cannot.

Remember that your muscles need sufficient time to recover from a weight-training session. Allow no less than 48 hours, but no more than 96 hours, between training sessions, so your body can recover from the workout and you avoid overtraining. Workouts on consecutive days do more harm than good because the body can't recover that quickly. Two or three 30-minute training sessions a week should be sufficient for building strength and endurance. Strength training twice a week at greater intensity and for a longer duration can be as effective as working out three times a week. However, your muscles will begin to atrophy if you let more than

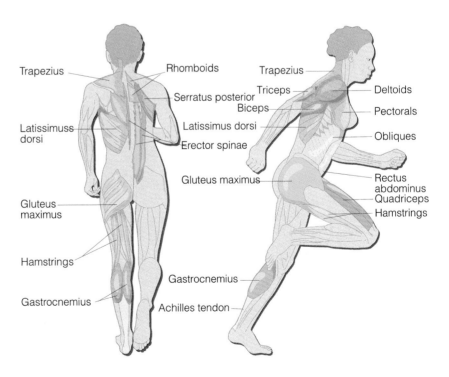

▲ **Figure 4-4** Primary Muscle Groups
Different exercises can strengthen and stretch different muscle groups.

three or four days pass without exercising them. For total fitness, you may want to schedule aerobic workouts for your days off from weight training.

## Flexibility

Flexibility is the characteristic of body tissues that determines the range of motion achievable without injury at a joint or group of joints. There are two types of flexibility: static and dynamic. **Static flexibility**—the type most people think of as flexibility—refers to the ability to assume and maintain an extended position at one end point in a joint's range of motion. **Dynamic flexibility,** by comparison, involves movement. It is the ability to move a joint quickly and fluidly through its entire range of motion with little resistance. The static flexibility in the hip joint determines whether you can do a split; dynamic flexibility would enable you to perform a split leap.

Static flexibility depends on many factors, including the structure of a joint and the tightness of the muscles, tendons, and ligaments attached to it. Dynamic flexibility is influenced by static flexibility, but also depends on additional factors, such as strength, coordination, and resistance to movement.

Genetics, age, gender, and body composition all influence how flexible you are. Girls and women tend to be more flexible than boys and men, to a certain extent because of hormonal and anatomical differences. The way females and males use their muscles and the activities they engage in can also have an effect. Over time, the natural elasticity of muscles, tendons, and joints decreases in both genders, resulting in stiffness.

## The Benefits of Flexibility

Just as cardiorespiratory fitness benefits the heart and lungs and muscular fitness builds endurance and strength, a stretching program produces unique benefits, including enhancement of the ability of the respiratory, circulatory, and neuromuscular systems to cope with the stress and pressures of our high-pressure world. Among the other benefits of flexibility are:

✔ **Prevention of injuries.** Flexibility training stretches muscles and increases the elasticity of joints. Strong, flexible muscles resist stress better than weak or inflexible ones. Adding flexibility to a training program for sports such as soccer, football, or tennis can reduce the rate of injuries by as much as 75 percent. In one study of competitive runners, weekly stretch-ing sessions significantly reduced the incidence of low back pain.

✔ **Relief of muscle strain.** Muscles tighten as a result of stress or prolonged sitting. If you study or work in one position for several hours, you'll often feel stiffness in your back or neck. Stretching helps relieve this tension and enables you to work more effectively.

✔ **Relaxation.** Flexibility exercises are great stress-busters that reduce mental strain, slow the rate of breathing, and reduce blood pressure.

✔ **Relief of soreness after exercise.** Many people develop delayed-onset muscle soreness (DOMS) one or two days after they work out. This may be the result of damage to the muscle fibers and supporting connective tissue. Some researchers theorize that stretching after exercise can decrease this aftereffect, although others contend that it produces only short-term benefits.

✔ **Improved posture.** Bad posture can create tight, stressed muscles. If you slump in your chair, for instance, the muscles in the front of your chest may tighten, causing those in the upper spine to over-stretch and become loose.

✔ **Better athletic performance.** Good flexibility allows for more efficient movement and exertion of more force through a greater range of motion, a special benefit for any activity, from gymnastics to golf, where positions beyond the normal range of motion are necessary to perform certain skills.

Flexibility can make everyday tasks, like bending over to tie a shoe or reaching up to a high shelf, easier and safer. It can also prevent and relieve the ankle, knee, back, and shoulder pain that many people feel as they get older. If you do other forms of exercise, flexibility lowers your risk of injury and may improve your performance. (See Figure 4-5.)

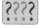 ## What Is the Difference Between Stretching and Warming Up?

Warming up means getting the heart beating, breaking a sweat, and readying the body for more vigorous activity. Stretching is a specific activity intended to elongate the muscles and keep joints limber, not simply a prelude to a game of tennis or a three-mile run.

For most sports, light to moderate activity, such as walking at gradually increasing intensity, is a better warm-up than stretching. One of the best times to stretch is after an aerobic workout. Your muscles will be warm, more flexible, and less prone to injury. In addition, stretching after aerobic activity can help a fatigued muscle return to its

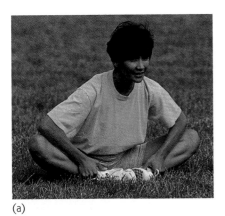
(a)

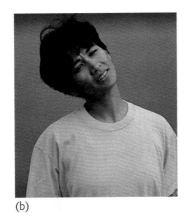
(b)

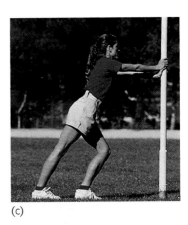
(c)

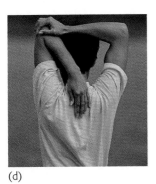
(d)

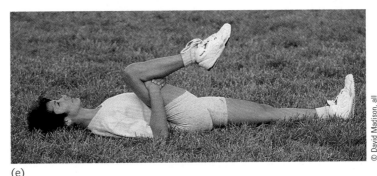
(e)

© David Madison, all

▲ **Figure 4-5** Some Simple Stretching Exercises
(a) *Foot pull for the groin and thigh muscles.* Sit on the ground and bend your legs so that the soles of your feet touch. Pull your feet closer as you press on your knees with your elbows. Hold for 10 seconds; repeat. (b) *Lateral head tilt.* Gently tilt your head to each side. Repeat several times. (c) *Wall stretch for the Achilles tendon.* Stand 3 feet from a wall or post with your feet slightly apart. Keeping your heels on the ground, lean into the wall. Hold for 10 seconds; repeat. (d) *Triceps stretch for the upper arm and shoulder.* Place your right hand behind your neck and grasp it above the elbow with your left hand. Gently pull the elbow back. Repeat with the left elbow. (e) *Knee-chest pull for lower back muscles.* Lying on your back, clasp one knee and pull it toward your chest. Hold for 15–30 seconds; repeat with the other knee.

## STRATEGIES FOR PREVENTION

### How to Avoid Stretching Injuries

▲ Never stretch to the point of pain. You should feel the pull of your muscles, but no sharp pain.

▲ Start small. Work the muscles of the smaller joints in the arms and legs first and then work the larger joints like the shoulders and hips.

▲ Stretch individual muscles before you stretch a group of muscles. For instance, stretch the ankle, knee, and hip before a stretch that works all three.

▲ Don't make quick, jerky movements while stretching. Since a slow stretch provokes less of a reaction from the stress receptors, the muscles can safely stretch farther than usual.

normal resting length and possibly helps reduce delayed muscle soreness.

## Sports Safety

Whenever you work out, you don't want to risk becoming sore or injured. Starting slowly when you begin any new fitness activity is the smartest strategy. Keep a simple diary to record the time and duration of each workout. First get accustomed to an activity and then begin to work harder or longer. In this way, you strengthen your musculoskeletal system so you're less likely to be injured, you lower the cardiovascular risk, and you build the exercise habit into your schedule.

Even seasoned athletes should listen to their bodies. If you develop aches and pains beyond what you might expect from an activity, stop. Never push to the point of fatigue. If you do, you could end up with sprained or torn muscles.

## ???? How Can I Prevent Sports Injuries?

Both genders are equally likely to suffer an exercise-related injury. An estimated one in four women and one in three men discontinue their exercise programs because of injury.[37] The most common exercise-related injury sites are the knees, feet, back, and shoulders, followed by the ankles and hips. **Acute injuries**—sprains, bruises, and pulled muscles—are the result of sudden trauma, such as a fall or collision. **Overuse injuries** are the result of overdoing a repetitive activity, such as running. When one particular joint is overstressed (such as a tennis player's elbow or a swimmer's shoulder), tendinitis, an inflammation at the point where the tendon meets the bone, can develop. Other overuse injuries include muscle strains and aches and stress fractures, which are hairline breaks in a bone, usually in the leg or foot.

To prevent injuries and other exercise-related problems before they happen, use common sense and take appropriate precautions, including the following:

✔ Get proper instruction and, if necessary, advanced training from knowledgeable instructors.
✔ Make sure you have good equipment and keep it in good condition. Know how to check and do at least basic maintenance on the equipment yourself. Always check your equipment prior to each use (especially if you're renting it).
✔ Always make sure that stretching and exercises are preventing, not causing, injuries.
✔ Use reasonable protective measures, including wearing a helmet when cycling or skating.
✔ For some sports, such as boating, always go with a buddy.
✔ Take each outing seriously—even if you've dived into this river a hundred times before, even if you know this mountain like you know your own backyard. Avoid the unknown under adverse conditions (for example, hiking unfamiliar terrain during poor weather or kayaking a new river when water levels are unusually high or low) or when accompanied by a beginner whose skills may not be as strong as yours.
✔ Never combine alcohol or drugs with any sport.

## Thinking of Temperature

Prevention is the wisest approach to heat problems. Always dress appropriately for the weather and be aware of the health risks associated with temperature extremes.

### Heeding Heat

Always wear as little as possible when exercising in hot weather. Choose loose-fitting, lightweight, white or light-colored clothes. Cotton is good because it absorbs perspiration. Never wear rubberized or plastic pants and jackets to sweat off pounds. These sauna suits will cause you to lose water only—not fat—and, because they don't allow your body heat to dissipate, they can be dangerous. On humid days, carry a damp washcloth to wipe off perspiration and cool yourself down. Be sure to drink plenty of fluids while exercising (especially water), and watch for the earliest signs of heat problems, including cramps, stress, exhaustion, and heatstroke.

### Coping with Cold

Protect yourself in cold weather (or cold indoor gyms) by covering as much of your body as possible, but don't overdress. Wear one layer less than you would if you were outside but not exercising. Don't use warm-up clothes of waterproof material because they tend to trap heat and keep perspiration from evaporating. Make sure your clothes are loose enough to allow movement and exercise of the hands, feet, and other body parts, thereby maintaining proper circulation. Choose dark colors that absorb heat. And because 40 percent or more of your body heat is lost through your head and neck, wear a hat, turtleneck, or scarf. Cover your hands and feet, too; mittens provide more warmth and protection than gloves.

### Overtraining

About half of all people who start an exercise program drop out within six months. One common reason is that they **overtrain**, pushing themselves to work too intensely too frequently. Signs of overdoing it include persistent muscle soreness, frequent injuries, unintended weight loss, nervousness, and an inability to relax. Overtraining for endurance sports like marathon running can damage the lungs and intensify asthma symptoms. If you're pushing too hard, you may find yourself unable to complete a normal workout or to recover after a normal workout.

If you develop any of the symptoms of overtraining, reduce or temporarily stop your workout sessions. Then gradually increase the intensity of your workouts. Allow 24 to 48 hours for recovery between workouts. Make sure you get adequate rest. Check with a physical education instructor, coach, or trainer to make sure your exercise program fits your individual needs.

 How fitness-conscious are people in your city?

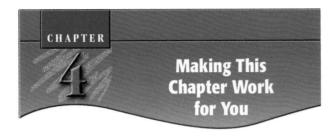

CHAPTER

**4**

**Making This Chapter Work for You**

1. Mary Ann takes a step aerobics class three times a week. Which component of physical fitness does her exercise routine emphasize?
   a. muscular strength and endurance
   b. flexibility
   c. cardiorespiratory fitness
   d. body composition

2. The benefits of regular physical activity include:
   a. decreased bone mass.
   b. lowered risk of shin splints.
   c. enhanced immune response.
   d. altered sleep patterns.

3. In the exercise pyramid, which activity does *not* help create a balanced exercise diet?
   a. walking the dog for 30 minutes
   b. playing golf for 30 minutes
   c. swimming for 30 minutes
   d. working on a computer game for 30 minutes

4. The three principles of exercise are:
   a. overload, specificity, and duration.
   b. overload, reversibility, and specificity.
   c. overload, progressive overloading, and FIT.
   d. frequency, intensity, and time.

5. To receive the cardiovascular benefits of exercise, at what percentage of your target heart rate must you exercise?
   a. 60 to 70
   b. 70 to 80
   c. 80 to 90
   d. 90 to 100

6. Which of the following best describes the primary benefit of aerobic exercise?
   a. It improves cardiorespiratory endurance.
   b. It helps condition your muscles, enabling them to work efficiently and reliably.
   c. It can enhance weight loss.
   d. It increases the range of motion of your joints.

7. An aerobic workout may consist of
   a. 5 minutes of brisk walking, 30 minutes of flexibility exercises, 5 minutes of brisk walking.
   b. 15 minutes of resistance exercises followed by 10 minutes of stretching.
   c. 10 minutes of sprints, 5 minutes of slow jogging, 5 minutes of stretching, and 10 minutes of sprints.
   d. 5 minutes of stretching, 5 minutes of brisk walking, 45 minutes of jogging, 5 minutes of slow walking, 5 minutes of stretching.

8. Which statement is true about isometric, isotonic, and isokinetic exercises?
   a. Isokinetic exercises usually involve pushing on an object, isotonic exercises involve pulling on an object, and isotonic exercises involve lifting an object.
   b. Isometric and isokinetic exercises can be done with free weights, but isotonic exercises require special resistance machines.
   c. Weight lifting is an isotonic exercise, pushing against the wall is an isometric exercise, and isokinetic exercises require special machines that move muscles through their range of motion.
   d. Isotonic exercises are much more effective at contracting muscles than isometric or isokinetic.

9. A regular flexibility program provides which of the following benefits?
   a. stronger heart and lungs
   b. relief of muscle strain and soreness
   c. increased strength and endurance
   d. increased bone mass and leaner muscles

10. To stay safe when exercising in hot weather, which of these is *not* a good idea?
    a. Wear loose-fitting, lightweight clothes.
    b. Carry a damp towel or cloth to cool yourself down.
    c. Drink plenty of fluids, especially water.
    d. Wear one layer more than you would if you were not exercising.

Answers to these questions can be found on page 415.

## Critical Thinking

1. Allison knows that exercise is good for her health, but she figures she can keep her weight down by dieting, and worry about her heart and health when she gets older. "I look good. I feel okay. Why should I bother exercising?" she asks. What would you reply?

2. When he started working out, Jeff simply wanted to stay in shape. But he felt so pleased with the way his body looked and responded that he kept doing more. Now he runs 10 miles a day (longer on weekends), lifts weights, works out on exercise equipment almost

every day, and plays racquetball or squash whenever he gets a chance. Is Jeff getting too much of a good thing? Is there any danger in his fitness program? What would be a more reasonable approach?

3. Your younger brother Andre is hoping to get a starting position on his high school football team.

Practices began in July. You are aware that a couple of other players have suffered heat-related incidences, but according to Andre, these players just weren't tough enough. What can you do to help your brother protect his health?

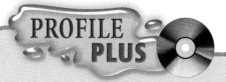

## PROFILE PLUS

Assess your current fitness levels and begin planning for a fitter future with these activities on your Profile Plus CD-ROM:

Exercise Prescription * Exercise Log * Cardiovascular Risk * Cardiorespiratory Endurance *Skill-Related

Fitness * Muscular Strength and Endurance Test * Heart Rate and Blood Pressure

## SITES & BYTES

### Shape Up America!
**www.shapeup.org**

This website provides information about safe weight management, healthy eating, and physical fitness. Special features include an online library, a body fat lab, a support center, and Shape Up and Drop 10 for personalized fitness and diet recommendations.

### Just Move.
**www.justmove.org**

At this website sponsored by the American Heart Association, after a free registration you can access an interactive exercise diary where you can keep track of your own exercise progress. In addition, an information resource called My Fitness provides recommendations for optimizing your exercise program to match your lifestyle, as well as a list of health and fitness resources.

### Georgia State University's Exercise and Physical Fitness Page
**www.gsu.edu/~wwwfit**

Sponsored by the Department of Kinesiology and Health at Georgia State University, this site features a series of links containing research-based exercise and fitness information, including how to get started on an exercise program and stay with it, aerobic exercises, strength training, flexibility, nutrition, and body composition.

Please note that links are subject to change. If you find a broken link, use a search engine such as www.yahoo.com and search for the website by typing in keywords.

**InfoTrac College Edition Activity**   Steve Stiefel. "Run to Build Muscle: Turn Your Cardio into a Resistance Workout and Get the Best of Both Worlds." *Men's Fitness*, May 2002, Vol. 18, No. 5, p. 38(3).

1. Describe one method of strengthening abdominal muscles while running.
2. Name and describe two ways to strengthen the muscles of the upper body while running.
3. What is an effective way to increase the muscle mass of the lower extremities while performing aerobic exercises?

You can find additional readings relating to fitness with InfoTrac College Edition, an online library of more than 900 journals and publications. Follow the instructions for accessing InfoTrac that were packaged with your textbook; then search for articles using a keyword search.

For additional links, resources, and suggested readings on InfoTrac, visit our Health & Wellness Resource Center at http://health.wadsworth.com.

## Key Terms

The terms listed here are used within the chapter on the page indicated. Definitions of the terms are in the Glossary at the end of this book.

| | | | |
|---|---|---|---|
| acute injuries 92 | dynamic flexbility 90 | muscular fitness 74 | progressive overloading 80 |
| aerobic exercise 74 | endorphins 78 | osteoporosis 78 | resting heart rate 82 |
| anaerobic exercise 82 | endurance 74 | overload principle 80 | reversibility principle 80 |
| body composition 75 | flexibility 75 | overloading 87 | specificity principle 80 |
| cardiorespiratory fitness 74 | isokinetic 89 | overtrain 92 | static flexibility 90 |
| | isometric 88 | overuse injuries 92 | strength 74 |
| conditioning 76 | isotonic 88 | physical fitness 74 | target heart rate 82 |

## References

1. Sparling, Phillip, and Teresa Snow. "Physical Activity Patterns in Recent College Alumni." *Research Quarterly for Exercise and Sport,* Vol. 73, No. 2, June 2002, p. 200.

2. "Biology Shows Women and Men Are Different." *Mayo Clinic Women's Healthsource,* September 2002.

3. Grubbs, Laurie, and Jason Carter. "The Relationship of Perceived Benefits and Barriers to Reported Exercise Behaviors in College Undergraduates." *Family and Community Health,* Vol. 25, No. 2, July 2002, p. 76.

4. "WHO Unmasks Another Killer: Inactivity." *Bulletin of the World Health Organization,* Vol. 80, No. 5, May 2002, p. 425.

5. Laukkanen, Jan, et al. "Mortality in Men." *Archives of Internal Medicine,* Vol. 161, No. 6, March 26, 2001, p. 825.

6. "How Fit You Are Determines Your Life Span." *Tufts University Health & Nutrition Letter,* Vol. 20, No. 5, July 2002, p. 6.

7. Palatini, P, et al. "Exercise Capacity and Mortality." *New England Journal of Medicine,* Vol. 347, No. 4 , July 25, 2002, p. 288.

8. Roberts, Shauna. "Why Exercise Matters." *Diabetes Forecast,* Vol. 55, No. 8, August 2002, p. 73.

9. "Heart Beat—Activity Keeps the Blood Flowing." *Harvard Heart Letter,* Vol. 12, No. 11, July 2002.

10. "Regular Physical Exertion May Fight Cancer As Well As Heart Disease." *Tufts University Health & Nutrition Letter,* Vol. 18, No. 7, September 2000.

11. "Exercise Lowers Levels of Blood Estrogen." *Women's Health Weekly,* August 8, 2002, p. 10.

12. Yonclas, Peter, et al. "Osteoporosis: How Much Exercise Is Enough for Bone Health?" *Consultant,* Vol. 42, No. 7, June 2002, p. 829(5).

13. "Exercise and Illness." *JOPERD—The Journal of Physical Education, Recreation & Dance,* Vol. 73, No. 6, August 2002, p. 19.

14. "Exercise Against Depression." *Harvard Mental Health Letter,* Vol. 17, No. 19, March 2001.

15. LeTourneau, Melanie. "Pump Up to Cheer Up." *Psychology Today,* May–June 2001, p. 27.

16. "Exercise As Psychotherapy." *Harvard Mental Health Letter,* Vol. 17, No. 3, September 2000.

17. Babyak, Michael, et al. "Exercise Treatment for Major Depression: Maintenance of Therapeutic Benefit at 10 Months." *Psychosomatic Medicine,* Vol. 62, No. 5, September–October 2000, pp. 633–638.

18. *National Blueprint: Increasing Physical Activity Among Adults Age 50 and Older.* Washington, DC: National Center for Chronic Disease Prevention and Health Promotion, May 1, 2001.

19. "Heart Lines—Walking and Gardening Beneficial for Heart Disease Patients." *Harvard Heart Letter,* Vol. 11, No. 8, April 2001.

20. "Easy Ways to Reduce the Risk of Heart Disease." *HealthFacts,* April 2001.

21. Panel on Macronutrients, Subcommittees on Upper Reference Levels of Nutrients and Interpretation and Uses of Dietary Reference Intakes, and the Standing Committee on the Scientific Evaluation of Dietary Reference Intakes. *Dietary Reference Intakes for Energy, Carbohydrates, Fiber, Fat, Protein and Amino Acids.* Washington, DC: National Academy of Sciences Press, 2002.

22. Wei, M, et al. "Relationship Between Low Cardiorespiratory Fitness and Mortality in Normal-Weight, Overweight, and Obese Men," *Journal of the American Medical Association,* Vol. 282, No. 16, October 27, 1999, p. 1547.

23. "Don't Sweat over How Much or What Type of Exercise . . . Just Do It." *American Family Physician,* Vol. 63, No. 10, May 15, 2001, p. 1899.

24. Ramadan, J., et al. "Low-Frequency Physical Activity Insufficient for Aerobic Conditioning Is Associated with Lower Body Fat Than Sedentary Conditions." *Nutrition,* Vol. 17, 2001, p. 225.

25. Lee, I-Min, et al. "Physical Activity and Coronary Heart Disease in Women: Is 'No Pain, No Gain' Passé?" *Journal of the American Medical Association,* Vol. 285, No. 11, March 21, 2001.

26. American College of Sports Medicine, www.acsm.org.

27. Burke, Edmund. "Heart Rate ABCs," *Better Nutrition,* Vol. 64, No. 8, August 2002, p. 48.

28. Manson, JoAnn, et al. "Walking Compared with Vigorous Exercise for the Prevention of Cardiovascular Events in Women." *New England Journal of Medicine,* Vol. 347, September 5, 2002, p. 716.

29. Lee, "Physical Activity and Coronary Heart Disease in Women."

30. "Heart Lines—Walking and Gardening Beneficial for Heart Disease Patients."

31. Yaffe, Kristin, et al. "A Prospective Study of Physical Activity and Cognitive Decline in Elderly Women." *Archives of Internal Medicine,* Vol. 161, No. 14, July 23, 2001, p. 1703.

32. Welch, Gregory. "Learning to Let Go." *American Fitness,* Vol. 19, No. 4, July 2001, p. 61.

33. "Orthopaedic Surgeons Offer Tips on How Not to 'Run' into Trouble This Spring." News release, American Academy of Orthopaedic Surgeons, May 5, 2001, http://orthoinfo.aaos.org.

34. Dibene, Julieanne. "10 Steps to Better Stepping." *American Fitness,* Vol. 19, No. 3, May 2001, p. 28.

35. Kraemer, William, et al. "Resistance Training Combined with Bench-Step Aerobics Enhances Women's Health Profile." *Medicine and Science in Sports and Exercise,* Vol. 33, No. 2, February 2001, p. 259.

36. "Buffed-Up Numbers." *Daybreak,* University of California, San Francisco, August 23, 2000.

37. Hootman, Jennifer, et al. "Epidemiology of Musculoskeletal Injuries Among Sedentary and Physically Active Adults." *Medicine and Science in Sports and Exercise,* Vol. 34, No. 5, May 2002, p. 838.

# Personal Nutrition

After studying the material in this chapter, you should be able to:

- **List** the basic nutrients necessary for a healthy body and **describe** their functions.
- **Describe** the Food Guide Pyramid and explain its significance.
- **Explain** current recommendations for food portions and servings.
- **Discuss** the purpose of the Dietary Reference Intakes and **explain** how to interpret the nutritional information provided on the food labels.
- **Compare** the advantages and disadvantages of various alternative diets and ethnic foods.
- **List** the food safety hazards and describe prevention measures.

We are indeed what we eat—and it shows in everything from our stamina and strength to the sheen in our hair and the glow in our cheeks. Eating well helps us live and feel well. As demonstrated by the science of **nutrition,** the field that explores the connections between our bodies and the foods we eat, our daily diet affects how long and how well we live. Sensible eating can provide energy for our daily tasks, protect us from many chronic illnesses, and may even extend longevity.

Many foods can serve as the building blocks of a healthy lifestyle. The latest guidelines for healthful eating—issued by the National Academy of Sciences' Institute of Medicine (IOM) in 2002—reflect this fact by allowing greater flexibility in putting together a diet tailored to individual activity levels and nutritional needs.[1] However, making good food choices isn't easy. Faced with a bewildering array of products in stores and restaurants and a blitz of advertising claims, you may well find it hard to select the foods that not only taste good but also are good for you.

This chapter can help. It translates the latest information on good nutrition into specific advice that you can use to nourish yourself as well as enjoy the pleasure of eating well.

# What You Need to Know About Nutrients

Every day your body needs certain **essential nutrients** that it cannot manufacture for itself. They provide energy, build and repair body tissues, and regulate body functions. The six classes of essential nutrients, which are discussed in this section, are water, protein, carbohydrates, fats, vitamins, and minerals (see Table 5-1 below).

Water makes up about 60 percent of the body and is essential for health and survival. Besides water, we also need energy to live, and we receive our energy from the carbohydrates, proteins, and fats in the foods we eat. These three essential nutrients are called **macronutrients,** because they are the nutrients required by the human body in the greatest amounts. The amount of energy that can be derived from the macronutrients is measured in **calories.** There are 9 calories in every gram of fat and 4 calories in every gram of protein or carbohydrate. The other two essential nutrients—the vitamins and minerals—are called **micronutrients** because our bodies need them in only very small amounts.

In 2002 the federal government, in the latest of a series of reports from the Institute of Medicine, issued its first standards for intakes of macronutrients. These standards are likely to lead to changes in everything from the Food Pyramid to nutrition labels, both discussed later in this chapter.[2]

Individuals' need for macronutrients depends on how much energy they expend. Because fats, carbohydrates, and protein can all serve as sources of energy, they can, to some extent, substitute for one another in providing calories. Adults, according to the new standards, should get 45 to 65 percent of calories from carbohydrates, 20 to 35 percent from fat, and 10 to 35 percent from protein. Children's fat intake should be slightly higher: 25 to 40 percent of their caloric intake.

## Water

Water, which makes up 85 percent of blood, 70 percent of muscles, and about 75 percent of the brain, performs many essential functions: It carries nutrients, maintains temperature, lubricates joints, helps with digestion, rids the body of waste through urine, and contributes to the production of sweat, which evaporates from the skin to cool the body. Research has correlated high fluid intake with a lower risk of kidney stones, colon cancer, and bladder cancer.

You lose about 64 to 80 ounces of water a day—the equivalent of eight to ten 8-ounce glasses—through perspiration, urination, bowel movements, and normal exhalation. You lose water more rapidly if you exercise, live in a

---

▼ **Table 5-1  The Essential Nutrients**

| | Functions | Sources |
|---|---|---|
| **Water** | Carries nutrients and removes waste; dissolves amino acids, glucose, and minerals; cleans body by removing toxins; regulates body temperature | Liquids, fruits, and vegetables |
| **Proteins** | Help build new tissue to keep hair, skin, and eyesight healthy; build antibodies, enzymes, hormones, and other compounds; provide fuel for body | Meat, poultry, fish, eggs, beans, nuts, cheese, tofu, vegetables, some fruits, pasta, breads, cereal, and rice |
| **Carbohydrates** | Provide energy | Grains, cereal, pasta, fruits, vegetables, nuts, milk, and sugars |
| **Fats** | | |
| **Saturated Fats** | Provide energy; trigger production of cholesterol (see Chapter 10) | Red meat, dairy products, egg yolks, and coconut and palm oils |
| **Unsaturated Fats** | Also provide energy, but trigger more "good" cholesterol production and less "bad" cholesterol production (see Chapter 10) | Some fish; avocados; olive, canola, and peanut oils; shortening; stick margarine; baked goods |
| **Vitamins** | Facilitate use of other nutrients; involved in regulating growth, maintaining tissue, and manufacturing blood cells, hormones, and other body components | Fruits, vegetables, grains, some meat and dairy products (see Table 5-2 on p. 102) |
| **Minerals** | Help build bones and teeth; aid in muscle function and nervous system activity; assist in various body functions including growth and energy production | Many foods (see Table 5-3 on p. 104) |

dry climate or at a high altitude, drink a lot of caffeine or alcohol (which increase urination), skip a meal, or become ill. To assure adequate water intake, nutritionists advise drinking a minimum of 64 ounces, enough so that your urine is not dark in color.

## Protein

Critical for growth and repair, **proteins** form the basic framework for our muscles, bones, blood, hair, and fingernails. Supplying 4 calories per gram, they are made of combinations of 20 **amino acids,** 9 of which we must get from our diet because the human body cannot produce them. These are called *essential amino acids.*

Animal proteins—meat, fish, poultry, and dairy products—are **complete proteins** that provide the nine essential amino acids. Grains, dry beans, and nuts are **incomplete proteins** that may have relatively low levels of one or two essential amino acids but fairly high levels of others. Combining incomplete proteins, such as beans and rice, ensures that the body gets sufficient protein.

Based on the latest data, the federal report reaffirms the previously established recommended level of protein intake: 0.8 gram per kilogram of body weight for adults. The panel did not set a tolerable upper intake level because of conflicting or inadequate data on the health risks of high-protein diets, although it did warn about this potential danger. The report also establishes age-based requirements for all nine of the essential amino acids found in dietary protein.

## Carbohydrates

**Carbohydrates** are organic compounds that provide our brains and bodies with *glucose,* their basic fuel. The major sources of carbohydrates are plants—including grains, veg-

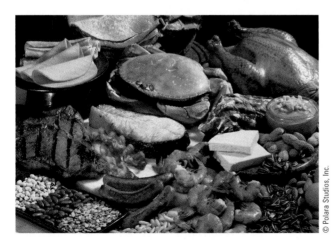

▲ Protein comes in many different forms.

etables, fruits, and beans—and milk. There are three types: *simple carbohydrates* (sugars), *complex carbohydrates* (starches), and *fiber.* All provide 4 calories per gram. The new federal report recommends that both adults and children consume at least 130 grams of carbohydrates each day, the minimum needed to produce enough glucose for the brain to function.[3]

### Simple Carbohydrates

**Simple carbohydrates,** include *natural sugars,* such as the lactose in milk and the fructose in fruit, and *added sugars,* including candy, soft drinks, fruit drinks, pastries, and other sweets. According to the federal report, added sugars should make up no more than 25 percent of total calories consumed. Those whose diets are higher in added sugars typically have lower intakes of other essential nutrients. Other nutritional advocacy groups, such as the Center for Science in the Public Interest, have challenged this recommendation and suggest a much lower 8 percent of calories, or about 40 grams of added sugar a day, for a person consuming 2,000 calories.

### Complex Carbohydrates

**Complex carbohydrates** are the foundation of a healthy diet and include grains, cereals, vegetables, beans, and nuts. Americans, however, get most of their complex carbohydrates from refined grains, which have been stripped of fiber and many nutrients.

Far more nutritious are whole grains, which are made up of all components of the grain: the *bran* (or fiber-rich outer layer), the *endosperm* (middle layer), and the *germ* (the nutrient-packed inner layer).[4] Increasing whole-grain consumption has become a public health priority, and several national health organizations have joined in recommending that Americans increase their consumption of whole-grain foods to at least three servings every day. Individuals who eat whole-grain products each day have about a 15 to 25 percent reduction in death from all causes, including heart disease and cancer.[5]

### Fiber

**Dietary fiber** is the nondigestible form of carbohydrates occurring naturally in plant foods, such as leaves, stems, skins, seeds, and hulls. **Functional fiber** consists of isolated, nondigestible carbohydrates that may be added to foods and that provide beneficial effects in humans. Total fiber is the sum of both.

The various forms of fiber enhance health in different ways: They slow the emptying of the stomach, which creates a feeling of fullness and aids weight control. They interfere with absorption of dietary fat and cholesterol, which lowers the risk of heart disease and stroke. In addition, fiber helps prevent constipation and diverticulosis (a painful inflammation of the bowel). The link between fiber and colon cancer is complex. Some studies have indicated that increased fiber intake reduces risk; a large-scale study of almost 90,000 women found no such correlation.[6]

The federal report on macronutrients set the first-ever recommendations for daily intake levels of total fiber (dietary plus functional fiber): 38 grams of total fiber for men and 25 grams for women. For men and women over 50 years of age, who consume less food, the recommendations are, respectively, 30 and 21 grams. The American Dietetic Association recommends 25 to 35 grams of dietary fiber a day, much more than the amount Americans typically consume.[7]

Good fiber sources include wheat and corn bran (the outer layer); leafy greens; the skins of fruits and root vegetables; oats, beans, and barley; and the pulp, skin, and seeds of many fruits and vegetables, such as apples and strawberries. Because sudden increases in fiber can cause symptoms like bloating and gas, experts recommend gradually adding more fiber to your diet with an additional serving or two of vegetables, fruit, or whole wheat bread.[8]

## Fats

Fats carry the fat-soluble vitamins A, D, E, and K; aid in their absorption in the intestine; protect organs from injury; regulate body temperature; and play an important role in growth and development. They provide 9 calories per gram—more than twice the amount in carbohydrates or proteins.

## Forms of Fat

**Saturated fats** and **unsaturated fats** are distinguished by the type of fatty acids in their chemical structures. Unsaturated fats, like oils, are likely to be liquid at room temperature and saturated fats, like butter, are likely to be solid. In general, vegetable and fish oils are unsaturated, and animal fats are saturated.

Olive, soybean, canola, cottonseed, corn, and other vegetable oils are unsaturated fats. Olive oil is considered a good fat and one of the best vegetable oils for salads and cooking. Used for thousands of years, this staple of the Mediterranean diet, discussed later in this chapter, has been correlated with a lower incidence of heart disease, including strokes and heart attacks. The omega-3 fatty acids in deep-water fish like salmon are unsaturated and may help lower the risk of cardiovascular disease.[9]

In contrast, saturated fats can increase the risk of heart disease and should be avoided as much as possible. In response to consumer and health professionals' demand for less saturated fat in the food supply, many manufacturers switched to partially hydrogenated oils.

The process of hydrogenation creates unsaturated fatty acids called **trans-fatty acids.** They are found in some margarine products and most foods made with partially hydrogenated oils, such as baked goods and fried foods. Even though trans-fatty acids are unsaturated, they appear similar to saturated fats in terms of raising cholesterol levels. Epidemiological studies have suggested a possible link between cardiovascular disease risk and high intakes of trans-fatty acids, and researchers have concluded that they are, gram for gram, twice as damaging as saturated fat. There is no safe level for trans-fatty acids, which occur naturally in meats as well as in foods prepared with partially hydrogenated vegetable oils. The federal panel recommends that trans-fatty acids be listed on food product labels so people can reduce their intake.

To cut down on both saturated and trans-fatty acids, choose soybean, canola, corn, olive, safflower, and sunflower oils, which are naturally free of trans-fatty acids and lower in saturated fats. Look for reduced-fat, low-fat, fat-free, and trans-fatty-acid–free versions of baked goods, snacks, and other processed foods.

 ## How Much Fat Is Okay?

Both high- and low-fat diets can be unhealthy. When people eat very low levels of fat and very high levels of carbohydrates, their levels of high-density lipoprotein, the so-called *good cholesterol*, declines. On the other hand, high-fat diets can lead to obesity and its related health dangers, discussed in Chapter 6.

The government's recommended range for fat intake is 20 to 35 percent. This is lower at the low end than most recommendations and somewhat higher at the high end than recommendations from the American Heart Association and American Cancer Society, which suggest no more than 30 percent of calories from fat.

 ## Why Should I Eat Fish?

Unsaturated fats known as *omega-3 fatty acids* make more molecules such as the prostaglandins that have proven beneficial for heart health. Because they are rich in omega-3 fatty acids, fish oils improve healthy blood lipids (fats), prevent blood clots, ward off age-related macular degeneration, and may lower blood pressure, especially in people with hypertension or atherosclerosis.

The American Heart Association recommends two 3-ounce servings of fatty fish, such as salmon, tuna, and sardines, every week. However, nutritionists do not recommend the use of fish oil supplements, which carry risks of their own: They can increase bleeding time, interfere with wound healing, worsen diabetes, and impair immune function. Since they are made from fish skins and livers, the supplements also may contain environmental contaminants.

## Vitamins and Minerals

**Vitamins,** which help put proteins, fats, and carbohydrates to use, are essential to regulating growth, maintaining tissue, and releasing energy from foods. Together with the enzymes in the body, they help produce the right chemical reactions at the right times. They're also involved in the manufacture of blood cells, hormones, and other compounds.

The body produces some vitamins, such as vitamin D, which is manufactured in the skin after exposure to sunlight. Other vitamins must be ingested. Vitamins A, D, E, and K are fat-soluble; they are absorbed through the intestinal membranes and stored in the body. The B vitamins and vitamin C are water-soluble; they are absorbed directly into the blood and then used up or washed out of the body in urine and sweat. They must be replaced daily. Table 5-2 summarizes key information about vitamins.

Carbon, oxygen, hydrogen, and nitrogen make up 96 percent of our body weight. The other 4 percent consists of **minerals** that help build bones and teeth, aid in muscle function, and help our nervous system transmit messages. Every day we need about a tenth of a gram (100 milligrams) or more of the major minerals: sodium, potassium, chloride, calcium, phosphorus, and magnesium. We also need about a hundredth of a gram (10 milligrams) or less of each of the trace minerals: iron (premenopausal women need more), zinc, selenium, molybdenum, iodine, copper, manganese, fluoride, and chromium. See Table 5-3 on p. 104 for a summary of mineral information.

## Other Substances in Food

### Antioxidants

**Antioxidants** are substances that prevent the harmful effects caused by oxidation within the body. They include vitamins C, E, and beta-carotene (a form of vitamin A), as well as compounds like carotenoids and flavonoids. All share a common enemy: renegade oxygen cells called free radicals released by normal metabolism, as well as by pollution, smoking, radiation, and stress.

Diets high in antioxidant-rich fruits and vegetables have been linked with lower rates of esophageal, lung, colon, and stomach cancer. Nevertheless, scientists have not proven conclusively that any specific antioxidant, particularly in supplement form, can prevent cancer.

### Phytochemicals

**Phytochemicals,** compounds that exist naturally in plants, serve many functions, including helping a plant protect itself from bacteria and disease. Some phytochemicals such as solanine, an insect-repelling chemical found in the leaves and stalks of potato plants, are natural toxins, but many are beneficial to humans. Flavonoids, found in apples, strawberries, grapes, onions, green and black tea, and red wine, may decrease atherosclerotic plaque and DNA damage related to cancer developments. Phytochemicals are associated with a reduced risk of heart disease, certain cancers, age-related macular degeneration, adult-onset diabetes, stroke, and other diseases. However, research has yet to show a cause-and-effect relationship between consumption of phytochemicals and prevention of a specific disease.

## Eating for Good Health

No one food can provide all the nutrients we need. To make sure you consume a healthful variety, the federal Dietary Guidelines suggest that you "let the Pyramid guide your food choices." The USDA's Food Guide Pyramid (see Figure 5-1 on p. 107), adopted in 1992, has five categories of foods. These categories are not considered nutritional equals. For the sake of good health, you need some food from all the groups every day, but in different amounts.

 College students often change the way they eat. In one recent survey, 59 percent of freshmen said their diet had changed since they began college. Two-thirds reported that they did not eat five fruits or vegetables daily; one-third no longer ate red meat.[10] In other studies, students of different ethnic backgrounds typically ate far less than the recommended amount of fruits and vegetables.[11] (See Student Snapshot: "How Freshmen Change the Way They Eat" on p. 106.) Even college athletes, bombarded with nutrition information from coaches, trainers, and popular sports magazines, often do not know the role of various nutrients or which foods or fluids can boost their performance.[12]

## Food Portions and Servings

Consumers often are confused by what a "*serving*" actually is, especially since many American restaurants have supersized the amount of food they put on their customers' plates. The average bagel has doubled in size in the last ten to fifteen years.[13] A standard fast-food serving of french fries is larger in the United States than in the United Kingdom. Very often a serving at a restaurant, in a cafeteria, or at home is much

▼ **Table 5-2  Key Information About Vitamins**

| Vitamin | Significant Sources | Chief Functions | Signs of Severe, Prolonged Deficiency | Signs of Extreme Excess |
|---|---|---|---|---|
| **Fat-Soluble** | | | | |
| Vitamin A | Fortified milk, cheese, cream, butter, fortified margarine, eggs, liver; spinach and other dark, leafy greens, broccoli, deep orange fruits (apricots, cantaloupes) and vegetables (squash, carrots, sweet potatoes, pumpkins) | Antioxidant, needed for vision, health of cornea, epithelial cells, mucous membranes, skin health, bone and tooth growth, hormone synthesis and regulation, immunity | Anemia, painful joints, cracks in teeth, tendency toward tooth decay, diarrhea, depression, frequent infections, night blindness, keratinization, corneal degeneration, rashes, kidney stones | Nosebleeds, bone pain, growth retardation, headaches, abdominal cramps and pain, nausea, vomiting, diarrhea, weight loss, overreactive immune system, blurred vision, pain in calves, fatigue, irritability, loss of appetite, dry skin, rashes, loss of hair, cessation of menstruation |
| Vitamin D | Fortified milk or margarine, eggs, liver, sardines; exposure to sunlight | Promotes calcium and phosphorus absorption | Abnormal growth, misshapen bones (bowing of legs), soft bones, joint pain, malformed teeth | Raised blood calcium, excessive thirst, headaches, irritability, loss of appetite, weakness, nausea, kidney stones, stones in arteries, mental and physical retardation |
| Vitamin E | Margarine, salad dressings, shortenings, green and leafy vegetables, wheat germ, whole-grain products, nuts, seeds | Antioxidant, needed for stabilization of cell membranes, regulation of oxidation reactions | Red blood cell breakage, anemia, muscle degeneration, weakness, difficulty walking, leg cramps, fibrocystic breast disease | Augments the effects of anticlotting medication; general discomfort |
| Vitamin K | Liver, green leafy vegetables, cabbage-type vegetables, milk | Needed for synthesis of blood-clotting proteins and a blood protein that regulates blood calcium | Hemorrhage | Interference with anticlotting medication; jaundice |
| **Water-Soluble** | | | | |
| Vitamin B$_6$ | Green and leafy vegetables, meats, fish, poultry, shellfish, legumes, fruits, whole grains | Part of a coenzyme needed for amino acid and fatty acid metabolism, helps make red blood cells | Anemia, smooth tongue, abnormal brain wave pattern, irritability, muscle twitching, convulsions | Depression, fatigue, impaired memory, irritability, headaches, numbness, damage to nerves, difficulty walking, loss of reflexes, weakness, restlessness |
| Vitamin B$_{12}$ | Animal products (meat, fish, poultry, milk, cheese, eggs) | Part of a coenzyme used in new cell synthesis, helps maintain nerve cells | Anemia, smooth tongue, fatigue, nervous system degeneration progressing to paralysis, hypersensitivity | None reported |

*(continued on next page)*

▼ **Table 5-2  Key Information About Vitamins—continued**

| Vitamin | Significant Sources | Chief Functions | Signs of Severe, Prolonged Deficiency | Signs of Extreme Excess |
|---|---|---|---|---|
| Vitamin C | Citrus fruits, cabbage-type vegetables, dark green vegetables, cantaloupe, strawberries, peppers, lettuce, tomatoes, potatoes, papayas, mangoes | Antioxidant, collagen synthesis (strengthens blood vessel walls, forms scar tissue, matrix for bone growth), amino acid metabolism, strengthens resistance to infection, aids iron absorption | Anemia, pinpoint hemorrhages, frequent infections, bleeding gums, loosened teeth, muscle degeneration and pain, hysteria, depression, bone fragility, joint pain, rough skin, blotchy bruises, failure of wounds to heal | Nausea, abdominal cramps, diarrhea, excessive urination, headache, fatigue, insomnia, rashes, aggravation of gout symptoms; deficiency symptoms may appear at first on withdrawal of high doses |
| Thiamin | Pork, ham, bacon, liver, whole grains, legumes, nuts; occurs in all nutritious foods in moderate amounts | Part of a coenzyme needed for energy metabolism, normal appetite function, and nervous system | Edema, enlarged heart, abnormal heart rhythms, heart failure, nervous/muscular system degeneration, wasting, weakness, pain, low morale, difficulty walking, loss of reflexes, mental confusion, paralysis | None reported |
| Riboflavin | Milk, yogurt, cottage cheese, meat, leafy green vegetables, whole-grain or enriched breads and cereals | Part of a coenzyme needed for energy metabolism, supports normal vision and skin health | Cracks at corner of mouth, magenta tongue, hypersensitivity to light, reddening of cornea, skin rash | None reported |
| Niacin | Milk, eggs, meat, poultry, fish, whole-grain and enriched breads and cereals, nuts, and all protein-containing foods | Part of a coenzyme needed for energy metabolism, supports skin health, nervous system, and digestive system | Diarrhea, black smooth tongue, irritability, loss of appetite, weakness, dizziness, mental confusion, flaky skin rash on areas exposed to sun | Diarrhea, heartburn, nausea, ulcer irritation, vomiting, fainting, dizziness, painful flush and rash, sweating, abnormal liver function, low blood pressure |
| Folate | Leafy green vegetables, legumes, seeds, liver, enriched bread, cereal, pasta, and grains | Part of a coenzyme needed for new cell synthesis | Anemia, heartburn, diarrhea, constipation, frequent infections, smooth red tongue, depression, mental confusion, fainting | Masks vitamin $B_{12}$ deficiency |
| Panothenic acid | Widespread in foods | Part of a coenzyme used in energy metabolism | Vomiting, intestinal distress, insomnia, fatigue | Water retention (rare) |
| Biotin | Widespread in foods | Used in energy metabolism, fat synthesis, amino acid metabolism, and glycogen synthesis | Abnormal heart action, loss of appetite, nausea, depression, muscle pain, weakness, fatigue, drying of facial skin, rash, loss of hair | None reported |

Source: Adapted from Sizer, Frances, and Eleanor Whitney. *Nutrition: Concepts and Controversies,* 8th ed. Belmont, CA: Wadsworth, 2000.

▼ **Table 5-3  Key Information About Essential Minerals**

| Mineral | Significant Sources | Chief Functions | Signs of Severe, Prolonged Deficiency | Signs of Extreme Excess |
|---|---|---|---|---|
| **Major Minerals** | | | | |
| Sodium | Foods processed with salt, cured foods (corned beef, ham, bacon, pickles, sauerkraut), table and sea salt, bread, milk, cheese, salad dressing | Needed to maintain acid-base balance in body fluids, helps regulate water in blood and body tissues, needed for muscle and nerve activity | Weakness, apathy, poor appetite, muscle cramps, headache, swelling | High blood pressure, kidney disease, heart problems |
| Potassium | Plant foods (potatoes, squash, lima beans, tomatoes, bananas, oranges, avocados), meats, milk and milk products, coffee | Needed to maintain acid-base balance in body fluids, helps regulate water in blood and body tissues, needed for muscle and nerve activity | Weakness, irritability, mental confusion, irregular heartbeat, paralysis | Irregular heartbeat, heart attack |
| Chloride | Foods processed with salt, cured foods (corned beef, ham, bacon, pickles, sauerkraut), table and sea salt, bread, milk, cheese, salad dressing | Aids in digestion, needed to maintain acid-base balance in body fluids, helps regulate water in the body | Muscle cramps, apathy, poor appetite, long-term mental retardation in infants | Vomiting |
| Calcium | Milk and milk products, broccoli, dried beans | Component of bones and teeth, needed for muscle and nerve activity, blood clotting | Weak bones, rickets, stunted growth in children, convulsions, muscle spasms, osteoporosis | Drowsiness, calcium deposits in kidneys, liver, and other tissues, suppression of bone remodeling, decreased zinc absorption |
| Phosphorus | Milk and milk products, meats, seeds, nuts | Component of bones and teeth, energy formation, needed to maintain the right acid-base balance of body fluids | Loss of appetite, nausea, vomiting, weakness, confusion, loss of calcium from bones | Loss of calcium from bones, muscle spasms |
| Magnesium | Plant foods (dried beans, tofu, peanuts, potatoes, green vegetables) | Component of bones and teeth, nerve activity, energy and protein formation | Stunted growth in children, weakness, muscle spasms, personality changes | Diarrhea, dehydration, impaired nerve activity |
| **Trace Minerals** | | | | |
| Iron | Liver, beef, pork, dried beans, iron-fortified cereals, prunes, apricots, raisins, spinach, bread, pasta | Aids in transport of oxygen, component of myoglobin, energy formation | Anemia, weakness, fatigue, pale appearance, reduced attention span, lowered resistance to infection, developmental delays in children | "Iron poisoning," vomiting, abdominal pain, blue coloration of skin, shock, heart failure, diabetes, decreased zinc absorption |
| Zinc | Meats, grains, nuts, milk and milk products, cereals, bread | Protein reproduction, component of insulin | Growth failure, delayed sexual maturation, slow wound healing, loss of taste and appetite; in pregnant women, low-birth-weight infants and preterm delivery | Nausea, vomiting, weakness, fatigue, susceptibility to infection, copper deficiency, metallic taste in mouth |
| Selenium | Meats and seafood, eggs, grains | Acts as an antioxidant in conjunction with vitamin E | Anemia, muscle pain and tenderness, Keshar disease, heart failure | Hair and fingernail loss, weakness, liver damage, irritability, garlic or metallic breath |

*(continued on next page)*

## ▼ Table 5-3  Key Information About Essential Minerals—continued

| Mineral | Significant Sources | Chief Functions | Signs of Severe, Prolonged Deficiency | Signs of Extreme Excess |
|---|---|---|---|---|
| Molybdenum | Dried beans, grains, dark green vegetables, liver, milk and milk products | Aids in oxygen transfer from one molecule to another | Rapid heartbeat and breathing, nausea, vomiting, coma | Loss of copper from the body, joint pain, growth failure, anemia, gout |
| Iodine | Iodized salt, milk and milk products, seaweed, seafood, bread | Component of thyroid hormones that helps regulate energy production and growth | Goiter, cretinism in newborns (mental retardation, hearing loss, growth failure) | Pimples, goiter, decreased thyroid function |
| Copper | Bread, potatoes, grains, dried beans, nuts and seeds, seafood, cereals | Component of enzymes involved in the body's utilization of iron and oxygen; functions in growth, immunity, cholesterol, and glucose utilization; brain development | Anemia, seizures, nerve and bone abnormalities in children, growth retardation | Wilson's disease (excessive accumulation of copper in the liver and kidneys); vomiting, diarrhea, tremors, liver disease |
| Manganese | Whole grains, coffee, tea, dried beans, nuts | Formation of body fat and bone | Weight loss, rash, nausea and vomiting | Infertility in men, disruptions in the nervous system, muscle spasms |
| Fluoride | Fluoridated water, foods, and beverages; tea; shrimp; crab | Component of bones and teeth (enamel) | Tooth decay and other dental diseases | Fluorosis, brittle bones, mottled teeth, nerve abnormalities |
| Chromium | Whole grains, liver, meat, beer, wine | Glucose utilization | Poor blood glucose control, weight loss | Kidney and skin damage |

Source: Adapted from Brown, Judith E. *Nutrition Now,* 3rd ed. Belmont, CA:Wadsworth, 2002.

larger than those referred to in the Food Guide Pyramid and on Nutrition Facts labels on packaged foods—and higher in calories.[14]

Most college students do not calculate portion sizes accurately.[15] One of the best ways to improve such estimates is by using three-dimensional food models. In a study of 380 undergraduates enrolled in an introductory nutrition course, students first estimated the amount of food in three dinners, each with varying portions of five foods (starchy food, cooked vegetables, salad, milk, and meat). After correcting their own estimates, students were asked to estimate portion sizes on a new display with different foods and amounts after one week, and then again after four weeks. Each day between these two tests, different food models were passed around in class. The accuracy of the students' estimates improved significantly afterward.[16]

The Food Guide Pyramid describes the total number of recommended *daily* servings of each of the food groups. It does *not* describe the size of an individual portion. (See Figure 5-1 on p. 107.)

The size of the daily serving is determined by four criteria:

✔ The amount of foods from a food group typically reported in surveys as consumed on one eating occasion.

✔ The amount of food that provides a comparable amount of key nutrients from that food group; for example, the amount of cheese that provides the same amount of calcium as a cup of milk.

✔ The amount of food recognized by most consumers or easily multiplied or divided to describe how much food is actually consumed.

✔ The amount traditionally used in previous food guides to describe servings.

A food-label *serving* is a specific amount of food that contains the quantity of nutrients described on the Nutrition Facts label. For many foods, the serving size in the Food Guide Pyramid and on the food label are the same (for example, half a cup of canned fruit or one slice of bread), but in other cases they differ. The Pyramid describes serving units for each food group in ways that consumers find easy to remember (for example, a cup of leafy raw vegetables), while the food label is meant to help consumers compare nutrient information on a number of food products within a category (for example, frozen dinner entrées containing foods from several food groups).

A *portion* is the amount of a specific food that an individual eats at one time. Portions can be bigger or smaller than the servings on food labels or in the Food Guide Pyramid. According to research by the USDA, portion sizes

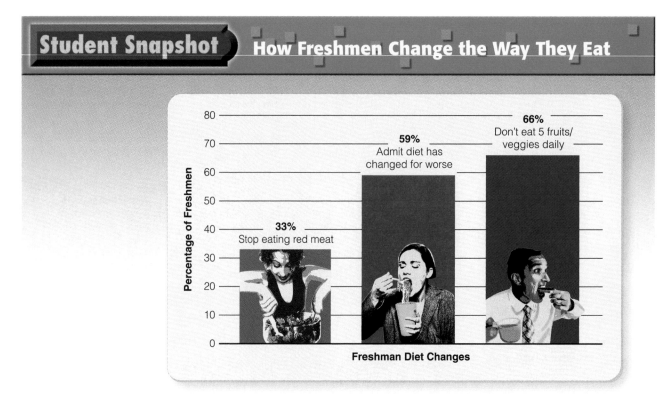

Source: Tufts University Longitudinal Health Study, 2002. "Freshman College Student Dining Habits."
*Food Service Director,* Vol. 15, No. 3, March 15, 2002, p. 1(1).

tend to be bigger for men than women, but to decrease for both genders with age. (See The X&Y Files: "Do Men and Women Have Different Nutritional Needs?" on p. 108.)

If you are trying to balance your diet or control your weight, it's important to keep track of the size of your portions so that you do not exceed the recommended serving. For instance, a 3-ounce serving of meat is about the size of a pack of playing cards. If you eat a larger amount, count it as more than one serving. (See Table 5-4.)

## Grains Group (6–11 servings a day)

Breads, cereals, rice, and pasta are the foundation of a healthy diet because they are a good source of complex carbohydrates. Both simple and complex carbohydrates (starches) have 4 calories per gram. The sugars in simple carbohydrates provide little more than a quick spurt of energy, whereas complex carbohydrates are rich in vitamins, minerals, and other nutrients.

A typical serving in this category might be one slice of bread, and 1 ounce of ready-to-eat cereal (or one-half cup of cooked cereal, rice, or pasta). Although many people

think of these foods as fattening, it's actually what you put on them, such as butter on a roll or cream sauce on pasta, that adds extra calories.

Here are suggestions for getting more grains in your diet:

- ✔ Add brown rice or barley to soups.
- ✔ Check labels of rolls and bread, and choose those with at least 2 to 3 grams of fiber per slice.
- ✔ Go for pasta power. Pasta has 210 calories per cooked cup and only 9 calories from fat. Like whole-grain breads, whole-grain pastas may provide more nutrients than those made with refined flour.

## Vegetables Group (3–5 servings a day)

Naturally low in fat and high in fiber, vegetables provide crucial vitamins (such as A and C) and minerals (such as iron and magnesium). A serving in this category consists of one cup of raw leafy vegetables, one-half cup of other vegetables (either cooked or raw), three-quarters cup of vegetable juice, or one potato or ear of corn. Since different

**Bread, Cereal, Rice, and Pasta Group (Grains Group)—whole grain and refined**
· 1 slice of bread
· About 1 cup of ready-to-eat cereal
· 1/2 cup of cooked cereal, rice, or pasta

**Vegetable Group**
· 1 cup of raw leafy vegetables
· 1/2 cup of other vegetables—cooked or raw
· 3/4 cup of vegetable juice

**Fruit Group**
· 1 medium apple, banana, orange, pear
· 1/2 cup of chopped, cooked, or canned fruit
· 3/4 cup of fruit juice

**Milk, Yogurt, and Cheese Group (Milk Group)[1]**
· 1 cup of milk[2] or yogurt[2]
· 1 1/2 ounces of a natural cheese[2] (such as Cheddar)
· 2 ounces of processed cheese[2] (such as American)

**Meat, Poultry, Fish, Dry Beans, Eggs, and Nuts Group (Meat and Beans Group)**
· 2–3 ounces of cooked lean meat, poultry, or fish
· 1/2 cup of cooked dry beans[3] or 1/2 cup of tofu counts as 1 ounce of lean meat
· 2 1/2-ounce soyburger or 1 egg counts as 1 ounce of lean meat
· 2 tablespoons of peanut butter or 1/3 cup of nuts counts as 1 ounce of meat

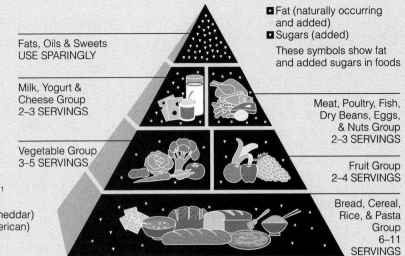

■ Fat (naturally occurring and added)
■ Sugars (added)
These symbols show fat and added sugars in foods

Fats, Oils & Sweets
USE SPARINGLY

Milk, Yogurt & Cheese Group
2–3 SERVINGS

Meat, Poultry, Fish, Dry Beans, Eggs, & Nuts Group
2–3 SERVINGS

Vegetable Group
3–5 SERVINGS

Fruit Group
2–4 SERVINGS

Bread, Cereal, Rice, & Pasta Group
6–11 SERVINGS

NOTE: Many of the serving sizes given above are smaller than those on the Nutritional Facts Label. For example, 1 serving of cooked cereal, rice, or pasta is 1 cup for the label but only 1/2 cup for the Pyramid.
[1] This includes lactose-free and lactose-reduced milk products. One cup of soy-based beverage with added calcium is an option for those who prefer a non-dairy source of calcium.
[2] Choose fat-free or reduced-fat dairy products most often.
[3] Dry beans, peas, and lentils can be counted as servings in either the meat and beans group or the vegetable group. As a vegetable, 1/2 cup of cooked, dry beans counts as 1 serving. As a meat substitute, 1 cup of cooked, dry beans counts as 1 serving (2 ounces of meat).

▲ **Figure 5-1** USDA's Food Guide Pyramid
This graphic demonstrates the daily food choices that make up a healthy diet: modest amounts of meat, dairy products, and fats; and a larger number of servings of foods containing grains and cereals.

Source: U.S. Department of Agriculture, *Dietary Guidelines for Americans, 2000.*

▼ **Table 5-4  How Many Servings Do You Need Each Day?**

| Food group | About 1,600 calories Children ages 2 to 6 years, women, some older adults | About 2,200 calories Older children, teen girls, active women, most men | About 2,800 calories Teen boys, active men |
|---|---|---|---|
| **Grains Group**—especially whole grain: Bread, Cereal, Rice, and Pasta Group | 6 | 9 | 11 |
| **Vegetable Group** | 3 | 4 | 5 |
| **Fruit Group** | 2 | 3 | 4 |
| **Milk Group**—preferably fat-free or lowfat: Milk, Yogurt, and Cheese Group | 2 or 3* | 2 or 3* | 2 or 3* |
| **Meat and Beans Group**—preferably lean or low fat: Meat, Poultry, Fish, Dry Beans, Eggs, and Nuts | 2, for a total of 5 ounces | 2, for a total of 6 ounces | 3, for a total of 7 ounces |

*The number of servings depends on your age. Older children and teenagers (ages 9 to 18 years) and adults over the age of 50 need 3 servings daily. Others need 2 servings daily. During pregnancy and lactation, the recommended number of milk group servings is the same as for nonpregnant women.

Source: Adapted from U.S. Department of Agriculture, Center for Nutrition Policy and Promotion. *The Food Guide Pyramid,* Home and Garden Bulletin Number 252, 1996.

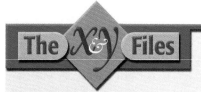

The X&Y Files

## Do Men and Women Have Different Nutritional Needs?

Men and women do not need to eat different foods, but their nutritional needs are different. Because most men are bigger and taller than most women, they consume more calories. Eating more means it's easier for them to get the nutrients they need, even though many don't make the wisest food choices.

Women, particularly those who restrict their caloric intake or are chronically dieting, are more likely to develop specific deficiencies. Calcium is one example. Women drink less milk than men, and many do not consume the recommended 800 to 1,200 milligrams of calcium daily. This deficiency increases the risk of bone-weakening osteoporosis.

Many women also get too little iron. Even in adolescence, girls are more prone to iron deficiency than boys; some suffer memory and learning impairments as a result. In adult women, menstrual blood loss and poor eating habits can lead to low iron stores, which puts them at risk for anemia. According to U.S. Department of Agriculture research, most women consume only 60 percent of the recommended 15 milligrams of iron per day. (The recommendation for men is 10 milligrams.) Regular blood tests can monitor a woman's iron status.

Here are some gender-specific strategies for better nutrition:

- Men should cut back on fat and meat in their diets, two things they eat too much.
- Women should increase their iron intake by eating meat (iron from animal sources is absorbed better than that from vegetable sources) or a combination of meat and vegetable iron sources together (for example, a meat and bean burrito). Those low in iron should consult a physician. Because large doses of iron can be toxic, iron supplements should be taken only with medical supervision.
- Women should consume more calcium-rich foods, including low-fat and nonfat dairy products, leafy greens, and tofu. Women who cannot get adequate amounts of calcium from their daily diet should take calcium supplements.
- Women who could become pregnant should take a multivitamin with 400 micrograms of folic acid, which helps prevent neural tube defects such as spina bifida. Folic acid is also useful to men because it may cut the risk of heart disease, stroke, and colon cancer.
- Both genders should increase their fruit and vegetable intake to ensure that they are getting adequate amounts of vitamins and fiber in their daily diet.

types of vegetables provide different nutrients, it's best to eat a variety. Dark green vegetables are especially good sources of vitamins and minerals; certain greens (such as collards, kale, turnip, and mustard) provide calcium and iron. Winter squash, carrots, and the plant family that includes broccoli, cabbage, kohlrabi, and cauliflower (the **crucifers**) are high in fiber, rich in vitamins, and excellent sources of **indoles,** chemicals that help lower cancer risk.

Here are ways to increase your vegetable intake:

- Make or order sandwiches with extra tomatoes or other vegetable toppings.
- Add extra vegetables whenever you're preparing soups and sauces.
- If you can't find fresh vegetables, use frozen. They contain less salt than canned veggies.
- Use raw vegetables for dipping, instead of chips.

## Fruits Group (2–4 servings a day)

Like whole grains and vegetables, fruits are excellent sources of vitamins, minerals, and fiber. Along with vegetables, fruits may protect against cancer; those who eat little

produce have a cancer rate twice that of people who eat the most fruits and vegetables. A serving consists of a medium apple, banana, or orange; a half-cup of chopped, cooked, or canned fruit; or three-quarters of a cup of fruit juice.

Try the following suggestions to get more fruit into your daily diet:

- Carry a banana, apple, or package of dried fruit with you as a healthy snack.
- Eat fruit for dessert or a snack. Try poached pears, baked apples, or fresh berries.
- Start the day with a daily double: a glass of juice and a banana or other fruit on cereal.
- Add citrus fruits (such as slices of grapefruit, oranges, or apples) to green salads, rice, or grains, and to chicken, pork, or fish dishes.

## Meat and Beans Group (2–3 servings a day)

Foods in the meat and bean group include meat, poultry, fish, tofu, dry beans (lentils, soy, kidney, black, etc.) and nuts. A serving in this category consists of 2 or 3 ounces of lean, cooked meat, fish, or poultry (roughly the size of an average hamburger or the amount of meat on half a medium chicken breast). An egg or one-half cup of cooked dry beans can substitute for 1 ounce of lean meat. One-third cup of nuts or 2 ounces of peanut butter count as 1 ounce of meat. Thus, one day's total protein intake might include an egg at breakfast; a serving of beans or 2 ounces of sliced chicken in a sandwich or 2 ounces of peanut butter in a sandwich at lunch; and 3 ounces of fish for dinner.

To pick the best protein, follow these recommendations:

✔ Choose the leanest meats, such as beef round or sirloin, pork tenderloin, or veal. Broil or roast instead of fry. Trim fat before cooking, which can lower the fat content of the meat you eat by more than 10 percent. Marinate low-fat cuts to increase tenderness.

✔ Cook stews, boiled meat, or soup stock ahead of time; refrigerate; and remove the hardened fat before using. Drain fat from ground beef after cooking.

✔ Watch out for processed chicken and turkey products; for example, bolognas and salamis made from turkey can contain 45 to 90 percent fat.

✔ Select small chickens when you shop: They're leaner than large ones. Broiler-fryers are lowest in fat, followed by roasters. Remove skin before eating poultry.

✔ Choose dry-roasted or raw nuts and low-fat peanut butter.

### ???? Are Eggs Good or Bad for Me?

Eggs, once America's favorite breakfast food, fell out of favor several years ago. The reason: A single egg yolk contains about 200 milligrams of **cholesterol,** the maximum amount that federal guidelines say you should eat in a day. (Egg whites, rich in protein, have no cholesterol.) There is ongoing debate over the risk of eggs to healthy individuals.[17]

Most people don't have to ban eggs from the breakfast table, but limit how often they are eaten. Avoid high-fat preparations like frying them in butter. If your diet is low in saturated fat, the kind found in meat and dairy products, the cholesterol in any eggs you eat will have less impact on your blood cholesterol levels than if you're eating a lot of high-fat foods.

## Milk Group (2–3 servings a day)

Most milk products—milk, yogurt, and cheese—are high in calcium, riboflavin, protein, and vitamins A and $B_{12}$. The Food Guide Pyramid recommends two servings of milk, yogurt, or cheese for most adults and three for women who are pregnant or breast-feeding. In addition, teenagers and young adults up to age 24 should also get three servings of milk products a day. Dairy products, such as milk and yogurt, are the best calcium sources, but be sure you choose products that are low-fat or, preferably, nonfat. A serving in this category consists of an 8-ounce cup of milk, one cup of plain yogurt, 1½ ounces of hard cheese, or 1 tablespoon of cheese spread. An 8-ounce glass of nonfat milk is a more nutritious choice than a tablespoon of a high-fat cheese spread.

A growing concern is the problem of lactose intolerance, or the inability to digest milk products, which is particularly common in nonwhite minority groups. In people who do not produce adequate amounts of the intestinal enzyme lactase, milk products travel through the stomach undigested and ferment in the small bowel, causing gas, cramps, and diarrhea. Overall, 25 percent of Americans have trouble digesting dairy products. Over-the-counter medicines can help, and many dairy products are available in special forms for the lactose-intolerant.

To make sure you get more milk with less fat, try the following:

✔ Gradually switch from whole milk to 2%-fat (reduced fat) milk, then to 1%-fat (low-fat) milk, then to nonfat (skim) milk.

✔ Substitute fat-free sour cream or nonfat plain yogurt for sour cream.

✔ Use part-skim or low-fat cheeses whenever possible.

✔ Note that cottage cheese is lower in calcium than most cheeses. Thus, one cup of cottage cheese counts as only one-half serving of milk.

## Fats, Oils, and Sweets (small amounts each day)

The Food Guide Pyramid places fats, oils, and sweets at the very top so that Americans will realize they should use them only in very small amounts. These foods supply calories but little or no vitamins or minerals.

Added sugars include sweeteners used in processing or at the table (such as jams, jellies, syrups, corn sweetener, molasses, fruit-juice concentrate, and the sugar in candy, cake, and cookies). These foods often are hidden in favorites—such as soft drinks (9 teaspoons of sugar per can), low-fat fruit yogurt (7 teaspoons per cup), fruit pie (6 teaspoons per serving), and catsup (a teaspoon in every tablespoon).

Try the following:

✔ Put a small, child-sized spoon in the sugar bowl.

✔ When you crave a sweet, reach for nature's candy: fruit.

✔ If you want a daily sweet, have it as dessert, when you'll eat less of it, rather than as a snack.

✔ Drink fruit juices and water instead of sugar-laden soft drinks.

## Nutritional Supplements

More than half of Americans regularly use nutritional supplements—vitamins, minerals, and botanical and biological substances that have not been approved for sale as drugs. There are serious questions about the safety and efficacy of these products.

Marketed as foods, supplements do not have to undergo the same rigorous testing required of drugs. They can carry *structure/function claims*—claims that a product may affect the structure or functioning of the body—but not claims that they can treat, diagnose, cure, or prevent a disease. For example, statements such as "helps maintain a healthy cholesterol level" are acceptable, while statements like "lowers cholesterol levels" are not.

The FDA has issued rules for nutritional supplement labeling. Labels must now include an information panel titled Supplement Facts (similar to the Nutrition Facts panel that appears on processed foods), a clear identity statement, and a complete list of ingredients. Specifically, the "Supplement Facts" panel must show the manufacturer's suggested dose/serving size; information on nutrients when they are present in significant levels (such as vitamins A and C, calcium, iron, and sodium) and the percent Daily Value where a reference has been established; and all other dietary ingredients present in the product, including botanicals and amino acids. Herbal products are identified by the common or usual name and the part of the plant used (such as root, stem, or leaf).

### Should I Take Vitamin Supplements?

Many health experts feel that the best way to make sure your body gets the vitamins and minerals it needs is to eat a wide variety of foods. If you rely on vitamin/mineral pills and fortified foods to make up for poor nutrition, you may shortchange yourself. See Table 5-5 for a summary of what we know about different supplements.

As scientists note, most health benefits and dangers stem from more than one source, so it's unlikely that changing any one nutrient will in itself produce great benefits—and may, by interfering with the complex balance of nutrients, do harm. In particular, the fat-soluble vitamins, primarily A and D, can build up in our bodies and cause serious complications, such as damage to the kidneys, liver, or bones. Large doses of water-soluble vitamins, including the B vitamins, may also be harmful. Excessive intake of vitamin $B_6$ (pyridoxine), often used to relieve premenstrual bloating, can cause neurological damage, such as numbness in the mouth and tingling in the hands. (An excessive amount in this case is 250 to 300 times the recommended dose.) High doses of vitamin C can produce stomachaches and diarrhea. Niacin, often taken in high doses to lower cholesterol, can cause jaundice, liver damage, and irregular heartbeats as well as severe, uncomfortable flushing of the skin. Table 5-2 provides more information about the effects of vitamin excess.

## Knowing What You Eat

Because of the Nutrition Labeling and Education Act, food manufacturers must provide information about fat, calories, and ingredients in large type on packaged food labels, and they must show how a food item fits into a daily diet of 2,000 calories. The law also restricts nutritional claims for terms such as *healthy, low-fat,* and *high-fiber.*

In evaluating food labels and product claims, keep in mind that while individual foods vary in their nutritional value, what matters is your total diet. If you eat too much of any one food—regardless of what its label states—you may not be getting the variety and balance of nutrients that you need.

### What Should I Look For on Nutrition Labels?

As Figure 5-2 on p. 112 shows, the Nutrition Facts on food labels present a wealth of information—if you know what to look for. The label focuses on those nutrients most clearly associated with disease risk and health: total fat, saturated fat, cholesterol, sodium, total carbohydrate, dietary fiber, sugar, and protein.

✔ **Calories.** Calories are the measure of the amount of energy that can be derived from food. Science defines a *calorie* as the amount of energy required to raise the temperature of 1 gram of water by one degree Celsius. In the laboratory, the caloric content of food is measured in 1,000-calorie units called *kilocalories.* The calorie referred to in everyday usage is actually the equivalent of the laboratory kilocalorie.

The Nutrition Facts label lists two numbers for calories: calories per serving and calories from fat per serving. This allows consumers to calculate how many calories they'll consume and to determine the percentage of fat in an item.

## ▼ Table 5-5 Do Nutritional Supplements Work?

| Supplement | Claims | What We Know |
|---|---|---|
| **Amino acids** | Increase muscle mass | No solid evidence that amino acid supplements promote muscle building. Little is known about the side effects of high doses of single or combination amino acid supplements. |
| **Beta-carotene** | Reduces your risk of cancer | Converts into vitamin A in the body. No evidence that beta-carotene supplements reduce cancer risk. |
| **B complex vitamins** | Provide energy; help relieve stress and may help reduce heart disease risk | No evidence that B vitamins relieve stress. Long thought to be nontoxic, but some B vitamins, such as $B_6$ and niacin, may have serious side effects when taken in very high doses. |
| **Vitamin C** | Prevents colds, certain cancers, and heart disease | Vitamin C supplements can lessen the severity of colds but not prevent them. Observational studies have shown that vitamin C may help prevent cancer and heart disease, but too few clinical trials have been conducted to substantiate those results. |
| **Calcium** | Prevents osteoporosis and colon cancer; reduces high blood pressure | Calcium plays a critical role in preventing osteoporosis if taken with vitamin D. Results of research on calcium's role in preventing colon cancer are still preliminary. It may help regulate blood pressure in some people, but there is no way of knowing who might benefit. |
| **Chromium picolinate** | Reduces body fat, builds muscle, and improves overall fitness | Scientists have found that this popular nutritional and dietary supplement causes DNA breakage and may be a cancer risk. |
| **Vitamin E** | Reduces the risk of heart disease and cancer | Supplements of 400–800 IU may protect against heart disease. Very few side effects have been reported, but high doses of vitamin E supplements should not be used by anyone taking anticoagulation medication. |
| **Niacin** | Helps lower cholesterol | Niacin, in the form of nicotinic acid, is an inexpensive alternative to cholesterol-lowering drugs but should be prescribed by a doctor. Side effects include flushing, itching, and gastrointestinal distress. Time-released niacin can be toxic to the liver. |
| **Zinc** | Boosts immunity, wards off colds, and improves sex drive | Zinc taken at the onset of a cold can lessen its severity. High doses of zinc, however, may *suppress* immune function. No evidence that zinc supplements affect sexual performance. |

✔ **Serving size.** Rather than the tiny portions manufacturers sometimes used in the past to keep down the number of calories per serving, the new labels reflect more realistic portions. Serving sizes, which have been defined for approximately 150 food categories, must be the same for similar products (for example, different brands of potato chips) and for similar products within a category (for example, snack foods such as pretzels, potato chips, and popcorn). This makes it easier to compare the nutritional content of foods.

✔ **Daily Values (DVs).** DVs refer to the total amount of a nutrient that the average adult should aim to get or not exceed on a daily basis. The DVs for cholesterol, sodium, vitamins, and minerals are the same for all adults. The DVs for total fat, saturated fat, carbohydrate, fiber, and protein are based on a 2,000-calorie daily diet—the amount of food ingested by many American men and active women.

✔ **Percent Daily Values (%DVs).** The goal for a full day's diet is to select foods that together add up to 100 percent of the DVs. The %DVs show how a particular food's nutrient content fits into a 2,000-calorie diet. Individuals who consume (or should consume) fewer than 2,000 total calories a day have to lower their DVs for total fat, saturated fat, and carbohydrates. For example, if their caloric intake is 10 percent less than 2,000 calories, they would lower the DV by 10 percent. Similarly, those who consume more than 2,000 calories should adjust the DVs upward.

✔ **Calories per gram.** The bottom of the food label lists the number of calories per gram for fat, carbohydrates, and protein.

People zero in on different figures on the food label—for example, calories if they're watching their weight, specific ingredients if they have food allergies. Among the useful items to check are the following:

✔ **Calories from fat.** Get into the habit of calculating the percentage of fat calories in a food before buying or eating it.

# Nutrition Facts

Serving Size 1/2 of package (21g)
Servings Per Container 2

**Amount Per Serving**

**Calories** 70   Calories from Fat 20

**% Daily Value***

| | |
|---|---|
| **Total Fat** 2.5g | **4%** |
| Saturated Fat 1.5g | **6%** |
| **Cholesterol** Less than 5mg | **1%** |
| **Sodium** 940mg | **39%** |
| **Total Carbohydrate** 12g | **4%** |
| Dietary Fiber 1g | **6%** |
| Sugars 4g | |
| **Protein** 2g | |

| | | | |
|---|---|---|---|
| Vitamin A 0% | • | Vitamin C 0% | |
| Calcium 6% | • | Iron 2% | |

*Percent Daily Values are based on 2,000 calorie diet. Your daily values may be higher or lower depending on your calorie needs:

| | | Calories: | 2,000 | 2,500 |
|---|---|---|---|---|
| Total Fat | Less than | | 65g | 80g |
| Sat Fat | Less than | | 20g | 25g |
| Cholesterol | Less than | | 300mg | 300mg |
| Sodium | Less than | | 2,400mg | 2,400mg |
| Total Carbohydrate | | | 300g | 375g |
| Dietary Fiber | | | 25g | 30g |

Calories per gram
Fat 9 • Carbohydrate 4 • Protein 4

**% Daily Value (%DV): Saturated Fat**
The %DV shows how the amount of saturated fat in a serving of this food—1.5 grams (g)—compares with 20 g, the DV for saturated fat for a 2,000-calorie diet. (1.5 g is about 6% of the DV for saturated fat.)

**% Daily Value (%DV): Cholesterol**
The %DV shows how the amount of cholesterol in this food— less than 5 milligrams (mg)— compares with 300 mg, the DV for cholesterol for all calorie levels. (Less than 5 mg is considered 1% of the DV for cholesterol.)

**% Daily Value (%DV): Dietary Fiber**
The %DV shows how the amount of fiber in this food— 1 gram (g)—compares with 25 g, the DV for fiber for a 2,000-calorie diet. (1 g is 6% of the DV for fiber.)

**% Daily Value (%DV): Iron**
The %DV shows how the amount of iron in this food compares with the DV for iron for all calorie levels—18 milligrams (mg). (This food contains 2% of the DV for iron.)

Larger packages may carry this expanded version of the label, which includes Daily Values (DVs) for these six nutrients based on both 2,000-calorie and 2,500-calorie diets. The DVs for other nutrients are not shown on the label.

▲ **Figure 5-2** Understanding Nutrition Labels
The Nutrition Facts label lists the essential nutrient content of packaged food as well as the amount of potentially harmful substances such as fat and sodium.

✔ **Total fat.** Since the average person munches on 15 to 20 food items a day, it's easy to overload on fat. Saturated fat is a figure worthy of special attention because of its reported link to several diseases.

✔ **Cholesterol.** Cholesterol is made by and contained in products of animal origin only. Many high-fat products, such as potato chips, contain 0 percent cholesterol because they're made from plants and are cooked in vegetable fats. However, the vegetable fats they contain can be processed and made into saturated fats that are more harmful to the heart than cholesterol.

✔ **Sugars.** There is no Daily Value for sugars because health experts have yet to agree on a daily limit. The figure on the label includes naturally present sugars, such as lactose in milk and fructose in fruit, as well as those added to the food, such as table sugar, corn syrup, or dextrose.

✔ **Fiber.** A "high-fiber" food has 5 or more grams of fiber per serving. A "good" source of fiber provides at least 2.5 grams. "More" or "added" fiber means at least 2.5 grams more per serving than similar foods—10 percent more of the DV for fiber.

✔ **Calcium.** "High" equals 200 milligrams (mg) or more per serving. "Good" means at least 100 mg, while "more" indicates that the food contains at least 100 mg more calcium—10 percent more of the DV—than the item usually would have.

✔ **Sodium.** Since many foods contain sodium, most of us routinely get more than we need. Read labels carefully to avoid excess sodium, which can be a health threat.

✔ **Vitamins.** A Daily Value of 10 percent of any vitamin makes a food a "good" source; 20 percent qualifies it as "high" in a certain vitamin.

Nutrition labeling for fresh produce, fish, meat, and poultry remains voluntary. Packages too small for a full-sized label must provide an address or phone number so consumers can obtain information from the manufacturer.

## Functional Foods

As the American Dietetic Association has noted, all foods are functional at some physiological level. However, the term *functional* generally applies to a food specifically created to have health-promoting benefits. The International Food Information Council defines functional foods as those "that provide health benefits beyond basic nutrition."[18]

Some manufacturers are adding herbs, such as the cold-fighter echinacea, to food products and promoting them as functional foods. However, the amounts added are often too low to have any effect, and many herb-sprinkled foods are high-sugared drinks and snack foods. These products have other dangers, including the use of low-quality or contaminated herbs and adverse drug and food interactions.[19]

## The Way We Eat

For centuries, Native Americans ate a diet of corn, beans, fish, game, wild greens, wild fruits, squash, and tomatoes. Over time the United States, a nation of immigrants, has imported a wide variety of ethnic cuisines. Although many people think of foods such as hamburgers, steak, potatoes, cheesecake, and ice cream as all-American favorites, in most cities across the country, all-American also includes dozens of different cultural cuisines.

## Dietary Diversity

 Whatever your cultural heritage, you have probably sampled Chinese, Mexican, Indian, Italian, and Japanese foods. If you belong to any of these ethnic groups, you may eat these cuisines regularly. Each type of ethnic cooking has its own nutritional benefits and potential drawbacks, yet all recommend eating more carbohydrate-rich grains, vegetables, and fruits, and less high-protein meat and dairy. None of these "all-American" cuisines endorses a high-protein diet as a healthy eating pattern.[20]

## African-American Diet

African-American cuisine traces some of its roots to food preferences from west Africa (for example, peanuts, okra, and black-eyed peas), as well as to traditional American foods, such as fish, game, greens, and sweet potatoes. Cajun cuisine, most closely associated with New Orleans, blends both African and French traditions in dishes such as gumbo (thick spicy soup), sausage, red beans, and seafood. African-American cooking uses many nutritious vegetables, such as collard greens and sweet potatoes, as well as legumes. However, some dishes include high-fat food products such as peanuts and pecans or involve frying, sometimes in saturated fat.

## Chinese Diet

The mainland Chinese diet, which is plant-based, high in carbohydrates, and low in fats and animal protein, is considered one of the healthiest in the world. The Food Guide Pagoda recommends plenty of cereals, vegetables, fruits, and beans, with physical activity balancing food intake.[21] However, Chinese food is prepared differently in America. Chinese restaurants here serve more meat and sauces than are generally eaten in China. According to laboratory tests of typical take-out dishes from Chinese restaurants, many have more fats and cholesterol than hamburger or egg dishes from fast-food outlets.

To eat healthfully when you choose Chinese cuisine, select boiled, steamed, or stir-fried dishes; mix entrées with steamed rice; and lift food out of a container with chopsticks or a fork and transfer it to serving bowls to leave excess sauce behind. Order wonton soup rather than egg rolls or pork spareribs. To avoid the cholesterol in egg yolks, steer away from egg foo yung and items made with lobster sauce. If you are prone to high blood pressure, watch out for the high sodium content of soy and other sauces, and of a seasoner called MSG (monosodium glutamate).

## French Diet

Traditional French cuisine, which includes rich, high-fat sauces and dishes, has never been considered healthful. Yet nutritionists have been stumped to explain the so-called French paradox. Despite a diet high in saturated fats, the French have had one of the lowest rates of coronary artery disease in the world.

Recent reports indicate that the French diet is changing. Until 1990 the French ate much less animal fat and had significantly lower blood cholesterol levels than Americans and Britons. Fat consumption in France has since risen as the French have begun eating more meat and fast foods, snacking more, eating fewer relaxed meals, exercising less, and drinking less wine.[22] They've also been getting fatter, and some researchers contend that their rates of heart

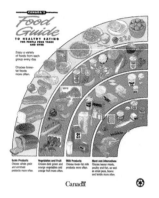
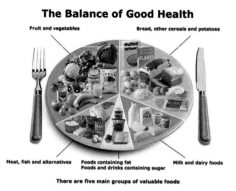

The Balance of Good Health

◀ Other countries use images other than a pyramid to present recommendations to eat more carbohydrate-rich grains, vegetables, and fruits. The United Kingdom and Mexico use plates. China and Korea use pagodas. Canada uses a rainbow.

disease will inevitably rise in the coming decades. The French diet increasingly resembles the American diet, but French portions tend to be one-third to one-half the size of American portions.

## Indian Diet

Many Indian dishes highlight healthful ingredients such as vegetables and legumes (beans and peas). However, many also use *ghee* (a form of butter) or coconut oil; both are rich in harmful saturated fats. The best advice in an Indian restaurant is to ask how each dish is prepared. Good choices include *daal* or *dal* (lentils), *karbi* or *karni* (chickpea soup), and *chapati* (tortilla-like bread). Hold back on *bhatura* (fried bread), coconut milk, and *samosas* (fried meat or vegetables in dough).

## Japanese Diet

The traditional Japanese diet is very low in fat, which may account for the low incidence of heart disease in Japan. Dietary staples include soybean products, fish, vegetables, noodles, and rice. A variety of fruits and vegetables are also included in many dishes. However, Japanese cuisine is high in salted, smoked, and pickled foods. Watch out for deep-fried dishes such as tempura, and salty soups and sauces (which you can ask for on the side). In a restaurant, ask for broiled entrées or nonfried dishes made with tofu, which has no cholesterol.

## Mediterranean Diet

Several years ago epidemiologists noticed something unexpected in the residents of regions along the Mediterranean Sea: a lower incidence of deaths from heart disease. They speculated that the plant-based Mediterranean diet, which is rich in fruits, vegetables, legumes, cereal, wine, and olive oil, may be the reason.

Subsequent research has confirmed that heart disease is much less common in countries along the Mediterranean than in other Western nations. No one knows exactly why.

As illustrated by the Mediterranean Food Pyramid (see Figure 5-3), the diet features lots of fruits and vegetables, legumes, nuts, and grains. Meat is used mainly as a condiment rather than as a main course, and fish, yogurt, and low-fat feta cheese are the predominant animal foods. The diet is relatively high in fat, but the main source is olive oil, an unsaturated fat.

## Mexican Diet

The cuisine served in Mexico features rice, corn, and beans, which are low in fat and high in nutrients. However, the dishes Americans think of as Mexican are far less healthful. Burritos, especially when topped with cheese and sour cream, are very high in fat. Although guacamole has a high fat content, it contains mostly monounsaturated fatty acids, a better form of fat.

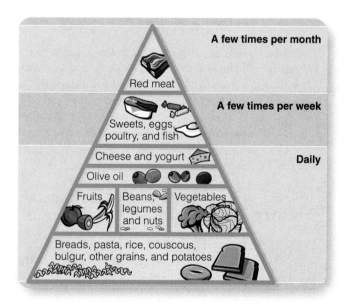

▲ **Figure 5-3** Mediterranean Food Pyramid
The Mediterranean diet relies heavily on fruits, vegetables, grain, and potatoes and includes considerable olive oil.

Source: Oldways Preservation & Exchange Trust. Reprinted by permission of the *New York Times.*

When eating at Mexican restaurants, ask that cheese and sour cream be served on the side. Avoid refried beans, which are usually cooked in lard. Hold back on guacamole, quesadillas, and enchiladas. Nutritious choices include rice, beans, and shrimp or chicken tostadas on unfried cornmeal tortillas.

## Southeast Asian Diet

A rich variety of fruits and vegetables—bamboo shoots, bok choy, cabbage, mangoes, papayas, cucumbers—provides a sound nutritional basis for this diet. In addition, most foods are broiled or stir-fried, which keeps fat low. However, coconut oil and milk, used in many sauces, are high in fat. The use of MSG and pickled foods means the sodium content is high. At Thai or Vietnamese restaurants, choose salads (*larb* is a chicken salad with mint) or seafood soup (*po tak*).

## ???? What Should I Know About Vegetarian Diets?

Not all vegetarians avoid all meats. Some, who call themselves *lacto-ovo-pesco-vegetarians,* eat dairy products, eggs, chicken, and fish, but not red meat. **Lacto-vegetarians** eat dairy products as well as grains, fruits, and vegetables; **ovo-lacto-vegetarians** also eat eggs. Pure vegetarians, called **vegans,** eat only plant foods; often they take vitamin $B_{12}$ supplements because that vitamin is normally found only in animal products. If they select their food with care, vegetarians can get sufficient amounts of protein, vitamin $B_{12}$, iron, and calcium without supplements (see Figure 5-4).

The key to getting sufficient protein from a vegetarian diet is understanding the concept of **complementary proteins.** Meat, poultry, fish, eggs, and dairy products are *complete proteins* that provide the nine essential amino acids—substances that the human body cannot produce itself. *Incomplete proteins,* such as legumes or nuts, may have relatively low levels of one or two essential amino acids, but fairly high levels of others. By combining complementary protein sources, you can make sure that your body makes the most of the nonanimal proteins you eat. Many cultures rely heavily on complementary foods for protein. In Middle Eastern cooking, sesame seeds and chickpeas are a popular combination; in Latin American dishes, beans and rice, or beans and tortillas; in Chinese cuisine, soy and rice.

Vegetarian diets have proven health benefits. Studies show that vegetarians' cholesterol levels are low, and vegetarians are seldom overweight. As a result, they're less apt to be candidates for heart disease than those who consume large quantities of meat. Vegetarians also have lower incidences of breast, colon, and prostate cancer; high blood pressure; and osteoporosis. When combined with exercise and stress reduction, vegetarian diets have helped reverse the buildup of harmful plaque within the blood vessels of the heart. (See Chapter 10 for further discussion of the connections between diet and heart disease.)

## Fast Food: Nutrition on the Run

On any given day, about 25 percent of adults in the United States go to a fast-food restaurant. The typical American consumes three hamburgers and four orders of french fries every week.[23] Not all fast foods are junk foods—that is, high in calories, sugar, salt, and fat, and low in beneficial nutrients. But while it's not all bad, fast food has definite disadvantages. A meal in a fast-food restaurant may cost twice as much as the same meal prepared at home and may provide half your daily calorie needs. The fat content of many items is extremely high. A Burger King Whopper

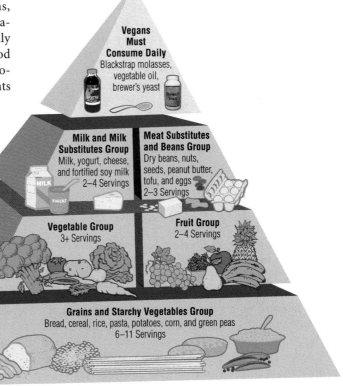

▲ **Figure 5-4** New York Medical College Vegetarian Pyramid
This version of the Food Guide Pyramid has been modified for use by vegetarians. Compare it to the Pyramid shown in Figure 5-1 on p. 107.

with cheese contains 723 calories and 48 grams of fat, 18 grams from saturated fat. A McDonald's Sausage McMuffin with egg has 517 calories and 33 grams of fat, 13 grams from saturated fat. Many fast-food chains have switched from beef tallow or lard to unsaturated vegetable oils for frying, but the total fat content of the foods remains the same.

At regular restaurants or cafeterias, you can usually get a better nutritional value for the calories you consume. For example, you can request that your entrée be baked or broiled without fat. You can also ask that fresh vegetables be steamed without salt or butter. When possible, ask for luncheon rather than dinner-sized portions.

## Food Safety

Increasingly, Americans are concerned not just with whether the food they eat is nutritious, but whether it's safe. Many unsuspected safety hazards have been identified by **food toxicologists,** specialists who detect toxins (potentially harmful substances) in food and treat the conditions they produce.

### Pesticides, Irradiation, and Genetic Engineering

Plants and animals naturally produce compounds that act as pesticides to aid in their survival. The vast majority of the pesticides we consume are therefore natural, not added by farmers or food processors. *Commercial pesticides* save billions of dollars of valuable crops from pests, but they also may endanger human health and life.

Fearful of potential risks in pesticides, many consumers are purchasing **organic** foods. The term *organic* refers to foods produced without the use of commercial chemicals at any stage. Independent groups now certify foods before they can be labeled organic. Foods that are truly organic are cleaner and have much lower levels of residues than standard commercial produce. There's no guarantee that the organic produce you buy at a grocery or health-food store is more nutritious than other produce. However, buying organic foods is one way in which you can work toward a healthier environment.

**Irradiation** is the use of radiation, either from radioactive substances or from devices that produce X rays, on food. It doesn't make the food radioactive. Its primary benefit is to prolong the shelf life of food. Like the heat in canning, irradiation can kill all the microorganisms that might grow in a food, and the sterilized food can then be stored for years in sealed containers at room temperature without spoiling. Are irradiated foods safe to eat? The best available answer is a qualified yes, because we don't have complete data yet.

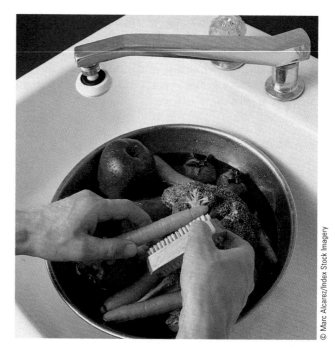

▲ Wash produce thoroughly in fresh water to remove dirt and any pesticide residue, scrubbing when necessary to clean off soil.

© Marc Alcarez/Index Stock Imagery

Genetically engineered foods—custom built to improve quality or remove unwanted traits—may become an important part of our diets in the future. By modifying the genetic makeup of plants, engineers will be able to produce apples that resist insects, raspberries that last longer, and potatoes that absorb less fat in cooking. Will these items be as tasty and healthful as foods grown the old-fashioned way? And will they have unforeseen health hazards? That's yet to be seen.

### Additives: Risks Versus Benefits

**Additives** are substances added to foods to lengthen storage time, change taste in a way the manufacturer thinks is better, alter color, or otherwise modify them to make them more appealing. The average American takes in approximately 160 pounds of food additives per year: more than 140 pounds of sweeteners, 15 pounds of table salt, and 5 to 10 pounds of all others.

Additives provide numerous benefits. Sodium and calcium propionate, sodium benzoate, potassium sorbate, and sulfur dioxide prevent the growth of bacteria, yeast, and mold in baked goods. BHA (butylated hydroxyanisole), BHT (butylated hydroxytoluene), propyl gallate, and vitamin E protect against the oxidation of fats (rancidity). Other additives include leavening agents, emulsifiers, stabilizers, thickeners, dough conditioners, and bleaching agents.

Some additives can pose a risk to eaters. For example, nitrites—used in bacon, sausages, and lunch meats to inhibit spoilage, prevent botulism, and add color—can react with other substances in your body or in food to form potentially cancer-causing agents called *nitrosamines.* In the last decade, the food industry has reduced the amount of nitrite used to cure foods, so there should be less danger than in the past. Sulfites, used to prevent browning, can produce severe, even fatal, allergic reactions in sensitive individuals. The FDA has required the labeling of sulfites in packaged foods and has banned the use of sulfites on fresh fruits and vegetables, including those in salad bars.

## ???? What Causes Food Poisoning?

*Salmonella* is a bacterium that contaminates many foods, particularly undercooked chicken, eggs, and sometimes processed meat. Eating contaminated food can result in salmonella poisoning, which causes diarrhea and vomiting. The CDC estimates 40,000 reported cases of salmonella poisoning a year; the actual number of cases could be anywhere from 400,000 to 4 million. The FDA has warned consumers about the dangers of unpasteurized orange juice because of the risk of salmonella contamination.

Another bacterium, *Campylobacter jejuni,* may cause even more stomach infections than salmonella. Found in water, milk, and some foods, Campylobacter poisoning causes severe diarrhea and has been implicated in the growth of stomach ulcers.

Bacteria can also cause illness by producing toxins in food. *Staphylococcus aureus* is the most common culprit. When cooked foods are cross-contaminated with the bacteria from raw foods and not stored properly, staph infections can result, causing nausea and abdominal pain anywhere from thirty minutes to eight hours after ingestion.

Even many healthy foods can pose dangers. The FDA has urged consumers to avoid eating raw sprouts because of the risk of getting sick. Sprouts, particularly alfalfa and clover, can be contaminated by salmonella or *E. coli* bacteria, which can cause nausea, diarrhea, and cramping in healthy adults. Children and senior citizens can experience serious symptoms that lead to kidney failure and compromised immune systems. The FDA advises people to either cook sprouts before eating them or request that they be left off sandwiches and other food ordered in restaurants. Homegrown sprouts can also present a risk if they come from contaminated seeds.

An uncommon but sometimes fatal form of food poisoning is **botulism,** caused by the *Clostridium botulinum* organism. Improper home-canning procedures are the most common cause of this potentially fatal problem.

There have been several outbreaks of listeriosis, caused by the bacteria **listeria,** commonly found in deli meats, hot dogs, soft cheeses, raw meat, and unpasteurized milk. At greatest risk are pregnant women, infants, and those with

---

## STRATEGIES FOR PREVENTION

### Protecting Yourself from Food Poisoning

▲ Clean food thoroughly. Wash produce thoroughly. Wash utensils, plates, cutting boards, knives, blenders, and other cooking equipment with very hot water and soap after preparing raw meat, poultry, or fish to avoid contaminating other foods or the cooked meat.

▲ Drink only pasteurized milk. Raw or unpasteurized milk increases the danger of microbial infections.

▲ Don't eat raw eggs. Since raw eggs can be contaminated with salmonella, don't use them in salad dressings, eggnog, or other dishes.

▲ Cook chicken thoroughly. About a third of all poultry sold contains harmful organisms. Thorough cooking eliminates any danger.

▲ Cook pork thoroughly. An internal temperature of 170° Fahrenheit must be reached to kill a parasite called *trichina* occasionally found in the muscles of pigs.

▲ Know how to store foods. Bacteria cannot survive in temperatures hotter than 140° Fahrenheit or colder than 40° Fahrenheit. The temperatures in between are a danger zone. If you must leave foods out—perhaps at a buffet or picnic—don't let them stay in the temperature danger zone for more than two hours. After that time, throw the food away.

▲ Stored food doesn't last forever. Refrigerate leftovers as soon as possible and use them within three days. If frozen, use leftovers within two to three months.

---

weakened immune systems. You can reduce your risk by cooking meats and leftovers thoroughly and by washing everything that may come into contact with raw meat.

## Food Allergies

Physicians disagree as to which foods are the most common triggers of food allergies. Cow's milk, eggs, seafood, wheat, soybeans, nuts, seeds, and chocolate have all been identified as culprits. The symptoms they provoke vary. One person might sneeze if exposed to an irritating food;

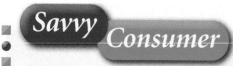

## Spotting Nutrition Misinformation

- Don't believe everything you read. A quick way to spot a bad nutrition self-help book is to look in the index for a diet to prevent or treat rheumatoid arthritis (none exists). If you find one, don't buy the book.

- Before you try any new nutritional approach, check with your doctor or a registered dietitian or call the American Dietetic Association's consumer hot line, (800)366-1655.

- Don't believe ads or advisers basing their nutritional recommendations on hair analysis, which is not accurate in detecting nutritional deficiencies.

- Be wary of anyone who recommends megadoses of vitamins or nutritional supplements, which can be dangerous. High doses of vitamin A, which some people take to clear up acne, can be toxic.

- Question personal testimonies about the powers of some magical-seeming pill or powder, and be wary of "scientific articles" in journals that aren't reviewed by health professionals.

- Be wary of any nutritional supplements sold in health stores or through health and bodybuilding magazines. These products may contain ingredients that have not been tested and proven safe.

---

another might vomit or develop diarrhea; others might suffer headaches, dizziness, hives, or a rapid heartbeat. Symptoms may not develop for up to 72 hours, making it hard to pinpoint which food was responsible.

If you suspect that you have a food allergy, see a physician with specialized training in allergy diagnosis. Medical opinion about the merits of many treatments for food allergies is divided. Once you've identified the culprit, the wisest and sometimes simplest course is to avoid it.

## Nutritional Quackery

The American Dietetic Association describes nutritional quackery as a growing problem for unsuspecting consumers. Because so much nutritional nonsense is garbed in scientific-sounding terms, it can be hard to recognize bad advice when you get it. One basic rule: If the promises of a nutritional claim sound too good to be true—they probably are. (See Savvy Consumer: "Spotting Nutrition Misinformation.")

If you seek the advice of a nutrition consultant, carefully check his or her credentials and professional associations. Because licensing isn't required in all states, almost anyone can use the label "nutritionist," regardless of qualifications. Be wary of diplomas from obscure schools and organizations that allow anyone who pays dues to join. (One physician obtained a membership for his dog!) A registered dietitian (R.D.), who has a bachelor's degree and specialized training (including an internship), and who passed a certification examination, is usually a member of the American Dietetic Association (ADA), which sets the standard for quality in diets. A nutrition expert with an M.D. or Ph.D. generally belongs to the ADA, the American

Institute of Nutrition, or the American Society of Clinical Nutrition; all have stringent membership requirements.

 How can eating fish twice a week help reduce cardiovascular disease?

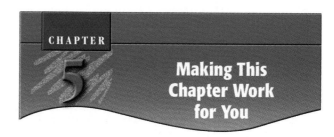

### Making This Chapter Work for You

1. The classes of essential nutrients include which of the following?
   a. amino acids, antioxidants, fiber, and cholesterol
   b. proteins, calcium, calories, and folic acid
   c. carbohydrates, minerals, fat, and water
   d. iron, whole grains, fruits, and vegetables

2. Which type of fat is *not* considered a threat to heart health?
   a. omega-3 fatty acids
   b. trans-fatty acids
   c. cholesterol
   d. saturated fats

3. Antioxidants
   a. are nutrients important in the production of hemoglobin.

b. are substances added to foods to make them more flavorful or physically appealing.

c. are suspected triggers of food allergies.

d. are substances that prevent the harmful effects of free radicals.

4. Which of the following is true about the Food Guide Pyramid?

a. It advises that, on a daily basis, you eat the same amounts of food from each of the food groups represented in the Pyramid.

b. The foods at the top of the pyramid are considered to be the most nutritionally essential.

c. According to the Pyramid, one should eat six to eleven servings of bread, cereals, rice, and pasta every week.

d. The Pyramid advises no more than two to three servings daily of dairy foods, and two to three servings daily of meat and other high-protein foods.

5. Which statement about essential nutrients is *false?*

a. Carbohydrates provide body cells with glucose.

b. Fats are necessary for the growth and repair of body cells.

c. Water is an essential nutrient but doesn't provide any energy.

d. Vitamins are necessary for the body to manufacture blood cells and hromones.

6. Food labels on packaged food include all of the following *except*

a. total weight of the package.

b. total amount of nutrients contained in the food.

c. the percent of nutrient Daily Values provided in the food.

d. serving size.

7. Which of the following statements is true?

a. The Chinese diet, which is high in fats and low in carbohydrates, leads to high incidence of obesity and heart disease.

b. The French diet is considered to be healthful because the food is high in saturated fats.

c. The Mediterranean diet is rich in fruits, vegetables, wine, and olive oil and may help prevent heart disease.

d. Mexican and African-American recipes often include MSG, which is unhealthy for people with high blood pressure.

8. Some vegetarians may

a. include chicken and fish in their diets.

b. avoid vitamin $B_{12}$ supplements if they eat only plant foods.

c. eat only legumes or nuts because these provide complete proteins.

d. have high cholesterol levels because of the saturated fats in fruits and vegetables.

9. Food hazards include all the following *except*

a. nitrites

b. raw eggs

c. pesticides

d. refrigerated leftovers used within 3 days

10. Common causes of foodborne infections include which of the following?

a. the influenza virus

b. salmonella and *E. coli* bacteria

c. additives

d. irradiation

Answers to these questions can be found on page 415.

## Critical Thinking

1. Which alternative or ethnic diet do you think has the best-tasting food? Which is the most healthy? Why?

2. Is it possible to meet nutritional requirements on a limited budget? Have you ever been in this situation? What would you recommend to someone who wants to eat healthfully on $30 a week?

3. Consider the number of times a week you eat fast food. How much money would you have saved it you had eaten home-prepared meals. Which fast foods could you have selected that would have provided more nutritional value?

4. Scientists are using genetic engineering to develop improved foods: tomatoes that won't bruise easily, cows that will produce more milk, corn that will grow larger ears. Some consumer advocates argue that these items shouldn't be put on the market because they haven't been studied carefully enough. What do you think of these foods? Would you eat them?

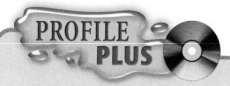

## PROFILE PLUS

Find the nutrient values of the food you are eating and plan a diet that supports a healthy lifestyle with this activity on your Profile Plus CD-ROM:

Nutrient Analysis and Diet Planning

## SITES & BYTES

### Nutrition.gov
www.nutrition.gov

This excellent online source for comprehensive nutrition information includes dietary guidelines, the Food Pyramid, food labels, education programs, nutritional supplements, healthy diets, health management, food safety, a description on how the body uses nutrients found in food, biotechnology, research, and current nutrition news.

### USDA Center for Nutrition Policy and Promotion
www.usda.gov/cnpp

This interactive site sponsored by the United States Center for Nutrition Policy and Promotion features the Interactive Health Eating Index, an online dietary assessment that enables you to receive a personalized score on the overall quality of your diet, on a daily basis, based on the recommendations of the Food Guide Pyramid. This tool provides you with information on total fat, cholesterol, sodium, and other nutrients. You can also download a series of brochures featuring dietary guidelines as well as healthy recipes.

### Nutrient Analysis Tool
www.nat.uiuc.edu

This site, provided as a public service by the Food Science and Human Nutrition Department at the University of Illinois, features a free nutrient analysis interactive program that calculates the amount of calories, carbohy-

drates, protein, fat, vitamins, minerals, and fiber in the foods that make up your daily diet.

Please note that links are subject to change. If you find a broken link, use a search engine such as www.yahoo.com and search for the website by typing in keywords.

### InfoTrac College Edition Activity
Wendy C. Reinhardt and Patricia B. Brevard. "Integrating the Food Guide Pyramid and Physical Activity Pyramid for Positive Dietary and Physical Activity Behaviors in Adolescents." *Journal of the American Dietetic Association,* Vol. 102, No. 3, March 2002, p. S96 (4).

1.   What were the objectives of the intervention curriculum and how did they relate to the two types of pyramid guidelines?

2.   What were the limitations of this study?

3.   What professional organizations have partnered to publish posters containing both the Food Guide Pyramid and the Physical Activity Pyramid? What are the long-term goals of this partnership?

You can find additional readings related to nutrition with InfoTrac College Edition, an online library of more than 900 journals and publications. Follow the instructions for accessing InfoTrac that were packaged with your textbook; then search for articles using a keyword search.

For additional links, resources, and suggested readings on InfoTrac, visit our Health & Wellness Resource Center at http://health.wadsworth.com.

## Key Terms

The terms listed here are used within the chapter on the page indicated. Definitions of the terms are in the Glossary at the end of this book.

## References

1. Panel on Micronutrients, Subcommittees on Upper Reference Levels of Nutrients and Interpretation and Uses of Dietary Reference Intakes, and the Standing Committee on the Scientific Evaluation of Dietary Reference Intakes. *Dietary Reference Intakes for Energy, Carbohydrates, Fiber, Fat, Protein and Amino Acids.* Washington, DC: National Academy of Sciences Press, 2002.

2. Ibid.

3. Ibid.

4. Harder, B. "Wholesome Grains: Insulin Effects May Explain Healthful Diet." *Science News,* Vol. 161, No. 20, May 18, 2002, p. 308.

5. Webb, Densie. "Whole Grains Boast Phytochemicals (Not Just Fiber) to Fight Diseases." *Environmental Nutrition,* Vol. 24, No. 2, February 2001, p. 1.

6. Panel on Micronutrients.

7. "Position of the American Dietetic Association: Health Implications of Dietary Fiber." *Journal of the American Dietetic Association,* Vol. 102, No. 7, July 2002, p. 993.

8. "Eating More Fiber Doesn't Have to Be Uncomfortable." *Tufts University Health & Nutrition Letter,* Vol. 20, No. 5, July 2002, p. 7.

9. "Evidence for Fish/Heart Health Connection Strengthens Even More." *Tufts University Health & Nutrition Letter,* Vol. 20, No. 4, June 2002, p. 3.

10. "Freshman College Student Dining Habits." *Food Service Director,* Vol. 15, No. 3, March 15, 2002, p. 1.

11. Evans, Alexandra, et al. "Fruit and Vegetable Consumption Among Mexican-American College Students." *Journal of the American Dietetic Association.* Vol. 100, No. 11, November 2000, p. 1399.

12. "Nutrition Knowledge of Collegiate Athletes." *Nutrition Research Newsletter,* Vol. 21, No. 4, April 2002, p. 3.

13. Glanz, Karen. "Reducing Chronic Diseases Risk Through Nutrition." *Facts of Life: Issue Briefing for Health Reporters,* Vol. 5, No. 9, November 2000, p. 2.

14. Warshaw, Hope. "Nutrition Tips: On Estimating Portion Sizes." *Diabetes Forecast,* Vol. 55, No. 5, May 2002, p. 55.

15. Knaust, Gretchen, and Irene Foster. "Estimation of Food Guide Pyramid Serving Sizes by College Students." *Family and Consumer Sciences Research Journal,* Vol. 29, No. 2, December 2000, p. 101.

16. Brown, C. Hsing-Kuan. "A Food Display Assignment and Handling Food Models Improves Accuracy of College Students' Estimates of Food Portions." *Journal of the American Dietetic Association,* Vol. 100, No. 9, September 2000, pp. 1063–1064.

17. Weggemans, Rianne, et al. "Dietary Cholesterol from Eggs Increases the Ratio of Total Cholesterol to High-Density Lipoprotein Cholesterol in Humans: A Meta-Analysis." *American Journal of Clinical Nutrition,* Vol. 73, No. 5, May 2001, p. 885.

18. Reyes, Sonia. "Fast, Functional Fare Fills the Bill." *Brandweek,* Vol. 42, No. 23.

19. McCaffree, Jim. "Herbal Foods: Health and Happiness on a Corn Flake?" *Journal of the American Dietetic Association,* Vol. 101, No. 4, April 2001, p. 398.

20. "Whether Pyramid, Plate, or Pagoda, All Countries Recommend Less Protein and More Carbohydrate." *Tufts University Health & Nutrition Letter,* Vol. 20, No. 4, June 2002, p. 6.

21. "Dietary Guidelines and the Food Guide Pagoda." *Journal of the American Dietetic Association,* Vol. 100, No. 8, August 2000.

22. de Lorgeril, Michel, and Patricia Salen. "Wine, Ethanol, Platelets, and Mediterranean Diet." *Lancet,* Vol. 353, No. 9158, March 27, 1999.

23. Schlosser, Eric. *Fast Food Nation.* New York: Simon & Schuster, 2001.

# CHAPTER 6

# Eating Patterns and Problems

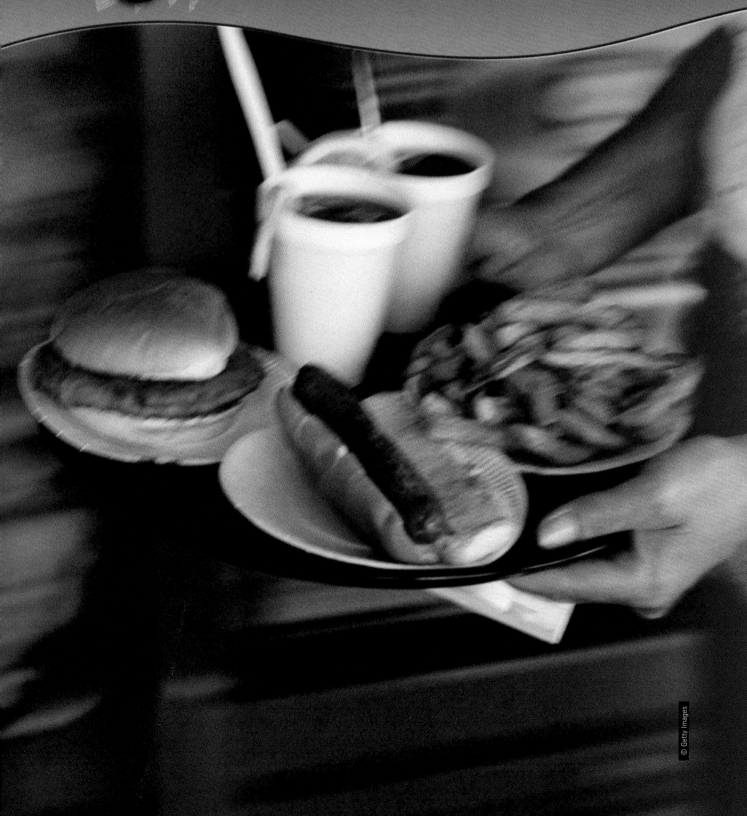

After studying the material in this chapter, you should be able to:

- **Define** body mass index (BMI) and **describe** the different methods of estimating body mass.
- **Identify** several factors that influence food consumption.
- **Identify** and **describe** the symptoms and dangers associated with eating disorders.
- **Define** obesity and **describe** its relationship to genetics, lifestyle, and major health problems.
- **Assess** various approaches to weight loss.
- **Design** a personal plan for sensible weight management.

America is turning into the land of the large. An estimated 34 percent of American adults between the ages of 20 and 74 are overweight; 27 percent—50 million people—are obese. About 14 percent of adolescents are overweight, almost triple the percentage of two decades ago.[1] Obese Americans now outnumber daily smokers and heavy drinkers.[2]

Ironically, as average weights have increased, the quest for thinness has become a national obsession. In a society where slimmer is seen as better, anyone who is less than lean may feel like a failure. Individuals who are overweight or embarrassed by their appearance often assume that they would be happier, sexier, or more successful in thinner bodies. And so they diet. Each year, 15 to 35 percent of Americans go on diets, but no matter how much they lose, 90 to 95 percent regain extra pounds within five years.

This chapter explores our national preoccupation with slimness; explains Body Mass Index (BMI); examines unhealthy eating patterns and eating disorders; tells what obesity is and why excess pounds are dangerous; shows why fad diets don't work; and offers guidelines for how to control weight safely, sensibly, and permanently.

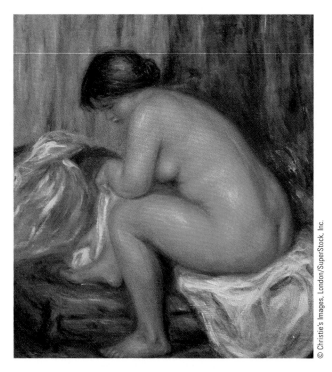

▲ "Thinner is better" is not the global standard, and in past centuries, the fuller figure was considered healthy and beautiful. This painting by Renoir from the late 1880s shows the feminine ideal of the time.

© Christie's Images, London/SuperStock, Inc.

## Body Image

Throughout most of history, bigger was better. The great beauties of centuries past, as painted by such artistic masters as Rubens and Renoir, were soft and fleshy, with rounded bellies and dimpled thighs. Culture often shapes views of beauty and health.

 Many developing countries still regard a full figure, rather than a thin one, as the ideal. Fattening huts, in which brides-to-be eat extra food to plump up before marriage, still exist in some African cultures. Among certain Native American tribes of the Southwest, if a girl is thin at puberty, a fat woman places her foot on the girl's back so she will magically gain weight and become more attractive.

Influenced by the media, many Americans are paying more attention to their body images than ever before—and at a younger age. In a study of high school girls, those who regularly read women's health and fitness magazines, which may present unrealistic physical ideals, were more likely to go on low-calorie diets, take pills to suppress their appetites, use laxatives, or force themselves to vomit after eating.[3] In other research, girls who watched a lot of television and expressed concern about slimness and popularity were more dissatisfied with their bodies than girls involved in sports.[4] Boys' body images also are influenced by media images depicting superstrong, highly muscular males.[5]

 African-American women often have more positive attitudes toward their bodies, feeling more satisfied with their weight and seeing themselves as more attractive. However, there are no significant differences between African-American women who diet and white women who diet in terms of self-esteem and body dissatisfaction.

 College students of different ethnic and racial backgrounds, including Asians, express as much—and sometimes more—concern about their body shape and weight as whites.[6] Men and women are prone to different distortions in body image. Women tend to see themselves as overweight, whether or not they are; men perceive themselves as underweight, even when their weights are normal or above normal.[7] In one recent study of university students, African-American and Caucasian men were similiar in their ideals for body size and in their perceptions of their own shapes. As shown in Student Snapshot: "Body Dissatisfaction in African-American and White Students," both African-American and white women perceived themselves as smaller than they actually were and desired an even smaller body size. However, the African-American women were more accepting of larger size.[8]

As men and women age, their attitudes about their bodies change. In a study comparing college students, parents, and grandparents, older men and women were more dissatisfied with their appearance than younger people. Women were more concerned with aging than men, but there were no gender differences in overall body dissatisfaction.[9]

## ???? What Should I Weigh?

Many factors determine what you weigh: heredity, eating behavior, food selection, and amount of daily exercise. For any individual of a given height, there is no single best weight, but a range of healthy weights. The federal government and medical experts have replaced ideal weight tables with a better measure—body mass index.

### Body Mass Index

**Body mass index (BMI)**, a ratio between weight and height, is a mathematical formula that correlates with body fat. The BMI numbers apply to both men and women. (See Table 6-1 on p. 126.)

You can also calculate your body mass index by following these three simple steps:

1.   Multiply your weight in pounds by 703.

## Student Snapshot

### Body Dissatisfaction in African-American and White Students

In a study of 630 undergraduates, both African-American and white women perceived themselves to be smaller than they actually were—and wished to be even smaller. However, the white students saw themselves and desired to be considerably smaller than the African-American women. Both African-American and white men rated the silhouette depicting a BMI of 20 as the most desirable.

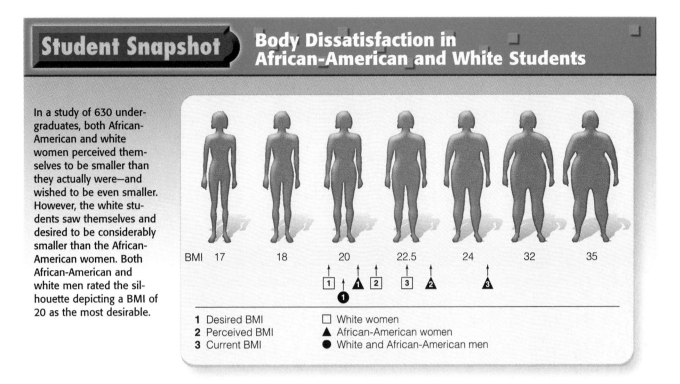

BMI   17      18      20      22.5      24      32      35

1 Desired BMI          □ White women
2 Perceived BMI        ▲ African-American women
3 Current BMI          ● White and African-American men

Source: "Body Dissatisfaction Among College Students," *Nutrition Research Newsletter,* Vol. 21, No. 3, March 2002, p. 9.

2. Multiply your height in inches by itself.
3. Divide the first number by the second and then round up to the nearest whole number. This is your body mass index.

Doctors use BMI to determine whether a person is at risk for weight-related diseases like diabetes. However, using BMI as an assessment tool has limitations. Muscular individuals, including athletes and body builders, may be miscategorized as overweight or obese because they have greater lean muscle mass. BMI also does not reliably reflect body fat, an independent predictor of health risk, and is not useful for growing children, women who are pregnant or nursing, or the elderly. In addition, BMI, which was developed in Western nations, may not accurately indicate the risk of obesity-related diseases in Asian men and women.[10]

If your BMI is high, you may be at increased risk of developing certain diseases, including hypertension, cardiovascular disease, adult-onset diabetes (type 2), sleep apnea, and osteoarthritis. (Being Overweight or Obese in this chapter discusses the health risks associated with a high BMI.)

## Body Composition Assessment

Knowing your body composition can provide useful information about body fat and health. Ideal body fat percentages for men range from 7 to 25 percent and for women from 16 to 35 percent. Methods of assessing body composition include:

✔ **Waist size.** Among those with BMIs over 25, men with waists larger than 40 inches and women with waists larger than 35 inches are at greater risk of heart disease. The danger increases along with the waistline. According to one study, women with waists of 30 inches run twice the risk of heart disease as slimmer women. At 38 inches, the risk is three times higher compared to women with waists of 28 inches or less.[11]

✔ **Waist-to-hip ratio (WHR).** A WHR greater than 1 for men or .85 for women is considered a signal of high risk for disease; a WHR of .90 to 1 for men or .80 to .85 for women indicates moderately high risk; a WHR less than .90 for men or less than .80 for women indicates lower risk.

### ▼ Table 6-1  Body Mass Index (BMI)

Find your height along the lefthand column and look across the row until you find the number that is closest to your weight. The number at the top of that column identifies your BMI. The area shaded in green represents healthy weight ranges.

| Height | 18 | 19 | 20 | 21 | 22 | 23 | 24 | 25 | 26 | 27 | 28 | 29 | 30 | 31 | 32 | 33 | 34 | 35 | 36 | 37 | 38 | 39 | 40 |
|---|---|---|---|---|---|---|---|---|---|---|---|---|---|---|---|---|---|---|---|---|---|---|---|
| | | | | | | | | | | Body Weight (pounds) | | | | | | | | | | | | | |
| 4'10" | 86 | 91 | 96 | 100 | 105 | 110 | 115 | 119 | 124 | 129 | 134 | 138 | 143 | 148 | 153 | 158 | 162 | 167 | 172 | 177 | 181 | 186 | 191 |
| 4'11" | 89 | 94 | 99 | 104 | 109 | 114 | 119 | 124 | 128 | 133 | 138 | 143 | 148 | 153 | 158 | 163 | 168 | 173 | 178 | 183 | 188 | 193 | 198 |
| 5'0" | 92 | 97 | 102 | 107 | 112 | 118 | 123 | 128 | 133 | 138 | 143 | 148 | 153 | 158 | 163 | 168 | 174 | 179 | 184 | 189 | 194 | 199 | 204 |
| 5'1" | 95 | 100 | 106 | 111 | 116 | 122 | 127 | 132 | 137 | 143 | 148 | 153 | 158 | 164 | 169 | 174 | 180 | 185 | 190 | 195 | 201 | 206 | 211 |
| 5'2" | 98 | 104 | 109 | 115 | 120 | 126 | 131 | 136 | 142 | 147 | 153 | 158 | 164 | 169 | 175 | 180 | 186 | 191 | 196 | 202 | 207 | 213 | 218 |
| 5'3" | 102 | 107 | 113 | 118 | 124 | 130 | 135 | 141 | 146 | 152 | 158 | 163 | 169 | 175 | 180 | 186 | 191 | 197 | 203 | 208 | 214 | 220 | 225 |
| 5'4" | 105 | 110 | 116 | 122 | 128 | 134 | 140 | 145 | 151 | 157 | 163 | 169 | 174 | 180 | 186 | 192 | 197 | 204 | 209 | 215 | 221 | 227 | 232 |
| 5'5" | 108 | 114 | 120 | 126 | 132 | 138 | 144 | 150 | 156 | 162 | 168 | 174 | 180 | 186 | 192 | 198 | 204 | 210 | 216 | 222 | 228 | 234 | 240 |
| 5'6" | 112 | 118 | 124 | 130 | 136 | 142 | 148 | 155 | 161 | 167 | 173 | 179 | 186 | 192 | 198 | 204 | 210 | 216 | 223 | 229 | 235 | 241 | 247 |
| 5'7" | 115 | 121 | 127 | 134 | 140 | 146 | 153 | 159 | 166 | 172 | 178 | 185 | 191 | 198 | 204 | 211 | 217 | 223 | 230 | 236 | 242 | 249 | 255 |
| 5'8" | 118 | 125 | 131 | 138 | 144 | 151 | 158 | 164 | 171 | 177 | 184 | 190 | 197 | 203 | 210 | 216 | 223 | 230 | 236 | 243 | 249 | 256 | 262 |
| 5'9" | 122 | 128 | 135 | 142 | 149 | 155 | 162 | 169 | 176 | 182 | 189 | 196 | 203 | 209 | 216 | 223 | 230 | 236 | 243 | 250 | 257 | 263 | 270 |
| 5'10" | 126 | 132 | 139 | 146 | 153 | 160 | 167 | 174 | 181 | 188 | 195 | 202 | 209 | 216 | 222 | 229 | 236 | 243 | 250 | 257 | 264 | 271 | 278 |
| 5'11" | 129 | 136 | 143 | 150 | 157 | 165 | 172 | 179 | 186 | 193 | 200 | 208 | 215 | 222 | 229 | 236 | 243 | 250 | 257 | 265 | 272 | 279 | 286 |
| 6'0" | 132 | 140 | 147 | 154 | 162 | 169 | 177 | 184 | 191 | 199 | 206 | 213 | 221 | 228 | 235 | 242 | 250 | 258 | 265 | 272 | 279 | 287 | 294 |
| 6'1" | 136 | 144 | 151 | 159 | 166 | 174 | 182 | 189 | 197 | 204 | 212 | 219 | 227 | 235 | 242 | 250 | 257 | 265 | 272 | 280 | 288 | 295 | 302 |
| 6'2" | 141 | 148 | 155 | 163 | 171 | 179 | 186 | 194 | 202 | 210 | 218 | 225 | 233 | 241 | 249 | 256 | 264 | 272 | 280 | 287 | 295 | 303 | 311 |
| 6'3" | 144 | 152 | 160 | 168 | 176 | 184 | 192 | 200 | 208 | 216 | 224 | 232 | 240 | 248 | 256 | 264 | 272 | 279 | 287 | 295 | 303 | 311 | 319 |
| 6'4" | 148 | 156 | 164 | 172 | 180 | 189 | 197 | 205 | 213 | 221 | 230 | 238 | 246 | 254 | 263 | 271 | 279 | 287 | 295 | 304 | 312 | 320 | 328 |
| 6'5" | 151 | 160 | 168 | 176 | 185 | 193 | 202 | 210 | 218 | 227 | 235 | 244 | 252 | 261 | 269 | 277 | 286 | 294 | 303 | 311 | 319 | 328 | 336 |
| 6'6" | 155 | 164 | 172 | 181 | 190 | 198 | 207 | 216 | 224 | 233 | 241 | 250 | 259 | 267 | 276 | 284 | 293 | 302 | 310 | 319 | 328 | 336 | 345 |

**Underweight (<18.5)**  **Healthy Weight (18.5–24.9)**  **Overweight (25–29.9)**  **Obese (≥30)**

Source: Reprinted from "The Body Test" (1988). © Dietitians of Canada.

✔ **Skinfold fat measurement.** A caliper is used to measure the amount of skinfold. The usual sites include the chest, abdomen, and thigh for men, and the tricep, hip, and thigh for women. Various equations determine body fat percentage, including calculations that take into account age, gender, race, and other factors.

✔ **Hydrostatic (underwater) weighing.** According to the Archimedes Principle, a body immersed in a fluid is buoyed by a force equal to the weight of the displaced fluid. Since muscle has a higher density than water and fat has a lower density, fat people tend to displace less water than lean people. This method, also known as hydrodensitometry, is expensive and complex.

✔ **Dual-energy X-ray absorptiometry (DXA).** X rays are used to quantify the skeletal and soft tissue components of body mass. The test requires just 10 to 20 minutes, and radiation dosage is low (800 to 2,000 times lower than a typical chest X ray). Some researchers believe that DXA will supplant hydrostatic testing as the standard for body composition assessment.

✔ **Home body fat analyzers.** Handheld devices and stand-on monitors sold online and in specialty stores promise to make measuring your body fat percentage as easy as finding your weight. None has been extensively tested.

## ??? How Many Calories Do I Need?

**Calories** are the measure of the amount of energy that can be derived from food. How many calories you need depends on your gender, age, body-frame size, weight, percentage of body fat, and your **basal metabolic rate (BMR)**—the number of calories needed to sustain your body at rest. Your activity level also affects your calorie requirements. (See Table 6-2.) Regardless of whether you consume fat, protein, or carbohydrates, if you take in more calories than required to maintain your size and don't work them off in some sort of physical activity, your body will convert the excess to fat.

## Hunger, Satiety, and Set Point

Why do you wake up starving? Why does your stomach rumble during a late afternoon lecture? The simple answer is **hunger:** the physiological drive to consume food. More than a dozen different signals may influence and control our desire for food. Researchers at the National Institutes of Health have discovered appetite receptors within the hypothalamus region of the brain that specifically respond to hunger messages carried by chemicals. Hormones, including insulin and stress-related epinephrine (adrenaline), may also stimulate or suppress hunger. Recent studies show that hunger activates parts of the brain involved with emotions, thinking, and feeling. Even the size of our fat cells may affect how hungry we feel.

**Appetite**—the psychological desire to eat—usually begins with the fear of the unpleasant sensation of hunger. We learn to avoid hunger by eating a certain amount of food at certain times of the day, just as dogs in a laboratory learn to avoid electric shocks by jumping at the sound of a warning bell. But appetite is easily led into temptation. In one famous experiment, psychologists bought bags of high-calorie goodies (peanut butter, marshmallows, chocolate-chip cookies, and salami) for their test rats. The animals ate so much on this supermarket diet that they gained more weight than any laboratory rats ever had before. The snack-food diet that fattened up these rats was particularly high in fats. Biologists speculate that creamy, buttery, or greasy foods may cause internal changes that increase appetite and, consequently, weight.

We stop eating when we feel satisfied; this is called **satiety,** a feeling of fullness and relief from hunger. According to the **set-point theory,** each individual has an unconscious control system for regulating appetite and satiety to keep body fat at a predetermined level, or *set point.* If our fat stores fall too low, our appetite gnaws at us, so we eat more. Physical activity, which dampens the appetite in the short run, is the only way to lower the set point for the long term.

## Unhealthy Eating Behavior

Unhealthy eating behavior takes many forms, ranging from not eating enough to eating too much too quickly. Its roots are complex. In addition to media and external pressures, a family history can play a role. Researchers have linked a specific gene to some cases of anorexia nervosa, but most believe that a variety of factors, including stress and culture, combine to cause disordered eating.[12]

About a third of female athletes in every sport show symptoms of disordered eating or eating disorders.[13] Girls and adolescent females who participate regularly in sports are at risk for disordered eating, menstrual dysfunction, and decreased bone mineral density, according to the American Academy of Pediatrics. The combination of these three disorders is known as the *female athlete triad.*[14]

Sooner or later many people don't eat the way they should. They may skip meals, thereby increasing the likelihood that they'll end up with more body fat, a higher weight, and a higher blood cholesterol level. They may live on diet foods, but consume so much of them that they gain weight anyway. Some even engage in more extreme eating behavior: Dissatisfied with almost all aspects of their appearance, they continuously go on and off diets, eat compulsively, or binge on high-fat treats.[15] Such behaviors can be warning signs of potentially serious eating disorders that should not be ignored.

| ▼ Table 6-2 | Daily Energy Requirements (in Calories) for People of Various Sizes and Levels of Activity | |
| --- | --- | --- |
| | **Sedentary** | **Active** |
| **5'1", 98 to 132 pounds** | | |
| Women | 1,688 to 1,834 | 2,104 to 2,290 |
| Men | 1,919 to 2,167 | 2,104 to 2,290 |
| **5'5", up to 150 pounds** | | |
| Women | 1,816 to 1,982 | 2,267 to 2,477 |
| Men | 2,068 to 2,349 | 2,490 to 2,842 |
| **5'9", 125 to 169 pounds** | | |
| Women | 1,948 to 2,134 | 2,434 to 2,670 |
| Men | 2,222 to 2,538 | 2,683 to 3,078 |
| **6'1", 139 to 188 pounds** | | |
| Women | 2,083 to 2,290 | 2,605 to 2,869 |
| Men | 2,382 to 2,736 | 2,883 to 3,325 |

Source: Panel on Micronutrients, Subcommittees on Upper Reference Levels of Nutrients and Interpretation and Uses of Dietary Reference Intakes, and the Standing Committee on the Scientific Evaluation of Dietary Reference Intakes. *Dietary Reference Intakes for Energy, Carbohydrates, Fiber, Fat, Protein and Amino Acids (Macronutrients):* Washington, DC: National Academy of Sciences Press, 2002.

# Disordered Eating in College Students

College students—particularly women, including varsity athletes—are at risk for unhealthy eating behaviors. The prevalence of disordered eating symptoms and eating disorders has increased dramatically in the last 20 years.

In a recent survey at a large, public, rural university in the mid-Atlantic states, 17 percent of the women were struggling with disordered eating. Younger women (ages 18 to 21) were more likely than older students to have an eating disorder. In this study, eating disorders did not discriminate, equally affecting women of different races (white, Asian, African-American, American Indian, and Hispanic), religions, athletic involvement, and living arrangements (on or off campus, with roommates, boyfriends, or family). Although the students viewed eating disorders as both mental and physical problems, and felt that individual therapy would be most helpful, all said that they would first turn to a friend for help.[16] In another study of 1,620 students, amost 11 percent of the women and 4 percent of the men were at risk for eating disorders. About 17 percent of the women and 10 percent of the men said concerns about weight interfered with their academic work. Women in sororities were at slightly increased risk of an eating disorder compared with those in dormitories.[17]

In a study of Australian male undergraduates, one in four men worried about shape and weight; one in five displayed attitudes and behaviors characteristic of disordered eating and eating disorders. (See Table 6-3.) None ever sought treatment, even if the students recognized they had a problem. The reason, the researchers theorized, may be that the young men hesitated to seek treatment for an illness stigmatized as a problem that affects only women. Some men exercised extremely intensively almost every day, even if ill or injured. None felt they had a problem with excessive exercise.[18]

The unique demands and stressors of the transition to college do not increase the likelihood of disordered eating for all freshmen. One study that followed more than 100 undergraduate women through their freshman year found that those who reported the most body dissatisfaction and unhealthy eating patterns at the beginning of the first semester were most likely to experience more eating problems, such as losing control of their eating when feeling strong emotions. The strongest predictor that eating symptoms would get worse over the freshman year was not BMI or weight, but body dissatisfaction.[19]

The most common weight-related problem on campuses may be gaining weight, particularly in the first year away from home. As many students discover, it's easy to

### ▼ Table 6-3  Eating Behavior and Concerns About Body Weight and Exercise of Australian Male College Students

| Behavior or Concern | Percentage Reporting "a lot" or "a great deal" |
|---|---|
| **Eating behavior** | |
| Follow rules about eating for any reason | 23 |
| Follow rules about eating for weight/shape | 20 |
| Limit what eat for weight/shape | 20 |
| Eat only 1 or 2 meals each day | 19 |
| Try to avoid eating liked foods for weight/shape | 18 |
| **Body weight/shape concern** | |
| Worry about shape and weight | 25 |
| Shape important for self-esteem | 16 |
| Feel fat | 12 |
| Unhappy about shape | 10 |
| Seriously want to lose weight | 9 |
| Feel inhibited about my weight | 9 |
| Afraid of gaining weight and becoming fat | 8 |
| Unhappy about weight | 8 |
| Feel distressed if had to be weighed regularly | 7 |
| Thinking of food affects concentration on other things | 3 |
| **Exercise concerns** | |
| Exercise important for self-esteem | 48 |
| Distressed if not exercise as much as wanted | 34 |
| Exercise to feel good | 33 |
| Exercise for weight and shape | 33 |
| Follow rules about exercising | 27 |
| Worry about exercise | 14 |

Source: O'Dea, Jennifer, and Suzanne Abraham. "Eating and Exercise Disorders in Young College Men." *Journal of American College Health,* Vol. 50, No. 4, May 2002, p. 273.

gain weight on campuses, which are typically crammed with vending machines, fast-food counters, and cafeterias serving up hearty meals. But the infamous *freshman 15,* the extra pounds acquired in the first year at college, seems to be a myth.[20] Several studies have documented much lower weight gains, ranging from 2.45 to 7 pounds. In one recent study of changes in both weight and body fat, freshman estimated that they had gained an average of 4.1 pounds. In fact, while their weights fluctuated from a gain of 15 pounds to a loss of 15 pounds, the average change was a loss of 1.5 pounds. (See Table 6-4.) Among the 60 percent of freshmen who did put on weight, the average gain was 4.6 pounds.[21]

Even international students may gain weight and body fat after arriving on American campuses. Ohio University

| ▼ Table 6-4 The Myth of the Freshman 15: Changes in Weight and Body Fat During Freshman Year | | | |
|---|---|---|---|
| In this study of 44 freshmen at a small Midwestern liberal arts college, weight change ranged from a loss of 15 pounds to a gain of 15 pounds. The average change in weight was a loss of 1.5 pounds. | | | |
| Change in Weight (Pounds) | Percentage of Students | Change in Body Fat | Percentage of Students |
| +10 to +15 | 6.8 | +2 to +5 percent | 6.8 |
| +5 to +9.5 | 22.7 | +0.5 to +1.9 percent | 15.9 |
| +.5 to +4.5 | 29.6 | No change | 34.1 |
| No change | 4.6 | −1.9 to +0.5 | 29.6 |
| −0.5 to +4.5 | 22.7 | −5 to −2 | 13.6 |
| −5 to 9.5 | 6.8 | | |
| −10 to −15 | 6.8 | | |

Source: Graham, Melody, and Amy Jones. "Freshman 15: Valid Theory or Harmful Myth?" *Journal of American College Health,* Vol. 50, No. 4, January 2002, p. 171.

researchers found that after 20 weeks, foreign students, who had incorporated foods high in fat, salt, and sugar into their diets, gained about 3 pounds on average and their percentage of body fat rose by about 5 percent.[22]

## Extreme Dieting

About half of girls attempt to control their weight by dieting.[23] In a year-long study of teenagers, both parents and the media had the most influence on the development of weight concerns and weight control practices, including dieting, among adolescents and preadolescents.[24]

Extreme dieters go beyond cutting back on calories or increasing physical activity. They become preoccupied with what they eat and weigh. Although their weight never falls below 85 percent of normal, their weight loss is severe enough to cause uncomfortable physical consequences, such as weakness and sensitivity to cold. Technically, these dieters do not have anorexia nervosa (discussed later in the chapter), but they are at increased risk for it.

Extreme dieters may think they know a great deal about nutrition, yet many of their beliefs about food and weight are misconceptions or myths. For instance, they may eat only protein because they believe complex carbohydrates, including fruits and breads, are fattening. When they're anxious, angry, or bored, they focus on food and their fear of fatness. Dieting and exercise become ways of coping with any stress in their lives.

Sometimes nutritional education alone can help change this eating pattern. However, many avid dieters who deny that they have a problem with food may need counseling (which they usually agree to only at their family's insistence) to correct dangerous eating behavior and prevent further complications.

## Compulsive Overeating

People who eat compulsively cannot stop putting food in their mouths. They eat fast and they eat a lot. They eat even when they're full. They may eat around the clock rather than at set meal times, often in private because of embarrassment over how much they consume.

Some mental health professionals describe compulsive eating as a food addiction that is much more likely to develop in women. According to Overeaters Anonymous (OA), an international 12-step program, many women who eat compulsively view food as a source of comfort against feelings of inner emptiness, low self-esteem, and fear of abandonment.

The following behaviors may signal a potential problem with compulsive overeating:

✔ Turning to food when depressed or lonely, when feeling rejected, or as a reward.
✔ A history of failed diets and anxiety when dieting.
✔ Thinking about food throughout the day.
✔ Eating quickly and without pleasure.
✔ Continuing to eat even when you're no longer hungry.
✔ Frequent talking about food, or refusing to talk about food.
✔ Fear of not being able to stop eating once you start.

Recovery from compulsive eating can be challenging because people with this problem cannot give up entirely the substance they abuse. Like everyone else, they must eat. However, they can learn new eating habits and ways of dealing with underlying emotional problems. An OA survey found that most of its members joined to lose weight but later felt the most important effect was their improved emotional, mental, and physical health. As one woman put it, "I came for vanity but stayed for sanity."

## Binge Eating

**Binge eating**—the rapid consumption of an abnormally large amount of food in a relatively short time—often occurs in compulsive eaters. Individuals with a binge-eating disorder typically eat a larger-than-ordinary amount of food during a relatively brief period, feel a lack of control over eating, and binge at least twice a week for at least a six-month period.[25] During most of these episodes, binge eaters experience at least three of the following:

✔ Eating much more rapidly than usual.
✔ Eating until they feel uncomfortably full.
✔ Eating large amounts of food when not feeling physically hungry.
✔ Eating large amounts of food throughout the day with no planned mealtimes.
✔ Eating alone because they are embarrassed by how much they eat and by their eating habits.

In a review of the research on dieting, eating disorders, and weight problems, the National Task Force on the Prevention and Treatment of Obesity found that moderate restriction of calories, combined with behavioral approaches, does not cause binge eating or eating disorders in overweight adults who do not already have a binge eating problem.[26]

Binge eaters may spend up to several hours eating, and consume 2,000 or more calories worth of food in a single binge—more than many people eat in a day. After such binges, they usually do not induce vomiting, use laxatives, or rely on other means (such as exercise) to control weight. They simply get fatter. As their weight climbs, they become depressed, anxious, or troubled by other psychological symptoms to a much greater extent than others of comparable weight.[27]

About 2 percent of Americans—some 5 million in all—may be binge eaters. This unhealthy eating behavior is most common among young women in college and, increasingly, in high school. There is a strong connection between women who binge and feelings of marked rejection from their fathers.[28] People who binge may require professional help to change their behavior. Treatment includes education, behavioral approaches, cognitive therapy, and psychotherapy. As they recognize the reasons for their behavior and begin to confront the underlying issues, those who seek help usually are able to resume normal eating patterns.

## Eating Disorders

According to the American Psychiatric Association, patients with **eating disorders** display a broad range of symptoms that occur along a continuum between those of anorexia nervosa and those of bulimia nervosa.[29] The best known eating disorders are anorexia nervosa, which affects fewer than 1 percent of adolescent women, and bulimia nervosa, which strikes 2 to 3 percent. Many more young women do not have the characteristic symptoms of these disorders but are preoccupied with their weight or experiment with unhealthy forms of dieting. (See Table 6-5 for major risk factors.)

The American Psychiatric Association has developed practice guidelines for the treatment of patients with eating disorders, which include medical, psychological, and behavioral approaches. One of the most scientifically supported is cognitive-behavioral therapy, described in Chapter 3.[30]

## ???? Who Develops Eating Disorders?

Eating disorders affect an estimated 5 to 10 million women and 1 million men. Most people with these problems are young (from ages 14 to 25), white, and affluent, with perfectionistic personalities. According to the Eating Disorders Awareness and Prevention Group of Seattle, 5 to 7 percent of American undergraduates suffer from eating disorders.[31]

 Despite past evidence that eating disorders were primarily problems for white women, they are increasing among men and members of different ethnic and racial groups.[32] (See The X&Y Files: "Men, Women, and Weight.") In the few

---

▼ **Table 6-5   Major Risk Factors for Eating Disorders**

**Biological**
Dieting
Obesity/overweight/pubertal weight gain

**Psychological**
Body image/dissatisfaction/distortions
Low self-esteem
Obsessive-compulsive symptoms
Childhood sexual abuse

**Family**
Parental attitudes and behaviors
Parental comments regarding appearance
Eating-disordered mothers
Misinformation about ideal weight

**Sociocultural**
Peer pressure regarding weight/eating
Media: TV, magazines
Distorted images: toys
Elite athletes as an at-risk group

Source: White, Jane. "The Prevention of Eating Disorders: A Review of the Research on Risk Factors with Implications for Practice." *Journal of Child and Adolescent Psychiatric Nursing,* Vol. 13, No. 2, April 2000.

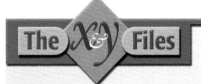 

## Men, Women, and Weight

Women have long been bombarded by the media with idealized images of female bodies that bear little resemblance to the way most women look. Increasingly, more advertisements and men's magazines are featuring idealized male bodies. Sleek, strong, and sculpted, they too do not resemble the bodies most men inhabit. The gap between reality and ideal is getting bigger for both genders.

In the last decade, numerous studies have shown that women in *Playboy* centerfolds and Miss America pageants weigh less than they did in the 1970s. In one analysis, 29 percent of *Playboy* centerfolds and 17 percent of Miss America pageant winners had BMIs below 17.5, one of the criteria for anorexia nervosa and a definite indication of being severely underweight.

As beauty pageant queens and female models have been shrinking, the men featured in *Playgirl* centerfolds have been bulking up. Their BMIs are higher than in the past, as are the BMIs of a sample of Canadian and American men between the ages of 18 and 24. Researchers do not know if the higher BMIs are the result of an increase in lean body mass or body fat. Their theory: The models have become more muscular over time, accounting for their high BMIs, while real guys may simply have gotten fatter.

When college men and women step on a scale or look in a mirror, they react in different ways. In a study of 525 undergraduates, the women failed to see themselves as underweight, even when they were, and perceived themselves as overweight, even when they were not. Many of the women who considered themselves normal weight nonetheless desired to be thinner. Men in the study generally saw themselves as underweight, even when they were not. Most desired to be heavier, though not obese. Women yearning to be thinner and men wanting to be heavier were equally likely to experience what the researchers dubbed *social physique anxiety*.

Women are more prone to unhealthy eating and eating disorders than men, but the incidence among men is increasing. Men and women with these problems share many psychological similarities and experience similar symptoms. However, men are more likely to have other psychiatric disorders and are less likely to seek professional treatment. Some feel that eating disorders fall under the category of "women's diseases." Others may not recognize the symptoms because eating disorders have long been assumed to plague only women.

studies of eating disorders in minority college students that have been completed, African-American female undergraduates had a slightly lower prevalence of eating disorders than whites. Asian Americans reported fewer symptoms of eating disorders but more body dissatisfaction, more concerns about shape, and more intense efforts to lose weight.

In one recent study, researchers analyzed the importance of BMI in evaluating eating disorders in different ethnic groups. The BMIs of Hispanics are generally higher than those of whites, and more Hispanics are categorized as overweight. Asians, as a group, weigh less than whites. In the study, college women with higher BMIs were most concerned about their weight and shape—regardless of their ethnic backgrounds. Data on Hispanics, Asians, and whites of similar weights show equivalent concern about their weight.[33]

In a recent study of Iranian-born young women living in Teheran (Iran) and Los Angeles, those in Teheran were more concerned about their weight than the California women, even though most had little access to images from the Western media and were obliged to wear clothes that hid the shape of their body. They also were as dissatisfied with their body and as likely to have symptoms of disordered eating as those in the United States.[34]

Male and female athletes are vulnerable to eating disorders, because of either the pressure to maintain ideal body weight or to achieve a weight that might enhance their performance. Many female athletes, particularly those participating in sports or activities that emphasize leanness (such as gymnastics, distance running, diving, figure skating, and classical ballet) have subclinical eating disorders that could undermine their nutritional status and energy levels. However, there is often little awareness or recognition of their disordered eating.

If someone you know has an eating disorder, let your friend know you're concerned and that you care. Don't criticize or make fun of his or her eating habits. Encourage your friend to talk about other problems and feelings, and suggest that he or she talk to the school counselor or someone at the mental health center, the family doctor, or another trusted adult. Offer to go along if you think that will make a difference.

## Anorexia Nervosa

Although *anorexia* means "loss of appetite," most individuals with **anorexia nervosa** are, in fact, hungry all the time. For them, food is an enemy—a threat to their sense of self, identity, and autonomy. In the distorted mirror of their mind's eye, they see themselves as fat or flabby even at a normal or below-normal body weight. Some simply feel fat; others think that they are thin in some places and too fat in others, such as the abdomen, buttocks, or thighs.

The incidence of anorexia nervosa has increased in the last three decades in most developed countries. An estimated 0.5 to 1 percent of young women in their late teens and early twenties develop anorexia. According to the American Psychiatric Association's Work Group on Eating Disorders, cases are increasing among males, minorities, women of all ages, and possibly preteens.

In the *restricting* type of anorexia, individuals lose weight by avoiding any fatty foods, and by dieting, fasting, and exercising. Some start smoking as a way of controlling their weight. In the *binge-eating/purging* type, they engage in binge eating, purging (through self-induced vomiting, laxatives, diuretics, or enemas), or both. Obsessed with an intense fear of fatness, they may weigh themselves several times a day, measure various parts of their body, check mirrors to see if they look fat, and try on different items of clothing to see if they feel tight.[35]

## Bulimia Nervosa

Individuals with **bulimia nervosa** go on repeated eating binges and rapidly consume large amounts of food, usually sweets, stopping only because of severe abdominal pain or sleep, or because they are interrupted. Those with *purging* bulimia induce vomiting or take large doses of laxatives to relieve guilt and control their weight. In *nonpurging* bulimia, individuals use other means, such as fasting or excessive exercise, to compensate for binges.

An estimated 1 to 3 percent of adolescent and young American women develop bulimia. Some experiment with bingeing and purging for a few months and then stop when they change their social or living situation. Others develop longer-term bulimia. Among males, this disorder is about one-tenth as common. The average age for developing bulimia is 18.

Most mental health professionals treat bulimia with a combination of nutritional counseling, psychodynamic

▲ Anorexia nervosa is complex in its cause and in its treatment, which usually requires medical, nutritional, and behavioral therapies.

© Richard T. Nowitz/CORBIS

### STRATEGIES FOR PREVENTION

#### Do You Have an Eating Disorder?

Physicians have developed a simple screening test for eating disorders, consisting of the following questions:

▲ Do you make yourself sick because you feel uncomfortably full?

▲ Do you worry you have lost control over how much you eat?

▲ Have you recently lost more than 14 pounds in a three-month period?

▲ Do you believe yourself to be fat when others say you are too thin?

▲ Would you say that food dominates your life?

Score one point for every "yes." A score of two or more is a likely indication of anorexia nervosa or bulimia nervosa.

Source: Miller, Karl. "Treatment Guideline for Eating Disorders." *American Family Physician*, Vol. 62, No. 1, July 1, 2000.

therapy, cognitive-behavioral therapy, individual or group psychotherapy, and medication.[36] The drug most often prescribed is an antidepressant such as fluoxetine (Prozac). About 70 percent of those who complete treatment programs reduce their bingeing and purging, although flare-ups are common in times of stress.

# Being Overweight or Obese

The federal government has developed clinical guidelines that have changed the definition of what it means to be overweight or obese by focusing on body composition. Based on the most extensive review ever of the scientific evidence, the guidelines shift focus away from body weight—the numbers on the scale—to body mass index (BMI), waist circumference, and individual risk factors for diseases and conditions associated with obesity.

The guidelines define **overweight** as a BMI of 25 to 29.9 and **obesity** as a BMI of 30 and above. (See Table 6-1.) As noted earlier, very muscular people may have a high BMI yet not be overweight or obese.

The risk for cardiovascular and other diseases rises significantly in individuals with BMIs above 25; the risk of premature death increases when BMI reaches 30 or above. As BMI levels rise, average blood pressure and total cholesterol levels increase, while high-density lipoprotein, the "good" form of cholesterol, decreases. Men in the highest obesity category have more than twice the risk of hypertension, high blood cholesterol, or both compared with men whose BMIs are in the healthy range. Women in the highest obesity category have four times the risk.

 Although more people in certain regions of the country are likely to be heavy, obesity affects all racial and ethnic groups. A third of white American women are obese, as are nearly 50 percent of African-American and Hispanic women. In some Native American communities, up to 70 percent of all adults are dangerously overweight. Differences in metabolic rates may be one factor.[37]

## Apples Versus Pears

The **waist-to-hip ratio,** which considers the distribution of weight and the location of excess fat, also is important. Excess weight around the abdominal area, creating an apple-shaped silhouette, is associated with increased cardiovascular risk for both men and women.[38] (See Figure 6-1.) A waist circumference of more than 40 inches in men and more than 35 inches in women signifies an increased risk in those with BMIs over 25.[39]

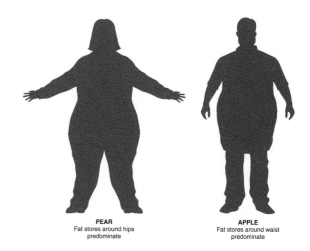

**PEAR**
Fat stores around hips predominate

**APPLE**
Fat stores around waist predominate

▲ **Figure 6-1** Pear-Shaped Versus Apple-Shaped Bodies

Many women accumulate excess pounds in their hips and thighs, giving them a pear shape. This fat, stored primarily for special purposes such as pregnancy and nursing, is more difficult to lose.

When men and women diet, men lose more visceral fat located around the abdominal area. This weight loss produces more cardiovascular benefits for men, including a decrease in triglycerides (fats circulating in the blood) and an increase in the "good" form of cholesterol, high-density lipoprotein (HDL).[40]

## ???? What Causes Obesity?

Are some people fated to be fat? Scientists have identified a gene for a protein that signals the brain to halt food intake or to step up metabolic rate to make use of extra calories. If this gene is defective or malfunctions, it could contribute to weight problems. The discovery of a genetic predisposition to excess weight could explain, at least in part, why children with obese parents tend to be obese themselves, especially if both parents are obese.[41]

A protein named *leptin* also may play a role. When laboratory mice are injected with high doses of leptin, they initially decrease their food intake, increase their metabolic rate, and become much thinner. Eventually, the body adapts to the high levels of leptin and becomes resistant to its effects. However, human studies have had contradictory results.[42] Some researchers suggest that increased leptin does not cause, but is caused by, obesity. A hormone called *ghrelin,* secreted primarily from the stomach, is also believed to play a role in the long-term regulation of body weight. The concentration of ghrelin in a person's blood rises rapidly before a meal and falls once food is eaten.[43]

Scientists now realize that obesity is a complex and serious disorder with multiple causes, including:

✔ **Developmental factors.** Some obese people have a high number of fat cells, others have large fat cells, and the most severely obese have both a high number and large fat cells. Whereas the size of fat cells can increase at any time in life, the number is set during childhood, possibly the result of genetics or overfeeding at a young age.

✔ **Social determinants.** In affluent countries, people in lower socioeconomic classes tend to be more obese. For reasons unknown, those in the upper classes, who can afford as much food as they want, tend to be leaner. Education may be a factor.

✔ **Physical activity.** Obesity tends to go with a sedentary lifestyle. In countries where many people tend to work at physically demanding jobs, obesity is rare. Physical activity prevents obesity by increasing caloric expenditure, decreasing food intake, and increasing metabolic rate.

✔ **Emotional influences.** Obese people are neither more nor less psychologically troubled than others. Psychological problems, such as irritability, depression, and anxiety, are more likely to be the result of obesity than the cause. However, emotions do play a role in weight problems. Just as some people reach for a drink or a drug when they're upset, others cope by overeating, bingeing, or purging.

✔ **Lifestyle.** People who watch more than three hours of TV a day are twice as likely to be obese as those who watch less than an hour. Even those who log between one and two hours are fatter than those who watch just one. Researchers don't know if TV watching causes obesity or if obese people watch more TV, but they have found that the more TV people watch, the less physically active and fit they are.

## Dangers of Obesity

Obesity is a culprit in approximately 280,000 deaths in the United States every year and in many serious health problems (see Figure 6-2), adding an estimated $31 billion to health-care costs every year.[44] Obesity has long been singled out as a major health threat that increases the risk of many chronic diseases. During ten years of tracking the health of middle-aged men and women, the incidence of diabetes, gallstones, hypertension, heart disease, and colon cancer increased with the degree of overweight in both sexes. Those with BMIs of 35 or more were approximately 20 times more likely to develop diabetes. Individuals who were overweight but not obese, with BMIs between 25 and 29.9, were significantly more likely than leaner women to develop gallstones, high blood pressure, high cholesterol, and heart disease.[45] Overweight men were also more likely to suffer strokes.

Overweight individuals who have surgery are more likely to develop complications. Even relatively small amounts of excess fat—as little as 5 pounds—can add to the dangers in those already at risk for hypertension and diabetes. According to a new study supported by the National Heart, Lung, and Blood Institute, being overweight, even if not obese, increases the risk of heart failure.[46] Obesity also causes alterations in various measures of immune function.[47]

Obesity now is considered a greater threat to a healthy heart than smoking. People who both smoke and are obese are at especially high risk of cardiovascular disease. Although some smokers have felt that they couldn't lose weight until they stopped smoking, researchers have found that weight loss among smokers is possible and beneficial, leading to a reduction in other risk factors, such as lower blood pressure and lower cholesterol.[48] Health educators also are targeting teenage dieters, who are more likely to begin smoking, often to help control their weight.[49]

Researchers estimate that the effects of obesity on health are the equivalent of twenty years of aging.[50] However, as discussed in Chapter 4, activity levels are critically important. Fat-and-fit people who exercise regularly are at less risk of dying prematurely than leaner sedentary men and women. Unfortunately, many heavy Americans are inactive and in increased danger of dying of all causes, particularly heart disease and cancer.

In our calorie-conscious and thinness-obsessed society, obesity also affects quality of life, including sense of

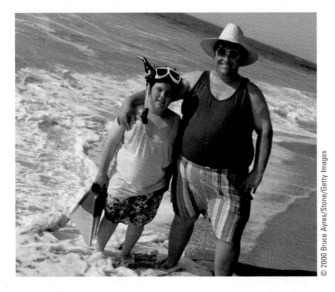

▲ Heredity plays a role in the tendency toward obesity, but so do environment and behavior.

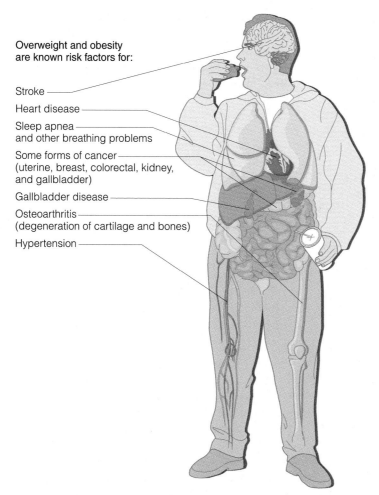

Overweight and obesity
are known risk factors for:

Stroke

Heart disease

Sleep apnea
and other breathing problems

Some forms of cancer
(uterine, breast, colorectal, kidney,
and gallbladder)

Gallbladder disease

Osteoarthritis
(degeneration of cartilage and bones)

Hypertension

Obesity is associated with:

High blood cholesterol

Urinary stress incontinence

Complications of pregnancy

Menstrual irregularities

Hirsutism (excess facial and body hair)

Psychological disorders such as depression

Increased risk during surgery

▲ **Figure 6-2** Dangers of Obesity

vitality and physical pain.[51] Many see it as a heavy psychological burden, a sign of failure, laziness, or inadequate willpower. Overweight men and women often blame themselves for becoming heavy, and feel guilty and depressed as a result. In fact, the psychological problems once considered the cause of obesity may be its consequence.

Does obesity lead to a shorter life? The answer is far from clear—and intensely controversial. Studies have shown that overweight middle-aged men and women have a higher risk of dying from all causes, especially from heart disease and certain cancers, than those who are normal weight or underweight. The risk rises if they develop diabetes.[52] Among men who have smoked, the risk of dying is almost two times higher for those with the highest body weight than for those with the lowest body weight. Researchers have found an association between greater body mass index and higher death rates.[53]

## ???? How Can I Overcome a Weight Problem?

Each year an estimated 15 to 35 percent of Americans go on a diet, but no matter how much weight they lose, 95 percent gain it back within five years. Most dieters cut back on food, not because they want to feel better, but because they want to look better. Those who drastically reduce their food intake and make weight loss a major part of their lives may be jeopardizing their physical and psychological well-being.

The best approach to a weight problem depends on how overweight a person is. For extreme obesity, medical treatments, including surgery, may be necessary to overcome the danger to a person's health and life. People who are moderately or mildly obese can lose weight through different approaches, including behavioral modification (monitoring food intake, altering eating style, avoiding eating "triggers," and similar strategies); cognitive therapy (changing thoughts or beliefs that lead to overeating); and social support (participating in groups such as Overeaters Anonymous). The keys to overcoming obesity are acknowledging biological limits, addressing individual differences, altering unrealistic expectations, setting limits, and learning coping skills to provide self-nurturing without relying on food.[54]

## Severe Obesity

A BMI higher than 40 (or higher than 35 for those with other conditions) indicates a life-threatening condition. Because of the medical dangers they face, some severely obese men and women, as a last resort, may undergo surgery to reduce the volume of their stomachs and to tighten the passageway from the stomach to the intestine. Others opt for a gastric bubble, a soft, polyurethane sac placed in the stomach to make the person feel full while following a low-calorie diet. It is not yet clear whether people who lose weight with this bubble will be able to keep it off.

## Mild to Moderate Obesity

For individuals with a BMI of 30 to 39, doctors recommend a six-month trial of lifestyle therapy, including a supervised diet and exercise. The initial goal should be a 10 percent reduction in weight, an amount that reduces obesity-related risks. With success and if warranted, individuals can attempt to lose more weight.

## Overweight

Rather than going on a low-calorie diet, people with BMIs of 25 to 29 should cut back moderately on their food intake and concentrate on developing healthy eating and exercise habits. Many moderately to mildly overweight people turn to national organizations such as Weight Watchers or to other commercial weight-loss groups. Most of these programs offer behavior-modification techniques, inspirational lectures, and carefully designed nutritional programs, but dropout rates are high. As many as half the members drop out in six weeks.

## Practical Guide to Weight Management

No diet—high-protein, low-fat, or high-carbohydrate—can produce permanent weight loss. Successful weight management, the American Dietetic Association has con-

cluded, "requires a lifelong commitment to healthful lifestyle behaviors emphasizing sustainable and enjoyable eating practices and daily physical activity."[55] Studies have shown that successful dieters were highly motivated, monitored their food intake, increased their activity, set realistic goals, and received social support from others. Another key to long-term success is tailoring any weight-loss program to an individual's gender, lifestyle, and cultural, racial, and ethnic values. You also have to do your homework; look into the claims of promoters of diet programs. (See Savvy Consumer: "Weight-Loss Consumer Bill of Rights.")

## Customize Your Weight-Loss Plan

"If there's one thing we've learned in decades of research into weight management, it's that the one-diet-fits-all approach doesn't work," says clinical psychologist David Schlundt of Vanderbilt University.[56] The key is recognizing the ways you tend to put on weight and developing strategies to overcome them. Here are some examples:

✔ Do you simply like food and consume lots of it? If so, keep a diary of everything you put in your mouth and tally up your daily total in calories and fat grams. The numbers may stun you. Look for the source of most of the calories—probably high-fat foods such as whole milk, chocolate, cookies, fried foods, potato chips, steaks—and cut down on how much and how often you eat them. Also watch portion sizes. A cup of cooked grains or vegetables is the size of a small fist; a teaspoon of butter or margarine is a thumb print.

✔ Do you eat when you're bored, sad, frustrated, or worried? If so, you may be especially susceptible to cues that trigger eating. "People get in the habit of using food to soothe bad feelings or cope with boredom," says Schlundt. "Sometimes the real issue is a self-esteem or body-image problem." Dealing with these concerns is generally more helpful in the long run than dieting.

✔ Do you graze, nibbling on snacks rather than eating regular meals? If so, limit yourself to low-calorie, low-fat foods, like carrots, celery, grapes, or air-popped popcorn. Take sips of water regularly to freshen your mouth. Even if you're having only a few crackers or carrots, put them on a plate, and try to eat in the same place, preferably while seated. This helps you break the habit of putting food in your mouth without thinking.

## Avoid Diet Traps

Whatever your eating style, there are only two effective strategies for losing weight: eating less and exercising more. Unfortunately, most people search for easier alternatives

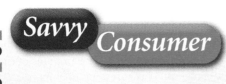

## Weight-Loss Consumer Bill of Rights (An Example)

**Warning:** Rapid weight loss may cause serious health problems. Rapid weight loss is weight loss of more than 1½ to 2 pounds per week or weight loss of more than 1 percent of body weight per week after the second week of participation in a weight-loss program.

Consult your personal physician before starting any weight-loss program.

Only permanent lifestyle changes, such as making healthful food choices and increasing physical activity, promote long-term weight loss and successful maintenance.

Qualifications of the weight-loss provider should be available upon request.

**You have a right to:**

- Ask questions about the potential health risks of this program and its nutritional content, psychological support, and educational components.

- Receive an itemized statement of the actual or estimated price of the weight-loss program, including extra products, services, supplements, examinations, and laboratory tests.

- Know the actual or estimated duration of the program.

- Know the name, address, and qualifications of the dietitian or nutritionist who has reviewed and approved the weight-loss program.

Source: Whitney, Eleanor, and Sharon Rolfes. *Understanding Nutrition,* 9th ed. Belmont, CA: Wadsworth/Thomson Learning, 2002, p. 277.

---

that almost invariably turn into dietary dead ends. Four common traps to avoid are diet foods, the yo-yo diet, the very low-calorie diet, and diet pills.

## Diet Foods

According to the Calorie Control Council, 90 percent of Americans choose some foods labeled "light." But even though these foods keep growing in popularity, Americans' weight keeps rising. There are several reasons: Many people think choosing a food that's lower in calories, fat-free, or light gives them a license to eat as much as they want. What they don't realize is that many foods that are low in fat are still high in sugar and calories. Refined carbohydrates, rapidly absorbed into the bloodstream, raise blood glucose levels. As they fall, appetite increases.

What about the artificial sweeteners and fake fats that appear in many diet products? Nutritionists caution to use them in moderation, and not to substitute them for basic foods, such as grains, fruits, and vegetables. Foods made with fat substitutes may have fewer grams of fat, but they don't necessarily have significantly fewer calories. Many people who consume reduced-fat, fat-free, or sugar-free sodas, cookies, chips, and other snacks often cut back on more nutritious foods, such as fruits and vegetables. They also tend to eat more of the low- or no-fat foods so that their daily calorie intake either stays the same or actually increases.

## The Yo-Yo Syndrome

On-and-off-again dieting, especially by means of very low-calorie diets (under 800 calories a day), can be self-defeating and dangerous. Some studies have shown that weight cycling may make it more difficult to lose weight or keep it off. (See Figure 6-3.) Repeated cycles of rapid weight loss followed by weight gain may even change food preferences. Chronic crash dieters often come to prefer foods that combine sugar and fat, such as cake frosting.

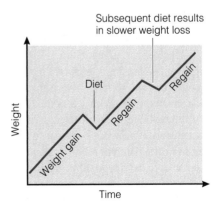

▲ **Figure 6-3** Weight-Cycling Effect of Repeated Dieting
Each round of dieting is typically followed by a rebound leading to a greater weight gain.

To avoid the yo-yo syndrome and overcome its negative effects: Exercise. Researchers at the University of Pennsylvania found that when overweight women who also exercised went off a very low-calorie diet, their metabolism did not stay slow but bounced back to the appropriate level for their new, lower body weight. The reason may be exercise's ability to preserve muscle tissue. The more muscle tissue you have, the higher your metabolic rate.

## Very Low-Calorie Diets

Any diet that promises to take pounds off fast can be dangerous. For reasons that scientists don't fully understand, rapid weight loss is linked with increased mortality. Most risky are very low-calorie diets that provide fewer than 800 calories a day. Whenever people cut back drastically on calories, they immediately lose several pounds because of a loss of fluid. As soon as they return to a more normal way of eating, they regain this weight.

On a very low-calorie diet, as much as 50 percent of the weight you lose may be muscle (so you'll actually look flabbier). Because your heart is a muscle, it may become so weak that it no longer can pump blood through your body. In addition, your blood pressure may plummet, causing dizziness, light-headedness, and fatigue. You may develop nausea and abdominal pain. You may lose hair. If you're a woman, your menstrual cycle may become irregular, or you may stop menstruating altogether. As you lose more water, you also lose essential vitamins, and your metabolism slows down. Even reaction time slows, and crash dieters may not be able to respond as quickly as usual.

Once you go off an extreme diet—as you inevitably must—your metabolism remains slow, even though you're no longer restricting your food intake. The human body appears to alter its energy use to compensate for weight loss. These metabolic changes may make it harder for people to maintain a reduced body weight after dieting.

## ???? Do High-Protein, Low-Carbohydrate Diets Work?

After trying the low-fat diets popular in the 1980s and 1990s, many Americans weighed more than ever. High-protein, low-carbohydrate diets, such as the Atkins diet and sugar busters, have emerged as the first diet fad of the twenty-first century. These diets appeal to many people because they can eat as much protein as they want, including steaks, eggs, and fatty foods they'd long been told to shun, as long as they strictly limit their carbohydrates.

The American College of Sports Medicine, the American Dietetic Association, and other professional groups have challenged these diets. As they note, no scientific evidence proves that a diet providing more than the 10 to 15 percent protein recommended by federal guidelines enhances health or athletic performance. The American Heart Association has issued scientific advisory warnings that high-protein diets consisting of large amounts of meat are potentially dangerous because they may increase the risk of heart diseases, diabetes, stroke, kidney and liver disease, and cancer.[57] Although it is possible to lose weight on a high-protein diet, the reason is the same as with other quick weight-loss diets: low calorie count.

## Diet Pills and Products

In their search for a quick fix to weight problems, millions of people have tried often-risky remedies. In the 1920s, some women swallowed patented weight-loss capsules that turned out to be tapeworm eggs. In the 1960s and 1970s, addictive amphetamines were common diet aids. In the 1990s, appetite suppressants known as fen-phen (*fen* referring to fenfluramine [Pondimin] or dexfenfluramine [Redux], appetite depressants; and *phen* referring to phentermine, a type of amphetamine) became popular. They were taken off the market after being linked to heart valve probems.

More weight-loss drugs have won FDA approval, including Meridia (sibutramine) and Xenical (orlistat). Both are intended only for people with a BMI of at least 30 or a BMI of 27 with additional risk factors. Although available only by prescription, Xenical and Meridia are being marketed over the Internet to anyone who fills out a computerized form reviewed by a company doctor. As a result, many people are taking this medication without medical supervision. Such misuse could cause health risks.

The search for the perfect diet drug continues—with plenty of economic incentives for drug makers. By some estimates, the potential market for weight-loss pills totals at least $5 billion. Other diet products, including diet sodas and low-fat foods, also are a very big business. Many people rely on meal replacements, usually shakes or snack bars, to lose or keep off weight. If used appropriately—as actual replacements rather than supplements to regular meals and snacks—they can be a useful strategy for weight loss. Yet people who use these products aren't necessarily sure to slim down. In fact, people who consume such products often gain weight because they think that they can afford to add high-calorie treats to their diet.

## Exercise: The Best Solution

You may think that exercise will make you want to eat more. Actually, it has the opposite effect. The combination of exercise and cutting back on calories may be the most effective way of taking weight off and keeping it off. According to the National Weight Control Registry, a data-

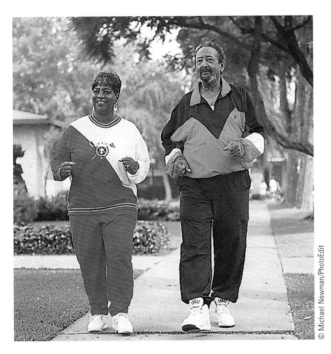

▲ The most effective and healthful way to manage your weight is to combine dietary changes with regular physical exercise.

base of people who have kept off a minimum of 30 pounds for more than five years, most successful weight losers both restrict how much they eat and increase their physical activity.

Exercise has other benefits: It increases energy expenditure, builds up muscle tissue, burns off fat stores, and stimulates the immune system. Exercise also may reprogram metabolism so that more calories are burned during and after a workout. (See Chapter 4 for a complete discussion of exercise.)

Moderate physical activity also can help control weight. Recent studies have found that everyday activities, such as walking, gardening, and heavy household chores, are as effective as a structured exercise program in maintaining or losing weight. Scientists use the acronym **NEAT**—for **non-exercise activity thermogenesis**—to describe such nonvolitional movements and have verified that this can be an effective way of burning calories. In a study of 16 nonobese adults, intentional exercise and metabolic rate had little effect on variations in weight gain, whereas NEAT did. One form of NEAT, fidgeting, turns out to play an important role in daily energy expenditure—and may be particularly useful in preventing weight gain after overeating.

Once you start an exercise program, keep it up. People who've started an exercise program during or after a weight-loss program are consistently more successful in keeping off most of the pounds they've shed.

## STRATEGIES FOR CHANGE

### Working Off Weight

▲ Get moving. Take the stairs instead of the elevator. Get off the bus a few blocks from your home and walk the rest of the way.

▲ Walk. Most people find it hard to make excuses for not walking 15 minutes every day. Once you start, increase gradually so that you go farther and faster.

▲ Exercise daily. You're more likely to lose and keep weight off if you exercise regularly. Try to burn 1,800 to 2,000 calories a week through exercise—the equivalent of 18 to 20 miles of walking or jogging.

▲ Get physical. There are more ways to burn calories than traditional exercise activities: Dancing, hiking, and gardening can all help you get in shape. Check your campus bulletin boards and newspapers for information on rock-climbing, kayaking, skiing, and other fun forms of working out.

 How do nutrients fuel the bodies of active teens?

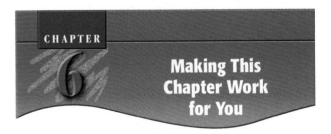

CHAPTER 6 **Making This Chapter Work for You**

1. The best way to determine whether you are a healthy weight is to
   a. measure your waist and hips.
   b. calculate your body mass index.
   c. check ideal weight tables.
   d. calculate your body fat percentage.

2. Body composition estimates can be obtained with which of the following methods?
   a. skinfold fat measurement
   b. home body fat analyzers

c. biofeedback analysis
d. basal metabolic rate measurement

3. According to the set-point theory:
   a. the physiological drive to consume food is stimulated by hormones
   b. body fat is maintained at a predetermined level by an unconscious control system.
   c. the psychological desire to eat is determined by the size of the hypothalamus.
   d. fat cells cannot increase in number beyond a genetically determined point.

4. Which of the following statements about body weight is *not* true?
   a. BMI is a mathematical formula that correlates with body fat.
   b. Daily energy requirements depend on your activity level.
   c. Only women have body weight and shape concerns.
   d. The infamous "freshman 15"—the 15 pounds that first-year students gain—turns out to be a myth.

5. Which of the following eating behaviors may be a warning sign of a serious eating disorder?
   a. vegetarianism
   b. compulsive food washing
   c. binge eating
   d. weight gain during the first year of college

6. Individuals with anorexia nervosa
   a. believe they are overweight even if they are extremely thin.
   b. typically feel full all the time, which limits their food intake.
   c. usually look overweight even though their body mass index is normal.
   d. have a reduced risk for heart-related abnormalities.

7. Bulimia nervosa is
   a. characterized by excessive sleeping followed by periods of insomnia.
   b. found primarily in older women who are concerned with the aging process.
   c. associated with the use of laxatives or excessive exercise to control weight.
   d. does not have serious health consequences.

8. Which of the following statements is *not* true?
   a. Obesity is a greater threat to heart health than smoking.
   b. Men who accumulate fat around their waist are at increased risk for cardiovascular risk.
   c. Individuals who are obese are neither more nor less psychologically troubled than people of normal weight.
   d. Children with an obese parent are more likely to be thin because of their embarrassment about the parent's appearance.

9. Weight management strategies that work include which of the following?
   a. Increase your activity level and eat less, aiming for a weekly weight loss of about 1½ pounds.
   b. Ask friends for recommendations for methods that helped them lose weight quickly.
   c. Practice good eating habits about 50 percent of the time so that you can balance your cravings with healthy food.
   d. Try a number of weight-loss diets to find the one that works best for you.

10. Which of the following statements is true?
    a. Very low-calorie diets increase metabolism, which helps burn calories more quickly.
    b. An individual eating low-calorie or fat-free foods can increase the serving sizes.
    c. High-protein, low-carbohydrate diets may increase the risk of heart disease.
    d. Yo-yo dieting works best for long-term weight loss.

Answers to these questions can be found on page 415.

## Critical Thinking

1. Do you think you have a weight problem? If so, what makes you think so? Is your perception based on your actual BMI measurement or on how you believe you look? If you found out that your BMI is within the ideal range, would that change your opinion about your body? Why or why not?

2. Different cultures have different standards for body weight and attractiveness. Within our society, men and women often seem to follow different standards. What influences have shaped your personal feelings about desired weight?

3. Suppose one of your roommates appears to have symptoms of an eating disorder. You have told him or her of your concerns, but your roommate has denied having a problem and brushed off your fears. What can you do to help this individual? Should you contact his or her parent? Why or why not?

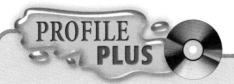

Discover the methods used for body composition assessment and the health risks associated with where you store fat, by participating in the following activities on your Profile Plus CD-ROM:

Body Composition * Weight and Health: Disease Risk

## SITES & BYTES

### National Eating Disorders Association
**www.nationaleatingdisorders.org**

The National Eating Disorders Association came into being in 2001, when Eating Disorders Awareness & Prevention joined forces with the American Anorexia Bulimia Association to create the largest eating disorders prevention and advocacy organization in the world. This site has abundant resources on all aspects of eating disorders, including information for both females and males; the latest information pertaining to prevention, health consequences, body image, statistics, and treatment; sources for referrals; and education curriculum resources.

### Something's Fishy Website on Eating Disorders
**www.something-fishy.org**

This comprehensive website features a wealth of information on all types of eating disorders, as well as current news, signs and symptoms, suggestions on how to help others, cultural issues, doctors and patients, prevention, online support, and an online newsletter.

### NHLBI Obesity Education Initiative
**www.nhlbi.nih.gov/about/oei/index.htm**

This site by the Obesity Education Initiative is sponsored by the National Heart, Lung, and Blood Institute (NHLBI) of the National Institutes of Health. The overall purpose of the initiative is to help reduce the prevalence of overweight and physical inactivity, thereby reducing the risk, morbidity, and mortality of coronary heart disease. The site features information on weight management and obesity for the general public and for health professionals. Interactive features include a BMI calculator, a menu planner, and treatment guidelines.

Please note that links are subject to change. If you find a broken link, use a search engine such as www.yahoo.com and search for the website by typing in keywords.

### InfoTrac College Edition Activity
Lyn Patrick. "Eating Disorders: A Review of the Literature with Emphasis on Medical Complications and Clinical Nutrition." *Alternative Medicine Review*, Vol. 7, No. 3, June 2002, p. 184 (19).

1. What psychiatric disorder has the highest overall mortality and is the leading cause of death in young women between the ages of 15 and 24?

2. What are some of the prevailing risk factors for the development of eating disorders?

3. What are common approaches to the treatment of anorexia nervosa and bulimia nervosa?

You can find additional readings relating to eating patterns and problems with InfoTrac College Edition, an online library of more than 900 journals and publications. Follow the instructions for accessing InfoTrac that were packaged with your textbook; then search for articles using a keyword search.

For additional links, resources, and suggested readings on InfoTrac, visit our Health & Wellness Resource Center at http://health.wadsworth.com.

## Key Terms

The terms listed here are used within the chapter on the page indicated. Definitions of the terms are in the Glossary at the end of the book.

anorexia nervosa  132
appetite  127
basal metabolic rate
   (BMR)  127
binge eating  130

body mass index (BMI)  124
bulimia nervosa  132
calorie  127
eating disorders  130
hunger  127

non-exercise activity
   thermogenesis
   (NEAT)  139
obesity  133
overweight  133

satiety  127
set-point theory  127
waist-to-hip ratio
   (WHR)  133

## References

1. National Institute of Diabetes & Digestive & Kidney Diseases, www.niddk.nih.gov.
2. Sturm, Roland, et al. "Datawatch: The Effects of Obesity, Smoking and Drinking on Medical Problems and Costs." *Journal of Health Affairs,* Vol. 21, No. 2, March 2002.
3. "Magazine Ideals Wrong." *Journal of the American Medical Association,* Vol. 286, No. 4, July 25, 2001, p. 409.
4. Tiggeman, Marika. "The Impact of Adolescent Girls' Life Concerns and Leisure Activities on Body Dissatisfaction, Disordered Eating, and Self-Esteem." *Journal of Genetic Psychology,* Vol. 162, No. 2, June 2001, p. 133.
5. Cohane, Geoffrey, and Harrison Pope. "Body Image in Boys: A Review of the Literature." *International Journal of Eating Disorders,* Vol. 29, No. 4, May 2001.
6. Arriaza, Ceceilia, and Traci Mann. "Ethnic Differences in Eating Disorders Among College Students: The Confounding Role of Body Mass Index." *Journal of American College Health,* Vol. 49, No. 6, May 2001, p. 309.
7. Lofton, Stacy, and Tim Bungum. "Attitudes and Behaviors Toward Weight, Body Shape, and Eating in Male and Female College Students." *Research Quarterly for Exercise and Sport,* Vol. 72, No. 1, March 2001, p. A-32.
8. "DiGioacchino, Rita, et al. "Body Dissatisfaction Among White and African American Male and Female College Students." *Eating Behaviors,* Vol. 2, December 2001, p. 39.
9. Cramer, M., and C. Murray. "Body Dissatisfaction Across Age and Gender: Function Vs. Appearance." *Gerontologist,* October 15, 2000, p. 202.
10. Choo, Vivien. "WHO Reassesses Appropriate Body-Mass Index for Asian Populations." *Lancet,* Vol. 360, No. 9328, July 20, 2002, p. 235.
11. "Use of Body Mass Index and Waist Circumference to Predict Risk of Chronic Disease." *Journal of the American Dietetic Association,* Vol. 101, No. 6, June 2001, p. 708.
12. McCaffree, Jim. "Eating Disorders: All in the Family?" *Journal of the American Dietetic Association,* Vol. 101, No. 6, June 2001, p. 622.
13. Nagel, Deborah, et al. "Evaluation of a Screening Test for Female College Athletes with Eating Disorders and Disordered Eating." *Journal of Athletic Training,* Vol. 35, No. 4, October–December 2000, p. 431.
14. "Young Female Athletes at Risk, Say U.S. Experts." *Lancet,* Vol. 356, No. 9234, September 16, 2000.
15. "Body Image Concerns," *Nutrition Research Newsletter,* Vol. 19, No. 5, May 2000.
16. Prouty, Ann, et al. "College Women: Eating Behaviors and Help-Seeking Preferences." *Adolescence,* Vol. 37, No. 146, Summer 2002, p. 353.
17. Roerr, Sharon, et al. "Eating Disorder a Risk in Sorority and Dorm Students." *Journal of the American College of Nutrition,* Vol. 21, August 2002, p. 307.
18. O'Dea, Jennifer, and Suzanne Abraham. "Eating and Exercise Disorders in Young College Men." *Journal of American College Health,* Vol. 50, No. 4, May 2002, p. 273.
19. Cooley, Eric, and Tamina Toray. "Disordered Eating in College Freshman Women: A Prospective Study." *Journal of American College Health,* Vol. 49, No. 5, March 2001, p. 229.
20. Keeling, Richard. "Fear, Shame and Health Promotion." *Journal of American College Health,* Vol. 50, No. 4, January 2002, p. 149.
21. Graham, Melody, and Amy Jones. "Freshman 15: Valid Theory or Harmful Myth?" *Journal of American College Health,* Vol. 50, No. 4, January 2002, p. 171.
22. Holben, David. "International Students Gain Fat and Weight from American Diet." Presentation, American Dietetic Association, October 18, 2000.
23. "Emergence of Dieting," *Nutrition Research Newsletter,* Vol. 19, No. 12, December 2000, p. 3.
24. Field, Alison, et al. "Peer, Parent, and Media Influences on the Development of Weight Concerns and Frequent Dieting Among Preadolescent and Adolescent Girls and Boys." *Pediatrics,* Vol. 107, No. 1, January 2001, p. 54.
25. "Nutrient Intake of Binge Eaters." *Nutrition Research Newsletter,* Vol. 20, No. 3, March 2001, p. 3.
26. "Dieting and Development of Eating Disorders in Overweight and Obese Adults." *Journal of the American Dietetic Association,* Vol. 101, No. 3, March 2001, p. 369.
27. "Attempting to Lose Weight, Restraint, and Binge Eating." *Nutrition Research Newsletter,* Vol. 20, No. 3, March 2001, p. 6.
28. LeTourneau, Melanie. "All in the Family." *Psychology Today,* Vol. 33, No. 4, July 2000.
29. Walling, Anne. "A New Screening Tool for Patients with Eating Disorders." *American Family Physician,* Vol. 61, No. 7, April 1, 2000.
30. Wilson, G., and Stewart Agras. "Practice Guidelines for Eating Disorders." *Behavior Therapy,* Vol. 32, No. 2, Spring 2001, p. 219.
31. Hubbard, Kim, et al. "Out of Control." *People,* April 23, 1999.
32. Woodside, D. Blake, et al. "Comparisons of Men with Full or Partial Eating Disorders, Men Without Eating Disorders, and Women with Eating Disorders in the Community." *American Journal of Psychiatry,* Vol. 158, April 2001, p. 570.
33. Arriaza and Mann, "Ethnic Differences in Eating Disorders Among College Students."
34. "Eating Disorders and Culture." *Harvard Mental Health Letter,* Vol. 18, No. 12, June 2002.

35. Sadovsky, Richard. "A Review of Anorexia Nervosa in Primary Care." *American Family Physician,* Vol. 65, No. 3, February 1, 2002, p. 478.

36. Wilson, Terence, et al. "Cognitive-Behavioral Therapy for Bulimia Nervosa: Time Course and Mechanisms of Change." *Journal of Consulting and Clinical Psychology,* Vol. 70, No. 2, April 2002, p. 267.

37. Weyer, Christian. "Basal Metabolic Rate in African-American Women." *Journal of Clinical Nutrition,* July 1999.

38. Seidell, Jacob, et al. "Abdominal Adiposity and Risk of Heart Disease." *Journal of the American Medical Association,* Vol. 281, No. 24, June 23, 1999.

39. "Fat Distribution Tied to Disease Risk." *Women's Health Weekly,* June 27, 2002, p. 16.

40. "Gender Difference in Weight Reduction." *Nutrition Research Newsletter,* Vol. 18, No. 2, February 1999.

41. Magid, Barry. "Is Biology Destiny After All?" *Journal of Psychotherapy Practice & Research,* Vol. 4, No. 1, Winter 1995.

42. Heymsfield, Steven, et al. "Recombinant Leptin for Weight Loss in Obese and Lean Adults." *Journal of the American Medical Association,* Vol. 282, No. 16, October 27, 1999.

43. Cummings, D., et al. "Plasma Ghrelin Levels After Diet-Induced Weight Loss or Gastric Bypass Surgery." *New England Journal of Medicine,* Vol. 346, No. 21, May 23, 2002, p. 1623.

44. Wang, Guijing, et al. "Economic Burden of Cardiovascular Disease Associated with Excess Body Weight in U.S. Adults." *American Journal of Preventive Medicine,* Vol. 23, No. 1, p. 1.

45. "Overweight, Obesity Threaten U.S. Health Gains." *FDA Consumer,* Vol. 36, No. 2, March–April, 2002, p. 8.

46. National Heart, Lung, and Blood Institute, www.nhlbi.nih.gov.

47. "Dangers Are Overlooked." *Medical Letter on the CDC & FDA,* August 12, 2001.

48. Wilson, K., et al. "Impact on Smoking Status on Weight Loss and Cardiovascular Risk Factors." *Journal of Epidemiology & Community Health,* Vol. 55, No. 3, March 2001, p. 213.

49. Austin, S. Bryn, and Steven Grotmaker. "Dieting and Smoking Initiation in Early Adolescent Girls and Boys: A Prospective Study." *American Journal of Public Health,* Vol. 91, No. 3, March 2001, p. 446.

50. Sturm, "Datawatch."

51. "Weight Change Affects Quality of Life." *JOPERD—The Journal of Physical Education, Recreation & Dance,* Vol. 71, No. 2, February 2000.

52. "Keeping Diabetes at Bay." *Nutrition Action Healthletter,* Vol. 28, No. 6, July 2001, p. 11.

53. "Weight Loss Can Decrease Mortality Risk." *Medical Letter on the CDC & FDA,* November 26, 2000.

54. Murphy, Dee. "Fit or Fad: A Dieting Decision." *Current Health 2,* Vol. 27, No. 7, March 2001, p. 16.

55. Cummings, Sue, et al. "Position of the American Dietetic Association: Weight Management." *Journal of the American Dietetic Association,* Vol. 102, No. 8, August 2002, pp. 11, 1145.

56. Schlundt, David. Personal interview.

57. "Secrets of Successful Dieters." *Harvard Women's Health Watch,* Vol. 9, No. 9, May 2002.

# Communication and Sexuality

**After studying the material in this chapter, you should be able to:**

- **Describe** the role verbal and nonverbal communication plays in forming and maintaining relationships.
- **Define** friendship and **explain** how friendship grows.
- **Discuss** the behavior and emotional expectations for friendship, dating, and intimate relationships.
- **Compare** and **contrast** romantic love and mature love.
- **Identify** the problems likely to affect long-term relationships, and **explain** how they can be prevented.
- **Describe** the male and female reproductive systems and the functions of the individual structures of each system.
- **Describe** conditions or issues unique to women's and men's sexual health.
- **Define** sexual orientation and **give** **examples** of sexual diversity.
- **List** the range of sexual behaviors practiced by adults.

We are born social. From our first days of life, we reach out to others, struggle to express ourselves, strive to forge connections. People make us smile, laugh, cry, hope, dream, pray. The fabric of our personalities and lives becomes richer as others weave through it the threads of their experiences.

We are also innately sexual. Our biological maleness or femaleness is an integral part of who we are, how we see ourselves, and how we relate to others. Among all of our involvements with others, sexual intimacy, or physical closeness, can be the most rewarding. Although sexual expression and experience can provide intense joy, they also can involve great emotional turmoil.

You are ultimately responsible for your sexual health and behavior. You make decisions that affect how you express your sexuality, how you respond sexually, and how you give and receive sexual pleasure. Yet most sexual activity involves another person. Therefore, your decisions about sex—more so than those you make about nutrition, drugs, or exercise—affect other people. Recognizing this fact is the key to responsible sexuality.

Sexual responsibility means learning about your relationships, your body, your partner's body, your sexual development and preferences, and the health risks associated with sexual activity. This chapter, an introduction to your social and sexual self, is an exploration of relationships

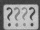

and sexual issues in today's world. It provides the information and insight you can use in making decisions and choosing behaviors that are responsible for all concerned.

## Personal Communication

Getting to know someone is one of life's greatest challenges and pleasures. When you find another person intriguing—as a friend, as a teacher, as a colleague, as a possible partner—you want to find out as much as you can about him or her, and you want to share more and more information about yourself. Roommates may talk for endless hours. Friends may spend years getting to know each other. Partners in committed relationships may delight in learning new things about each other.

Communication stems from a desire to know and a decision to tell. Each of us chooses what information about ourselves we want to disclose and what we want to conceal or keep private. But in opening up to others, we increase our own self-knowledge and understanding.

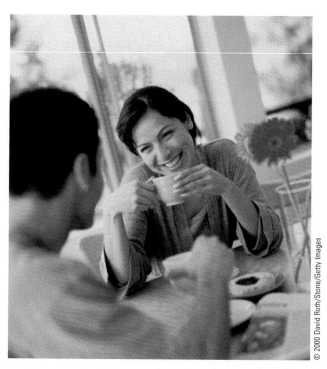

▲ Good communication is essential to a healthy and successful relationship.

### Talking and Listening

A great deal of daily communication focuses on facts: on the who, what, where, when, and how. Information is easy to convey and comprehend. Emotions are not. Some people have great difficulty saying "I appreciate you" or "I care about you," even though they are genuinely appreciative and caring. Others find it hard to know what to say in response and how to accept such expressions of affection.

Some people feel that relationships shouldn't require any effort, that there's no need to talk of responsibility between people who care about each other. Yet responsibility is implicit in our dealings with anyone or anything we value—and what can be more valuable than those with whom we share our lives? Friendships and other intimate relationships always demand an emotional investment, but the rewards they yield are great.

Sometimes people convey strong emotions with a kiss or a hug, a pat or a punch, but such actions aren't precise enough to communicate exact thoughts. Stalking out of a room and slamming the door may be clear signs of anger, but they don't explain what caused the anger or suggest what to do about it. You must learn how to communicate all feelings clearly and appropriately if you hope to become truly close to another person.

As two people build a relationship, they must sharpen their communication skills so they can discuss all the issues they may confront. They must learn how to communicate

anger as well as affection, sadness as well as joy—and they must listen as carefully as they speak.

Listening involves more than waiting for the other person to stop talking. Listening is an active process of trying to understand the other person's feelings and motivation. Effective listeners ask questions when they're not sure they understand the other person and prompt the other person to continue.

### Nonverbal Communication

More than 90 percent of communication may be nonverbal. While we speak with our vocal cords, we communicate with our facial expressions, tone of voice, hands, shoulders, legs, torsos, posture. "Body language is a very elementary level of communication that people react to without realizing why," observes Albert Mehrabian, a professor of psychology at the University of California, Los Angeles, and author of *Silent Messages*. "It's the building block upon which more advanced verbal forms of communication rest."[1]

Learning to interpret what people *don't* say can reveal more than what they *do* say. "Understanding nonverbal communication is probably the best tool there is for a good life of communicating, be it personally or professionally," says Marilyn Maple, an educator at the University of Florida. "It's one of the most practical skills you can develop. When you can consciously read what others are

## STRATEGIES FOR CHANGE

### How to Enhance Communication

▲ Use I statements. Describe what's going on with you. Say, "I worry about being liked" or "I get frustrated when I can't put my feelings into words." Avoid generalities such as "You never think about my feelings" or "Nobody understands me."

▲ Gently ask how the other person feels. If your friend or partner describes thoughts rather than feelings, ask for more adjectives. Was he or she sad, excited, angry, hurt?

▲ Become a very good listener. When another person talks, don't interrupt, ask why, judge, or challenge. Nod your head. Use your body language and facial expression to show you're eager to hear more.

▲ Respect confidences. Treat a friend's or partner's secrets with the discretion they deserve. Consider them a special gift entrusted to your care.

saying unconsciously, you can deal with issues before they become problems."[2]

Culture has a great deal of influence over body language. In some cultures, for example, establishing eye contact is considered hostile or challenging; in others, it conveys friendliness. A person's sense of personal space—the distance from others at which he or she feels most comfortable—varies in different societies.

Nonverbal messages also reveal something important about the individual. "Nonverbal messages come from deep inside of you, from your own sense of self-esteem," says Maple. "To improve your body language, you have to start from the inside and work out. If you're comfortable with yourself, it shows. People who have good self-esteem, who give themselves status and respect, who know who they are, have a relaxed way of talking and moving and always come across best."

## Forming Relationships

As children we first learn how to relate in our families. Our relationships with parents and siblings change dramatically as we grow toward independence. In college, students can choose to spend their leisure time socializing or engaging in solitary activities, like watching TV. Relationships between friends also change as they move or develop different interests; between lovers, as they come to know more about each other; between spouses, as they pass through life together; and between parents and children, as youngsters develop and mature. But throughout life, close relationships, tested and strengthened by time, allow us to explore the depths of our souls and the heights of our emotions.

## I, Myself, and Me

The way each of us perceives himself or herself affects all the ways we reach out and relate to others. If we feel unworthy of love, others may share that opinion. Self-esteem (discussed in Chapter 3) provides a positive foundation for our relationships with others. Self-esteem doesn't mean vanity or preoccupation with our own needs; rather, it is a genuine concern and respect for ourselves so that we remain true to our own feelings and beliefs. We can't know or love or accept others until we know and love and accept ourselves, however imperfect we may be.

If we're lacking in self-esteem, our relationships may suffer. According to research on college students by psychologists at the University of Texas, individuals with negative views of themselves seek out partners (friends, roommates, dates) who are critical and rejecting—and who confirm their low opinion of their own worth.[3]

## Friendship

Friendship has been described as "the most holy bond of society." Every culture has prized the ties of respect, tolerance, and loyalty that friendship builds and nurtures. An anonymous writer put it well:

*A friend is one who knows you as you are,*
*Understands where you've been,*
*Accepts who you've become,*
*And still gently invites you to grow.*

Friends can be a basic source of happiness, a connection to a larger world, a source of solace in times of trouble. Although we have different friends throughout life, often the friendships of adolescence and young adulthood are the closest we ever form. They ease the normal break from parents and the transition from childhood to independence.

Both teenage boys and girls see their same-sex friendships as important. However, girls rate the quality of their friendships more positively, express more positive emotions toward friends, share power more equally, and show less jealousy, particularly in friendships they describe as "satisfying" rather than "unsatisfying." From middle childhood into adulthood, girls and women continue to show more responsive and supportive behavior toward their female friends, disclose more, and disagree less than male friends.[4]

In the past, many people believed that men and women couldn't become close friends without getting romantically involved. But as the genders have worked together and come to share more interests, this belief has changed. Yet unique obstacles arise in male-female friendships, such as distinguishing between friendship and romantic attraction and dealing with sexual tension. However, men and women who overcome such barriers and become friends benefit from their relationship—but in different ways. For men, a friendship with a woman offers support and nurturance. What they report liking most is talking and relating to women, something they don't do with their male buddies. Women view their friendships with men as more light-hearted and casual, with more joking and less fear of hurt feelings. They especially like gaining insight into what guys really think.[5]

Friendship transcends all boundaries of distance and differences, and enhances feelings of warmth, trust, love, and affection between two people. It is a common denominator of human existence that cuts across major social categories: In every country, culture, and language, human beings make friends. Friendship is both a universal and a deeply satisfying experience.

"Wishing to be friends," Aristotle wrote, "is quick work, but friendship is a slowly opening fruit." The qualities that make a good friend include honesty, acceptance, dependability, empathy, and loyalty. To sustain a close friendship, both people must be able to see the other's perspective, anticipate each other's needs, and take each other's viewpoint into account.[6] More than anything else, good friends are there when we need them. They see us at our worst but never lose sight of our best. They share our laughter and tears, our triumphs and tragedies.

## Dating

A date is any occasion during which two people share their time. It can be a Friday night dance, a bicycle ride, a dinner for two, or a walk in the park. Friends and lovers go on dates; so do complete strangers. Some men date other men; some women date other women. We don't expect to love, or even like, everyone we date. Yet the people you date reveal something about the sort of person you are.

While in school, you may go out with people you meet in class or on campus. Some students form such close relationships that they are practically "joined at the hip." Others "hook up," connecting only for a one-time sexual encounter that might involve anything from kissing to intercourse. With more people remaining single longer, the search for a good date has become more complex. Singles bars have become less popular because of the dangers of excessive drinking and casual sex. Cafés, laundromats,

health clubs, and bookstores have become more acceptable as places to meet new people. Personal ads and cyberspace—the electronic web linking people through computers—are alternative ways to meet potential dates. (See Savvy Consumer: "Do's and Don'ts of Online Dating.")

Dating can do more than help you meet people. By dating, you can learn how to make conversation, get to know more about others as well as yourself, and share feelings, opinions, and interests. In adolescence and young adulthood, dating also provides an opportunity for exploring your sexual identity. Some people date for months and never share more than a good-night kiss. Others may fall into bed together before they fall in love or even "like."

Separating your emotional feelings about someone you're dating from your sexual desire is often difficult. The first step to making responsible sexual decisions is respecting your sexual values and those of your partner. If you care about the other person—not just his or her body—and the relationship you're creating, sex will be an important, but not the all-important, factor while you're dating.

Dating has potential dangers. As discussed in Chapter 14, approximately one in five female teens is physically and/or sexually abused by a dating partner.[7] Although the roots of such violence are complex, researchers have found a correlation between watching wrestling, with its high levels of vulgar language and physical and verbal abuse, and dating violence.[8]

Most longitudinal studies on dating relationships have shown little change in love over time, although love has been found to increase for individuals who advance to a deeper, more long-lasting commitment. Romantic partners in enduring relationships generally perceive their love, commitment, and satisfaction as increasing over time. A four-year study of romantic couples, all dating as the study began, found that those who remained together perceived that their love, satisfaction, and commitment had grown.[9]

## ???? What Causes Romantic Attraction?

What draws two people to each other and keeps them together: chemistry or fate, survival instincts or sexual longings? "Probably it's a host of different things," reports sociologist Edward Laumann, coauthor of *Sex in America,* a landmark survey of 3,432 men and women conducted by the National Opinion Research Center at the University of Chicago.[10] "But what's remarkable is that most of us end up with partners much like ourselves—in age, race, ethnicity, socioeconomic class, education."

Why? "You've got to get close for sexual chemistry to occur," says Laumann. "Sparks may fly when you see someone across a crowded room, but you only see a preselected group of people—people enough like you to be in the same room in the first place. This makes sense because initiating

## Savvy Consumer

### Do's and Don'ts of Online Dating

Forget personal ads and singles bars. If you're looking for love in the new millennium, the place more people are turning is cyberspace. Some estimate that thousands, perhaps millions of people, are using the Internet to find a companion.

E-mail flirtations can be fun, but they also entail some risks, particularly if you decide to go off-line and meet in person. Here are some guidelines:

- Be careful of what you type. Anything you put on the Internet can end up almost anywhere. To avoid embarrassment, don't say anything you wouldn't want to see in newspaper print.

- Don't give out your address, telephone number, or any other identifying information. The people you meet online are strangers, and you should keep your guard up.

- Don't "date" on an office or university computer. You could end up supplying your professors, classmates, or coworkers with unintentional entertainment. Also, many organizations and institutions consider e-mail messages company property.

- Remember that you have no way of verifying if a correspondent is telling the truth about anything— sex, age, occupation, marital status. If your online partner seems insincere or strange in any way, stop corresponding.

- If you decide to meet, make your first face-to-face encounter a double or group date, and make it somewhere public, like a café or museum. Don't plan a full-day outing. Coffee or a drink in a crowded place makes the best transition from e-mails.

- Make sure you tell a friend or family member your plans and have your own way of getting home. It's also a good idea to schedule the first meeting in the afternoon or early evening rather than later at night.

- Don't let your expectations run wild. Finding Mr. or Ms. Right is no easier in cyberspace than anywhere else, so be realistic about where your relationship might lead.

- Don't rely on the Internet as your only method of meeting people. Continue to get out in the real world and meet potential dates the old-fashioned ways.

a sexual relationship is very uncertain. We all have such trepidations about being too fat, too ugly, too undesirable. We try to lower the risk of rejection by looking for people more or less like us."

Scientists have tried to analyze the combination of factors that attracts two people to each other. In several studies of college students, four predictors ranked as the most important reasons for attraction: warmth and kindness, desirable personality, something specific about the person, and reciprocal liking.[11]

In his cross-cultural research, psychologist David Buss, author of *The Evolution of Desire,* found that men in 37 sample groups drawn from Africa, Asia, Europe, North and South America, Australia, and New Zealand rated youth and attractiveness as more important in a possible mate than did women. Women placed greater value on potential mates who were somewhat older, had good financial prospects, and were dependable and hardworking.[12]

The reason for this gender difference could be evolutionary. Throughout time, men have sought fertile females of "high reproductive value." Two outward signs of female fertility are youth and a more subtle factor: waist-to-hip ratio. When researchers analyzed the physical dimensions

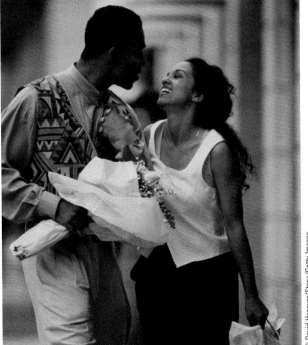

▲ Romantic attraction is characterized by a high level of emotional arousal, reciprocal liking, and mutual sexual desire.

of the women considered most attractive by men, those with the slimmest waists and roundest hips were consistently rated as most desirable. Women have had to look for mates who could provide greater security for their offspring. For them, a man's power, wealth, and status—which require more time to assess—mattered more than appearance. (See The X & Y Files: "Men, Women, and Marital Preferences.")

## Intimate Relationships

The term **intimacy**—the open, trusting sharing of close, confidential thoughts and feelings—comes from the Latin word for *within.* Intimacy doesn't happen at first sight, or in a day or a week or a number of weeks. Intimacy requires time and nurturing; it is a process of revealing rather than hiding, of wanting to know another and to be known by that other. (See Figure 7-1 for the elements of love.) Although intimacy doesn't require sex, an intimate relationship often includes a sexual relationship, heterosexual or homosexual.

All of our close relationships, whether they're with parents or friends, have a great deal in common. We feel we can count on these people in times of need. We feel they understand us and we understand them. We give and receive loving emotional support. We care about their happiness and welfare. However, when we choose one person above all others, there is something even deeper and richer—something we call *mature love.*

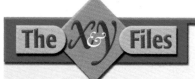

## The X & Y Files     Men, Women, and Marital Preferences

In a national survey of more than 13,000 adults researchers asked how willing they would be to marry an individual, based on education, income, age, and other factors. As shown in the table below, the women were significantly more willing than men to marry someone who was older, better educated, would earn more, and was not good-looking. The men were more willing than women to marry someone who had less education, was younger, wasn't likely to hold a steady job, and who would earn less. There were minor differences on items related to prior marriages, religion, and already having children.

| How Willing Would You Be to Marry Someone Who . . . | Women | Men |
| --- | --- | --- |
| had more education than you? | 5.82 | 5.22 |
| had less education than you? | 4.08 | 4.67 |
| was older than you by five or more years? | 5.29 | 4.15 |
| was younger than you by five or more years? | 2.80 | 4.54 |
| was not good-looking? | 4.42 | 3.41 |
| was not likely to hold a steady job? | 1.62 | 2.73 |
| would earn much less than you? | 3.76 | 4.60 |
| would earn much more than you? | 5.93 | 5.19 |
| had been married before? | 3.44 | 3.35 |
| was of a different religion? | 4.31 | 4.24 |
| already had children? | 3.11 | 2.84 |

Note: These responses are based on a 7-point scale, ranging from 1 ("not at all") to 7 ("very willing").

Source: Crooks, Robert, and Karla Baur. *Our Sexuality,* 8th ed. Pacific Grove, CA: Wadsworth, 2002, p. 190.

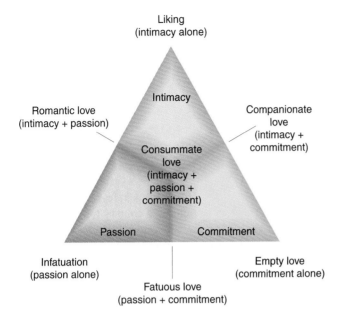

Liking
(intimacy alone)

Intimacy

Romantic love
(intimacy + passion)

Companionate
love
(intimacy +
commitment)

Consummate
love
(intimacy +
passion +
commitment)

Passion          Commitment

Infatuation
(passion alone)

Empty love
(commitment alone)

Fatuous love
(passion + commitment)

▲ **Figure 7-1** Sternberg's Love Triangle
The three components of love are intimacy, passion, and commitment. The various kinds of love are composed of different combinations of the three components.

## Mature Love

Social scientists have distinguished between *passionate love* (characterized by intense feelings of elation, sexual desire, and ecstasy) and *companionate love* (characterized by friendly affection and deep attachment). Often relationships begin with passionate love and evolve into a more companionate love. Sometimes the opposite happens and two people who know each other well discover that their friendship has caught fire and the sparks have flamed an unexpected passion.

A romantic relationship shows definite promise if:

✔ You feel at ease with your new partner.
✔ You feel good about your new partner when you're together and when you're not.
✔ Your partner is open with you about his or her life— past, present, and future.
✔ You can say no to each other without feeling guilty.
✔ You feel cared for, appreciated, and accepted as you are.
✔ Your partner really listens to what you have to say.

Mature love is a complex combination of sexual excitement, tenderness, commitment, and—most of all— an overriding passion that sets it apart from all other love relationships in one's life. This passion isn't simply a matter of orgasm, but also entails a crossing of the psychological boundaries between oneself and one's lover. You feel as if you're becoming one with your partner while simultaneously retaining a sense of yourself.

## When Love Ends

Breaking up is indeed hard to do. Sometimes two people gradually grow apart, and both of them realize that they must go their separate ways. More often, one person falls out of love first. It hurts to be rejected; it also hurts to inflict pain on someone who once meant a great deal to  you. In surveys, college students say it's more difficult to initiate a breakup than to be rejected. Those who decided to end a relationship reported greater feelings of guilt, uncertainty, discomfort, and awkwardness than those with whom they broke up. However, rejected students with high levels of jealousy are likely to feel a desire for vengeance that can lead to aggressive behavior.[13]

Research suggests that people do not end their relationships because of the disappearance of love. Rather a sense of dissatisfaction or unhappiness develops, which may then cause love to stop growing. The fact that love does not dissipate completely may be one reason why breakups are so painful. While the pain does ease over time, ending their relationship in a way that shows kindness and respect can help both parties. Your basic guideline should be to think of how you would like to be treated if someone were breaking up with you. Would it hurt more to find out from someone else? Would it be more painful if the person you cared for lied to you or deceived you, rather than admitted the truth? Saying "I don't feel the way I once did about you; I don't want to continue our relationship" is hard, but it's also honest and direct.

## ???? Is Living Together a Good Idea?

Although couples have always shared homes in informal relationships without any official ties, "living together," or **cohabitation,** has become more common, increasing by 80 percent in the last two decades. Often young people live together in a trial marriage, getting to know each other better to see whether they're compatible—although this does not necessarily lead to a more successful marriage. People who have been married and divorced may be content just sharing their lives with one another.

According to the U.S. Census Bureau, more than 4 million unmarried heterosexual couples live together, in contrast to only half a million 40 years ago. For many young adults, particularly children of divorced parents, living together seems like a good way to achieve some of the benefits of marriage as they get to know each other and find out if they're suited to each other. According to surveys, most young people say it is a good idea to live with a person before marrying.

That's not the case, argues a controversial report. Researchers for the National Marriage Project of Rutgers University in New Jersey reviewed all available research and concluded that living together is not a good way to prepare for marriage or to avoid divorce. They found that these unions, in comparison to marriages, tend to have more episodes of domestic violence toward women, and more physical and sexual abuse of children. Unmarried couples also report lower levels of happiness and well-being than married couples. Annual rates of depression among unmarried couples are more than three times those of married couples. The divorce rate among couples who eventually marry is also higher.[14]

According to the report, cohabitation is probably least harmful (though not necessarily helpful) when it is prenuptial—when both partners are definitely planning to marry, have formally announced their engagement, and have picked a wedding date. The longer two people live together without marrying, the more likely they are to have problems. The reason, the researchers suggest, is that individuals develop a *low-commitment ethic* that is the opposite of what is required for a successful marriage.[15]

Multiple living-together experiences also have a negative impact, both for an individual's own sense of well-being and for the likelihood of establishing a strong lifelong partnership. Rather than teaching people to have better relationships, repeated cohabiting is a strong predictor of the failure of future relationships.

Cohabitation poses particular risks to children. Since cohabiting parents break up at a much higher rate than married parents, children face a greater likelihood of a potentially devastating breakup.

Unmarried couples are gaining legal recognition. Some U.S. cities have domestic partnership laws that grant a variety of spousal rights—such as insurance benefits and bereavement leave—to partners, heterosexual or homosexual, who live together.

## Committed Relationships

Even though men and women today may have more sexual partners than in the past, most still yearn for an intense, supportive, exclusive relationship, based on mutual commitment and enduring over time. In our society, most such relationships take the form of heterosexual marriages, but partners of the same sex or heterosexual partners who never marry also may sustain long-lasting, deeply committed relationships. These couples are much like married people: They make a home, handle daily chores, cope with problems, celebrate special occasions, plan for the future— all the while knowing that they are not alone, that they are part of a pair that adds up to far more than just the sum of two individual souls.

## Marriage

*Like everything which is not the involuntary result of fleeting emotion but the creation of time and will, any marriage, happy or unhappy, is infinitely more interesting and significant than any romance, however passionate.*

**W. H. Auden**

Contemporary marriage has been described as an institution that everyone on the outside wants to enter and everyone on the inside wants to leave. About 56 percent of all American adults (111 million people) are married and living with their spouses. The marriage rate has dropped dramatically: A lower percentage of couples tied the knot in the 1990s than in previous decades. In fact, the national marriage rate has dropped over the last four decades to its lowest point ever.

Not only are fewer people getting married, but fewer marital partners describe themselves as "very happy" in their relationships. In a recent report on "the social health of marriage in America," researchers at Rutgers University found that more couples are choosing to live together outside of marriage or are putting off vows until later in life.[16] Young people also have grown disenchanted with the prospect of marriage. The percentage of teenagers who thought they would be happier married than not married has fallen over the last two decades.

Not too long ago, marriage was often a business deal, a contract made by parents for economic or political reasons when the spouses-to-be were still very young. In some countries, arranged marriages are still culturally acceptable. Even in America, certain ethnic groups, such as Asians who have recently immigrated to the United States, plan marriages for their children. In such arrangements, the marriage partners are likely to have similar values and expectations. However, the newlyweds also start out as strangers who may not even know whether they like—let alone love—each other. Sometimes arranged marriages do lead to loving unions; sometimes they trap both partners in loneliness and longing.

Most of today's marriages aren't arranged, but even in this day and age, partners often marry because they have to: One of every six brides is pregnant on her wedding day. Other young couples marry as a way to escape from their parents' homes and authority. But most people say they marry for one far-from-simple reason: love.

### Preparing for Marriage

With more than half of all marriages ending in divorce, there's little doubt that modern marriages aren't made in heaven. Are some couples doomed to divorce even before they swap "I do's"? Could counseling before a marriage increase its odds of success? According to recent research findings, the answer to both questions is yes.

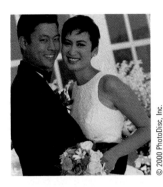 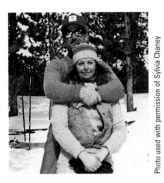

▲ A relationship is just as alive as the individuals who create it. With caring, it grows; with emotional nourishment, it blossoms; with commitment, it endures.

There have been government attempts to set requirements for couples who want to marry. Some states, such as Arizona and Louisiana, have established covenant marriages in which engaged couples are required to participate in premarital counseling. Utah allows counties to require counseling before issuing marriage licenses to minors and people who have been divorced. Florida requires high school students to take marriage education classes.[17]

## Finding Mr. or Ms. Right

Generally, men and women marry people from the geographical area they grew up in and from the same social background. Differences in religion and race can add to the pressures of marriage, but they also can enrich the relationship if they aren't viewed as obstacles. In our culturally diverse society, interracial and crosscultural marriages are becoming more common and more widely accepted, although the odds are much greater for partners of the same race to live together or marry.

 In a study of 75,000 couples who lived together and 480,000 married couples in the United States, researchers found that African Americans were 365 times more likely to marry a black than a nonblack spouse and 110 times more likely to cohabit with a black partner than someone of another racial group. Asians were 55 times more likely to marry another Asian and 17 times more likely to cohabit with another Asian. Hispanics were 12 times more likely to select a Hispanic spouse and nine times more likely to live with a Hispanic partner. Whites were about eight times more likely to marry another white person and five times more likely to cohabit with someone who is white rather than nonwhite.[18]

Some of the traits that appeal to us in a date become less important when we select a mate; others become key ingredients in the emotional cement holding two people together. According to psychologist Robert Sternberg of Yale University, the crucial ingredients for commitment are the following:

✔ Shared values.
✔ A willingness to change in response to each other.
✔ A willingness to tolerate flaws.
✔ A match in religious beliefs.
✔ The ability to communicate effectively.

The single best predictor of how satisfied one will be in a relationship, according to Sternberg, is not how one feels toward a lover, but the difference between how one would like the lover to feel and how the lover actually feels. Feeling that the partner you've chosen loves too little or too much is, as he puts it, "the best predictor of failure."[19]

## Premarital Assessments

There are scientific ways of predicting marital happiness. Some premarital assessment inventories identify strengths and weaknesses in many aspects of a relationship: realistic expectations, personality issues, communication, conflict resolution, financial management, leisure activities, sex, children, family and friends, egalitarian roles, and religious orientation. Couples who become aware of potential conflicts by means of such inventories may be able to resolve them through professional counseling. In some cases, they may want to reconsider or postpone their wedding.

## STRATEGIES FOR PREVENTION

### When to Think Twice About Getting Married

Don't get married if:

▲ You or your partner is constantly asking the other such questions as "Are you sure you love me?"

▲ You spend most of your time together disagreeing and quarreling.

▲ You're both still very young (under the age of 20).

▲ Your boyfriend or girlfriend has behaviors (such as nonstop talking), traits (such as bossiness), or problems (such as drinking too much) that really bother you and that you're hoping will change after you're married.

▲ Your partner wants you to stop seeing your friends, quit a job you enjoy, or change your life in some other way that diminishes your overall satisfaction.

Other common predictors of marital discord, unhappiness, and separation are:

✔ A high level of arousal during a discussion.
✔ Defensive behaviors such as making excuses and denying responsibility for disagreements.
✔ A wife's expressions of contempt.
✔ A husband's stonewalling (showing no response when a wife expresses her concerns).

By looking for such behaviors, researchers have been able to predict with better than 90 percent accuracy whether a couple will separate within the first few years of marriage.

## What Is the Current Divorce Rate?

About half of all marriages end in divorce, but the odds of a first marriage lasting are slightly better. According to an analysis of the most recent census data by the Centers for Disease Control and Prevention, about 43 percent of first marriages end in separation or divorce within 15 years. The older the bride, the better the chance the marriage will last. Nearly 60 percent of brides under age 18 eventually separate or divorce, compared with 36 percent of those age 20 or older. Women who marry and divorce young are more apt to wed again: 81 percent of those divorced before age 25 remarry within ten years, compared with 68 percent of those divorced at age 25 or older.

 Race also influences marriage and divorce rates. African-American couples are more likely to break up than white couples, and black divorcées are less likely to marry again. Researchers have found that African Americans place an equally high value on marriage. However, there is a smaller marriageable pool of black men for a variety of reasons, including a higher mortality rate.[20]

Even after their hopes for happiness with one spouse end, men and women still yearn to mesh two personalities, two life histories, and two persons' dreams into a marriage. Eighty percent of divorced men and women remarry, and the remarriage rate increases with the number of times an individual has been divorced. The remarriage rate after a second divorce is 90 percent; after a third divorce, it's even higher. However, more second, third, and fourth marriages fail than original unions.[21]

## Family Ties

America's families are growing—and changing. According to the Census Bureau, the number of households in the United States increased 15 percent from 1990 to 2000, with nonfamily households increasing about twice as much (23 percent) as family households (11 percent).[22] Married couples make up the majority of households, though by a smaller number than in 1990. (See Figure 7-2.) Family households headed by women with no husbands outnumber by almost three times households headed by men without wives. Women with children under 18 years head 7.2 percent of all households, up from 6.6 percent in 1990.

Although the number of people and households in the United States increased from 1990 to 2000, both average household size and family size decreased somewhat. Today the average family numbers 3.16 people. People living alone make up one in four households in the United States. One-person households are four times as common as nonfamily households with two or more people.

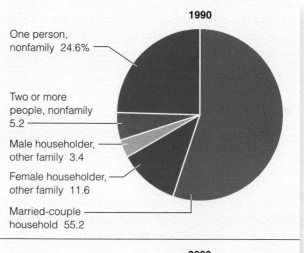

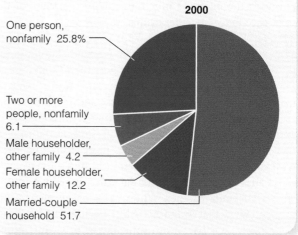

▲ **Figure 7-2** Comparison of Households by Type: 1990 and 2000
The percent of married-couple households has decreased while the number of other types of households has increased.

Source: U.S. Census Bureau.

Utah has the highest proportion of married-couple households (63 percent), followed by Idaho and Iowa. Only 23 percent of households in the District of Columbia are maintained by married couples. Massachusetts, Rhode Island, Louisiana, Mississippi, and Nevada also have less than half of their households maintained by married couples.

The number of households with unmarried partners increased from 3.2 million in 1990 to 5.5 million in 2000 (4.9 million consist of partners of the opposite sex). Unmarried partners account for 5.2 percent of all households, up from 3.5 percent in 1990. California has the largest number of nonmarried-partner households.

## Diversity Within Families

 The all-American **family**—as portrayed on television and in movies—is typically white and middle-class. But families of different cultures—Italian to Indian to Indonesian—reflect different traditions, beliefs, and values. Within African-American families, for instance, traditional gender roles are often reversed, with women serving as head of the household, a kinship bond uniting several households, and a strong religious commitment or orientation. In Chinese-American families, both spouses may work and see themselves as breadwinners, but the wife may not have an equal role in decision making. In Hispanic families, wives and mothers are acknowledged and respected as healers and dispensers of wisdom. At the same time, they are expected to defer to their husbands, who see themselves as the strong, protective, dominant head of the family. As time passes and families from different cultures become more integrated into American life, traditional gender roles and decision-making patterns often change, particularly among the youngest family members.

American families are diverse in other ways. *Multigenerational families,* with children, parents, and grandparents, make up 3.7 percent of households. They occur most often in areas where new immigrants live with relatives, where housing shortages or high costs force families to double up their living arrangements, or where high rates of out-of-wedlock childbearing force unwed mothers to live with their children in their parents' home.[23]

Three of every ten households consist of **blended families,** formed when one or both of the partners bring children from a previous union. In the future, social scientists predict, American families will become even more diverse, or pluralistic. But as norms or expectations about the configurations of families have changed, values or ideas about the intents and purposes of families have not. American families of every type still support each other and strive toward values such as commitment and caring.

Only recently has medical research devoted major scientific investigations to issues in women's health. Until about a decade ago, the National Institutes of Health routinely excluded women from experimental studies because of concerns about menstrual cycles and pregnancy. In clinical settings and with identical complaints, women are more likely than men to have their symptoms dismissed as psychological and not to be referred to a specialist. Some physicians are suggesting the creation of a new medical specialty (distinct from obstetrics and gynecology) that would be devoted to women's health, thereby providing more comprehensive care and overcoming the current gender gap in health services. A lack of health insurance is another barrier to adequate health care, particularly for low-income women.[24]

### Female Sexual Anatomy

As illustrated in Figure 7-3A, the **mons pubis** is the rounded, fleshy area over the junction of the pubic bones. The folds of skin that form the outer lips of a woman's genital area are called the **labia majora.** They cover soft flaps of skin (inner lips) called the **labia minora.** The inner lips join at the top to form a hood over the **clitoris,** a small elongated erectile organ and the most sensitive spot in the entire female genital area. Below the clitoris is the **urethral opening,** the outer opening of the thin tube that carries urine from the bladder. Below that is a larger opening, the mouth of the **vagina,** the canal that leads to the primary internal organs of reproduction. The **perineum** is the area between the vagina and the anus (the opening to the rectum and large intestine).

At the back of the vagina is the **cervix,** the opening to the womb, or **uterus** (see Figure 7-3B). The uterine walls are lined by a layer of tissue called the **endometrium.** Two **ovaries**—about the size and shape of almonds, with one on the left of the uterus and one on the right—contain egg cells called **ova** (singular, **ovum**). Extending outward and back from the upper uterus are the **fallopian tubes,** the canals that transport ova from the ovaries to the uterus. When an egg is released from an ovary, the fingerlike ends of the adjacent fallopian tube catch the egg and direct it into the tube.

### ???? What Is the Menstrual Cycle?

As shown in Figure 7-4 on p. 157, the hypothalamus monitors hormone levels in the blood and sends messages to the pituitary gland to release follicle-stimulating hormone (FSH) and luteinizing hormone (LH). In the ovaries, these

## A. External structure

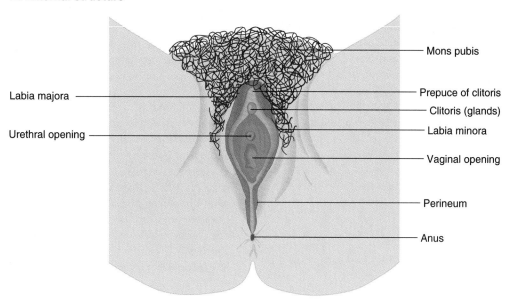

Mons pubis

Labia majora

Urethral opening

Prepuce of clitoris

Clitoris (glands)

Labia minora

Vaginal opening

Perineum

Anus

## B. Internal structure

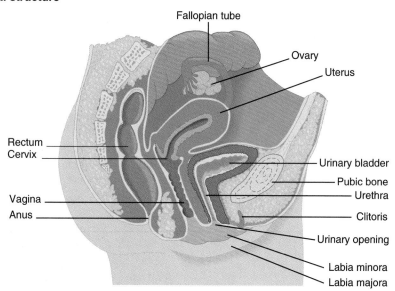

Fallopian tube

Ovary

Uterus

Rectum
Cervix

Urinary bladder

Pubic bone

Urethra

Vagina
Anus

Clitoris

Urinary opening

Labia minora
Labia majora

▲ **Figure 7-3** Female Sex Organs and Reproductive Structures

hormones stimulate the growth of a few of the immature eggs stored in every woman's body. Usually, only one ovum matures completely during each monthly cycle. As it does, the ovaries increase production of the female sex hormone **estrogen,** which in turn triggers the release of a larger surge of LH.

At midcycle, the increased LH hormone levels trigger **ovulation,** the release of the ovum from the ovary. Estrogen levels drop, and the remaining cells of the follicle then enlarge, change character, and form the **corpus luteum,** or yellow body. In the second half of the menstrual cycle, the corpus luteum secretes estrogen and larger

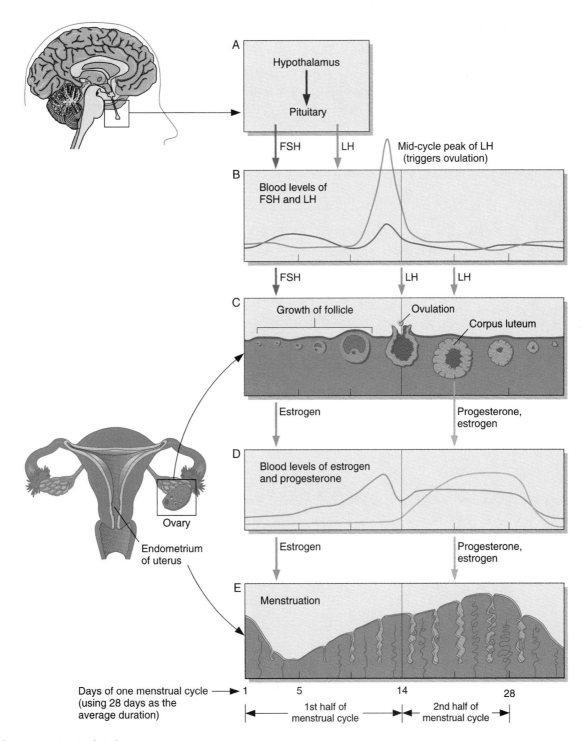

▲ **Figure 7-4** Menstrual Cycle
Levels of the hormones FSH and LH rise and then fall to stimulate the cycle. These changes affect the levels of the hormones estrogen and progesterone, which in turn react with LH and FSH. As a result of the increase in estrogen, the ovarian follicle matures and then ruptures, releasing the ova (eggs) into the fallopian tubes. The progesterone helps prepare the lining of the uterus to receive a fertilized egg. If a fertilized egg is deposited into the uterus, pregnancy begins. But if the egg is not fertilized, progesterone production decreases, and the uterine lining is shed (menstruation). At this point, both estrogen and progesterone levels have dropped, so the pituitary responds by producing FSH, and the cycle begins again.

amounts of **progesterone.** The endometrium (uterine lining) is stimulated by progesterone to thicken and become more engorged with blood in preparation for nourishing an implanted, fertilized ovum.

If the ovum is not fertilized, the corpus luteum disintegrates. As the level of progesterone drops, **menstruation** occurs—the uterine lining is shed during the course of a menstrual period. If the egg is fertilized and pregnancy occurs, the cells that eventually develop into the placenta secrete *human chorionic gonadotropin* (HCG), a messenger hormone that signals the pituitary not to start a new cycle. The corpus luteum then steps up its production of progesterone.

Many women experience physical or psychological changes, or both, during their monthly cycles. Usually the changes are minor, but more serious problems can occur.

## Premenstrual Syndrome

Women with **premenstrual syndrome (PMS)** experience bodily discomfort and emotional distress for up to two weeks, from ovulation until the onset of menstruation. Three to 15 percent of these women develop very severe symptoms. Because there are no consistent or objective ways of diagnosing premenstrual complaints, it's hard to know precisely how many women are affected. In some studies, as many as 40 to 45 percent of women have reported at least one PMS symptom.

Once dismissed as a psychological problem, PMS has been recognized as a very real physiological disorder that may be caused by a hormonal deficiency; abnormal levels of thyroid hormone; an imbalance of estrogen and progesterone; changes in brain chemicals; or social and environmental factors, particularly stress. The most common symptoms of PMS are mood changes, anxiety, irritability, difficulty concentrating, forgetfulness, impaired judgment, tearfulness, digestive symptoms (diarrhea, bloating, constipation), hot flashes, palpitations, dizziness, headache, fatigue, changes in appetite, cravings (usually for sweets or salt), water retention, breast tenderness, and insomnia.

For a diagnosis to be made, women—using a self-rating symptom scale or calendar—must report troubling premenstrual symptoms in the period before menstruation in at least two successive menstrual cycles. Treatments for PMS depend on specific symptoms. Diuretics (drugs that speed up fluid elimination) can relieve water retention and bloating. Relaxation techniques have led to a 60 percent reduction in anxiety symptoms. Sleep deprivation, or the use of bright light to adjust a woman's circadian or daily rhythm, also has proven beneficial. Behavioral approaches, such as exercise or charting cycles, help by letting women know when they're vulnerable.

Low doses of medications known as *selective serotonin-reuptake inhibitors* (SSRIs), such as fluoxetine (marketed as Prozac, Sarafem, and in generic forms), provide relief for symptoms such as tension, depression, irritability, and mood swings, even when taken only during the premenstrual phase rather than daily throughout the month.[25] Calcium supplements also may be beneficial.[26] Other treatments with some reported success include vitamins; exercise; less caffeine, alcohol, salt, and sugar; acupuncture; and stress management techniques such as meditation or relaxation training.[27]

## Premenstrual Dysphoric Disorder

**Premenstrual dysphoric disorder (PMDD),** which is not related to PMS, occurs in an estimated 3 to 5 percent of all menstruating women.[28] It is characterized by regular symptoms of depression (depressed mood, anxiety, mood swings, diminished interest or pleasure) during the last week of the menstrual cycle. Women with PMDD cannot function as usual at work, school, or home. They feel better a few days after menstruation begins. SSRIs, which are used to treat PMS, also are effective in relieving symptoms of PMDD.[29]

PMDD remains controversial, primarily for political reasons. Some women's advocacy groups oppose labeling women with menstruation-linked symptoms as mentally ill. Others contend that a diagnosis of PMDD simply recognizes the distress some women experience and may make it easier for them to obtain needed help.

## Menstrual Cramps

**Dysmenorrhea** is the medical name for the discomforts—abdominal cramps and pain, back and leg pain, diarrhea, tension, water retention, fatigue, and depression—that can occur during menstruation. About half of all menstruating women suffer from dysmenorrhea. The cause seems to be an overproduction of bodily substances called *prostaglandins,* which typically rise during menstruation.

Women who produce excessive prostaglandins have more severe menstrual cramps. During a cramp, the uterine muscles may contract too strongly or frequently, and temporarily deprive the uterus of oxygen, causing pain. Medications that inhibit prostaglandins can reduce menstrual pain, and exercise can also relieve cramps.

## Amenorrhea

Women may stop menstruating—a condition called **amenorrhea**—for a variety of reasons, including a hormonal disorder, drastic weight loss, strenuous exercise, or change in the environment. Boarding-school amenorrhea is common among young women who leave home for

## STRATEGIES FOR PREVENTION

### Preventing Premenstrual Problems

▲ Get plenty of exercise. Physically fit women usually have fewer problems both before and during their periods.

▲ Eat frequently and nutritiously. In the week before your period, your body doesn't regulate the levels of sugar, or glucose, in your blood as well as it usually does.

▲ Swear off salt. If you stop using salt at the table and while cooking, you may gain less weight premenstrually, feel less bloated, and suffer less from headaches and irritability.

▲ Cut back on caffeine. Coffee, colas, diet colas, chocolate, and tea can increase breast tenderness and other symptoms.

▲ Don't drink or smoke. Some women become so sensitive to alcohol's effects before their periods that a glass of wine hits with the impact of several stiff drinks. Nicotine worsens low blood sugar problems.

▲ Watch out for sweets. Premenstrual cravings for sweets are common, but try to resist. Sugar may pick you up, but later you'll feel worse than before.

school. Distance running and strenuous exercise also can lead to amenorrhea. The reason may be a drop in body fat from the normal range of 18 to 22 percent to a range 9 to 12 percent. To be considered amenorrhea, a woman's menstrual cycle is typically absent for three or more consecutive months. Prolonged amenorrhea can have serious health consequences, including a loss of bone density that may lead to stress fractures or osteoporosis.

In recent years scientists have discovered that the menstrual cycle actually begins in the brain with the production of gonadotropin-releasing hormone (GnRH). Each month a surge of GnRH sets into motion the sequence of steps that lead to ovulation, the potential for conception, and, if conception doesn't occur, menstruation. This understanding has led to the development of chemical mimics, or analogues, of GnRH—usually administered by nasal spray—that trigger ovulation in women who don't ovulate or menstruate normally.

## Toxic Shock Syndrome

This rare, potentially deadly bacterial infection primarily strikes menstruating women under the age of 30 who use tampons. Both *Staphylococcus aureus* and group A *Streptococcus pyogenes* can produce **toxic shock syndrome (TSS).** Symptoms include a high fever; a rash that leads to peeling of the skin on the fingers, toes, palms, and soles; dizziness; dangerously low blood pressure; and abnormalities in several organ systems (the digestive tract and the kidneys) and in the muscles and blood. Treatment usually consists of antibiotics and intense supportive care; intravenous administration of immunoglobulins that attack the toxins produced by these bacteria also may be beneficial.

Menstruating women should follow these guidelines to reduce their risk of TSS:

✔ Use sanitary napkins instead of tampons.
✔ If you do use tampons, check the box label for information on absorbency (which the FDA has required manufacturers to provide), and avoid superabsorbent brands.
✔ Change tampons every four to eight hours.
✔ Use napkins during the night or for some time during each day of menstrual flow.
✔ As menstrual flow decreases, switch to less-absorbent tampons, which are less likely to cause problems.[30]

## Men's Sexual Health

Because the male reproductive system is simpler in many ways than the females, it's often ignored—especially by healthy young men. However, just like women, men should make regular self-exams (including checking their penises, testes, and breasts, as described in Chapter 10) part of their routine.

### Male Sexual Anatomy

The visible parts of the male sexual anatomy are the **penis** and the **scrotum,** the pouch that contains the **testes** (see Figure 7-5). The testes manufacture **testosterone,** the hormone that stimulates the development of a male's secondary characteristics, and **sperm,** the male reproductive cells. Immature sperm are stored in the **epididymis,** a collection of coiled tubes adjacent to each testis.

The penis contains three hollow cylinders loosely covered with skin. The two major cylinders, the *corpora cavernosa,* extend side by side through the length of the penis. The third cylinder, the *corpus spongiosum,* surrounds the **urethra,** the channel for both seminal fluid and urine (see Figure 7-5).

## A. External structure

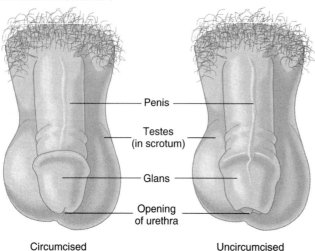

Penis

Testes
(in scrotum)

Glans

Opening
of urethra

Circumcised          Uncircumcised

## B. Internal structure

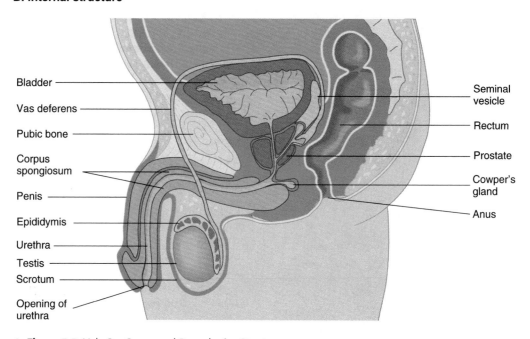

Bladder

Vas deferens

Pubic bone

Corpus
spongiosum

Penis

Epididymis

Urethra

Testis

Scrotum

Opening of
urethra

Seminal
vesicle

Rectum

Prostate

Cowper's
gland

Anus

▲ **Figure 7-5** Male Sex Organs and Reproductive Structures

When hanging down loosely, the average penis is about 3¾ inches long. During erection, its internal cylinders fill with so much blood that they become rigid, and the penis stretches to an average length of 6¼ inches. About 90 percent of all men have erect penises measuring between 5 and 7 inches in length. There is no relation, however, between penis size and female sexual satisfaction: A woman's vagina naturally adjusts during intercourse to the size of her partner's penis.

Inside the body are several structures involved in the production of seminal fluid, or **semen,** the liquid in which sperm cells are carried out of the body during ejaculation.

The **vas deferens** are two tubes that carry sperm from the epididymis into the urethra. The **seminal vesicles,** which make some of the seminal fluid, join with the vas deferens to form the **ejaculatory ducts.** The **prostate gland** produces some of the seminal fluid, which it secretes into the urethra during ejaculation. The **Cowper's glands** are two pea-sized structures on either side of the urethra (just below where it emerges from the prostate gland) and connected to it via tiny ducts. When a man is sexually aroused, the Cowper's glands often secrete a fluid that appears as a droplet at the tip of the penis. This fluid is not semen, although it occasionally contains sperm.

##  What Is Circumcision?

In its natural state, the tip of the penis is covered by a fold of skin called the *foreskin*. About 60 percent of baby boys in the United States undergo **circumcision,** the surgical removal of the foreskin. However, increasingly more parents are opting for the natural look.

An estimated 1.2 million newborn males are circumcised in the United States annually for reasons that vary from religious traditions to preventive health measures. Until the last half century, scientific evidence to support or repudiate routine circumcision was limited. The American Academy of Pediatrics (AAP) reviewed 40 years of data and concluded that although there are potential medical benefits, the data are not strong enough to recommend routine neonatal circumcision.[31] However, other experts, challenging this controversial view, argue that lack of circumcision increases the risk of sexually transmitted diseases, including HIV and syphilis.[32]

Boys who are not circumcised are four times as likely to develop urinary tract infections in their first year; however, such infections develop in only 1 percent of circumcised boys. Uncircumcised men are three times as likely to develop penile cancer, but the absolute risk is low. (Only about nine in every million American men ever gets cancer of the penis.) The drawbacks of circumcision include the risk of complications (which tend to be uncommon and minor) and pain. The AAP recommends that when circumcision is performed, analgesic creams or anesthetic shots be used to minimize discomfort.

Parents who choose not to have their sons circumcised should not attempt to retract the foreskin. This could lead to infection, bleeding, or scarring. As a boy gets older, gradual retraction of the foreskin during bath time helps it dilate, with full retraction possible by age two to four. There is little consensus on what impact the presence or absence of a foreskin has on sexual functioning or satisfaction.

Parents have mixed feelings about the decisions they make. In one study, families who did not have their sons circumcised were less satisfied with their decision. They were more likely to feel that they had not been adequately informed and to reconsider their decision.[33]

## Sexual Behavior

From birth to death, we are sexual beings. Our sexual identities, needs, likes, and dislikes emerge in adolescence and become clearer as we enter adulthood, but we continue to change and evolve throughout our lives. In men, sexual interest is most intense at age 18; in women, it reaches a peak in the thirties. Although age brings changes in sexual responsiveness, we never outgrow our sexuality.

##  How Sexually Active Are College Students?

Most unmarried college students are sexually active. In one recent study of college students attending four universities in a Southern state, 83 percent reported having had sexual intercourse.[34] Nationwide about 25 percent of female students and 60 percent of males report engaging in casual sex.[35]

According to the Kaiser Family Foundation's National Survey of Youth (Knowledge and Attitudes on Sexual Health), the majority of young people between the ages of 15 and 24 considered sexual health a "very big concern" for their age group. In the survey, 37 percent of those 15 to 17 years old and 80 percent of those 18 to 24 reported having sexual intercourse. Most—82 percent of the 15- to 17-year-olds and 74 percent of the 18- to 24-year-olds—said they wanted more information on sexual health. Survey participants reported learning about sex from various sources; friends and sex-education classes were the prime sources for "a lot" of sex-related information.[36] (See Student Snapshot: "Where Do Young Americans Learn About Relationships and Sexual Health?")

 College students see sexual activity as normal behavior for their peer group. When researchers at Pennsylvania State University conducted focus groups with undergraduates, most agreed that the majority of college students (80 to 90 percent, in their estimate) are sexually active and that alcohol and drug use make sexual activity more likely.[37]

Yet students' assumptions about their peers' behaviors may be grossly inaccurate. In one study, undergraduates believed that the "average" college student engaged

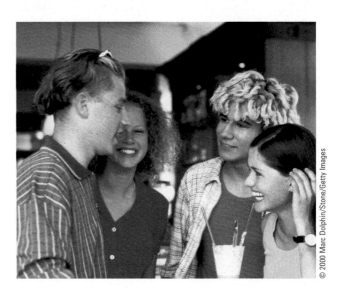

▲ During adolescence, sexuality develops rapidly. Teens explore different social and intimate relationships as they begin to develop a sexual identity.

© 2000 Marc Dolphin/Stone/Getty Images

## Student Snapshot ▸ Where Do Young Americans Learn About Relationships and Sexual Health?

| 18- to 24-year-olds | | Men | Women | Sexually Active | Not Sexually Active |
|---|---|---|---|---|---|
| **Friends** | | | | | |
| A lot | 47% | 44% | 48% | 48% | 42% |
| Some | 29% | 30% | 30% | 27% | 35% |
| Only a little | 16% | 17% | 15% | 16% | 15% |
| Nothing at all | 7% | 9% | 6% | 8% | 7% |
| **Sex-education classes** | | | | | |
| A lot | 40% | 46% | 45% | 43% | 50% |
| Some | 24% | 22% | 24% | 21% | 25% |
| Only a little | 17% | 16% | 15% | 17% | 12% |
| Nothing at all | 18% | 15% | 16% | 17% | 12% |
| **Boyfriends, girlfriends, partners** | | | | | |
| A lot | 39% | 35% | 34% | 41% | 20% |
| Some | 31% | 32% | 31% | 31% | 32% |
| Only a little | 18% | 19% | 20% | 18% | 22% |
| Nothing at all | 12% | 13% | 15% | 9% | 24% |
| **Media** | | | | | |
| A lot | 38% | 30% | 43% | 37% | 35% |
| Some | 35% | 37% | 33% | 34% | 37% |
| Only a little | 19% | 22% | 17% | 19% | 20% |
| Nothing at all | 8% | 10% | 7% | 9% | 7% |
| **Parents** | | | | | |
| A lot | 37% | 34% | 37% | 35% | 43% |
| Some | 27% | 31% | 29% | 29% | 32% |
| Only a little | 25% | 23% | 21% | 25% | 17% |
| Nothing at all | 11% | 11% | 8% | 11% | 7% |

*Numbers don't necessarily add up to 100 percent because some respondents said "don't know" or refused to answer.

Source: *The Sexual Health of Adolescents and Young Adults.* Menlo Park, CA: Henry J. Kaiser Family Foundation, 2002.

in HIV-risky sexual activity (such as intercourse without a condom) far more frequently than they did themselves. According to their self-reports, 14 percent of the students engaged in unprotected intercourse, 19 percent in oral sex, and 2 percent had sexual relations with someone they had just met. Yet they believed that much higher percentages of students—more than half in some cases—engaged in these behaviors, particularly if drunk or high.[38]

 Although different Asian cultures vary in their openness about sex, most consider sex outside marriage inappropriate, and they tend to value modesty and restrained sexuality. In several studies over recent decades, Asian-American college students tended to be more sexually conservative than their peers. In a survey of college students in southern California, Asian-American men and women were more

likely to be virgins than Caucasians. Those who were sexually active reported fewer lifetime sexual partners.[39]

 Students' sexual activity, particularly unsafe practices, often correlate with other risky behaviors. Researchers have found that students who have had multiple sexual partners are more likely to report binge drinking, drinking and driving, physical fighting, thinking about suicide, and marijuana use.[40]

A substantial proportion of college students—male and female—report that they engage in unwanted sexual activity. Sometimes this is the result of sexual coercion (a problem discussed in Chapter 14) or alcohol use.[41] However, some students admit to feigning desire and consenting to an unwanted sexual activity for various reasons, including satisfying a partner's needs, promoting intimacy, and avoiding relationship tension.

College students, even when well informed, do not always take precautions to reduce the risk of STDs. Often they believe that HIV and other infections simply couldn't happen to them, or they use misleading criteria in assessing risk. Some college students, especially men, rely too much on a potential partner's physical attractiveness and give less consideration to sexual history. Women tend to insist on safe-sex practices with a new partner, but as they become more seriously involved, they use protection less often—a potentially dangerous practice since knowing someone better doesn't make sex safer.

A study of 61 homosexual college men at a large mid-Atlantic state university found considerable concern about HIV infection. More than a quarter of the men had not engaged in homosexual activity. Of the 72 percent who had, some made dramatic changes in their sexual behavior because of their fear of HIV: 7 percent became celibate, and 14 percent no longer engaged in anal intercourse. About half limited the number of people with whom they had sex and reported being more selective in choosing partners; 36 percent refused to have sex without a condom.

## Sexual Diversity

Human beings are diverse in all ways—including sexual preferences and practices. Physiological, psychological, and social factors determine whether we are attracted to members of the same sex or the other sex. This attraction is our **sexual orientation.** Sigmund Freud argued that we all start off **bisexual,** or attracted to both sexes. But by the time we reach adulthood, most males prefer female sexual partners, and most females prefer male partners. **Heterosexual** is the term used for individuals whose primary orientation is toward members of the other sex. In virtually all cultures, some men and women are **homosexuals,** preferring partners of their own sex.

In our society, we tend to view heterosexuality and homosexuality as very different. In reality, these orientations are opposite ends of a spectrum of sexual preferences. Sex researcher Alfred Kinsey devised a seven-point continuum representing sexual orientation in American society. At one end of the continuum are those exclusively attracted to members of the other sex; at the opposite end are people exclusively attracted to members of the same sex. In between are varying degrees of homosexual, bisexual, and heterosexual orientation.

According to Kinsey's original data, 4 percent of men and 2 percent of women are exclusively homosexual. More recent studies have found lower numbers. For instance, in the University of Chicago's national survey, 2.8 percent of men and 1.4 percent of women defined themselves as homosexual. However, when asked if they'd had sex with a person of the same gender since age 18, about 5 percent of men and 4 percent of women said yes. When asked if they found members of the same gender sexually attractive, 6 percent of men and 5.5 percent of women said yes.

## Bisexuality

 Bisexuality—sexual attraction to both males and females—can develop at any point in one's life. In some cultures, bisexual activity is considered part of normal sexual experimentation. Among the Sabmia Highlanders in Papua New Guinea, for instance, boys perform oral sex on one another as part of the rites of passage into manhood.[42]

Some people identify themselves as bisexual even if they don't behave bisexually. Some are *serial* bisexuals—that is, they are sexually involved with same-sex partners for a while and then with partners of the other sex, or vice versa. An estimated 7 to 9 million men, about twice the number thought to be exclusively homosexual, could be described as bisexual during some extended period of their lives. The largest group are married, rarely have sexual relations with women other than their wives, and have secret sexual involvements with men.

Fear of HIV infection has sparked great concern about bisexuality, particularly among heterosexual women who worry about becoming involved with a bisexual man. About 20 to 30 percent of women with AIDS were infected by bisexual partners, and health officials fear that bisexual men who hide their homosexual affairs could transmit HIV to many more women.

## Homosexuality

Homosexuality—social, emotional, and sexual attraction to members of the same sex—exists in almost all cultures. Men and women homosexuals are commonly referred to as *gay;* women homosexuals are also called *lesbians.*

Homosexuality threatens and upsets many people, perhaps because homosexuals are viewed as different, or perhaps because no one understands why some people are heterosexual and others homosexual. *Homophobia* has led to an increase in *gay bashing* (attacking homosexuals) in many communities, including college campuses. Some blame the emergence of AIDS as a societal danger. However, researchers have found that fear of AIDS has not created new hostility but has simply given bigots an excuse to act out their hatred.

Violations of basic human rights for homosexuals remain common around the globe. Amnesty International has documented abuses ranging from exile to labor camps in China to social cleansing death squads in Colombia to the death penalty in Iran.

According to polls conducted by the Gallup Organization, American attitudes toward homosexuality

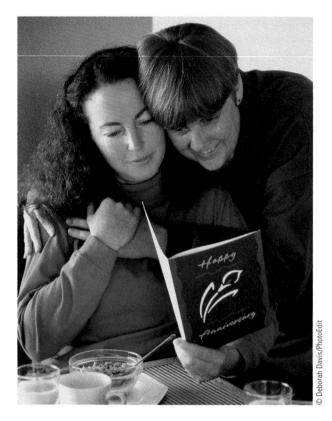

▲ Close-couple homosexual relationships are similar to stable heterosexual relationships.

have become more tolerant over time. In 1977, when pollsters asked Americans, "Do you think homosexual relations between consenting adults should or should not be legal?" 43 percent said they should be legal and 43 percent said they should not; 14 percent weren't sure. In 2001, 54 percent said yes, 42 percent said no, 4 percent weren't sure. The percentage of those saying that homosexuals should have equal rights in terms of job opportunities rose from 56 percent in 1977 to 85 percent in 2001. In 2001, 52 percent said that homosexuality should be considered an acceptable alternative lifestyle, up from 34 percent in 1982.[43]

## Roots of Homosexuality

Most mental health experts agree that nobody knows what causes a person's sexual orientation. Research has discredited theories tracing homosexuality to troubled childhoods or abnormal psychological development. Sexual orientation probably emerges from a complex interaction that includes biological and environmental factors.

For decades, behavioral and medical specialists have debated whether homosexuality is biologically or socially determined. Some say that sexual orientation is genetically determined. However, new research has cast doubt on the existence of a homosexuality gene. Others contend that prenatal hormones influence sexual preference. Today, questions and controversies persist about the roots and nature of sexual orientation.

## Homosexual Lifestyles

Extensive studies of male and female homosexuals have shown that only a minority have problems coping with their homosexuality. The happiest and best adjusted tend to be those in close-couple relationships, the equivalent of stable heterosexual partnerships. An estimated 3 to 5 million gays and lesbians have conceived children in heterosexual relationships; others have become parents through adoption or artificial insemination. These men and women describe their families as much like any other, and studies of lesbian mothers have found that their children are essentially no different from children of heterosexual couples in self-esteem, gender-related issues and roles, sexual orientation, and general development.[44]

 Different ethnic groups respond to homosexuality in different ways. To a greater extent than white homosexuals, gays and lesbians from ethnic groups tend to stay in the closet longer rather than risk alienation from their families and communities. Often they feel forced to choose between their gay and their ethnic identities.

# Sexual Activity

Part of learning about your own sexuality is having a clear understanding of human sexual behaviors. Understanding frees us from fear and anxiety, so that we may accept ourselves and others as the natural sexual beings we all are.

## Celibacy

A celibate person does not engage in sexual activity. Complete **celibacy** means that the person doesn't masturbate (stimulate himself or herself sexually) or engage in sexual activity with a partner. In partial celibacy, the person masturbates but doesn't have sexual contact with others. Many people decide to be celibate at certain times of their lives. Some don't have sex because of concerns about pregnancy or STDs; others haven't found a partner for a permanent, monogamous relationship. Many simply have other priorities, such as finishing school or starting a career, and realize that sex outside of a committed relationship is a threat to their physical and psychological well-being.

## STRATEGIES FOR CHANGE

### How to Say No to Sex

▲ First of all, recognize your own values and feelings. If you believe that sex is something to be shared only by people who've already become close in other ways, be true to that belief.

▲ If you're at a loss for words, try these responses: "I like you a lot, but I'm not ready to have sex." "You're a great person, but sex isn't something I do to prove I like someone." "I'd like to wait until I'm married to have sex."

▲ If you're feeling pressured, let your date know that you're uncomfortable. Be simple and direct. Watch out for emotional blackmail. If your date says, "If you really like me, you'd want to make love," point out that if he or she really likes you, he or she wouldn't try to force you to do something you don't want to do.

▲ If you're a woman, monitor your sexual signals. Men impute more sexual meaning to gestures (such as casual touching) that women perceive as friendly and innocent.

▲ Communicate your feelings to your date sooner rather than later. It's far easier to say, "I don't want to go to your apartment," than to fight off unwelcome advances once you're there.

▲ Remember that if saying no to sex puts an end to a relationship, it wasn't much of a relationship in the first place.

## Abstinence

The CDC defines **abstinence** as "refraining from sexual activities which involve vaginal, anal, and oral intercourse." Increasing numbers of adolescents and young adults are choosing to remain virgins and abstain from sexual intercourse until they enter a permanent, committed, monogamous relationship. About 2.5 million teens have taken pledges to abstain from sex. According to a major study, teens who do so are 34 percent less likely to have premarital sex than others, and are far older when they finally engage in intercourse.[45] The federal government, which has promoted abstinence as a means of preventing pregnancy and sexually transmitted diseases, funded abstinence education programs for two decades.[46] However, programs receiving no federal funding, such as the abstinence-only

program called Best Friends, also report success by providing teens with moral support and the facts on the real consequences of premarital sex.[47]

Many people who were sexually active in the past also are choosing abstinence because the risk of medical complications associated with STDs increases with the number of sexual partners a person has. Abstinence is the safest, healthiest option for many. However, there is confusion about what it means to abstain, and individuals who think they are abstaining may still be engaging in behaviors that put them at risk for HIV and STDs.

## Sex in Cyberspace

The Internet, designed for communication of very different sorts, has become a new medium for relationships, including those that might be described as sexual. In certain chat rooms, individuals can share explicit sexual fantasies or engage in the cyberspace equivalent of mutual fantasizing. In some ways, the Internet is the perfect venue for a safe form of sexual risk-taking. Individuals can assume any name, gender, race, or personality, and can pretend to lead lives entirely different from their actual existences. However, studies of individuals who had sexual intercourse with partners they met through the Internet found a greater risk for sexually transmitted diseases.[48]

Many see cybersex as a harmless way of adding an extra erotic charge to their daily lives. In some cases, individuals who meet in cybersex chat rooms develop what they come to think of as a meaningful relationship and arrange to meet in person. Sometimes these meetings are awkward; sometimes they do lead to a real-life romance. However, they rarely survive the intrusive reality of everyday existence and sometimes they end disastrously in disappointment or danger.

 In a study of 506 undergraduates at a public university in Texas, 43 percent had logged on to sexually explicit materials through the Internet, although only 2.9 percent said they did so frequently. About one in ten campus computer users logged on to sexually explicit websites from university computers; one in four home computer users searched for sexually explicit material. Male students were much more likely to have done so; curiosity about sex was their motivation for this behavior. Women were significantly more likely to have experienced sexual harassment while online. Asked about specific behaviors while online, 15 percent of the students reported masturbating online.[49] (See Figure 7-6.)

For some individuals, particularly gays and lesbians, the Internet provides the opportunity to join a virtual community. In addition to sexual exchanges, they can find access to information and resources that may not be available elsewhere. For adolescents struggling with gender identity or for closeted homosexuals, going online can be

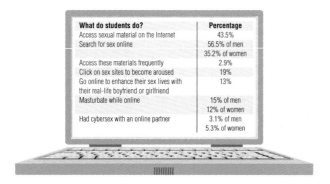

| What do students do? | Percentage |
|---|---|
| Access sexual material on the Internet | 43.5% |
| Search for sex online | 56.5% of men |
| | 35.2% of women |
| Access these materials frequently | 2.9% |
| Click on sex sites to become aroused | 19% |
| Go online to enhance their sex lives with | 13% |
| their real-life boyfriend or girlfriend | |
| Masturbate while online | 15% of men |
| | 12% of women |
| Had cybersex with an online partner | 3.1% of men |
| | 5.3% of women |

▲ **Figure 7-6** Cybersex on Campus
A study of more than 500 undergraduates found that many students use the Internet as a resource for a variety of sexual activities.

Source: Goodson, Patricia, et al. "Searching for Sexually Explicit Materials on the Internet: An Exploratory Study of College Students' Behavior and Attitudes." *Archives of Sexual Behavior*, Vol. 30, No. 3, April 2001, p. 101.

their only opportunity to be open about their sexuality. But they do face an increased risk of syphilis and HIV if they pursue a relationship off-line.[50]

## Masturbation

Not everybody masturbates, but most people do. Kinsey estimated that 7 out of 10 women and 19 out of 20 men masturbate (and admit they do). Their reason is simple: It feels good. **Masturbation** produces the same physical responses as sexual activity with a partner and can be an enjoyable form of sexual release.

Masturbation has been described as immature; unsocial; tiring; frustrating; and a cause of hairy palms, warts, blemishes, and blindness. None of these myths is true. Even Freud felt that masturbation was normal for children. Sex educators recommend masturbation to adolescents as a means of releasing tension and becoming familiar with their sexual organs. Throughout adulthood, masturbation often is the primary sexual activity of individuals not involved in a sexual relationship and can be particularly useful when illness, absence, divorce, or death deprives a person of a partner. In the University of Chicago survey, about 25 percent of men and 9 percent of women said they masturbate at least once a week.

White men and women have a higher incidence of masturbation than African-American men and women. Hispanic women have the lowest rate of masturbation, when compared with Hispanic men, white men and women, and black men and women. Individuals with a higher level of education are more likely to masturbate than those with less schooling, and people living with sexual partners masturbate more than those who live alone.

## Intercourse

Vaginal **intercourse,** or *coitus,* refers to the penetration of the vagina by the penis. (See Figure 7-7). This is the preferred form of sexual intimacy for most heterosexual couples, who may use a wide variety of positions. The most familiar position for intercourse in our society is the so-called missionary position, with the man on top, facing the woman. An alternative is the woman on top, either lying down or sitting upright. Other positions include lying side by side (either face to face or with the man behind the woman, his penis entering her vagina from the rear); lying with the man on top of the woman in a rear-entry position; and kneeling or standing (again, in either a face-to-face or rear-entry position). Many couples move into several different positions for intercourse during a single episode of lovemaking; others may have a personal favorite or may choose different positions at different times.

Sexual activity, including intercourse, is possible throughout a woman's menstrual cycle. However, some women prefer to avoid sex while menstruating because of uncomfortable physical symptoms, such as cramps, or concern about bleeding or messiness. Others use a diaphragm or cervical cap (see Chapter 8) to hold back menstrual flow. Since different cultures have different views on intercourse during a woman's menstrual period, partners should discuss their own feelings and try to respect each other's views. If they choose not to have intercourse, there are other gratifying forms of sexual activity.

Vaginal intercourse, like other forms of sexual activity involving an exchange of bodily fluids, carries a risk of sexually transmitted diseases, including HIV infection. In many other parts of the world, in fact, heterosexual intercourse is the most common means of HIV transmission. (See Chapter 9.)

## Oral-Genital Sex

Our mouths and genitals give us some of our most intense pleasures. Though it might seem logical to combine the two, some people are very uncomfortable with oral-genital sex. Some even consider it a perversion; it is against the law in many states and a sin in some religions. However, others find it normal and acceptable.

The formal terms for oral sex are **cunnilingus,** which refers to oral stimulation of the woman's genitals, and **fellatio,** oral stimulation of the man's genitals. For many couples, oral-genital sex is a regular part of their lovemaking. For others, it's an occasional experiment. Oral sex with a partner carrying a sexually transmitted disease, such as herpes or HIV infection, can lead to infection, so a condom should be used (with cunnilingus, a condom cut in half to lay flat can be used).

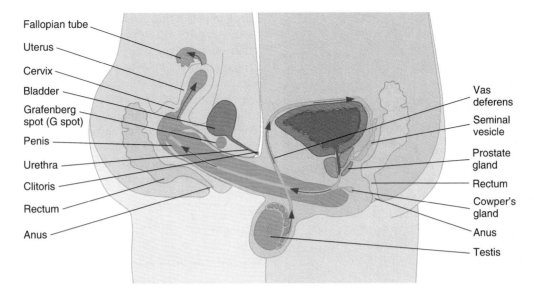

▲ **Figure 7-7** Cross-Sectional View of Sexual Intercourse
Sperm are formed in each of the testes and stored in the epididymis. When a man ejaculates, the sperm (in semen) travels up the vas deferens. (The prostate gland and seminal vesicles contribute components of the semen.) The semen is expelled from the penis through the urethra and deposited in the vagina, near the cervix. During sexual excitement and orgasm in a woman, the upper end of the vagina enlarges and the uterus elevates. After orgasm, these organs return to their normal states, and the cervix descends into the pool of semen.

 Different groups of the population have diverse views of oral sex. In one survey, more African-American than white men reported never having performed or received oral sex.[51]

## Anal Stimulation and Intercourse

Because the anus has many nerve endings, it can produce intense erotic responses. Stimulation of the anus by the fingers or mouth can be a source of sexual arousal; anal intercourse involves penile penetration of the anus. As with oral-genital sex, not everyone feels comfortable with anal stimulation and anal intercourse. An estimated 25 percent of adults have experienced anal intercourse at least once. However, anal sex involves important health risks, such as damage to sensitive rectal tissues and the transmission of various intestinal infections, hepatitis, and STDs, including HIV.

## Sexual Concerns

Many sexual concerns stem from myths and misinformation. There is no truth, for instance, behind these misconceptions: Men are always capable of erection, sex always involves intercourse, partners should experience simultaneous orgasms, and people who truly love each other always have satisfying sex lives.

Cultural and childhood influences can affect our attitudes toward sex. Even though America's traditionally puritanical values have eased, our society continues to convey mixed messages about sex. Some children, repeatedly warned of the evils of sex, never accept the sexual dimensions of their identity. Others, especially young boys, may be exposed to macho attitudes toward sex and feel a need to prove their virility. Young girls may feel confused by media messages that encourage them to look and act provocatively and a double standard that blames them for leading boys on. In addition, virtually everyone has individual worries. A woman may feel self-conscious about the shape of her breasts; a man may worry about the size of his penis; both partners may fear not pleasing the other.

The concept of sexual normalcy differs greatly in different times, cultures, or racial and ethnic groups. In certain times and places, only sex between a husband and wife has been deemed normal. In other circumstances, "normal" has been applied to any sexual behavior that does not harm others or produce great anxiety and guilt.

## Safer Sex

Having sex is never completely safe; the only 100 percent risk-free sexual choice is abstinence. If you choose to be sexually active, you can greatly reduce your risk by restricting sexual activity to the context of a mutually exclusive, monogamous relationship in which both partners know,

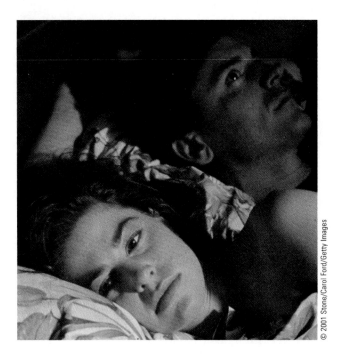

▲ Sexual problems can be difficult for partners to talk about, but lack of communication can create tension and anxiety.

© 2001 Stone/Carol Ford/Getty Images

time and place that is relaxed and comfortable. Arm yourself with facts so you can answer any questions or objections your partner raises. Start on a positive note—for instance, by saying how much you care for your partner and saying that this is the reason you want to discuss something important. This is the time for you to be honest about any STDs you might have had or still carry. Give your partner time to take in what you've said. If you find out about a partner's STD, you may feel a range of emotions. You also will need to acquire information about symptoms, treatment, and how the disease is spread.[53]

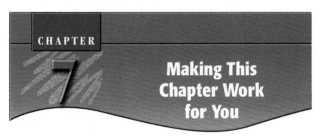

 What does research say about the connection between chat rooms and STDs?

CHAPTER

7

**Making This Chapter Work for You**

on the basis of laboratory testing, that neither has HIV antibodies or a sexually transmitted disease. Sober sex, in which both partners are not under the influence of drugs or alcohol, is more likely to be safer sex.

 In a study of college students, information on how many couples practice safer sex had unexpected effects. On the one hand, when students learn that the prevalence of safer sex is high, they see this as "normative" or typical, acceptable behavior. On the other hand, they conclude that because of this, their perceived risk is lower—so they are less likely to say they intend to use condoms the next time they engage in sex.[52]

Sex with a person who has never been exposed to HIV or to other STDs is safe (for you), regardless of what type of sexual activity you engage in. The only way of knowing for certain that a prospective partner doesn't have an STD or is not infected with HIV is through laboratory testing (see Chapter 9). Sex educators and health professionals strongly encourage couples to abstain from any sexual activity that puts them at risk for STDs until they both undergo medical examinations and testing for STDs. This process greatly reduces the danger of disease transmission and can also help foster a deep sense of mutual trust and commitment. Many campus and public health clinics provide exams or laboratory testing free of charge or on a sliding scale determined by your income.

Talking to a potential partner is the first step toward safer sex. Professionals offer advice on how to discuss a topic that makes many people uncomfortable: Choose a

1. In friendships and other intimate relationships, which of the following is *not* true?
   a. Friends can communicate feelings as well as facts.
   b. Listening is just as important as talking.
   c. Emotional investment is required but the rewards are great.
   d. There is no need to pay attention to nonverbal communication.

2. The characteristics of a good relationship include which of the following?
   a. trust
   b. financial stability
   c. identical interests
   d. physical attractiveness

3. When looking for a mate, the crucial ingredients for commitment include which of the following?
   a. shared values
   b. desire to make the relationship work
   c. willingness to tolerate flaws
   d. ability to communicate effectively

4. Partners in successful marital relationships
   a. are generally from the same social and ethnic background.
   b. usually lived together before marrying.
   c. were usually very young at the time of their marriage.
   d. have premarital agreements.

5. Which of the following statements about divorce is false?

a. The older the bride, the more likely the chance that the marriage will endure.

b. African-American couples are more likely to divorce than white couples.

c. About 25% of all marriages end in divorce.

d. The majority of divorced men and women remarry, even after multiple divorces.

6. Which of the following statements about menstruation and the menstrual cycle is true?

a. Distance running can lead to amenorrhea.

b. Premenstrual syndrome is a physiological disorder that usually results in amenorrhea.

c. Ovulation occurs at the end of the menstrual cycle.

d. Premenstrual syndrome is a physiological condition that is unrelated to premenstrual dysphoric disorder.

7. Which statement about male anatomy is *incorrect*?

a. The testes manufacture testosterone and sperm.

b. Sperm cells are carried in the liquid semen.

c. Cowper's glands secrete semen.

d. Circumcision is the surgical removal of the foreskin of the penis.

8. Young Americans learn about relationships and sexuality primarily from which of the following?

a. friends

b. sex-education classes

c. the media

d. their parents

9. Which of the following statements is true about sexual orientation?

a. Most individuals who identify themselves as bisexual are really homosexual.

b. Homosexuality is caused by a poor family environment.

c. Homosexual behavior is found only in affluent and well-educated cultures.

d. African-American, Hispanic, and Asian cultures tend to be less accepting of homosexuality than the white community.

10. According to the Centers for Disease Control and Prevention, abstinence is defined as

a. refraining from all sexual behaviors that result in arousal.

b. refraining from all sexual activities that involve vaginal, anal, and oral intercourse.

c. having sexual intercourse with only one partner.

d. refraining from drinking alcohol before sexual activity.

Answers to these questions can be found on page 415.

## Critical Thinking

1. While our society has become more tolerant, marriages between people of different religious and racial groups still face special pressures. What issues might arise if a Christian marries a Jewish or Muslim man or woman? What about the issues facing partners of different races? How could these issues be resolved? What are your own feelings about mixed marriages? Would you date someone of a different religion or race? Why or why not?

2. What are your personal criteria for a successful relationship? Develop a brief list of factors you consider important, and support your choices with examples or experiences from your own life.

3. Bill told his girlfriend, Anita, that he has never taken any sexual risks. But when she suggested that they get tested for STDs, he became furious and refused. Now Anita says she doesn't know what to believe. Could Bill be telling the truth, or is he hiding something? If he is telling the truth, why is Bill so upset? Anita doesn't want to take any risks, but she doesn't want to lose him either. What would you advise her to say or do? What would you advise Bill to say or do?

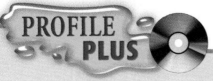

## PROFILE PLUS

Caring communication is the key to most healthy relationships. Assess the degree of good communication in your intimate relationship with this activity on your Profile Plus CD-ROM:

How Strong is the Communication and Affection in Your Relationship?

# SITES & BYTES

## International Society for the Study of Personal Relationships
www.isspr.org

This site contains information for professionals and educators on interpersonal relationship dynamics. Features include current news articles on relationships, calendar of upcoming conferences, lists of publications, and links to other professional organizations.

## Go Ask Alice
www.goaskalice.columbia.edu/Cat6.html

This site, created by Columbia University's Health Education program, features answers to questions pertaining to relationships, sexuality, and sexual health.

## Sexuality Information and Education Council of the United States (SIECUS)
www.siecus.org

This site features sexual education information for youth, parents, and teachers. The site also provides numerous fact sheets on topics ranging from abstinence to birth control, and on issues that target specific groups (for example, adolescents or homosexuals).

## InfoTrac College Edition Activity
Eli Coleman. "Promoting Sexual Health and Responsible Sexual Behavior: An Introduction." *Journal of Sex Research,* Vol. 39, No. 1, February 2002, p. 3 (4).

1. According to the authors, what is the definition of *sexual health?* Why is it difficult to construct a universally acceptable definition?

2. Besides the biologic concepts of sex, what other components describe *sexuality*?

3. According to the World Health Organization, what are five overarching goals and corresponding strategies useful to promote sexual health?

You can find additional readings related to communication and to sexuality with InfoTrac College Edition, an online library of more than 900 journals and publications. Follow the instructions for accessing InfoTrac that were packaged with your textbook; then search for articles using a keyword search.

For additional links, resources, and suggested readings on InfoTrac, visit our Health & Wellness Resource Center at http://health.wadsworth.com.

# Key Terms

The terms listed here are used within the chapter on the page indicated. Definitions of the terms are in the Glossary at the end of the book.

| | | | |
|---|---|---|---|
| abstinence 165 | endometrium 155 | mons pubis 155 | seminal vesicles 160 |
| amenorrhea 158 | epididymis 159 | ovaries 155 | sexual orientation 163 |
| bisexual 163 | estrogen 156 | ovulation 156 | sperm 159 |
| blended family 155 | fallopian tubes 155 | ovum (ova) 155 | testes 159 |
| celibacy 164 | family 155 | penis 159 | testosterone 159 |
| cervix 155 | fellatio 166 | perineum 155 | toxic shock syndrome |
| circumcision 161 | heterosexual 163 | premenstrual dysphoric | (TSS) 159 |
| clitoris 155 | homosexual 163 | disorder (PMDD) 158 | urethra 159 |
| cohabitation 151 | intercourse 166 | premenstrual syndrome | urethral opening 155 |
| corpus luteum 156 | intimacy 150 | (PMS) 158 | uterus 155 |
| Cowper's glands 160 | labia majora 155 | progesterone 158 | vagina 155 |
| cunnilingus 166 | labia minora 155 | prostate gland 160 | vas deferens 160 |
| dysmenorrhea 158 | masturbation 166 | scrotum 159 | |
| ejaculatory duct 160 | menstruation 158 | semen 160 | |

# References

1. Mehrabian, Albert. Personal interview.

2. Maple, Marilyn. Personal interview.

3. Swann, William, et al. "Socialization Patterns of Depressed and Non-Depressed College Students." *Journal of Abnormal Psychology,* Vol. 104, 1992.

4. Brendgen, Mara, et al. "The Relations Between Friendship Quality, Ranked-Friendship Preference, and Adolescents' Behavior with Their Friends." *Merrill-Palmer Quarterly,* Vol. 47, No. 3, July 2001, p. 395.

5. Chatterjee, Camille. "Can Men and Women Be Friends?" *Psychology Today,* September–October, 2001, p. 61.

6. Gard, Caroline. "The Secrets to Making Lasting Friendships." *Current Health 2,* Vol. 27, No. 2, October 2000.

7. Silverman, Jay, et al. "Dating Violence Against Adolescent Girls and Associated Substance Use, Unhealthy Weight Control, Sexual Risk Behavior, Pregnancy, and Suicidality." *Journal of the American Medical Association,* Vol. 286, No. 5, August 1, 2001, p. 572.

8. DuRant, Robert. "Watching Wrestling Positively Associated with Date Fighting." Presentation, American Academy of Pediatrics Meeting, Baltimore, April 2001.

9. Sprecher, Susan. "Insiders' Perspectives on Reasons for Attraction to a Close Other." *Social Psychology Quarterly,* Vol. 61, No. 4, December 1998.

10. Laumann, Edward. Personal interview.

11. Sprecher. "Insiders' Perspectives on Reasons for Attraction to a Close Other."

12. Buss, David. *The Evolution of Desire.* New York: Basic Books, 1994.

13. Sommers, Jennifer, and Stephen Vodanovich. "Vengeance Scores Among College Students: Examining the Role of Jealously and Forgiveness." *Education,* Vol. 121, No. 1, Fall 2000.

14. Jabusch, Willard. "The Myth of Cohabitation: Cohabiting Couples Lack Both Specialization and Commitment in Their Relationships." *America,* Vol. 183, No. 10, October 7, 2000.

15. Ibid.

16. Popenoe, David. *The State of Our Unions: The Social Health of Marriage in America.* Piscataway, NJ: Rutgers, 2000.

17. Kantrowitz, Barbara, and Pat Wingert. "Unmarried, with Children." *Newsweek,* May 28, 2001, p. 46.

18. Crooks, Robert, and Karla Baur. *Our Sexuality,* 8th ed. Pacific Grove, CA: Wadsworth, 2002.

19. Sternberg, Robert. Personal interview.

20. Bramlett, Matthew, and William Mosher. "Love and Marriage." *Forecast,* Vol. 21, No. 10, July 2, 2001, p. 11. Also available at www/cdc.gov/nchs/data/ad/ad323.pdf.

21. Popenoe, *The State of Our Unions.*

22. U.S. Census Bureau.

23. Ibid.

24. Wyn, Roberta, et al. "Falling Through the Cracks: Health Insurance Coverage of Low-Income Women." Menlo Park, CA: Henry J. Kaiser Family Foundation, February 2001.

25. Dimmock, Paul, et al. "Efficacy of Selective Serotonin-Reuptake Inhibitors in Premenstrual Syndrome: A Systematic Review." *Lancet,* Vol. 356, No. 9236, September 30, 2000.

26. "Calcium for PMS, Bone Health." *Contemporary OB/GYN,* Vol. 46, No. 5, May 2001, p. 151.

27. "New Treatment Approved for Severe Premenstrual Symptoms." *FDA Consumer,* Vol. 34, No. 5, September 2000.

28. Steiner, Meir. "Recognition of Premenstrual Dysphoric Disorder and Its Treatment." *Lancet,* Vol. 356, No. 9236, September 30, 2000.

29. "Premenstrual Mood Disturbance." *Harvard Medical Health Letter,* Vol. 17, No. 12, June 2001.

30. Swayze, Sonia. "Preventing Problems from Tampon Use." *Nursing,* Vol. 31, No. 7, July 2001, p. 28.

31. "Just the Facts . . . Circumcision." American Academy of Pediatrics, www.aap.org/mrt/factscir.htm

32. Schoen, Edgar et al. "New Policy on Circumcision—Cause for Concern." *Pediatrics,* Vol. 105, No. 3, March 2000.

33. Adler, Robert, et al. "Circumcision: We Have Heard from the Experts; Now Let's Hear from the Parents." *Pediatrics,* Vol. 107, No. 2, February 2001, p. 395.

34. Kelley, R. Mark. "Sexual Behaviors of College Students Attending Four Universities in a Southern State." *Research Quarterly for Exercise and Sport,* Vol. 72, No. 1, March 2001, p. A-31.

35. Bon, Rebecca, et al. "Normative Perceptions in Relation to Substance Use and HIV-Risky Sexual Behaviors of College Students." *Journal of Psychology,* Vol. 135, No. 2, March 2001, p. 165.

36. "The Sexual Health of Adolescents and Young Adults." Menlo Park, CA: Henry J. Kaiser Family Foundation, 2002.

37. Luquis, R., et al. "College Students' Perceptions of Substance Use and Sexual Behaviors." *Research Quarterly for Exercise and Sport,* Vol. 72, No. 1, March 2001, p. A-33.

38. Bon, "Normative Perceptions in Relation to Substance Use and HIV-Risky Sexual Behaviors of College Students."

39. Okazaki, Sumie. "Influences of Culture on Asian Americans' Sexuality." *Journal of Sex Research,* Vol. 39, No. 1, February 2002, p. 34.

40. Ogletree, Roberta, et al. "Associations Between Lifetime Sexual Partners and Health Risk Behaviors in a Representative Sample of United States College Students." *Research Quarterly for Exercise and Sport,* Vol. 72, March 2001.

41. Ullman, Sarah, et al. "Alcohol and Sexual Assault in a National Sample of College Women." *Journal of Interpersonal Violence,* Vol. 14, No. 6, June 1999.

42. Crooks, Robert, and Karla Baur. *Our Sexuality,* 8th ed. Pacific Grove, CA: Wadsworth, 2002.

43. McKay, Alexander. "American Attitudes Toward Homosexuality Continue to Become More Tolerant." *Canadian Journal of Human Sexuality,* Vol. 9, No. 3, Fall 2000, p. 212.

44. Baugher, Shirley. "Same Sex Relationships." *Journal of Family and Consumer Sciences,* Vol. 92, No. 3, May 2000.

45. "Better Than Condoms in a Cookie Jar." *American Enterprise,* Vol. 12, No. 3, April 2001, p. 10.

46. Sonfield, Adam, and Rachel Gold. "States' Implementation of the Section 510 Abstinence Education Program." *Family Planning Perspectives,* Vol. 33, No. 4, July 2001, p. 166.

47. Edwards, Catherine. "Teens Really Need 'Best Friends.'" *Insight on the News,* Vol. 17, No. 28, July 30, 2001, p. 18.

48. Toomey, Kathleen, and Richard Rothenberg, "Sex and Cyberspace—Virtual Networks Leading to High-Risk Sex." *Journal of the American Medical Association,* Vol. 284, No. 4, July 26, 2000.

49. Goodson, Patricia, et al. "Searching for Sexually Explicit Materials on the Internet: An Exploratory Study of College Students' Behavior and Attitudes." *Archives of Sexual Behavior,* Vol. 30, No. 2, April 2001, p. 101.

50. McFarlane, M., et al. "The Internet as a Newly Emerging Risk Environment for Sexually Transmitted Diseases." *Journal of the American Medical Association,* Vol. 384, No. 4, July 26, 2000.

51. Crooks and Baur, *Our Sexuality.*

52. Buunk, Bram, et al. "The Double-Edged Sword of Providing Information About the Prevalence of Safer Sex." *Journal of Applied Social Psychology,* Vol. 32, No. 4, 2002, p. 684.

53. "It's Your (Sex) Life." Menlo Park, CA: Henry J. Kaiser Family Foundation, 2002.

# Reproductive Choices

After studying the material in this chapter, you should be able to:

- **Describe** the process of human conception.
- **List** the major options available for contraception, and **identify** the advantages and risks of each.
- **Describe** the commonly used abortion methods.
- **Discuss** the physiological effects of pregnancy on a woman and **describe** fetal development.
- **Describe** the three stages of labor and the birth process.
- **Give examples** of infertility treatments.

s human beings, we have a unique power: the ability to choose to conceive or not to conceive. No other species on Earth can separate sexual activity and pleasure from reproduction. However, simply not wanting to get pregnant is never enough to prevent conception nor is wanting to have a child always enough to get pregnant. Both desires require individual decisions and actions.

Anyone who engages in vaginal intercourse must be willing to accept the consequences of that activity—the possibility of pregnancy and responsibility for the child who might be conceived—or take action to avoid those consequences. Although many people are concerned about the risks associated with contraception, using birth control is safer and healthier than not using it. According to the Population Reference Bureau, the use of contraceptives, including oral contraceptives, saves millions of lives each year. Some forms of contraception also reduce the risk of sexually transmitted diseases.

This chapter provides information on conception, birth control, abortion, infertility, and the processes by which a new human life develops and enters the world.

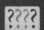

# Conception

The equation for making a baby is quite simple: One sperm plus one egg equals one fertilized egg, which can develop into an infant. But the processes that affect or permit **conception** are quite complicated. The creation of sperm, or **spermatogenesis,** starts in the male at puberty, and the production of sperm is regulated by hormones. Sperm cells form in the seminiferous tubules of the testes and are passed into the epididymis, where they are stored until ejaculation (see Figure 8-1); a single male ejaculation may contain 500 million sperm. Each sperm released into the vagina during intercourse moves on its own, propelling itself toward its target, an ovum.

To reach its goal, the sperm must move through the acidic secretions of the vagina, enter the uterus, travel up the fallopian tube containing the ovum, then fuse with the nucleus of the egg (**fertilization**). Just about every sperm produced by a man in his lifetime fails to accomplish its mission.

There are far fewer human egg cells than there are sperm cells. Each woman is born with her lifetime supply of ova, and between 300 and 500 eggs eventually mature and leave her ovaries during ovulation. As discussed in

Chapter 7, every month, one or the other of the woman's ovaries releases an ovum to the nearby fallopian tube. It travels through the fallopian tube until it reaches the uterus, a journey that takes three to four days. An unfertilized egg lives for about 24 to 36 hours, disintegrates, and, during menstruation, is expelled along with the uterine lining.

Even if a sperm, which can survive in the female reproductive tract for two to five days, meets a ripe egg in a fallopian tube, its success is not assured. It must penetrate the layer of cells and a jellylike substance that surround each egg. Every sperm that touches the egg deposits an enzyme that dissolves part of this barrier. When a sperm bumps into a bare spot, it can penetrate the egg membrane and merge with the egg. (See Figure 8-2.) The fertilized egg travels down the fallopian tube, dividing to form a tiny clump of cells called a **zygote.** When it reaches the uterus, about a week after fertilization, it burrows into the endometrium, the lining of the uterus. This process is called **implantation.**

Conception can be prevented by **contraception.** Some contraceptive methods prevent ovulation or implantation, and others block the sperm from reaching the egg. Some methods are temporary; others permanently alter one's fertility.

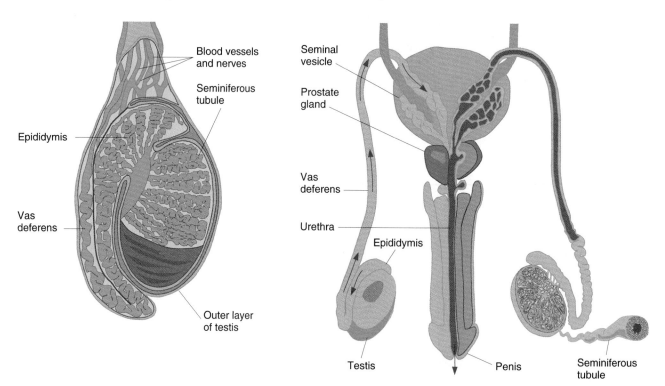

▲ **Figure 8-1** The Testes
Spermatogenesis takes place in the testes. Sperm cells form in the seminiferous tubules and are stored in the coils of the epididymis. Eventually, the sperm drain into the vas deferens, ready for ejaculation.

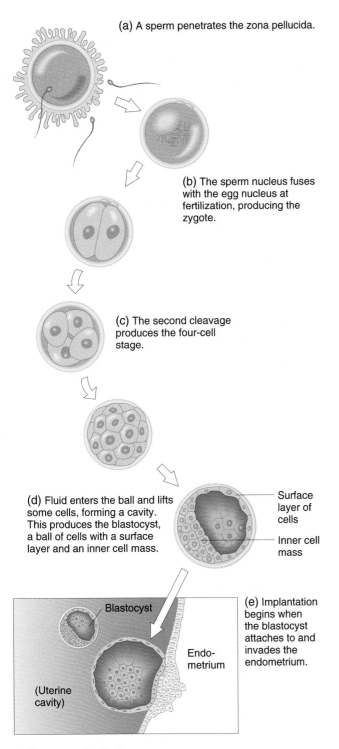

(a) A sperm penetrates the zona pellucida.

(b) The sperm nucleus fuses with the egg nucleus at fertilization, producing the zygote.

(c) The second cleavage produces the four-cell stage.

(d) Fluid enters the ball and lifts some cells, forming a cavity. This produces the blastocyst, a ball of cells with a surface layer and an inner cell mass.

Surface layer of cells

Inner cell mass

Blastocyst

(e) Implantation begins when the blastocyst attaches to and invades the endometrium.

Endo-metrium

(Uterine cavity)

▲ **Figure 8-2** Fertilization
(a) The efforts of hundreds of sperm may allow one to penetrate the ovum's corona radiata, an outer layer of cells, and then the zona pellucida, a thick inner membrane. (b) The nuclei of the sperm and the egg cells merge, and the male and female chromosomes in the nuclei come together, forming a zygote. (c) The zygote divides into two cells, then four cells, and so on. (d) As fluid enters the ball, cells form a ball of cells called a blastocyst. (e) The blastocyst implants itself in the endometrium.

# Birth Control Basics

A heterosexual woman in Western countries spends 90 percent of her reproductive years trying to prevent pregnancy and 10 percent of these years trying to become or being pregnant. Today birth control is safer, more effective, and more convenient than in the past—yet none of today's contraceptives is 100 percent safe, 100 percent effective, or 100 percent convenient. And even protection that is effective 95 percent of the time (which, some contend, is the best available in real-life use) isn't as good as it may sound. With just a 5 percent failure rate, statistically speaking, seven in ten women who want no more than two children would have to undergo one or more abortions in order to achieve their desired family size. See Table 8-1, which shows the use of contraception around the world.

Ideally, two partners should decide together which form of birth control to use. However, female methods account for 63 percent of all contraceptive methods reported by women between ages 15 and 44.[1] According to a national poll, more than 70 percent of men and women said men were "not responsible enough" to choose a birth control method. Both sexes believed that men were uninvolved because they "don't care" and because they consider birth control the "female's responsibility."[2] Lack of male involvement may account for 40 percent of each year's unwanted pregnancies.

Another barrier to birth control is cost. Although Medicaid contributes one of every two public dollars spent for family planning in the United States, many health insurers have not covered the cost of reversible methods of birth control—a policy that may be changing.[3] However, even when birth control is affordable and available, many college students do not use it consistently.

If you are engaging in sexual activity that could lead to conception, you have to be realistic about your situation. This may mean assuming full responsibility for your reproductive ability, whether you're a man or a woman. The more you know about contraception, the more likely you are to use birth control. You also have to recognize the risks associated with various methods of contraception. If you're a woman, the risks are chiefly yours. Although most women never experience any serious complications, it's important to be aware of the potential for long-term risks. Risks that are acceptable to others may not be acceptable to you.

 In one recent study at a Western college, undergraduates were more likely to report "almost always" using a reliable, proven method of birth control after completing an introductory health course.[4]

▼ **Table 8-1  Global Use of Contraception**

| Method of Contraception | Regularly Used by (Approximate) | Most Popular in These Places |
|---|---|---|
| Sterilization | 200 million | Asia, Latin America |
| Intrauterine device (IUD) | 110 million | China, Arab states |
| The pill | 70 million | Latin America, United States, Europe |
| Injectable methods | 10 million | Sub-Saharan Africa |
| Implants | 1.5 million | Indonesia |
| Condom | >25 million | Worldwide |

## How Do I Choose a Birth Control Method?

When it comes to deciding which form of birth control to use, there's no one "right" decision. In a study of contraceptive decisionmaking among African-American, Hispanic, and European-American women ages 18 to 50, those who made contraceptive decisions alone were older, single, African American, used pregnancy prevention, or had histories of sexually transmitted diseases and unintended pregnancies. Older African-American women were more likely to choose no contraception. Among contraceptive users, African Americans used effective methods of pregnancy, but not disease prevention. Women who had a history of sexually transmitted diseases and younger, more educated women were more likely to use methods that prevent both pregnancy and disease.[5]

Good decisions are based on sound information. You should consult a physician or family-planning counselor if you have questions or want to know how certain methods might affect existing or familial medical conditions, such as high blood pressure or diabetes. Table 8-2 presents your contraceptive choices. As the table indicates, contraception doesn't always work. When you evaluate any contraceptive, always consider its *effectiveness* (the likelihood that it will indeed prevent pregnancy). The **failure rate** refers to the number of pregnancies that occur per year for every 100 women using a particular method of birth control.

The reliability of contraceptives in actual, real-life use is much lower than those reported in national surveys or clinical trials. In general, failure rates are highest among cohabiting and other unmarried women, very poor families, black and Hispanic women, adolescents, and women in their twenties. Teenagers whose partners are three or more years older are less likely to use contraceptives regularly. Unmarried adolescent women who are living with a partner have an average failure rate of about 31 percent in the first year of contraceptive use, regardless of method of birth control, compared with a failure rate of 7 percent among married women aged 30 and older. The annual failure rate among black women is about 19 percent, regardless of family income. Among Hispanic women, the overall failure rate is 10 percent, but it is higher among poorer women than more affluent ones.

Some couples use withdrawal or **coitus interruptus,** removal of the penis from the vagina before ejaculation, to prevent pregnancy, even though this is not a reliable form of birth control. About half the men who have tried coitus interruptus find it unsatisfactory, either because they don't know when they're going to ejaculate or because they can't withdraw quickly enough. Also, the Cowper's glands, two pea-sized structures located on each side of the urethra, often produce a fluid that appears as drops at the tip of the penis any time from arousal and erection to orgasm. This

### STRATEGIES FOR PREVENTION

**Choosing a Contraceptive**

Your contraceptive needs may change throughout your life. To decide which method to use now, you need to know:

▲ How well will it fit into your lifestyle?

▲ How convenient will it be?

▲ How effective will it be?

▲ How safe will it be?

▲ How affordable will it be?

▲ How reversible will it be?

▲ Will it protect against sexually transmitted diseases?

Source: "Facts About Birth Control." www.plannedparenthood.org.

▼ **Table 8-2  Your Contraceptive Choices**

| Method | Effectiveness (Percentage) | Protection Against STDs | Cost |
|---|---|---|---|
| Abstinence | 100 | complete | none |
| Sterilization | 99.5–99.9 | none | $1,000–$2,500 for tubal sterilization; $240–$520 for vasectomy |
| Intrauterine device | 98–99 | none | $250–$400 for exam, insertion, and follow-up visit |
| Diaphragm, cervical cap | 80–90 for women who have not had a child; 60–80 for women who have had a child | limited | $35–$125 for exam; $13–$25 for diaphragm or cap |
| Combined hormonal methods | | | |
| The pill | 95–99.95 | none | $35–$125 for initial exam; $15–$35 for monthly packet of pills |
| The monthly shot (Lunelle) | 99 | none | $35–$125 for initial exam; $30–$35 for monthly injection |
| The ring (NuvaRing) | 95–99 | none | $35–$125 for initial exam; $30–$35 for month's supply of rings |
| The patch (Ortho Evra) | 95–99 | none | $35–$125 for initial exam; $$30–$35 for monthly supply of patches |
| Progestin-only methods | | | |
| The contraceptive implant | 99.95 | none | $500–$750 for exam, implant, and insertion; $100–$200 for removal |
| The quarterly shot (Depo-Provera) | 99.7 | none | $20–$40 for visits to clinic; $30–$75 for injection |
| Progestin-only birth control pill | 95 | none | $35–$125 for initial exam; $15–$35 for monthly pills |
| Over-the-counter methods | | | |
| Male condom | 86 (lowest estimate) | good | 50 cents and up per condom |
| Female condom | 79 (lowest estimate) | good | $2.50 per condom |
| Vaginal spermicide | 72 (lowest estimate) | none | $8 per applicator kit of foam or jelly, $4–$8 per refill |
| Periodic abstinence and fertility awareness methods | N/A | none | $5–$8 for temperature kits |

Sources: Planned Parenthood, Association of Reproductive Health Professionals..

fluid can contain active sperm and, in infected men, human immunodeficiency virus (HIV).

As many as 3 million unintentional pregnancies each year in the United States are the result of contraceptive failure, either from problems with the drug or device itself or from improper use. Partners can lower the risk of unwanted pregnancy by using backup methods—that is, more than one form of contraception simultaneously. Emergency or after-intercourse contraception (discussed later in this chapter) could prevent as many as 2.3 million unwanted pregnancies each year.[6]

Even college students aware of the risks associated with unprotected sexual intercourse often do not practice safe-sex behaviors. There are many reasons, ranging from the influence of sex and alcohol to embarrassment about buying condoms. Generally, the ability to talk about a desire to use condoms has been found to be associated with a greater use of condoms. However, a recent survey of college students found that a significant percentage of both men and women either tried to dissuade a potential partner from condom use or had a sexual partner who'd tried to discourage condom use.

Both men and women generally used the same arguments against condoms: that sex felt better without them, that the woman wouldn't get pregnant, and that neither would get a sexually transmitted disease.[7] (See Student Snapshot: "Condoms on Campus.")

The bottom line is that it takes two people to conceive a baby, and two people should be involved in deciding *not* to conceive a baby. In the process, they can also enhance their skills in communication, critical thinking, and negotiating.

## Abstinence and Outercourse

The contraceptive methods discussed in this chapter are designed to prevent pregnancy as a consequence of vaginal intercourse. Couples who choose abstinence make a very different decision—to abstain from vaginal intercourse and other forms of sexual activity (any in which ejaculation occurs near the vaginal opening) that could result in conception.

For many individuals, abstinence represents a deliberate choice regarding their bodies, minds, spirits, and sexuality. People choose abstinence for various reasons, including waiting until they are ready for a sexual relationship or until they find the "right" partner, respecting religious or moral values, enjoying friendships without sexual involvement, recovering from a breakup, or preventing pregnancy and sexually transmitted disease.

Abstinence is the only form of birth control that is 100 percent effective and risk-free. It is also an important, increasingly valued lifestyle choice. A growing number of individuals, including some who have been sexually active in the past, are choosing abstinence until they establish a relationship with a long-term partner.

Abstinence offers special health benefits for women. Those who abstain until their twenties and engage in sex with fewer partners during their lifetime are less likely to get sexually transmitted diseases, to suffer infertility, or to develop cervical cancer. However, some people find it difficult to abstain for long periods of time. There also is a risk that people will abruptly end their abstinence without being prepared to protect themselves against pregnancy or infection.[8]

Individuals who choose abstinence from vaginal intercourse often engage in activities sometimes called *outercourse,* such as kissing, hugging, sensual touching,

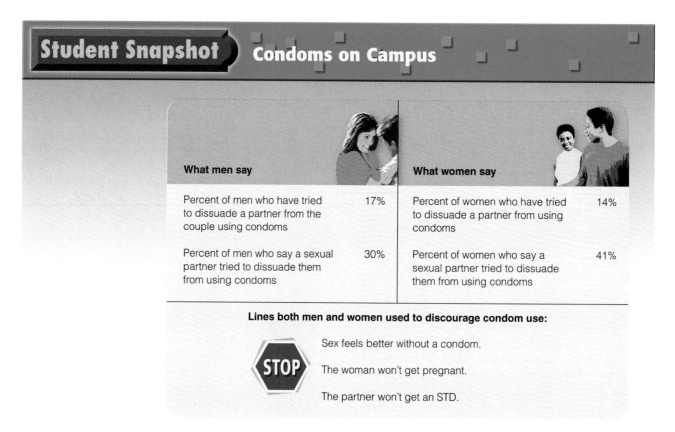

**Student Snapshot** **Condoms on Campus**

**What men say**

| | |
|---|---|
| Percent of men who have tried to dissuade a partner from the couple using condoms | 17% |
| Percent of men who say a sexual partner tried to dissuade them from using condoms | 30% |

**What women say**

| | |
|---|---|
| Percent of women who have tried to dissuade a partner from using condoms | 14% |
| Percent of women who say a sexual partner tried to dissuade them from using condoms | 41% |

**Lines both men and women used to discourage condom use:**

**STOP**

Sex feels better without a condom.

The woman won't get pregnant.

The partner won't get an STD.

Sources: Oncale, Renee, and Bruce King. "Comparisons of Men's and Women's Attempts to Dissuade Sexual Partners from the Couple Using Condoms." *Archives of Sexual Behavior,* Vol. 30, No. 4, August 2001, p. 379.

and mutual masturbation. Outercourse is nearly 100 percent effective as a contraceptive measure, but pregnancy is possible if there is genital contact. If the man ejaculates near the vaginal opening, sperm can swim up into the vagina and fallopian tubes to fertilize an egg. Except for oral-genital and anal sex, outercourse also may lower the risk of contracting sexually transmitted diseases. It is an effective form of safe sex as long as no body fluids are exchanged.

Some couples routinely restrict themselves to outercourse; others temporarily choose such sexual activities when it is inadvisable for them to have vaginal intercourse—for example, after childbirth. Other benefits: Outercourse has no medical or hormonal side effects; it may prolong sex play and enhance orgasm, and it can be used when no other methods are available.[9]

## Prescription Contraceptives

The most effective and most widely used methods of birth control in the United States include oral contraceptives, hormonal implants and injections, the intrauterine device, the diaphragm, and the cervical cap. The newest prescription contraceptives are the contraceptive ring and the contraceptive patch. All are reversible and available only from health professionals.

### Birth Control Pill

*The pill*—the popular term for **oral contraceptives**—is the method of birth control preferred by unmarried women and by those under age 30, including college students. Women 18 to 24 years old are most likely to choose oral contraceptives. In use for 40 years, the pill is one of the most researched, tested, and carefully followed medications in medical history—and one of the most controversial.[10] The impact of the pill has been enormous. By virtually eliminating the risk of pregnancy, the pill encouraged women's careers. It also altered the marriage market by enabling young men and women to delay marriage while not having to delay sex.[11]

Although many women incorrectly think that the risks of the pill are greater than those of pregnancy and childbirth, long-term studies show that oral contraceptive use does not increase mortality rates. Oral contraceptives significantly reduce the risk of ovarian and endometrial cancer and produce no increase in serious disease, including breast cancer, diabetes, multiple sclerosis, rheumatoid arthritis, and liver disease.[12] There is an increased risk of blood clots and pulmonary embolism for smokers and women who used earlier types of oral contraceptives.[13]

Three types of oral contraceptives are widely used in the United States: the constant-dose combination pill, the multiphasic pill, and the progestin-only pill. The **constant-dose combination** or **monophasic pill** releases two hormones, synthetic estrogen and progestin, which play important roles in controlling ovulation and the menstrual cycle, at constant levels throughout the menstrual cycle.

The **multiphasic pill** mimics normal hormonal fluctuations of the natural menstrual cycle by providing different levels of estrogen and progesterone at different times of the month. Multiphasic pills reduce total hormonal dose and side effects. Both constant-dose combination and multiphasic pills block the release of hormones that would stimulate the process leading to ovulation. They also thicken and alter the cervical mucus, making it more hostile to sperm, and they make implantation of a fertilized egg in the uterine lining more difficult. Multiphasic pills may heighten a woman's sex drive.

The **progestin-only pill,** or **minipill,** contains a small amount of progestin and no estrogen. Unlike women who take constant-dose combination pills, those using minipills probably ovulate at least occasionally. The minipills make the mucus in the cervix so thick and tacky, however, that sperm can't enter the uterus. Minipills also may interfere with implantation by altering the uterine lining.

The FDA has approved a new oral contraceptive, Yasmin, the first birth control pill that contains a type of progestin called *drospirenone*. As with other oral contraceptives, the most frequent side effects associated with Yasmin are headache, menstrual disorder, breast pain, abdominal pain, and nausea.[14]

**Advantages** Birth control pills have several advantages: They are extremely effective. Among women who miss no pills, only 1 in 1,000 becomes pregnant in the first year of use. They are reversible, so a woman can easily stop using them. They do not interrupt sexual activity. Women on the pill have more regular periods, less cramping, and fewer tubal, or ectopic, pregnancies (discussed later in this chap-

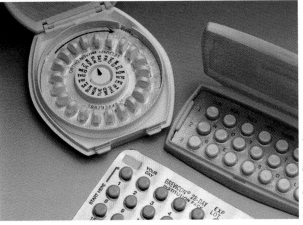

▲ Various types of birth control pills contain different hormones and combinations of hormones.

ter). After five years of use, the pill halves the risk of endometrial and ovarian cancer.

In a major study in 2002, scientists at the Centers for Disease Control and Prevention and the National Institutes of Health looked at more than 9,200 women ages 35 to 64 and found that the pill does not raise the risk of breast cancer, even among women who started taking it early or who have close relatives with the disease.[15] This held true regardless of a woman's race, weight, whether she had started taking contraceptives before age 20, took the early higher-dose oral contraceptives, or had a family history of breast cancer.[16] The pill also reduces the risk of benign breast lumps, ovarian cysts, iron-deficiency anemia, and pelvic inflammatory disease (PID). In actual use, the failure rate is 1 to 5 percent for estrogen/progesterone pills and 3 to 10 percent for minipills. Some physicians suggest that in the future women may use the pill to regulate their menstrual cycle.[17]

**Disadvantages**  The pill does not protect against HIV infection and other sexually transmitted diseases, so condoms and spermicide should also be used.[18] In addition, the hormones in oral contraceptives may cause various side effects, including spotting between periods, weight gain or loss, nausea and vomiting, breast tenderness, and decreased sex drive. Some women using the pill report emotional changes, such as mood swings and depression. Oral contraceptives can interact with other medications and diminish their effectiveness; women should inform any physician providing medical treatment that they are taking the pill.

Current birth control pills contain much lower levels of estrogen than early pills. As a result, the risk of heart disease and stroke among users is much lower than it once was; the danger may be lowest with the minipill. Yet a risk of cardiovascular problems is still associated with use of the pill, primarily for women over 35 who smoke and those with other health problems, such as high blood pressure. Heart attacks strike an estimated 1 in 14,000 pill users between the ages of 30 and 39, and 1 in 1,500 between the ages of 40 and 44. Strokes occur five times more frequently among women taking oral contraceptives, and clots in the veins develop in 1 of every 500 previously healthy women. (See Savvy Consumer: "Evaluating the Health Risks of Birth Control Methods.")

**Before Using Oral Contraceptives**  Before starting on the pill, you should undergo a thorough physical examination that includes the following tests:

- Routine blood pressure test.
- Pelvic exam, including a Pap smear.
- Breast exam.
- Blood test.
- Urine sample.

Let your doctor know about any personal or family incidence of high blood pressure or heart disease, diabetes, liver dysfunction, hepatitis, unusual menstrual history, severe depression, sickle-cell anemia, cancer of the breast, ovaries, or uterus, high cholesterol levels, or migraine headaches.

**How to Use Oral Contraceptives**  An estimated 2 million women worldwide become unintentionally pregnant every year because they do not use the pill as

---

## Savvy Consumer

### Evaluating the Health Risks of Birth Control Methods

For individuals with certain medical conditions, specific types of birth control can pose a health risk. To be safe, follow these guidelines:

- **High blood pressure** (180/110 mmHg or higher): Avoid birth control pills and injectables containing estrogen, which may increase your risk of a heart attack or stroke.

- **Episodes of depression:** Avoid products that contain progestin, such as Depo-Provera, contraceptive implants, and the minipill. In some women with depression, progestin may worsen depressive symptoms. Also, check with your doctor if you are taking an antidepressant medication; it may affect or be affected by oral contraceptives and you may require a different dose.

- **Seizure disorder:** Avoid low-dose birth control pills. Some antiseizure medications, such as Dilantin, accelerate liver metabolism of all substances, including oral contraceptives, and make them less effective.

- **Ectopic pregnancy:** Avoid IUDs. Although IUDs do not cause ectopic pregnancies, if your fallopian tubes have been scarred by a previous ectopic gestation, you're more likely to have another ectopic pregnancy if you use an IUD.

- **Hepatitis** (discussed in Chapter 9): Avoid birth control pills or injectables containing estrogen, which is metabolized in the liver, an organ damaged by hepatitis.

directed.[19] The pill usually comes in 28-day packets: 21 of the pills contain the hormones, and 7 are "blanks," included so that the woman can take a pill every day, even during her menstrual period. If a woman forgets to take one pill, she should take it as soon as she remembers. However, if she forgets during the first week of her cycle or misses more than one pill, she should rely on another form of birth control until her next menstrual period.

Even if you experience no discomfort or side effects while on the pill, see a physician at least once a year for an examination, which should include a blood pressure test, a pelvic, and a breast exam. Notify your doctor at once if you develop severe abdominal pain, chest pain, coughing, shortness of breath, pain or tenderness in the calf or thigh, severe headaches, dizziness, faintness, muscle weakness or numbness, speech disturbance, blurred vision, a sensation of flashing lights, a breast lump, severe depression, or yellowing of your skin.

Generally, when a woman stops taking the pill, her menstrual cycle resumes the next month, but it may be irregular for the next couple of months. However, 2 to 4 percent of pill users experience prolonged delays. Women who become pregnant during the first or second cycle after discontinuing use of the pill may be at greater risk of miscarriage; they also are more likely to conceive twins. Most physicians advise women who want to conceive to change to another method of contraception for three months after they stop taking the pill.

## Contraceptive Ring

The first contraceptive vaginal ring, the NuvaRing, became available in 2002. Once in place, the NuvaRing releases a low dose of estrogen and progestin into the surrounding tissue. The ring contains a lower amount of hormones than birth control pills.

The flexible plastic 2-inch ring compresses so a woman can easily insert it. Each ring stays in place for three weeks, then is removed for the fourth week of the menstrual cycle. Like the pill and the patch, the ring works by preventing ovulation.

**Advantages** Women have no need for a daily pill, a fitting by a doctor, or the use of a spermicide. A woman's ability to become pregnant returns quickly once she stops using the ring.

**Disadvantages** There were increased complaints of vaginal discharge, irri-

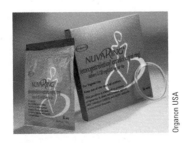

▲ The NuvaRing releases estrogen and progestin, preventing ovulation.

tation, or infection. Women cannot use oil-based vaginal medicine to treat yeast infections while the ring is in place, or a diaphragm or cervical cap for a backup method of birth control.

## Contraceptive Patch

The first *transdermal* (through-the-skin) contraceptive, the Ortho Evra, became available in 2002. Embedded in its adhesive layer are two hormones, a low-dose estrogen and a progestin, that are slowly released when the 1¾-square-inch patch is applied to the skin of the upper arm, abdomen, back, or buttocks.

Rather than taking a daily pill, a woman replaces the patch every seven days for three consecutive weeks. The fourth week is patch-free. In clinical studies, about 5 percent of women had at least one patch detach from their skin; about 2 percent discontinued use because of skin irritation.[20]

Clinical studies have shown that the patch is as effective as the low-dose birth control pill in preventing pregnancy and less likely to cause breakthrough bleeding or spotting.[21]

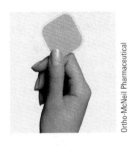

▲ The hormones in Ortho Evra are slowly released when the patch is applied to the skin.

**Advantages** A woman does not have to remember to take a daily pill and can become pregnant quickly once she stops its use.

**Disadvantages** Users have an increased risk of blood clots, heart attack, and stroke. Cigarette smoking increases the risk of serious cardiovascular side effects. The patch may be less effective in women who weigh more than 198 pounds.[22] Wearers of contact lenses may experience a change in vision or be unable to continue to wear lenses.

## Contraceptive Implants

Hormonal implants, placed under the skin, deliver a constant low dose of progestin. Norplant, consisting of six thin silicone rubber capsules containing a synthetic form of progestin, was the first such implant available in the United States. Approximately 9 million women used this method before it was taken off the market. Newer contraceptive implants use several progestins in one or two capsules. The Implanon, a single capsule that has been used for several years in Europe and Canada, provides contraceptive protection for at least three years.

Contraceptive implants work primarily by suppressing ovulation, but they also thicken the cervical mucus (which inhibits sperm migration), inhibit the development and growth of the uterine lining, and limit secretion of progesterone during the second or luteal half of the menstrual cycle. The best candidates for implants are women who desire reversible long-term contraception, those who don't want to insert or ingest a contraceptive, those who cannot take estrogen-containing oral contraceptives, those who would face high medical risks if they did become pregnant, and those who are undecided about sterilization.[23] Adolescents using Norplant were considerably less likely than pill users to become pregnant unintentionally, even after one unintended pregnancy.[24]

**Advantages** A five-year study of some 8,000 users of Norplant in eight developing countries found no significant increases in cancer or in cardiovascular problems, such as stroke or blood clots, in Norplant users compared to women using nonhormonal methods.[25]

Contraceptive implants may be most effective in women who weigh less than 110 pounds and somewhat less effective in those weighing more than 154 pounds. However, even in heavier women, implants are more effective than oral contraceptives. Like the pill, they may reduce the risk of endometrial and ovarian cancer. They also protect against ectopic pregnancy.

For sexually active adolescents and young adults, who often do not consistently use birth control pills and other forms of contraception, the primary advantage of implants is long duration of action and the fact that they do not need to remember to use it. However, in clinical studies, teenagers reported more side effects with implants than with oral contraceptives.

**Disadvantages** Contraceptive implants do not protect against STDs, so condoms and spermicides should also be used.

Common side effects include menstrual irregularities, spotting, and amenorrhea; these are most likely to occur in the first year of use. Other possible complications include ovarian cysts, headaches, acne, weight changes, breast discharge, nausea, and hair growth. Because contraceptive implants do not include estrogen (as birth control pills do), there is no risk of clotting or high blood pressure. However, women with acute liver disease, unexplained vaginal bleeding, breast cancer, or blood clots in the lungs, legs, or eyes should not use them.

**How to Use Contraceptive Implants** Implants are not advised for women who are pregnant, have unexplained vaginal bleeding, are breast-feeding or have given birth in the last six weeks, have ever had breast cancer, have had certain rare kinds of headache, or are sensitive to the ingredients in implants.[26]

A qualified health-care professional, using a local anesthetic, implants a capsule with a needle under the skin of a woman's upper arm. The simple surgical procedure generally takes about a minute for one capsule. Once in place, the

capsule can be felt and may be visible, particularly in slender women. Complications can occur during removal; the most common are bruising, slight bleeding, and pain at the removal site. After removal, fertility generally returns within one or two menstrual cycles. According to various studies, most former users of Norplant began ovulating again within seven weeks of implant removal, and most of those who wished to conceive did so within one year.

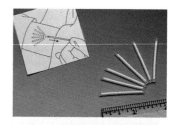
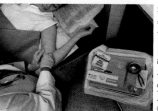

▲ Norplant implants were surgically placed in a woman's arm.

## Contraceptive Injectables

One injection of Depo-Provera, a synthetic version of the natural hormone progesterone, provides three months of contraceptive protection. This long-acting hormonal contraceptive raises levels of progesterone, thereby simulating pregnancy. The pituitary gland doesn't produce FSH and LH, which normally cause egg ripening and release. The endometrial lining of the uterus thins, preventing implantation of a fertilized egg.

A monthly injectable contraceptive that combines estrogen and progestin, Lunelle, proved highly effective and safe in initial studies. Side effects are similar to those of hormonal contraceptives, including weight gain, acne, and irregular bleeding.[27] Some batches of prefilled syringes of Lunelle were recalled in 2002 because of concerns that the doses might not be sufficient to prevent pregnancy.

**Advantages** The main advantage is that women do not need to take a daily pill. Because Depo-Provera contains only

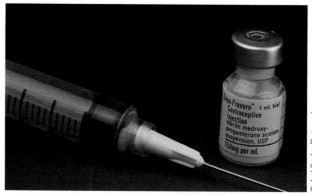

▲ Depo-Provera is given by injection every 12 weeks.

progestin, it can be used by women who cannot take oral contraceptives containing estrogen (such as those who've had breast cancer). Depo-Provera also may have some protective action against endometrial and ovarian cancer.

**Disadvantages**  Injectable contraceptives provide no protection against HIV and other STDs. Depo-Provera causes menstrual irregularities in most users, and in a small percentage of users it causes a delayed return of fertility, excessive endometrial bleeding, and other side effects, including decreased libido, depression, headaches, dizziness, weight gain, frequent urination, and allergic reactions. Long-term use may lead to significantly reduced bone density.

**How to Use Injectable Contraceptives**  Women must receive an injection of Depo-Provera once every 12 weeks, ideally within five days of the beginning of menstruation. Lunelle must be injected once a month.

## Intrauterine Device

The **intrauterine device (IUD)** is a small piece of molded plastic, with a nylon string attached, that is inserted into the uterus through the cervix. It prevents pregnancy by interfering with implantation. Once widely used, IUDs became less popular after most brands were removed from the market because of serious complications such as pelvic infection and infertility. The currently available IUDs have not been shown to increase the risk of such problems for women in mutually monogamous relationships. (See Figure 8-3.)

According to manufacturers' estimates, about 2 percent of American women using contraception currently rely on IUDs. Throughout the world more than 25 million IUDs have been distributed in 70 countries. Progestaser System is a T-shaped device containing progesterone, which prevents implantation; it must be replaced every year.

The Copper T (Paragard) contains copper, which interferes with the growth of a fertilized egg by causing biochemical reactions with the uterine lining. The Copper T remains effective for ten years, making it the longest-acting reversible contraceptive available to women in the United States. Its cumulative failure rate is 2.6.

The newest IUD, Mirena intrauterine system, consists of a polyethylene T-shaped device surrounded by a sleeve containing the progestin levonorgestrel, which is released directly to the lining of the uterus. Mirena, which has been used by more than 1.4 million women in Europe, Asia, and Latin America, contains no estrogen and is 99 percent effective in preventing pregnancy for up to five years.[28]

**Advantages**  The IUD is highly effective and easy to reverse. According to recent analyses, the Copper T is the cheapest and most cost-effective form of birth control. Current models cause fewer complications than the pill. The IUD does not interrupt sexual activity.

IUDs were long believed to increase the risk of pelvic inflammatory disease, which can lead to scarring and infertility. More recent research has shown that although IUD users are more likely to develop PID than nonusers, it is an uncommon complication. The greatest risk of PID occurs during the first few weeks following insertion; it falls at about 20 days.[29]

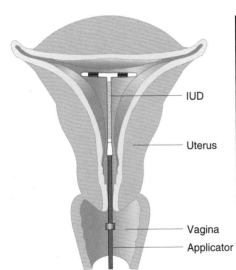

IUD

Uterus

Vagina

Applicator

The IUD is placed in the uterus.

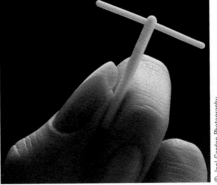

Progestaser system

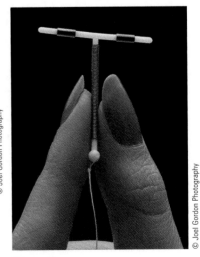

Copper T

© Joel Gordon Photography

▲ **Figure 8-3** Intrauterine Device (IUD)
The IUD is effective and cost-efficient for preventing pregnancy, although some women may expel the device. The IUD does not offer protection against STDs.

**Disadvantages**   Many gynecologists recommend other forms of birth control for childless women who someday may want to start a family. Women who have never given birth and have used an IUD for an extended period of time may find it more difficult to conceive after discontinuing its use.[30] In addition, women with many sexual partners, who are at highest risk of PID, are not good candidates for this method.[31]

During insertion of an IUD, women may experience discomfort, cramping, bleeding, or pain, which may continue for a few days or longer. The hormonal IUD causes less excess bleeding and cramping than the Copper T. An estimated 2 to 20 percent of users expel an IUD within a year of insertion.

If a woman using an IUD does become pregnant, the IUD is removed to reduce the risk of miscarriage (which can be as high as 50 percent). In addition, physicians generally offer a therapeutic abortion to the pregnant patient because of the serious risks (including infection, premature delivery, and possibly a higher rate of birth defects) of continuing the pregnancy.

**How to Use an IUD**   A physician inserts an IUD during a woman's period, when the cervix is slightly softened and dilated. Antibiotics may be prescribed to lower any risk of infection. An IUD can be removed at any time during her cycle. A woman should check regularly, particularly after each menstrual period, for the nylon string attached to the IUD, because she may not otherwise notice if an IUD has been expelled.

## Diaphragm

The **diaphragm** is a bowl-like rubber cup with a flexible rim that is inserted into the vagina to cover the cervix and prevent the passage of sperm into the uterus during sexual intercourse. (See Figure 8-4.) When used with a spermicide, the diaphragm is both a physical and a chemical barrier to sperm. The effectiveness of the diaphragm in preventing pregnancy depends on strong motivation (to use it faithfully) and a precise understanding of its use. If diaphragms with spermicide are used consistently and carefully, they can be 95 to 98 percent effective. Without a spermicide, the diaphragm is not effective.

**Advantages**   Diaphragms have become increasingly popular, most likely because of concern about the side effects of hormonal contraceptives. Many women feel that using a diaphragm makes them more knowledgeable and comfortable about their bodies.

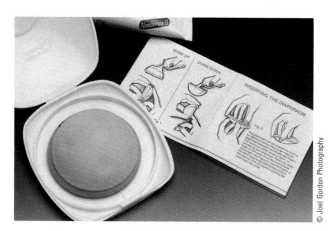

© Joel Gordon Photography

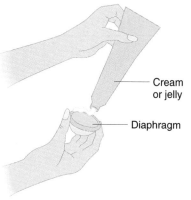

Cream or jelly
Diaphragm

Squeeze spermicide into dome of diaphragm and around the rim.

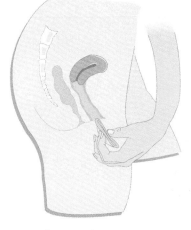

Squeeze rim together; insert jelly-side up.

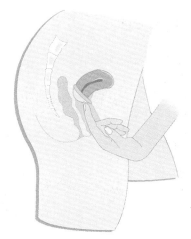

Check placement to make certain cervix is covered.

▲ **Figure 8-4** Diaphragm
When used correctly and consistently and with a spermicide, the diaphragm is effective in preventing pregnancy and STDs. It must be fitted by a health-care professional.

**Disadvantages** Some people find that the diaphragm is inconvenient and interferes with sexual spontaneity. The spermicidal cream or jelly is messy, detracts from oral-genital sex, and can cause irritation. A poorly fitted diaphragm may cause discomfort during sex; some women report bladder discomfort, urethral irritation, or recurrent cystitis as a result of diaphragm use.

**How to Use a Diaphragm** Diaphragms are fitted and prescribed by a qualified health-care professional in diameter sizes ranging from 2 to 4 inches (50 to 105 millimeters). The diaphragm's main function is to serve as a container for a spermicidal (sperm-killing) foam or jelly, which is available at pharmacies without a prescription. A diaphragm should remain in the vagina for at least six hours after intercourse to ensure that all sperm are killed. If intercourse occurs again during this period, additional spermicide must be inserted with an applicator tube.

The key to proper use of the diaphragm is having it available. A sexually active woman should keep it in the most accessible place—her purse, bedroom, bathroom. Before every use, a diaphragm should be checked for tiny leaks (hold up to the light or place water in the dome). A health-care provider should check its fit and condition every year when the woman has her annual Pap smear. Oil-based lubricants will deteriorate the latex of the diaphragm and should not be used with one.

## Cervical Cap

Like the diaphragm, the **cervical cap,** combined with spermicide, serves as both a chemical and physical barrier blocking the path of the sperm to the uterus. The rubber or plastic cap is smaller and thicker than a diaphragm and resembles a large thimble that fits snugly around the cervix. (See Figure 8-5.) It is about as effective as a diaphragm (95 to 98 percent).

**Advantages** Women who cannot use a diaphragm because of pelvic-structure problems or loss of vaginal muscle tone can often use the cap. Also, the cervical cap is less messy and does not require additional applications of spermicide if intercourse occurs more than once within several hours.

**Disadvantages** A cervical cap is more difficult to insert and remove, and may damage the cervix. Some women find it uncomfortable to wear. In the past, only four sizes of conventional cervical caps were available, and about 25 percent of women had difficulty getting a proper fit. Newer products, such as Lea's Shield, come in one size and are designed to fit all women.[32]

Some cap users have developed abnormal Pap smears within three months of beginning this birth control method. Doctors recommend a Pap smear before beginning and after three months of cervical cap use.[33]

**How to Use a Cervical Cap** Like the diaphragm, the cervical cap is fitted by a qualified health-care professional. For use, the woman fills it one-third to two-thirds full with spermicide and inserts it by holding its edges together and sliding it into the vagina. The cup is then pressed onto the cervix. (Most women find it easiest to do so while squatting or in an upright sitting position.) The cap can be inserted up to 6 hours prior to intercourse and should not be removed for at least 6 hours afterward. It can be left in

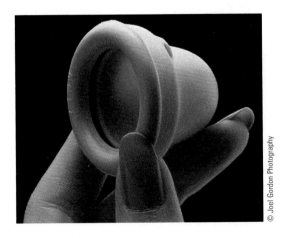

© Joel Gordon Photography

▲ **Figure 8-5** Cervical Cap
This device is very similar to the diaphragm and may work better for some women. It is smaller than the diaphragm and covers only the cervix.

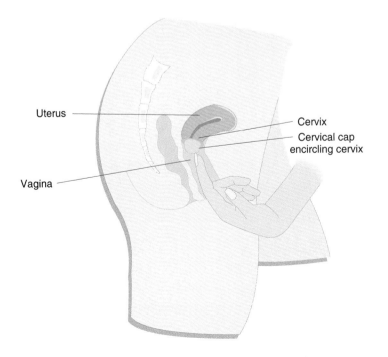

Uterus
Vagina
Cervix
Cervical cap encircling cervix

place up to 24 hours. Pulling on one side of the rim breaks the suction and allows easy removal. Oil-based lubricants should not be used with the cap because they can deteriorate the latex.

# Nonprescription Contraceptives

As their name implies, **barrier contraceptives,** available without a prescription, block the meeting of egg and sperm by means of a physical barrier (a condom, a diaphragm, or a cervical cap), or a chemical one (vaginal spermicide in jellies, foams, creams, suppositories, or film). These forms of birth control have become increasingly popular because they can do more than prevent conception—they can also help reduce the risk of STDs.

## Male Condom

The male **condom** covers the erect penis and catches the ejaculate, thus preventing sperm from entering the woman's reproductive tract. (See Figure 8-6.) Most are made of thin surgical latex or sheep membrane; a new type is made of polyurethane, which is thinner, stronger, more heat-sensitive, and more comfortable than latex. Condoms with a spermicidal lubricant (nonoxynol-9) kill most sperm on contact and are thus more effective than other brands.

Although the theoretical effectiveness rate for condoms is 97 percent, the actual rate is only 80 to 85 percent. The condom can be torn during the manufacturing process or during its use; testing by the manufacturer may not be as strenuous as it could or should be. Careless removal can also decrease the effectiveness of condoms. However, the major reason that condoms have such a low actual effectiveness rate is that couples don't use them each

and every time they have sex. Users who have little experience with condoms—who are young, single, or childless, or who engage in risky behaviors—are more likely to have condoms break.[34]

Condoms are second only to the pill in popularity among college-age adults. Condom use has increased in the last decade. Approximately one in five women ages 15 to 44 who used contraception rely on their partner's use of condoms as their primary method of birth control.[35]

More teens also are using condoms but not consistently. (See the X&Y Files: "Sex, Lies, and Condom Use"). From one-third to one-half of sexually active teens report using condoms for every act of intercourse. However, condom use decreases as teens get older, with fewer males ages 18 and 19 using condoms than those 15 to 17 years old. Teenage girls report less frequent use of condoms than males.[36]

For girls, being from an intact family and having a mother with higher educational achievement are associated with greater condom use at first intercourse. Black adolescents, teens with more educated parents, and teens who were older at first intercourse also had greater condom use. The less similar adolescents are to their partners—whether because of a difference in age, grade, or school—the less likely adolescents are to use condoms and other contraceptive methods.[37]

According to the National Longitudinal Study of Adolescent Health, one-fifth to one-half of sexually active adolescents share common misconceptions about condoms.[38] Many believe that there is no space at the tip of a condom or think that Vaseline can be used with condoms; some say that lambskin protects against HIV better than latex. None of these is true.[39] Television advertising of condoms, which has been controversial in the past, may help correct such misinformation. According to a recent study, nine in ten Americans surveyed endorsed condom adver-

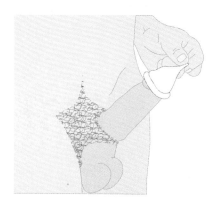

Pinch or twist the tip of the condom, leaving one-half inch at the tip to catch the semen.

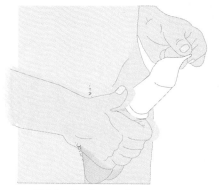

Holding the tip, unroll the condom.

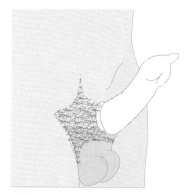

Unroll the condom until it reaches the pubic hairs.

▲ **Figure 8-6** Male Condom
Condoms effectively reduce the risk of pregnancy as well as STDs. Using them consistently and correctly are important factors.

## Sex, Lies, and Condom Use

In a series of focus groups with 92 sexually active, young, ethnically and racially diverse individuals, ages 15 to 20, in five American cities, researchers focused on their views and motivations for sex and for condom use. Most found it difficult to believe that people their age used condoms every single time they had sex. Although they acknowledged that everyone is at risk for sexually transmitted diseases, the young people saw their own risk as minimal.

The genders had very different motives both for engaging in sex and for using condoms. In the interviews, young women said they engaged in sexual relations because of a desire for physical intimacy and a committed relationship. They generally reported having sex only with men they cared for and deeply trusted, and expected that these men would be honest and forthright about their sexual history. This trust played a significant role in their decision whether to insist on condom use.

In contrast, few of the young men said relationships were an important dimension of their sexual involvements. Their primary motivation was a desire for physical and sexual satisfaction. Most said they were not interested in commitment and viewed emotional expectations as a complication of becoming sexually involved with a woman. The young men also admitted to making judgments about types of girls. To them, young women they didn't care about were "sluts" with whom they used a condom for their own protection.

Which partner determined whether a couple would use a condom? In these interviews, the answer was the women—if they chose to do so. Regardless of race or ethnicity, many of the young women were adamant in demanding that their partners use condoms—and many young men said they would not challenge such a demand out of fear of losing the opportunity for sex. Men often expected potential partners to want to use condoms and described themselves as "suspicious" of women who did not.

Both sexes named two primary reasons for using condoms: preventing pregnancy and protecting against sexually transmitted diseases. Young women saw an unwanted pregnancy as an occurrence that would be disruptive, expensive, and could "ruin" their lives and their parents' lives. Young men saw condom use as a way of protecting themselves against emotional entanglements and paternity issues.

The young people were most strongly motivated to use condoms when they did not know a potential sexual partner well or were at the earliest stages of sexual involvement with others. Nearly all said they solicited information about a potential partner's sexual history from this person or from friends. Rather than directly asking about the number of past partners, they more often relied on feelings and visual observations. Some admitted to lying when asked about their own sexual experience in order to avoid being seen as promiscuous. Once a couple had sex without a condom, both partners—but especially women—found it awkward to resume condom use because doing so would imply a lack of trust.

---

tising on TV, either freely, like any other product, or at restricted times.

**Advantages** Condoms made of latex or polyurethane, especially when used with spermicides containing nonoxynol-9, can help reduce the risk of certain STDs, including syphilis, gonorrhea, chlamydia, and herpes. They appear to lower a woman's risk of pelvic inflammatory disease (PID) and may protect against some parasites that cause urinary tract and genital infections. Public health officials view condoms as the best available defense against HIV infection. They are available without a prescription or medical appointment, and their use does not cause harmful side effects. Some men appreciate the slight blunting of sensation they experience when using a condom because it helps prolong the duration of intercourse before ejaculation.

**Disadvantages** Condoms are not 100 percent effective in preventing pregnancy or STDs, including infection with HIV or HPV (human papilloma virus, discussed in Chapter 9). For anyone, heterosexual or homosexual, not in a monogamous relationship with a mutually exclusive, healthy partner, condoms can reduce the risks of sexual involvement, but they cannot eliminate them. Condoms may have manufacturing defects, such as pin-size holes, or they may break or slip off during intercourse.

The main objections to condoms include odor, lubrication (too much or too little), rips or breaks, access, disposal, feel, taste, and difficulty opening the packages. Some couples feel that putting on a condom interferes with sexual spontaneity; others incorporate it into their sex play. Some men dislike the reduced penile sensitivity or will not use them because they believe they interfere with sexual pleasure. Others cannot sustain an erection while putting on a condom. A small number are allergic to latex condoms.

**How to Use a Condom** Most physicians recommend prelubricated, spermicide-treated American-made latex or

## Female Condom

The female condom, made of polyurethane, consists of two rings and a polyurethane sheath, and is inserted into the vagina with a tampon-like applicator. (See Figure 8-7.) Once in place, the device loosely lines the walls of the vagina. Internally, a thickened rubber ring keeps it anchored near the cervix. Externally, another rubber ring, 2 inches in diameter, rests on the labia and resists slippage.

Although not widely used in the West, the female condom is gaining acceptance in Africa, Asia, and Latin America. Properly used, it is believed to be as good or better than the male condom for preventing infections, including HIV, because it is stronger and covers a slightly larger area.[40] However, it is slightly less effective at preventing pregnancy.

**Advantages**    The female condom gives women more control in reducing their risk of pregnancy and STDs. It does not require a prescription or medical appointment. One size fits all.

**Disadvantages**    The failure rate for the female condom is higher than for other contraceptives. The statistical fail-

polyurethane condoms, not membrane condoms ("natural" or "sheepskin"). Before using a condom, check the expiration date, and make sure it's soft and pliable. If it's yellow or sticky, throw it out. Don't check for leaks by blowing up a condom before using it; you may weaken or tear it.

The condom should be put on at the beginning of sexual activity, before genital contact occurs. (See Figure 8-6.) There should be a little space at the top of the condom to catch the semen. Wait until just before intercourse to apply spermicide. Any vaginal lubricant should be water-based. Petroleum-based creams or jellies (such as Vaseline, baby oil, massage oil, vegetable oils, or oil-based hand lotions) can deteriorate the latex. After ejaculation, the condom should be held firmly against the penis so that it doesn't slip off or leak during withdrawal. Couples engaging in anal intercourse should use a water-based lubricant as well as a condom, but should never assume the condom will protect them from HIV infection or other STDs.

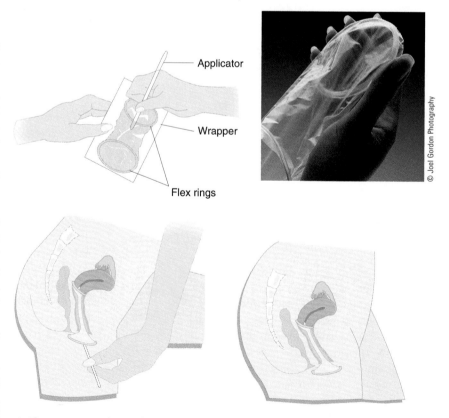

Applicator

Wrapper

Flex rings

© Joel Gordon Photography

▲ **Figure 8-7** Female Condom
This device is less effective than the male condom for preventing pregnancy and STDs (since no spermicide is used). Like the male condom, this method does not require a prescription.

ure rate is 12.2 percent, which means that 12 of every 100 women using the device could expect to get pregnant during a six-month period. In clinical trials, the actual failure rate was even higher—20.6 percent. Since it does not have spermicide on it, the female condom does not provide as much risk-reduction against STDs as male condoms with spermicide. Women complained that the condom, which retails for $2 to $3, was too expensive, difficult to use, squeaked, and looked odd.

**How to Use a Female Condom**  As illustrated in Figure 8-7, a woman removes the condom and applicator from the wrapper and inserts the condom slowly by gently pushing the applicator toward the small of the back. When properly inserted, the outer ring should rest on the folds of skin around the vaginal opening, and the inner ring (the closed end) should fit against the cervix. The condom should be used with a spermicide and a water-based lubricant.

The female condom can be washed and reused several times and still meet the standards set by the Food and Drug Administration (FDA), according to the study conducted in South Africa in which a sample of women washed, dried and relubricated female condoms up to seven times.[41]

## Vaginal Spermicide

The various forms of **vaginal spermicide** include chemical foams, creams, jellies, vaginal suppositories, and gels. (See Figure 8-8.) Some creams and jellies are made for use with a diaphragm; others can be used alone. Several vaginal suppositories claim high effectiveness, but no American studies have confirmed these claims. In general, failure rates for vaginal suppositories are as high as 10 to 25 percent.

**Advantages**  Conscientious use of a spermicide together with another method of contraception, such as a condom, can provide safe and effective birth control and reduce the risk of some vaginal infections, pelvic inflammatory disease, and STDs. The side effects of vaginal spermicides are minimal.

**Disadvantages**  Even though spermicides can be applied in less than a minute, couples may feel that they interfere with sexual spontaneity. Some people are irritated by the chemicals in spermicides, but often a change of brand solves this problem. Others find foam spermicides messy or feel they interfere with oral-genital contact. Spermicidal suppositories that do not dissolve completely can feel gritty.

**How to Use a Vaginal Spermicide**  The various types of spermicide come with instructions that should be followed carefully for maximum protection. Contraceptive vaginal suppositories take about 20 minutes to dissolve and

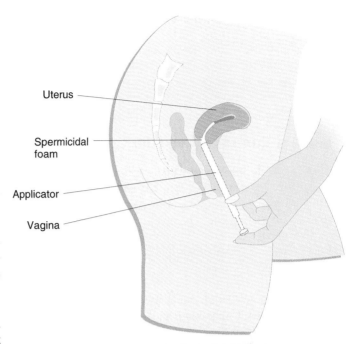

Uterus

Spermicidal foam

Applicator

Vagina

© Joel Gordeon Photography

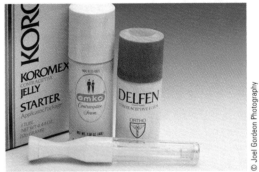

▲ **Figure 8-8** Vaginal Spermicides
These various creams, foams, and jellies are available without a prescription and have minimal side effects. They are most effective in preventing pregnancy and STDs when used together with a condom.

cover the vaginal walls. Foam, inserted with an applicator, goes into place much more rapidly. You must apply additional spermicide before each additional intercourse. After sex, women should shower rather than bathe to prevent the spermicide from being rinsed out of the vagina, and they should not douche for at least six hours.

## Contraceptive Sponge

The nonprescription Today Sponge is a soft, disposable polyurethane sponge permeated with a spermicide. On the market from 1983 to 1995, the Today Sponge was one of the most popular contraceptive options for women. It was taken off the market because of problems at the product's sole manufacturing plant, including bacterial contamination of water and sanitizing equipment.

Although the original manufacturer sold the manufacturing rights and it was approved by the FDA, the Today Sponge has not become available as expected. A similar device, the Protectaid Sponge, is available in Canada. An estimated 6.4 million women have used the sponge at some time.

## Vaginal Contraceptive Film

Available from pharmacies without a prescription, the 2-inch-by-2-inch thin film known as **vaginal contraceptive film (VCF)** is laced with spermicide. (See Figure 8-9.) Once folded and inserted into the vagina, it dissolves into a stay-in-place gel. Its theoretical effectiveness is similar to that of other forms of spermicide; paired with a condom, it is almost 100 percent effective.

**Advantages**   VCF film can be used by people allergic to foams and jellies. Unlike foams and jellies, it dissolves gradually and almost unnoticeably.

**Disadvantages**   Some people feel that insertion, even though it takes only seconds, interrupts sexual spontaneity.

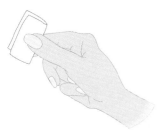

1. Remove the square of film from the convenient sealed envelope and fold it in half.

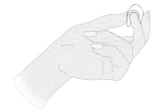

2. Make sure your fingers are dry. Place film on your second or third finger.

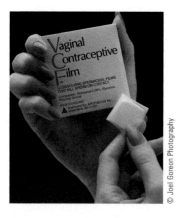
© Joel Goreon Photography

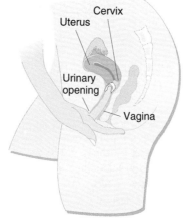

Cervix
Uterus
Urinary opening
Vagina

3. With one swift movement, place the film high in your vagina against the cervix.

▲ **Figure 8-9** How to Use Vaginal Contraceptive Film (VCF)
This thin film is laced with spermicide. Its effectiveness is similar to other vaginal spermicides, and it is most effective paired with a condom.

**How to Use Vaginal Contraceptive Film**   Place one square of VCF on your second or third finger, then insert high into the vagina, near the cervix. VCF is effective for one hour. One film should be used for each act of intercourse.

## Periodic Abstinence and Fertility Awareness Methods

Awareness of a woman's cyclic fertility can help in both conception and contraception. The different methods of birth control based on a woman's menstrual cycle are sometimes referred to as *natural family planning* or *fertility awareness methods.* They include the cervical mucus method, the calendar method, and the basal-body-temperature method (all described below). New fertility monitors that use saliva for testing can improve the accuracy of these methods.

**Advantages**   Birth control methods based on the menstrual cycle involve no expense, no side effects, and no need for prescriptions or fittings. On the days when the couple can have intercourse, there is nothing to insert, swallow, or check. In addition, abstinence during fertile periods complies with the teachings of the Roman Catholic Church.

**Disadvantages**   During times of possible fertility (usually eight or nine days a month), couples must abstain from vaginal intercourse or use some form of contraception. Conscientious planning and scheduling are essential. Women with irregular cycles may not be able to rely on the calendar method. Others may find the mucus or temperature methods difficult to use. For all these reasons, this approach to birth control is less reliable than many others. In theory, the overall effectiveness rate for the various fertility awareness methods is 80 percent. In practice, of every 100 women using one of these methods for a year, 24 become pregnant. However, using a combination of the basal-body-temperature method and the cervical mucus method may be 90 to 95 percent effective in preventing pregnancy. (See Figure 8-10.)

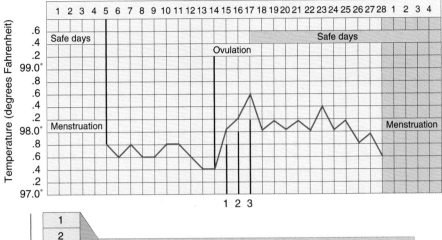

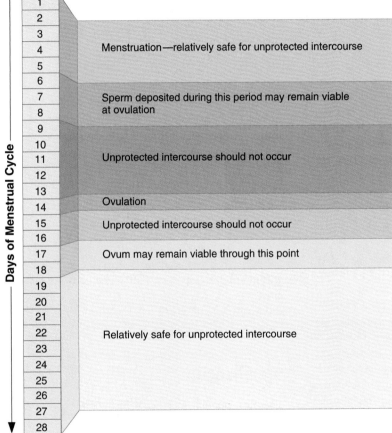

▲ **Figure 8-10** Fertility Awareness Methods
These methods are based on a woman's menstrual cycle and involve charting basal body temperature (top), careful calculation of the menstrual cycle (bottom), or careful observations of cervical mucus. Use of other contraceptive methods during fertile days or periods of abstinence are a necessary part of these methods.

## Cervical Mucus Method

This method, also called the **ovulation method,** is based on the observation of changes in the consistency of the mucus in the vagina. In the first days after menstruation, the vagina feels dry because of a decline in hormone production, indicating a safe period for unprotected intercourse. Within a few days, estrogen levels rise, and the mucus begins to thin out and becomes less cloudy: The fertile period begins. At peak estrogen levels, the mucus is smooth, stretchable, and slippery (like raw egg white), and very clear. Mucus with these characteristics is usually observed within 24 hours of ovulation and lasts one to two days, signaling maximum fertility. The mucus becomes sticky and cloudy again three days thereafter, and the second safe period begins. Most women using this method have to refrain from unprotected intercourse for about 9 days of each 28-day menstrual cycle.

## Calendar Method

This approach, often called the **rhythm method,** involves counting the days after menstruation begins to calculate the estimated day of ovulation. Ideally, a woman first keeps a chart of her monthly cycles for about a year so she knows the average length of her cycle. The first day of menstruation is day one. She counts the number of days until the last day of her cycle, which is the day before menstrual flow begins. To determine the starting point of the period during which she should avoid unprotected intercourse, she subtracts 18 from the number of days in her shortest cycle. For instance, if her shortest cycle was 28 days, day 10 would be her first high-risk day. To calculate when she can again have unprotected intercourse, she subtracts 10 from the number of days in her longest cycle. If her longest cycle is 31 days, she could resume intercourse on day 21. Other forms of sexual activity can continue from day 10 to day 21. This method requires careful timing to avoid the possible meeting of a ripe egg and active sperm in the woman's fallopian tube.

## Basal–Body-Temperature Method

In this method the woman measures her **basal body temperature,** the body temperature upon waking in the morning, using a specially calibrated rectal thermometer, which is more precise than an oral one. She records her temperature on a chart. (See Figure 8-10.) The basal body temperature remains relatively constant from the beginning of the menstrual cycle to ovulation. After ovulation, however, the basal body temperature rises by more than 0.5 degree Fahrenheit. The woman knows that her safe period has begun when her temperature has been elevated for three consecutive days. After eight to ten months, she should have a sense of her ovulatory pattern, in addition to knowing her daily readings.

## ???? What Is Emergency Contraception?

**Emergency contraception (EC)** is the use of a method of contraception to prevent unintended pregnancy after unprotected intercourse or the failure of another form of contraception, such as a condom breaking or slipping off. Medical researchers do not fully understand how EC works. Emergency contraception pills (ECPs) may inhibit or delay ovulation, prevent union of sperm and ovum, or alter the endometrium so a fertilized ovum cannot implant itself. The copper-bearing intrauterine device (IUD) is also an EC option.[42]

There are two types of emergency contraceptive pills. Combined ECPs use estrogen and progestin, the same hormones used in ordinary birth control pills. A brand called Preven is specifically packaged for emergency use, but several other brands can be used as well. Combined ECPs reduce the risk of unintended pregnancy by 75 to 88 percent.[43] The second type of ECP contains only the hormone progestin and is packaged under the brand name Plan B. It has proven more effective than the first type, reducing the risk of pregnancy by 89 percent, with a lower risk of nausea and vomiting.

Although ECPs are sometimes called *morning-after pills,* it is not necessary to wait until the morning after. A woman can start the pills right away or up to three days after unprotected sex. Therapy is more effective the earlier it is initiated, ideally within 24 hours. The second dose is generally taken 12 hours after the first dose. Each dose may consist of 1, 2, 4, or 5 pills, depending on the brand. Most women can safely use them, even if they cannot use birth control pills as their regular method of birth control. (Although ECPs use the same hormones as birth control pills, not all brands of birth control pills can be used for emergency contraception.) Some women may experience spotting or a full menstrual period a few days after taking

ECs, depending on where they were in their cycle when they began therapy. Most women have their next period at the expected time.

Another alternative is the copper IUD, which can be inserted by a physician up to five days after ovulation to prevent pregnancy. IUDs are more effective at preventing pregnancy than hormonal ECPs and reduce the risk of pregnancy by 99 percent. However, they are not used as commonly as hormonal methods for EC. Once inserted, the IUD can provide highly effective continuous contraceptive protection for 10 years.

The American College of Obstetricians and Gynecologists (ACOG) estimates that emergency contraception has the potential to reduce by half the 3 million unintended pregnancies each year in the United States.[44] Along with other women's health groups, ACOG supports over-the-counter availability for ECP and has recommended that physicians offer women of reproductive age an advance prescription for use in any future emergency.[45]

Despite its safety and effectiveness, emergency contraception has not been widely used. Many physicians do not regularly discuss it with patients, and many Americans are unaware of this option.[46] There have been campaigns to inform Americans of after-intercourse options, including setting up a website: www.NOT-2-LATE.com.

 In a recent national survey of colleges and universities, slightly more than half—52.2 percent—of student health centers offer emergency contraception. Private institutions, as well as those with a high proportion of commuter students, were less likely to do so than large public schools. Half of the schools that offered ECP had begun doing so within the previous five years. The primary benefit they cited was pregnancy prevention. Student health centers in the Midwest and South are less likely to offer ECP than those in the Northeast.[47]

## Sterilization

The most popular method of birth control among married couples in the United States is **sterilization** (surgery to end a person's reproductive capability). Each year an estimated 1 million men and women in the United States undergo sterilization procedures. Fewer than 25 percent ever seek reversal.

**Advantages** Sterilization has no effect on sex drive in either men or women. Many couples report that their sexual activity increases after sterilization because they're free from the fear of pregnancy or the need to deal with contraceptives.

**Disadvantages** Sterilization should be considered permanent and should be used only if both individuals are sure they want no more children. Although sterilization doesn't usually create psychological or sexual problems, it can worsen existing problems, particularly marital ones. Couples should discuss sterilization, with each other and with a physician, to understand fully the possible physical and emotional consequences. Although a link between vasectomy and an increased risk of prostate cancer was reported, the most recent research did not find a correlation.

## Male Sterilization

In men, the cutting of the vas deferens, the tube that carries sperm from one of the testes into the urethra for ejaculation, is called **vasectomy.** During the 15- or 20-minute office procedure, done under a local anesthetic, the doctor makes small incisions in the scrotum, lifts up each vas deferens, cuts them, and ties off the ends to block the flow of sperm. (See Figure 8-11.) Sperm continue to form, but they are broken down and absorbed by the body.

The man usually experiences some local pain, swelling, and discoloration for about a week after the procedure. More serious complications, including the formation of a blood clot in the scrotum (which usually disappears without treatment), infection, and an inflammatory reaction, occur in a small percentage of cases. The National Institute of Child Health and Human Development, in a 15-year follow-up study of nearly 5,000 men, found that sterilization poses no increased danger of heart disease, even decades after the procedure. The pregnancy rate among the wives of men who've had vasectomies is about 15 in 10,000 women per year. Most result from a couple's failure to wait several weeks after the operation, until all sperm stored in each vas deferens have been ejaculated, before having unprotected coitus.

Sometimes men want to reverse their vasectomies, usually because they want to have children with a new spouse. Although anyone who chooses to have a vasectomy should consider it permanent, surgical reversal (*vasovasostomy*) is sometimes successful. New microsurgical techniques have led to annual pregnancy rates for the wives of men undergoing vasovasostomies of about 50 percent, depending on such factors as the doctor's expertise and the time elapsed since the vasectomy.

## Female Sterilization

Female sterilization procedures modify the fallopian tubes, which each month normally carry an egg from the ovaries to the uterus. These operations may soon surpass the pill as the first contraceptive choice among women. The two terms used to describe female sterilization are **tubal ligation** (the cutting or tying of the fallopian tubes) and **tubal occlusion** (the blocking of the tubes). The tubes may be cut or sealed with thread, a clamp, or a clip, or by coagulation (burning) to prevent the passage of eggs from the

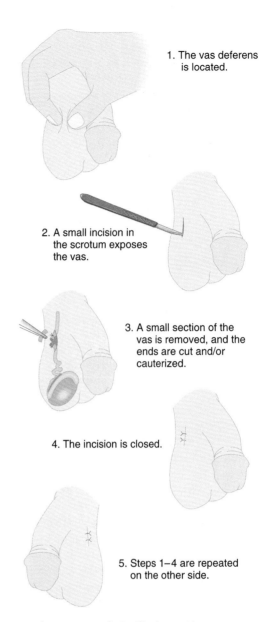

1. The vas deferens is located.

2. A small incision in the scrotum exposes the vas.

3. A small section of the vas is removed, and the ends are cut and/or cauterized.

4. The incision is closed.

5. Steps 1–4 are repeated on the other side.

▲ **Figure 8-11** Male Sterilization, or Vasectomy

ovaries. (See Figure 8-12.) They can also be blocked with bands of silicone.

The procedures used for sterilization are laparotomy, laparoscopy, and colpotomy. **Laparotomy** involves making an abdominal incision about 2 inches long and cutting the tubes. A laparotomy usually requires a hospital stay and up to several weeks of recovery. It leaves a scar and carries the same risks as all major surgical procedures: the side effects of anesthesia, potential infection, and internal scars. In a **minilaparotomy,** an incision about an inch long is made just above the pubic hairline. The tubes may be tied, cut, plugged, or sealed by electrical coagulation. The operation can be performed by a skilled physician in 10 to 30 minutes, usually under local anesthesia, and the woman can

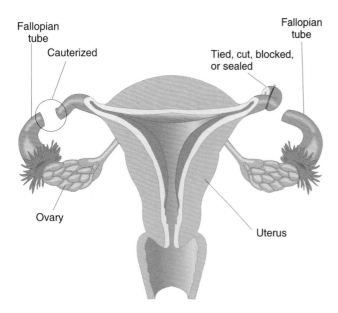

Fallopian tube

Cauterized

Fallopian tube

Tied, cut, blocked, or sealed

Ovary

Uterus

▲ **Figure 8-12** Female Sterilization, or Tubal Ligation

generally go home the same day. The failure (pregnancy) rate is only 1 in 1,000.

Tubal ligation or occlusion can also be performed with the use of **laparoscopy,** commonly called *belly-button* or *band-aid surgery.* This procedure is done on an outpatient basis and takes 15 to 30 minutes. A lighted tube called a *laparoscope* is inserted through a half-inch incision made right below the navel, giving the doctor a view of the fallopian tubes. Using surgical instruments that may be inserted through the laparoscope or through other tiny incisions, the doctor then cuts or seals the tubes, most commonly by electrical coagulation. The possible complications are similar to those of minilaparotomy, as is the failure rate.

In a **colpotomy,** the fallopian tubes are reached through the vagina and cervix. This procedure leaves no external scar, but is somewhat more hazardous and less effective. A **hysterectomy** (removal of the uterus) is a major surgical procedure that is too dangerous to be used as a method of sterilization, unless there are other medically urgent reasons for removing the uterus.

## Abortion

Each year an estimated 5.4 million pregnancies occur in the United States. More than half of unintended pregnancies end in induced abortions.[48] Abortion rates vary greatly around the world. The U.S. abortion rate, which declined through most of the last decade, still remains higher than that of many Western countries, including Canada, Great Britain, the Netherlands, and Sweden. Although there is no one single or simple explanation for this difference, researchers focus on America's high rate of unintended pregnancies. In many nations with fewer unwanted pregnancies and lower abortion rates, contraceptives are generally easier and cheaper to obtain, and early sex education strongly emphasizes their importance.

No woman in any country ever elects to be in a situation where she has to consider abortion. But if faced with an unwanted pregnancy, many women consider *elective abortion* as an option. Every year 3 out of every 100 American women between the ages of 15 and 44 choose to terminate a pregnancy. According to federal data, 43 percent of American women undergo an abortion by age 45.

These women do not fit neatly into any particular category. About 80 percent are unmarried. Most—70 percent—intend to have children, but not at this point in time. Many cannot afford a baby. Some feel unready for the responsibility; others fear that another child would jeopardize the happiness and security of their existing family.

About 55 percent of women who undergo abortion are under age 25; only 22 percent are older than age 30. Unmarried pregnant women are six times more likely to have abortions than married ones; poor women are three times more likely to abort a pregnancy than women in higher economic groups. White women account for 63 percent of abortions, yet nonwhite women (who make up a smaller proportion of the population) are twice as likely to have an abortion as white women. Catholic women are more likely than Protestant women to have abortions, but women with no religious affiliations have a higher abortion rate than those who belong to a particular religion.

## Thinking Through the Options

A woman faced with an unwanted pregnancy—often alone, unwed, and desperate—can find it extremely difficult to decide what to do. The political debate over the right to life almost always is secondary to practical and emotional matters, such as the quality of her relationship with the baby's father, their capacity to provide for the child, the impact on any children she already has, and other important life issues.

Giving up her child for adoption is an option for women who do not feel abortion is right for them. Because the number of would-be adoptive parents greatly exceeds the number of available newborns, some women considering adoption may feel pressured by offers of money from couples eager to adopt. Others, particularly minority women, may feel cultural pressures to keep a child—regardless of their age, economic situation, or ability to care for an infant. Advocates of adoption reform are pressing for mandatory counseling for all pregnant women considering adoption (available now in agency-arranged, but not private, adoptions) and for extending the period of time during which a new mother can change her mind about giving up her child for adoption.

In deciding whether or not to have an abortion, women report asking themselves many questions, including the following:

- How do I feel about the man with whom I conceived this baby? Do I love him? Does he love me? Is this man committed to staying with me?
- What sort of relationship, if any, have we had or might we have in the future?
- If I continue the pregnancy and give birth, could I love the baby?
- Who can help me gain perspective on this problem?
- Have I thought about adoption? Do I think I could surrender custody of my baby? Would it make a difference if the adoption process were open and I could know the adoptive parents?
- If I keep my child, can I perperly care for him or her?
- How would the birth of another baby affect my other children?
- Do I have marketable skills, an education, an adequate income? Would I be able to go to school or keep my job if I have a child? Who would help me?
- Would this child be born with serious abnormalities? Would it suffer or thrive?
- How does each option fit with what I believe is morally correct? Could I emotionally handle each option?

Answering these questions honestly and objectively may help women as they think through the realities of their situation.

## Medical Abortion

The term **medical abortion** describes the use of drugs, also called *abortifacients,* to terminate a pregnancy. In 2000 the abortion pill mifepristone (Mifeprex), formerly known as RU-486, became available for use in the United States. Mifepristone, which is 97 percent effective in inducing abortion, blocks progesterone, the hormone that prepares the uterine lining for pregnancy. Two days after taking this compound, a woman takes a prostaglandin to increase uterine contractions. The uterine lining is expelled along with the fertilized egg. (See Figure 8-13.) Women have compared the discomfort of this experience to severe menstrual cramps. Common side effects include excessive bleeding, nausea, fatigue, abdominal pain, and dizziness. About 1 woman in 100 requires a blood transfusion.

Other agents used in medical abortion are methotrexate, widely used to treat certain cancers and arthritis, and misoprostol (Cytotec), primarily prescribed in the United States to prevent gastrointestinal ulcers. Methotrexate interferes with the ability of cells to multi-

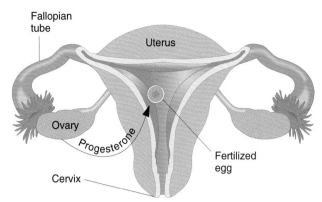

Progesterone, a hormone produced by the ovaries, is necessary for the implantation and development of a fertilized egg.

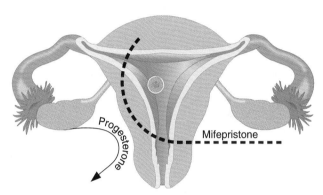

Step 1. Taken early in pregnancy, mifepristone blocks the action of progesterone and makes the body react as if it isn't pregnant.

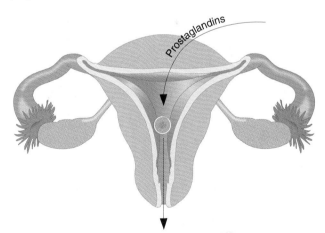

Step 2. Prostaglandins, taken two days later, cause the uterus to contract and the cervix to soften and dilate. As a result, the fertilized egg is expelled in 97 percent of the cases.

▲ **Figure 8-13** Medical Abortion
Mifepristone works by blocking the action of progesterone.

ply and divide, which halts development of an embryo or placenta. Misoprostol causes the uterus to contract, which helps expel a fertilized egg. Although misoprostol has been used in combination with mifespristone, researchers are investigating whether it can be used alone to terminate pregnancy.[49]

Although condemned by right-to-life advocates, abortion medications may in time lower the public profile of pregnancy termination. They are not painless, cheap, or equally available to all, but they do offer women a chance to carry through on their personal choice in greater privacy and safety. In a recent study, women who had a medical abortion reported a significantly higher level of satisfaction than those undergoing a surgical abortion.[50]

Medical abortion does not require anesthesia, can be performed very early in pregnancy, and may feel more private. However, women experience more cramping and bleeding during medical abortion than during surgical abortion, and bleeding lasts for a longer period.[51]

## Other Abortion Methods

More than half of all abortions (54 percent) are performed within the first 8 weeks of pregnancy. Only about 1 percent of abortions occur after 20 weeks. Medically, first-trimester abortion is less risky than childbirth. However, the likelihood of complications increases when abortions are performed in the second trimester (the second three-month period) of pregnancy.[52]

The vast majority of abortions performed in the United States today are surgical.[53] **Suction curettage,** usually done from 7 to 13 weeks after the last menstrual period, involves the gradual dilation (opening) of the cervix, often by inserting into the cervix one or more sticks of *laminaria* (a sterilized seaweed that absorbs moisture and expands, thus gradually stretching the cervix). Some women feel pressure or cramping with the laminaria in place. Occasionally, the laminaria itself starts to bring on a miscarriage.

At the time of abortion, the laminaria is removed, and dilators are used to further enlarge the cervical opening, if needed. The physician inserts a suction tip into the cervix, and the uterine contents are drawn out via a vacuum system. (See Figure 8-14.) A *curette* (a spoon-shaped surgical instrument used for scraping) is used to check for complete removal of the contents of the uterus. With suction curettage, the risks of complication are low. Major complications, such as perforation of the uterus, occur in fewer than 1 in 100 cases.

For early second-trimester abortions, physicians generally use a technique called **dilation and evacuation (D and E),** in which they open the cervix and use medical instruments to remove the fetus from the uterus. D and E procedures are performed under local or general anesthesia.

To induce abortion from week 16 to week 20, prostaglandins (natural substances found in most body tissues) are administered as vaginal suppositories or injected into the amniotic sac by inserting a needle through the abdominal wall. They induce uterine contractions, and the

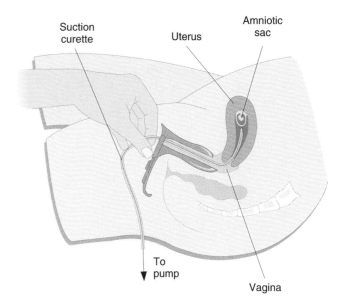

▲ **Figure 8-14** Suction Curettage
The contents of the uterus are extracted through the cervix with a vacuum apparatus.

fetus and placenta are expelled within 24 hours. Injecting saline or urea solutions into the amniotic sac can also terminate the pregnancy by triggering contractions that expel the fetus and placenta. Sometimes vaginal suppositories or drugs that help the uterus contract are used. Complications from abortion techniques that induce labor include nausea, vomiting, diarrhea, tearing of the cervix, excessive bleeding, and possible shock and death.

**Hysterotomy** involves surgically opening the uterus and removing the fetus. This is generally done from week 16 to week 24 of the pregnancy, primarily in emergency situations when the woman's life is in danger, or when other methods of abortion are considered too risky. However, late pregnancy abortions increase the risk of spontaneous abortion or premature labor in subsequent pregnancies and should be avoided if possible.

## What Is the Psychological Impact of Abortion?

Many assume that abortion must be psychologically devastating, that women who abort a fetus sooner or later develop what some have termed *post-abortion trauma syndrome.* In her studies at the University of Chicago, psychiatrist Nada Stotland found that there is no such thing. The primary emotion of women who have just had an abortion, she discovered, is relief. Although many women also express feelings of sadness or guilt, their anxiety levels eventually drop until they are lower than they were immediately before the abortion.[54]

Nonetheless, although psychologists consider the mental-health risks minimal compared to those of bearing an unwanted child, this does not mean women who have abortions never have regrets. In one recent study, nearly one in five women reported sadness, dissatisfaction, and regret about her abortion two years later.[55] But a feeling—even one as painful as loss, sadness, or guilt—is not a syndrome, and a woman's responses to abortion often change with passing days, weeks, months, or years. Anniversaries—of conception, of the date a woman found out she was pregnant, of the abortion, of the delivery date—can trigger memories and a sense of loss, but most women deal with these and move on with their lives.

The best predictor of psychological well-being after abortion is a woman's emotional well-being prior to pregnancy. At highest risk are women who have had a psychiatric illness, such as an anxiety disorder or clinical depression, prior to an abortion, and those whose abortions occurred among complicated circumstances (such as a rape, or coercion by parents or a partner). The vast majority of women manage to put the abortion into perspective as one of many life events.

## Politics of Abortion

Abortion is one of the most controversial political, religious, and ethical issues of our time. The issues of when life begins, a woman's right to choose, and an unborn child's right to survival are among the most divisive Americans face. Abortions were legal in the United States until the 1860s. For decades after that, women who decided to terminate unwanted pregnancies did so by attempting to abort themselves or by obtaining illegal abortions—often performed by untrained individuals using unsanitary and unsafe procedures. In the late 1960s, some states changed their laws to make abortions legal. In 1973, the U.S. Supreme Court, following a 1970 ruling on the case of *Roe v. Wade* by the New York Supreme Court, said that an abortion in the first trimester of pregnancy was a decision between a woman and her physician, and was protected by privacy laws. The Court further ruled that abortion during the second trimester could be performed on the basis of health risks and that abortion during the final trimester could be performed only for the sake of the mother's health.

Since then, several laws have restricted the availability of legal abortions for low-income women. In 1989, the U.S. Supreme Court narrowed the interpretation of *Roe v. Wade* by upholding a law that sharply restricted publicly funded abortions and required doctors to test if a fetus more than 20 weeks old could survive. In 1992, in *Planned Parenthood v. Casey,* the Court upheld the right to legalized abortion but gave states the right to restrict abortion as long as they did not place an "undue burden" on a woman. This limited the availability of abortion to young, rural, and low-income women. In 2000, in *Sternberg v. Carhart,* the U.S. Supreme Court struck down Nebraska's ban on "partial

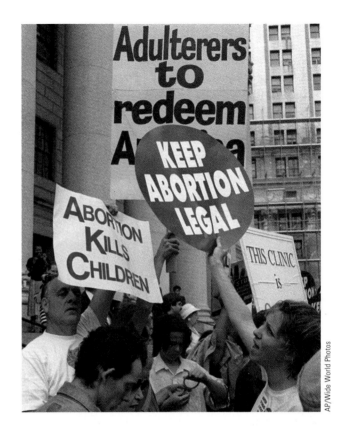

▲ The controversy over abortion has resulted in countless demonstrations and encounters between pro-choice and pro-life supporters.

birth abortions," a term abortion opponents use for dilation and extraction, a second-trimester surgical procedure.

The debate over abortion continues to stir passionate emotions, with pro-life supporters arguing that life begins at conception and that abortion is therefore immoral, and pro-choice advocates countering that an individual woman should have the right to make decisions about her body and health. The controversy over abortion has at times become violent: Physicians who performed abortions have been shot and killed; abortion clinics have been bombed, wounding and killing patients and staff members.

Although the majority of Americans continue to support abortion, many feel that it should be more restricted and difficult to obtain. While 61 percent of Americans say abortion should be permitted during the first three months of pregnancy, only 15 percent support second-trimester abortions and 7 percent feel that abortions in the last trimester should be legal.

## Pregnancy

In the last half century, pregnancy rates have generally declined, although the absolute number of births has risen.[56] The average age of mothers has risen, but about 70 percent of babies are still born to women in their twenties. Mothers are now averaging slightly fewer than two children each. Not every married couple is opting for parenthood.

Of course, you don't have to be part of a couple to want or to conceive a child. The number of never-married, college-educated, career women who are becoming single parents has risen dramatically. They want children—with or without an ongoing relationship with a man—and may feel that, because of their age, they can't delay getting pregnant any longer.

## Preconception Care: A Preventive Approach

The time *before* a child is conceived can be crucial in assuring that an infant is born healthy, full-size, and full-term. Women who smoke, drink alcohol, take drugs, eat poorly, are too thin or too heavy, suffer from unrecognized infections or illnesses, or are exposed to toxins at work or home may start pregnancy with one or more strikes against them and their unborn babies. The best chance for lowering the infant mortality rate and preventing birth defects is before pregnancy. **Preconception care**—the enhancement of a woman's health and well-being prior to conception in order to ensure a healthy pregnancy and baby—includes risk assessment (evaluation of medical, genetic, and lifestyle risks), health promotion (such as teaching good nutrition), and interventions to reduce risk (such as treatment of infections and other diseases, and assistance in quitting smoking or drug use).

## How a Woman's Body Changes During Pregnancy

The 40 weeks of pregnancy transform a woman's body. At the beginning of pregnancy, the woman's uterus becomes slightly larger, and the cervix becomes softer and bluish due to increased blood flow. Progesterone and estrogen trigger changes in the milk glands and ducts in the breasts, which increase in size and feel somewhat tender. The pressure of the growing uterus against the bladder causes a more frequent need to urinate. As the pregnancy progresses, the woman's skin stretches as her body shape changes, her center of gravity changes as her abdomen protrudes, and her internal organs shift as the baby grows. (See Figure 8-15.) Pregnancy is typically divided into three-month periods called trimesters.

## How a Baby Grows

Silently and invisibly, over a nine-month period, a fertilized egg develops into a human being. When the zygote reaches

the uterus, it's still smaller than the head of a pin. Once nestled into the spongy uterine lining, it becomes an **embryo.** The embryo takes on an elongated shape, rounded at one end. A sac called the **amnion** envelops it (see photo, Figure 8-15). As water and other small molecules cross the amniotic membrane, the embryo floats freely in the absorbed fluid, cushioned from shocks and bumps. At nine weeks the embryo is called a **fetus.**

A special organ, the **placenta,** forms. Attached to the embryo by the umbilical cord, it supplies the growing baby with fluid and nutrients from the maternal bloodstream and carries waste back to the mother's body for disposal. (See Figure 8-16.)

## Emotional Aspects of Pregnancy

Almost all prospective parents worry about their ability to care for a helpless newborn. By talking openly about their feelings and fears, however, they can strengthen the bonds between them, so that they can work together as parents as well as partners. Psychological problems, such as depression, can occur during pregnancy. The availability of social support and other resources for coping with stress can make a great difference in the potential impact of emotional difficulties.

The physiological changes of pregnancy can affect a woman's mood. In early pregnancy, she may feel weepy, irritable, or emotional. As the pregnancy continues, she may become calmer and more energetic. Men, too, feel a range of intense emotions about the prospect of having a child: pride, anxiety, hope, fears for their unseen child and for the woman they love. Although many men want to be as supportive as possible, they may think that they have to be strong and calm—and may therefore pull away from their wives. The more involved fathers become in preparing for birth, the closer they feel to their partners and babies afterward.

## Complications of Pregnancy

In about 10 to 15 percent of all pregnancies, there is increased risk of some problem, such as a baby's failure to grow normally. **Perinatology,** or maternal-fetal medicine, focuses on the special needs of high-risk mothers and their unborn babies. Perinatal centers, with state-of-the-art equipment and 24-hour staffs of specialists in this field, have been set up around the country. Several of the most frequent potential complications of pregnancy are discussed below.

### Ectopic Pregnancy

Any woman who is of childbearing age, has had intercourse, and feels abdominal pain with no reasonable cause

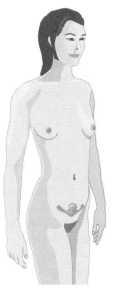
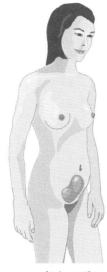

### First Trimester

Increased urination because of hormonal changes and the pressure of the enlarging uterus on the bladder.

Enlarged breasts as milk glands develop.

Darkening of the nipples and the area around them.

Nausea or vomiting, particularly in the morning.

Fatigue.

Increased vaginal secretions.

Pinching of the sciatic nerve, which runs from the buttocks down through the back of the legs, as the pelvic bones widen and begin to separate.

Irregular bowel movements.

Before conception                    At 4 months

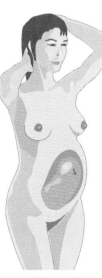
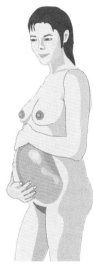

### Second Trimester

Thickening of the waist as the uterus grows.

Weight gain.

Increase in total blood volume.

Slight increase in size and change in position of the heart.

Darkening of the pigment around the nipple and from the navel to the pubic region.

Darkening of the face.

Increased salivation and perspiration.

Secretion of colostrum from the breasts.

Indigestion, constipation, and hemorrhoids.

Varicose veins.

At 9 months

At 7 months

### Third Trimester

Increased urination because of pressure from the uterus.

Tightening of the uterine muscles (called Braxton-Hicks contractions).

Shortness of breath because of increased pressure by the uterus on the lungs and diaphragm.

Heartburn and indigestion.

Trouble sleeping because of the baby's movements or the need to urinate.

Descending ("dropping") of the baby's head into the pelvis about two to four weeks before birth.

Navel pushed out.

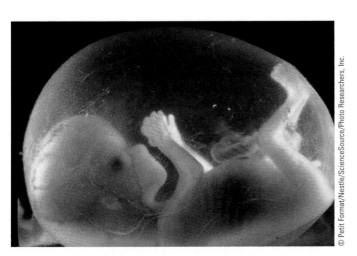

© Petit Format/Nestle/ScienceSource/Photo Researchers, Inc.

▲ **Figure 8-15** Physiological Changes of Pregnancy

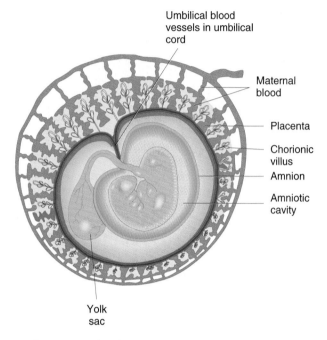

Umbilical blood vessels in umbilical cord

Maternal blood

Placenta

Chorionic villus

Amnion

Amniotic cavity

Yolk sac

▲ **Figure 8-16** The Placenta
The placenta supplies the growing embryo with fluid and nutrients from the maternal bloodstream and carries waste back for disposal.

may have an **ectopic pregnancy.** In this type of pregnancy, the fertilized egg remains in the fallopian tube instead of traveling to the uterus. Ectopic, or tubal, pregnancies have increased dramatically in recent years, now accounting for 2 percent of all reported pregnancies. STDs, particularly chlamydia infections (discussed in Chapter 9), have become a major cause of ectopic pregnancy. Other risk factors include previous pelvic surgery, particularly involving the fallopian tubes; pelvic inflammatory disease; infertility; and use of an IUD.

## Miscarriage

About 10 to 20 percent of pregnancies end in **miscarriage,** or spontaneous abortion, before the 20th week of gestation. Major genetic disorders may be responsible for 33 to 50 percent of pregnancy losses. The most common cause is an abnormal number of chromosomes.[57] About 0.5 to l percent of women suffer three or more miscarriages, possibly because of genetic, anatomic, hormonal, infectious, or autoimmune factors.[58] An estimated 70 to 90 percent of women who miscarry eventually become pregnant again.

## Infections

The infectious disease most clearly linked to birth defects is **rubella** (German measles). All women should be vaccinated against this disease at least three months prior to conception,

to protect themselves and any children they may bear. (See Chapter 9 for more on immunization.) The most common prenatal infection today is *cytomegalovirus.* This infection produces mild flulike symptoms in adults but can cause brain damage, retardation, liver disease, cerebral palsy, hearing problems, and other malformations in unborn babies.

STDs, such as syphilis, gonorrhea, and genital herpes, can be particularly dangerous during pregnancy if not recognized and treated. If a woman has a herpes outbreak around the date her baby is due, her physician will deliver the baby by caesarean section to prevent infecting the baby. HIV infection endangers both a pregnant woman and her unborn baby, and all pregnant women and new mothers should be aware of the HIV epidemic, the risks to them and their babies, and the availability of anonymous testing.

## Premature Labor

Approximately 10 percent of all babies are born too soon (before the 37th week of pregnancy). According to researchers, prematurity is the main underlying cause of stillbirth and infant deaths within the first few weeks after birth. Bed rest, close monitoring, and, if necessary, medications for at-risk women can buy more time in the womb for their babies. But women must recognize the warning signs of **premature labor**—dull, low backache; a feeling of tightness or pressure on the lower abdomen; and intestinal cramps, sometimes with diarrhea. Low-birthweight premature babies face the highest risks, but comprehensive, enriched programs can reduce developmental and health problems.

# Childbirth

A generation ago, delivering a baby was something a doctor did in a hospital. Today parents can choose from an almost bewildering array of birthing options. The first decision parents-to-be face is choosing a birth attendant, who can be a physician or a nurse-midwife. Certified nurse-midwives in the United States deliver more than 90,000 babies a year, mostly in hospitals and birth centers. Their approach is based on the belief that the typical pregnant woman can deliver her baby naturally without technological intervention. Lay midwives have a similar orientation but less formal training; only a handful of states permit lay midwives to deliver babies.

When interviewing physicians or midwives, look for the following:

✔ Experience in handling various complications.
✔ Extensive prenatal care.
✔ A commitment to be at the mother's side for the entire labor in order to quickly spot complications and provide assistance.

✔ A compatible philosophy toward childbirth and medical interventions.

## Preparing for Childbirth

The most widespread method of childbirth preparation is **psychoprophylaxis,** or the **Lamaze method.** Fernand Lamaze, a French doctor, instructed women to respond to labor contractions with prelearned, controlled breathing techniques. As the intensity of each contraction increases, the laboring woman concentrates on increasing her breathing rate in a prescribed way. Her partner coaches her during each contraction and helps her cope with discomfort.

Women who have had childbirth preparation training tend to have fewer complications and require fewer medications. However, painkillers or anesthesia are always an option if labor is longer or more painful than expected. The lower body can be numbed with an **epidural block,** which involves injecting an anesthetic into the membrane around the spinal cord, or a **spinal block,** in which the injection goes directly into the spinal canal. General anesthesia is usually used only for emergency caesarean births.

## ???? What Is Childbirth Like?

There are three stages of **labor.** The first starts with *effacement* (thinning) and *dilation* (opening up) of the cervix. Effacement is measured in percentages, and dilation in centimeters or finger-widths. Around this time, the amniotic sac of fluids usually breaks, a sign that the woman should call her doctor or midwife.

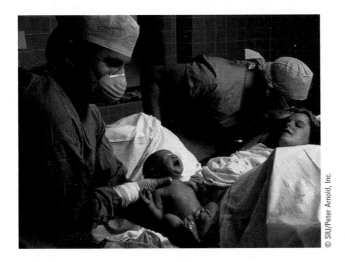

© SIU/Peter Arnold, Inc.

▲ Fathers are routinely present at the birth of their children and often act as birth coaches after both parents train in Lamaze techniques.

The first contractions of the early, or *latent,* phase of labor are usually not uncomfortable; they last 15 to 30 seconds, occur every 15 to 30 minutes, and gradually increase in intensity and frequency. The most difficult contractions come after the cervix is dilated to about 8 centimeters, as the woman feels greater pressure from the fetus. The first stage ends when the cervix is completely dilated to a diameter of 10 centimeters (or five finger-widths) and the baby is ready to come down the birth canal. (See Figure 8-17.) For women having their first baby, this first stage of labor averages 12 to 13 hours. Women having another child often experience shorter first-stage labor.

When the cervix is completely dilated, the second stage of labor occurs, during which the baby moves into the vagina, or birth canal, and out of the mother's body. As this stage begins, women who have gone through childbirth preparation training often feel a sense of relief from the acute pain of the transition phase and at the prospect of giving birth.

This second stage can take up to an hour or more. Strong contractions may last 60 to 90 seconds and occur every two to three minutes. As the baby's head descends, the mother feels an urge to push. By bearing down, she helps the baby complete its passage to the outside.

As the baby's head appears, or *crowns,* the doctor may perform an *episiotomy*—an incision from the lower end of the vagina toward the anus to enlarge the vaginal opening. The purpose of the episiotomy is to prevent the baby's head from causing an irregular tear in the vagina, but routine episiotomies have been criticized as unnecessary. Women may be able to avoid this procedure by trying different birthing positions or having an attendant massage the perineal tissue.

Usually the baby's head emerges first, then its shoulders, then its body. With each contraction, a new part is born. However, the baby can be in a more difficult position, facing up rather than down, or with the feet or buttocks first (a **breech birth**), and a caesarean birth may then be necessary.

In the third stage of labor, the uterus contracts firmly after the birth of the baby and, usually within five minutes, the placenta separates from the uterine wall. The woman may bear down to help expel the placenta, or the doctor may exert gentle external pressure. If an episiotomy has been performed, the doctor sews up the incision. To help the uterus contract and return to its normal size, it may be massaged manually, or the baby may be put to the mother's breast to stimulate contraction of the uterus.

## Caesarean Birth

In a **caesarean delivery** (also referred to as a *caesarean section*), the doctor lifts the baby out of the woman's body through an incision made in the lower abdomen and uterus. The most common reason for caesarean birth is *failure to progress,* a vague term indicating that labor has gone on too long and may put the baby or mother at risk.

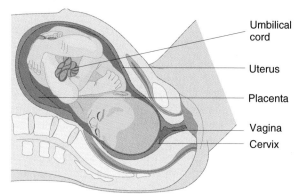

Umbilical
cord

Uterus

Placenta

Vagina
Cervix

1. The cervix is partially dilated, and the
   baby's head has entered the birth canal.

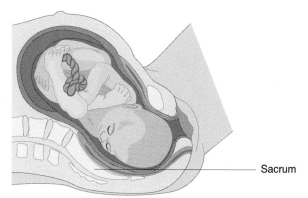

Sacrum

2. The cervix is nearly completely dilated. The baby's head
   rotates so that it can move through the birth canal.

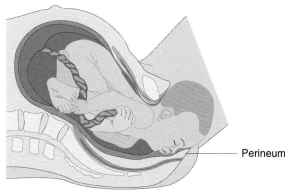

Perineum

3. The baby's head extends as it reaches
   the vaginal opening, and the head and the rest
   of the body pass through the birth canal.

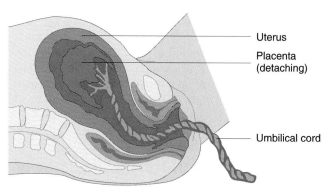

Uterus

Placenta
(detaching)

Umbilical cord

4. After the baby is born, the placenta detaches from
   the uterus and is expelled from the woman's body.

▲ **Figure 8-17**  Birth

Other reasons include the baby's position (if feet or buttocks are first) and signs that the fetus is in danger.

Thirty years ago, only 5 percent of babies born in America were delivered by caesarean birth; the current rate is 22.6 percent, substantially higher than in most other industrialized countries. About 36 percent of caesarean sections are performed because the woman has had a previous caesarean birth. However, four of every five women who have had caesarean births *can* have successful vaginal deliveries in subsequent pregnancies.

Caesarean birth involves abdominal surgery, so many women feel more physical discomfort after a caesarean than a vaginal birth, including nausea, pain, and abdominal gas. Women who have had a caesarean section must refrain from strenuous activity, such as heavy lifting, for several weeks.

### After the Birth

Hospital stays for new mothers are shorter than in the past. The average length of stay is now only 2.6 days for a vagi-

nal delivery and 4.1 days after a caesarean birth. A primary reason has been pressure to reduce medical costs. Obstetricians have voiced concern that the rush to release new mothers may jeopardize their well-being and the health of their babies, who are more likely to require emergency care for problems such as jaundice. The American College of Obstetricians and Gynecologists and the American Academy of Pediatrics recommend that women remain in the hospital two days after a vaginal delivery and four days after a caesarean birth.

### Infertility

The World Health Organization defines **infertility** as the failure to conceive after one year of unprotected intercourse. Western societies regard infertility as a medical rather than social problem. In other regions, such as Africa's infertility belt, involuntary childlessness is more complex, a consequence of other problems such as AIDS and famine.[59] The main causes of infertility are ovulation problems, tubal damage, or sperm dysfunction. Less common causes are endometriosis, cervical factors, or coital difficulties. Even after intensive investigation, 10 to 20 percent of couples have unexplained infertility in which no cause can be demonstrated.

Of the couples who marry this year, 1 in 12 won't be able to conceive a child, and 10 percent of couples already married won't be able to have additional children. The percentage of women seeking infertility services rose from 12 to 15 percent since the 1980s.[60] Infertility is a problem of the couple, not of the individual man or woman. In 40 percent of cases, infertility is caused by female problems, in 40 percent by male problems, in 10 percent by a combination of male and female problems, and in 10 percent by unexplained causes. A thorough diagnostic workup can reveal a cause for infertility in 90 percent of cases.

In women, the most common causes of subfertility or infertility are age, abnormal menstrual patterns, suppression of ovulation, and blocked fallopian tubes. A woman's fertility peaks between ages 20 and 30 and then drops quickly: by 20 percent after 30, by 50 percent after 35, and by 95 percent after 40. In a survey of 1,168 professional women in the United States, 42 percent of those over 40 were childless—only 14 percent by choice.[61]

Male subfertility or infertility is usually linked to either the quantity or the quality of sperm, which may be inactive, misshapen, or insufficient (less than 20 million sperm per milliliter of semen in an ejaculation of 3 to 5 milliliters). Sometimes the problem is hormonal or a blockage of a sperm duct. Some men suffer from the inability to ejaculate normally, or from retrograde ejaculation, in which some of the semen travels in the wrong direction, back into the body of the male.

Infertility can have an enormous emotional impact. Often, the wife begins to worry first because infertility touches on a core aspect of femininity. Many women long to experience pregnancy and childbirth and feel great loss if they cannot conceive. Their self-esteem may be diminished, and they may become obsessed with success and outcome. Women in their thirties and forties fear that their biological clock is running out of time. Men may be confused and surprised by the intensity of their partner's emotions. Most are more concerned about their wife than about having a baby, but they feel helpless and frustrated in their husbandly role of fixing matters for the wife. Although they both need each other's support more than ever, they may pull away from each other because of their sadness and a sense of losing control over their lives.

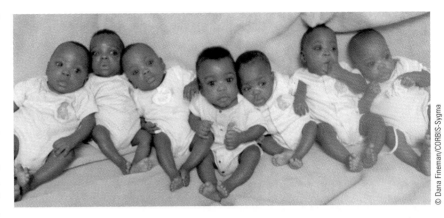

▲ Fertility drugs can increase the chances of multiple births.

The treatment of infertility has become a $2 billion a year enterprise in the United States. The odds of successful pregnancy range from 30 to 70 percent, depending on the specific cause of infertility. One result of successful infertility treatments has been a boom in multiple births, including quintuplets and sextuplets. Some obstetricians have urged less aggressive treatment for infertility to avoid such high-risk multiple births.

## Artificial Insemination

Since the 1960s, **artificial insemination**—the introduction of viable sperm into the vagina by artificial means—has led to an estimated 250,000 births in the United States, primarily in couples in which the husband was infertile. However, some states do not recognize such children as legitimate; others do, but only if the woman's husband gave his consent for the insemination.

## Assisted Reproductive Technology

New approaches to infertility include microsurgery, sometimes with lasers, to open destroyed or blocked egg and sperm ducts; new hormone preparations to induce ovulation; and the use of balloons, inserted through the cervix and inflated, to open blocked fallopian tubes (a procedure called *balloon tuboplasty*). Less than 1 percent of live births are the result of artificial reproductive technology (ART).[62]

Among the most well-known techniques to overcome fertility problems is *in vitro fertilization (IVF),* which involves removing the ova from a woman's ovary and placing the woman's egg and her mate's sperm in a laboratory dish for fertilization. If the fertilized egg cell shows signs of development, within several days it is returned to the woman's uterus, the egg cell implants itself in the lining of the uterus, and the pregnancy continues as normal. The success rate varies but is generally less than 20 percent, and the costs are high.

 Are emergency contraceptives like the morning-after pill safe? Should they be made available over the counter?

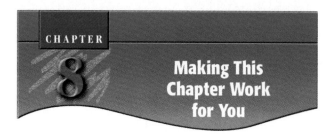

**CHAPTER 8**

**Making This Chapter Work for You**

1. Conception occurs
   a. when a fertilized egg implants in the lining of the uterus.
   b. when sperm is blocked from reaching the egg.
   c. when a sperm fertilizes the egg.
   d. after the uterine lining is discharged during the menstrual cycle.

2. Factors to consider when choosing a contraceptive method include all of the following *except*
   a. cost.
   b. failure rate.
   c. effectiveness in preventing sexually transmitted diseases.
   d. preferred sexual position.

3. When used correctly, which is the most effective non-hormonal contraceptive method?
   a. Copper T intrauterine device
   b. condom
   c. spermicide
   d. diaphragm

4. Which of the following contraceptive choices offers the best protection against STDs?
   a. condom alone
   b. condom plus spermicide
   c. abstinence
   d. withdrawal plus spermicide

5. Which statement about prescription contraceptives is *not* true?
   a. Prescription contraceptives do not offer protection against STDs.
   b. Some prescription contraceptives contain estrogen and progestin, and some contain only progestin.
   c. The contraceptive ring must be changed every week.

   d. IUDs prevent pregnancy by preventing or interfering with implantation.

6. Which of the following statements is true about sterilization?
   a. In women, the most frequently performed sterilization technique is hysterectomy.
   b. Many couples experience an increase in sexual encounters after sterilization.
   c. Vasectomies are easily reversed with surgery.
   d. Sterilization is recommended for single men and women who are unsure about whether they want children.

7. The incidence of abortion is
   a. highest in women older than 30 and who have several children.
   b. lower in the United States than in countries where birth control education begins early and contraceptives are easier and cheaper to obtain.
   c. higher in affluent women, who can afford the procedure, than in poor women.
   d. higher in Catholic women than in Protestant women.

8. In the third trimester of pregnancy,
   a. the woman experiences shortness of breath as the enlarged uterus presses on the lungs and diaphragm.
   b. the embryo is now called a fetus.
   c. the woman should begin regular prenatal checkups.
   d. the woman should increase her activity level to ensure that she is fit for childbirth.

9. During childbirth,
   a. breech birth can be prevented by practicing the Lamaze method.
   b. the cervix thins and dilates so that the baby can exit the uterus.
   c. the intensity of contraction decreases during the second stage of labor.
   d. the placenta is expelled immediately before the baby's head appears.

10. Which of the following statements is true about infertility?
    a. Infertility is most often caused by female problems.
    b. In men, infertility is usually caused by a combination of excess sperm production and an ejaculation problem.
    c. In vitro fertilization involves introducing sperm into the vagina with a long needle.
    d. Less than 1 percent of live births are the result of artificial reproductive technology.

Answers to these questions can be found on page 415.

## Critical Thinking

1. After reading about the various methods of contraception, which do you think would be most effective for you? What factors enter into your decision (convenience, risks, effectiveness, etc.)?

2. In Wyoming, a pregnant woman went to the police station to report that her husband had beaten her. Instead of charges being brought against him, she was arrested for intoxication and charged with abusing her fetus by drinking. Across the country, other women who use hard drugs or alcohol while pregnant or whose newborns test positive for drugs have been arrested and put on trial for abusing their unborn children. Prosecutors argue that they are defending the innocent victims of substance abuse. Some health officials, on the other hand, argue that addicted women need help, not punishment. What do you think? Why?

3. Suppose that you and your partner were told that your only chance of having a child is by using fertility drugs. After taking the drugs, you and your partner are informed that there are seven fetuses. Would you carry them all to term? What if you knew that the chances of them all surviving were very slim and that eliminating some of them would improve the odds for the others? What ethical issues do cases like these raise?

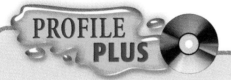

## PROFILE PLUS

Make informed choices about your method of birth control. Discover which method is best for you with this activity on your Profile Plus CD-ROM.

Which Contraceptive Method is Best for You?

## SITES & BYTES

**American Society for Reproductive Medicine**
**www.asrm.org**

This professional site features information for patients, health professionals, and the media on a variety of topics, including contraception and infertility. The site contains fact sheets, annual meeting information, and information about current clinical trials.

**National Women's Health Information Center**
**www.4woman.gov**

This site, by the U.S. Public Health Office on Women's Health, features current women's health topics and press releases, as well as information on screening and immunization schedules, violence, smoking cessation, prevention, pregnancy, disabilities, and body image. Also, there is information for health professionals and an online newsletter.

**Planned Parenthood**
**www.plannedparenthood.org**

This site features current health information pertaining family planning, including emergency contraception, as well as pregnancy, sexually transmitted diseases, safer sex, and political action.

### InfoTrac College Edition Activity

Erica Lumiere. "New No-Hassle Birth Control: A New Generation of Patches, Pills, and Devices Is Hitting the Market, Making Birth Control Easier to Take Than the Pill—and Just As Effective." *Marie Claire,* Vol. 9, No. 4, April 2002, p. 225 (1).

1. What are the advantages and disadvantages of Lunelle?

2. Compare the advantages and disadvantages of the Nuvaring compared to the Ortho Evra skin patch.

3.  How does the new hormonal IUD Mirena work?

You can find additional readings related to contraception and reproduction with InfoTrac College Edition, an online library of more than 900 journals and publications. Follow the instructions for accessing InfoTrac College Edition that were packaged with your textbook; then search for articles using a keyword search.

For additional links, resources, and suggested readings on InfoTrac, visit our Health & Wellness Resource Center at http://health.wadsworth.com.

## Key Terms

The terms listed here are used within the chapter on the page indicated. Definitions of the terms are in the Glossary at the end of the book.

amnion 198
artificial insemination 203
barrier contraceptives 186
basal body temperature 192
breech birth 201
caesarean delivery 201
cervical cap 185
coitus interruptus 176
colpotomy 194
conception 174
condom 186
constant-dose combination
  pill 179
contraception 174
diaphragm 184
dilation and evacuation
  (D and E) 196

ectopic pregnancy 200
embryo 198
emergency contraception
  (EC) 192
epidural block 201
failure rate 176
fertilization 174
fetus 198
hysterectomy 193
hysterotomy 196
implantation 174
infertility 202
intrauterine device
  (IUD) 183
labor 201
Lamaze method 201
laparoscopy 194

laparotomy 193
medical abortion 195
minilaparotomy 193
minipill 179
miscarriage 200
monophasic pill 179
multiphasic pill 179
oral contraceptives 179
ovulation method 191
perinatology 198
placenta 198
preconception care 198
premature labor 200
progestin-only pill 179
psychoprophylaxis 201
rhythm method 191
rubella 200

spermatogenesis 174
spinal block 201
sterilization 192
suction curettage 196
tubal ligation 193
tubal occlusion 193
vaginal contraceptive film
  (VCF) 190
vaginal spermicide 189
vasectomy 193
zygote 174

## References

1.  Darroch, Jacqueline. "The Pill and Men's Involvement in Contraception." *Family Planning Perspective*, Vol. 32, No. 2, March 2000.
2.  Steinhauer, Jennifer. "Men Avoiding Obligation for Birth Control." *New York Times*, May 25, 1995.
3.  Gold, Rachel Benson, and Cory Richards. *Medicaid Support for Family Planning in the Managed Care Era.* New York: Alan Guttmacher Institute, 2001, p. 10.
4.  Murray, Steven, and Jessica L. Miller. "Birth Control and Condom Usage Among College Students." *Research Quarterly for Exercise and Sport*, Vol. 71, No. 1, March 2000.
5.  Wyatt, Gail, et al. "Factors Affecting HIV Contraceptive Decision-Making Among Women." *Sex Roles: A Journal of Research*, April 2000.
6.  Pennachio, Dorothy. "New Approaches to Emergency Contraception." *Patient Care*, Vol. 35, No. 5, March 15, 2001, p. 19.
7.  Oncale, Renee, and Bruce King. "Comparisons of Men's and Women's Attempts to Dissuade Sexual Partners from the Couple Using Condoms." *Archives of Sexual Behavior*, Vol. 30, No. 4, August 2001, p. 379.
8.  "Is Abstinence Right for You?" www.plannedparenthood.org.
9.  "Facts About Birth Control." www.plannedparenthood.org.
10. "Hormonal Contraception Forty Years after Approval of 'The Pill.'" *Kaiser Family Foundation Issue Update*, June 2002, p. 1.
11. Goldin, Claudia, and Lawrence Katz. "The Power of the Pill: Oral Contraceptives and Women's Career and Marriage Decisions." *Journal of Political Economy*, Vol. 110, No. 4, August 2002, p. 730.
12. Kemmeren, Jeanet, et al. "Third Generation Oral Contraceptives and Risk of Venous Thrombosis: Meta-Analysis." *British Medical Journal*, Vol. 323, No. 7305, July 21, 2001.
13. Ibid.
14. Schwetz, Bernard. "New Oral Contraceptive." *Journal of the American Medical Association*, Vol. 286, No. 5, August 1, 2001, p. 527.
15. Davidson, N. and K. Helzsouer. "Good News About Oral Contraceptives." *New England Journal of Medicine*, Vol. 346, June 27, 2002, p. 2078.

16. Marchbanks, P., et al. "Oral Contraceptives and the Risk of Breast Cancer." *New England Journal of Medicine,* Vol. 346, June 27, 2002, p. 2025.

17. Nelson, Anita. "Whose Pill Is It Anyway." *Family Planning Perspectives,* Vol. 32, No. 2, March 2000.

18. Guillebaud, John. "Will the Pill Become Obsolete in This Century?" *Family Planning Perspectives,* Vol. 32, No. 2, March 2000.

19. "Helping Women Use the Pill." *Population Reports,* Vol. 28, No. 2, Summer 2000.

20. "First Contraceptive Skin Patch Is Applied Only Once Weekly." *RN,* Vol. 65, No. 2, February 2002, p. 85.

21. Ditrich, Richard, et al. "Transdermal Contraception." *American Journal of Obstetrics and Gynecology,* Vol. 186, No. 1, January 2002, p. 15.

22. "Does Weight Play a Role in Effectiveness?" *Contraceptive Technology Update,* Vol. 23, No. 7, July 2002, p. 81.

23. "Norplant Implant Deemed Safe, Effective." *Contraceptive Technology Update,* Vol. 22, No. 6, June 2001, p. 64.

24. Stevens-Simon, Catherine, et al. "A Village Would Be Nice But . . . It Takes a Long-Acting Contraceptive to Prevent Repeat Adolescent Pregnancies." *American Journal of Preventive Medicine,* Vol. 21, No. 1, 2001, pp. 60–65.

25. Meirik, Olav, et al. "Safety and Efficacy of Levonorgestrel Implants, Intrauterine Devices, and Sterilization." *Obstetrics & Gynecology,* Vol. 97, No. 4, April 2001.

26. "Facts About Birth Control."

27. Kupecz, Deborah. "Lunelle: A New Contraceptive Alternative." *Nurse Practitioner,* Vol. 26, No. 6, June 2001, p. 55.

28. Vernarec, Emil. "This Non-Estrogen IUD Is Effective for Five Years." *RN,* Vol. 64, No. 3, March 2001, p. 98.

29. "The IUD and PID: What Are the Risks? *Contraceptive Technology Update,* Vol. 22, No. 6, June 2001, p. 68. "Rediscovering the Benefits of the IUD." *Contraceptive Technology Update,* Vol. 22, No. 1, January 2001, p. 5.

30. Hirozawa, A. "A First Pregnancy May Be Difficult to Achieve After Long-Term Use of an IUD." *Family Planning Perspectives,* Vol. 33, No. 4, July 2001, p. 181.

31. Hollander, Dore. "IUD Ifs, Ands and Buts." *Family Planning Perspectives,* Vol. 34, No. 2, March–April 2002, p. 60.

32. Greydanus, Donald, et al. "Contraception in the Adolescent: An Update." *Pediatrics,* Vol. 107, No. 3, March 2001, p. 562.

33. Ibid.

34. Murray and Miller, "Birth Control and Condom Usage Among College Students."

35. Michaels Opinion Research. "In the Heat of the Moment." Menlo Park, CA: Henry J. Kaiser Family Foundation, June 2001.

36. "Condom Use by Adolescents." *Pediatrics,* Vol. 107, No. 6, June 2001, p. 463.

37. Ford, Kathleen, et al. "Characteristics of Adolescents' Sexual Partners and Their Association with Use of Condoms and Other Contraceptive Methods." *Family Planning Perspectives,* Vol. 33, No. 3, May 2001, p. 100.

38. "Condom Misconceptions Abound Among Sexually Active Adolescents." *Medical Letter on the CDC and FDA,* May 27, 2001.

39. "Perceived Versus Actual Knowledge About Correct Condom Use Among U.S. Adolescents: Results from a National Study." *Journal of Adolescent Health,* Vol. 28, No. 5, May 2001, p. 415.

40. "Study of Female Condom Aims to Combat AIDS Worldwide." *AIDS Weekly,* November 13, 2000.

41. Hollander, D. "Female Condoms Remain Structurally Sound After Being Washed and Reused As Many As Seven Times." *Family Planning Perspectives,* Vol. 33, No. 4, July 2001, p. 186.

42. Grimes, David, et al. "New Approaches to Emergency Contraception." *Contemporary OB/GYN,* Vol. 46, No. 6, June 2001, p. 89.

43. "Emergency OCs: A Long-Kept Secret," *University of California, Berkeley, Wellness Letter,* Vol. 18, No. 11, August 2002, p. 6.

44. "Statement Supporting the Availability of Over-the-Counter Emergency Contraception." *American College of Obstetricians and Gynecologists,* March 2001.

45. Gardner, Jacqueline, et al. "Increasing Access to Emergency Contraception Through Community Pharmacies." *Family Planning Perspectives,* Vol. 33, No. 4, July 2001.

46. Golden, Neville, et al. "Emergency Contraception: Pediatricians' Knowledge, Attitudes, and Opinions." *Pediatrics,* Vol. 107, No. 2, February 2001, p. 287.

47. McCarthy, Susan. "Availability of Emergency Contraceptive Pills at University and College Student Health Centers." *Journal of American College Health,* Vol. 51, No. 1, July 2002, p. 15.

48. "Abortion in the United States." Menlo Park, CA: Henry J. Kaiser Family Foundation, May 2001.

49. "Mifepristone: An Early Abortion Option." Menlo Park, CA: Henry J. Kaiser Family Foundation, May 2001.

50. Hollander, D. "Most Abortion Patients View Their Experience Favorably, But Medical Abortion Gets a Higher Rating Than Surgical." *Family Planning Perspectives,* Vol. 32, No. 5, September 2000.

51. "Mifepristone: An Early Abortion Option."

52. "Chemical Abortion Vs. Surgical." *Insight on the News,* Vol. 17, No. 4, January 29, 2001, p. 16.

53. "Abortion Policy and Politics." Menlo Park, CA: Henry J. Kaiser Family Foundation, May 2001.

54. Stotland, Nada. *Abortion: Facts and Feelings.* Washington, D.C.: American Psychiatric Press, 1998.

55. Bower, B. "Study Explores Abortion's Mental Aftermath." *Science News,* Vol. 158, No. 8, August 19, 2000.

56. "Births, Marriages, Divorces, and Deaths." *National Vital Statistics Reports,* Vol. 49, No. 6, August 22, 2001.

57. Cohen, Jon. "Sorting Out Chromosome Errors." *Science,* Vol. 296, June 21, 2002, p. 2164.

58. Moore, Peter. "Tackling Autoantibody-Linked Pregnancy Loss." *Lancet,* Vol. 350, No. 9073, July 26, 1997. Cowchock, Susan. "Autoantibodies and Pregnancy Loss." *New England Journal of Medicine,* Vol. 337, No. 3, July 17, 1997.

59. Inhorn, Marcia, and Frank van Balen. *Infertility Around the Globe.* Berkeley: University of California Press, 2002.

60. Stephen, Elizabeth, and Aniani Chandra. "Use of Infertility Services in the United States." *Family Planning Perspectives,* Vol. 32, No. 3, May 2000.

61. Hewlett, Sylvia. *Creating a Life: Professional Women and the Quest for Children.* New York: Miramax Books, 2002.

62. Centers for Disease Control and Prevention. "Use of Assisted Reproductive Technology." *Journal of the American Medical Association,* Vol. 287, No. 12, March 27, 2002, p. 1521.

63. Gottlieb, Scott. "Assisted Reproduction Increases Risk of Birth Defects, Study Says." *British Medical Journal,* Vol. 324, No. 7338, March 16, 2002, p. 633.

# Protecting Yourself from Infectious Diseases

Throughout history, infectious diseases have claimed more lives than any military conflict or natural disaster. Although modern medicine has won many victories against the agents of infection, we remain vulnerable to a host of infectious illnesses. Drug-resistant strains of tuberculosis and *Staphylococcus* bacteria challenge current therapies. And scientists warn of the potential danger of new emerging viruses and of the use of infectious agents as weapons of war and terrorism.

Some of today's most common and dangerous infectious illnesses spread primarily through sexual contact, and their incidence has skyrocketed. The federal government estimates that 65 million Americans have a sexually transmitted disease.[1] These diseases cannot be prevented in the laboratory. Only you, by your behavior, can prevent and control them.

This chapter is a lesson in self-defense against all forms of infection. The information it provides can help you boost your defenses, recognize and avoid enemies, protect yourself from sexually transmitted diseases, and realize when to seek help.

# Understanding Infection

We live in a sea of microbes. Most of them don't threaten our health or survival; some, such as the bacteria that inhabit our intestines, are actually beneficial. Yet in the course of history, disease-causing microorganisms have claimed millions of lives. The twentieth century brought the conquest of infectious killers such as cholera and scarlet fever. Although modern science has won many victories against the agents of infection, infectious illnesses remain a serious health threat.

Infection is a complex process, triggered by various **pathogens** (disease-causing organisms) and countered by the body's own defenders. Physicians explain infection in terms of a **host** (either a person or a population) that contacts one or more agents in an environment. A **vector**—a biological or physical vehicle that carries the agent to the host—provides the means of transmission.

## Agents of Infection

The types of microbes that can cause infection are viruses, bacteria, fungi, protozoa, and helminths (parasitic worms).

### Viruses

The tiniest pathogens—**viruses**—are also the toughest; they consist of a bit of nucleic acid (DNA or RNA, but never both) within a protein coat. Unable to reproduce on its own, a virus takes over a body cell's reproductive machinery and instructs it to produce new viral particles, which are then released to enter other cells.

The most common viruses are these types:

✔ Rhinoviruses and adenoviruses, which get into the mucous membranes and cause upper-respiratory tract infections and colds.

✔ Influenza viruses, which can change their outer protein coats so dramatically that individuals resistant to one strain cannot fight off a new one.

✔ Herpes viruses, which take up permanent residence in the cells and periodically flare up.

✔ Papilloma viruses, which cause few symptoms in women and almost none in men, but may be responsible, at least in part, for a rise in the incidence of cervical cancer among younger women.

✔ Hepatitis viruses, which cause several forms of liver infection, ranging from mild to life threatening.

✔ Slow viruses, which give no early indication of their presence but can produce fatal illnesses within a few years.

✔ Retroviruses, which are named for their backward (*retro*) sequence of genetic replication compared to

other viruses. One retrovirus, human immunodeficiency virus (HIV), causes acquired immune deficiency syndrome (AIDS).

✔ Filoviruses, which resemble threads and are extremely lethal.

The problem in fighting viruses is that it's difficult to find drugs that harm the virus and not the cell it has commandeered. **Antibiotics** (drugs that inhibit or kill bacteria) have no effect on viruses. **Antiviral drugs** don't completely eradicate a viral infection, although they can decrease its severity and duration. Because viruses multiply very quickly, antiviral drugs are most effective when taken before an infection develops or in its early stages.

## Bacteria

Simple one-celled organisms, **bacteria** are the most plentiful microorganisms as well as the most pathogenic. Most kinds of bacteria don't cause disease; some, like *Escherichia coli* that aid in digestion, play important roles within our bodies. Even friendly bacteria, however, can get out of hand and cause acne, urinary tract infections, vaginal infections, and other problems.

Bacteria harm the body by releasing either enzymes that digest body cells or toxins that produce the specific effects of such diseases as diphtheria or toxic shock syndrome. In self-defense the body produces specific proteins (called *antibodies*) that attack and inactivate the invaders. Tuberculosis, tetanus, gonorrhea, scarlet fever, and diphtheria are examples of bacterial diseases.

Because bacteria are sufficiently different from the cells that make up our bodies, antibiotics can kill them without harming our cells. Antibiotics work only against specific types of bacteria. If your doctor thinks you have a bacterial infection, tests of your blood, pus, sputum, urine, or stool can identify the particular bacterial strain.

## Fungi

Single-celled or multicelled organisms, **fungi** consist of threadlike fibers and reproductive spores. These plants, lacking chlorophyll, must obtain their food from organic material, which may include human tissue. Fungi release enzymes that digest cells and are most likely to attack hair-covered areas of the body, including the scalp, beard, groin, and external ear canals. They also cause athlete's foot. Treatment consists of antifungal drugs.

## Protozoa

These single-celled, microscopic animals release enzymes and toxins that destroy cells or interfere with their function. Diseases caused by **protozoa** are not a major health problem in this country, primarily because of public health measures. Around the world, however, some 2.24 billion people (more than 40 percent of the world's population) are at risk for acquiring malaria—a protozoan-caused disease. Up to 3 million die from this disease annually. Many more come down with amoebic dysentery. Treatment for protozoa-caused diseases consists of general medical care to relieve the symptoms, replacement of lost blood or fluids, and drugs that kill the specific protozoan.

The most common disease caused by protozoa in the United States is *giardiasis,* an intestinal infection caused by microorganisms in human and animal feces. It has become a threat at day-care centers, as well as among campers and hikers who drink contaminated water. Symptoms include nausea, lack of appetite, gas, diarrhea, fatigue, abdominal cramps, and bloating. Many people recover in a month or two without treatment. However, in some cases the microbe causes recurring attacks over many years. Giardiasis can be life-threatening in small children and the elderly, who are especially prone to severe dehydration from diarrhea. Treatment usually consists of antibiotics.

## Helminths (Parasitic Worms)

Small parasitic worms that attack specific tissues or organs and compete with the host for nutrients are called **helminths.** One major worldwide health problem is *schistosomiasis,* a disease caused by a parasitic worm, the fluke, that burrows through the skin and enters the circulatory system. Infection with another helminth, the tapeworm, may be contracted from eating undercooked beef, pork, or fish containing larval forms of the tapeworm. Helminthic diseases are treated with appropriate medications.

## How Do You Catch an Infection?

The major vectors, or means of transmission, for infectious disease are animals and insects, people, food, and water.

## Animals and Insects

Disease can be transmitted by house pets, livestock, and wild animals. Insects also spread a variety of diseases. The housefly may spread dysentery, diarrhea, typhoid fever, or trachoma (an eye disease rare in the United States but common in other parts of the world). Other insects, including mosquitoes, ticks, mites, fleas, and lice, can transmit such diseases as malaria, yellow fever, encephalitis, dengue fever (a growing threat in Mexico), and Lyme disease.

A new threat in the United States is West Nile virus (WNV). First spotted in a sick crow in 1999, West Nile virus has spread to 111 species of birds, including the bald

---

### STRATEGIES FOR PREVENTION

**Protecting Yourself from Insect-Borne Diseases**

▲ Apply insect repellent containing DEET (N,N-diethyl-meta-toluamide), which provides the longest-lasting protection against bites, when you're outdoors.

▲ When possible, wear long-sleeved clothes and long pants treated with repellents containing permethrin or DEET since mosquitoes may bite through thin clothing. Do not apply repellents containing permethrin directly to exposed skin. If you spray your clothing, there is no need to spray repellent containing DEET on the skin under your clothing.

▲ Consider staying indoors at dawn, dusk, and in the early evening, which are peak mosquito-biting times.

▲ Limit the number of places available for mosquitos to lay their eggs by eliminating standing water sources from around your home.

Source: Centers for Disease Control and Prevention, www.cdc.gov.

---

eagle. WNV can be transmitted by a mosquito that feeds on an infected bird and then bites a human. WNV also can be transmitted through transplanted organs and possibly from blood products. By the end of 2002, the CDC reported more than 3,775 positively confirmed cases of West Nile virus and 216 deaths.[2]

WNV interferes with normal central nervous system functioning and causes inflammation of brain tissue. Symptoms include fever, body aches, brain swelling, coma, and paralysis. Less than 1 percent of those infected with WNV develop severe illness. Among these, 3 to 15 percent die, with the highest mortality rate among the elderly. An antiviral drug, interferon, which might lessen the symptoms and duration of the illness in infected patients, is undergoing testing.[3]

## People

The people you're closest to can transmit pathogens through the air, through touch, or through sexual contact. To avoid infection, stay out of range of anyone who's coughing, sniffling, or sneezing, and don't share food or dishes. Carefully wash your dishes, utensils, and hands, and abstain from sex or make self-protective decisions about sexual partners. (See "Sexually Transmitted Diseases" later in this chapter.)

## Food

Every year foodborne illnesses strike millions of Americans, sometimes with fatal consequences. Bacteria account for two-thirds of foodborne infections, and thousands of suspected cases of infection with *Escherichia coli* bacteria in under-cooked or inadequately washed food have been reported.

Every year as many as 4 million Americans have a bout with *Salmonella* bacteria, which have been found in about a third of all poultry sold in the United States. These infections can be serious enough to require hospitalization and can lead to arthritis, neurological problems, and even death. Consumers can greatly reduce the number of salmonella infections by proper handling, cooking, and refrigeration of poultry.

A deadly food disease, *botulism,* is caused by certain bacteria that grow in improperly canned foods. Although its occurrence is rare in commercial products, botulism is a danger in home canning. Another uncommon threat is *trichinosis,* caused by the larvae of a parasitic roundworm in uncooked meat. This infection, which causes nausea, vomiting, diarrhea, fever, thirst, profuse sweating, weakness, and pain, can be avoided by thoroughly cooking meat.

## Water

Waterborne diseases, such as typhoid fever and cholera, are still widespread in less developed areas of the world. They have been rare in the United States, although outbreaks caused by inadequate water purification have occurred.

## The Process of Infection

If someone infected with the flu sits next to you on a bus and coughs or sneezes, tiny viral particles may travel into your nose and mouth. Immediately the virus finds or creates an opening in the wall of a cell, and the process of infection begins. During the **incubation period,** the time between invasion and the first symptom, you're unaware of the pathogen multiplying inside you. In some diseases, incubation may go on for months, even years; for most, it lasts several days or weeks.

The early stage of the battle between your body and the invaders is called the *prodromal period.* As infected cells die, they release chemicals that help block the invasion. Other chemicals, such as *histamines,* cause blood vessels to dilate, thus allowing more blood to reach the battleground. During all of this, you feel mild, generalized symptoms, such as headache, irritability, and discomfort. You're also highly contagious. At the height of the battle—the typical

illness period—you cough, sneeze, sniffle, ache, feel fever-ish, and lose your appetite.

Recovery begins when the body's forces gain the advantage. With time, the body destroys the last of the invaders and heals itself. However, the body is not able to develop long-lasting immunity to certain viruses, such as colds, flu, or HIV.

## How Your Body Protects Itself

Various parts of your body safeguard you against infectious diseases by providing **immunity,** or protection, from these health threats. Your skin, when unbroken, keeps out most potential invaders. Your tears, sweat, skin oils, saliva, and mucus contain chemicals that can kill bacteria. Cilia, the tiny hairs lining your respiratory passages, move mucus, which traps inhaled bacteria, viruses, dust, and foreign matter, to the back of the throat, where it is swallowed; the digestive system then destroys the invaders.

When these protective mechanisms can't keep you infection-free, your body's immune system, which is on con-stant alert for foreign substances that might threaten the body, swings into action. The immune system includes structures of the lymphatic system—the spleen, thymus gland, lymph nodes, and lymph vessels—that help filter impurities from the body. (See Figure 9-1.) More than a dozen different types of white blood cells are concentrated in the organs of the lymphatic system or patrol the entire body by way of the blood and lymph vessels. The two basic types of immune mechanisms are humoral and cell-mediated.

**Humoral immunity** refers to the protection provided by antibodies, proteins derived from white blood cells called *B lymphocytes* or B cells. Humoral immunity is most effective during bacterial or viral infections. An *antigen* is any substance that enters the body and triggers production of an antibody. Once the body produces antibodies against a specific antigen—the mumps virus, for instance—you're protected against that antigen for life. If you're again exposed to mumps, the antibodies previously produced prevent another episode of the disease.

But you don't have to suffer through an illness to acquire immunity. Inoculation with a vaccine containing synthetic or weakened antigens can give you the same pro-tection. The type of long-lasting immunity in which the body makes its own antibodies to a pathogen is called *active immunity.* Immunity produced by the injection of **gamma globulin,** the antibody-containing part of the blood from another person or animal that has developed antibodies to a disease, is called *passive immunity.*

The various types of T cells are responsible for **cell-mediated immunity.** T cells are lymphocytes manufac-tured in the bone marrow and carried to the thymus for

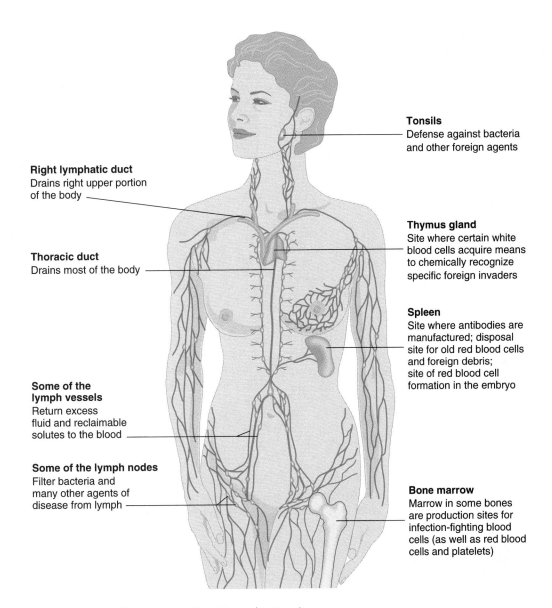

**Tonsils**
Defense against bacteria
and other foreign agents

**Right lymphatic duct**
Drains right upper portion
of the body

**Thoracic duct**
Drains most of the body

**Thymus gland**
Site where certain white
blood cells acquire means
to chemically recognize
specific foreign invaders

**Spleen**
Site where antibodies are
manufactured; disposal
site for old red blood cells
and foreign debris;
site of red blood cell
formation in the embryo

**Some of the
lymph vessels**
Return excess
fluid and reclaimable
solutes to the blood

**Some of the lymph nodes**
Filter bacteria and
many other agents of
disease from lymph

**Bone marrow**
Marrow in some bones
are production sites for
infection-fighting blood
cells (as well as red blood
cells and platelets)

▲ **Figure 9-1** The Human Lymphatic System and Its Functions
The lymphatic system helps filter impurities from the body.

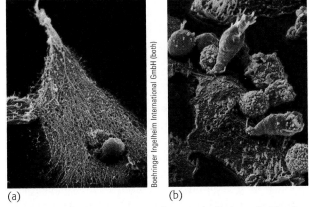

Boehringer Ingelheim International GmbH (both)

(a)                              (b)

▲ Types of lymphocytes. (a) B cell covered with bacteria. The B
cells function in humoral immunity by producing antibodies.
(b) T cells attack a cancer cell. The T cells function in cell-
mediated immunity.

maturation. Cell-mediated immunity mainly protects
against parasites, fungi, cancer cells, and foreign tissue (see
photos at left). Thousands of different T cells work
together to ward off disease. Different T cells have differing
functions, including the activation of other immune cells,
help in antibody-mediated responses, and the suppression
of lymphocyte activity.

## Immune Response

Attacked by pathogens, the body musters its forces and fights.
Sometimes the invasion is handled like a minor border skir-
mish; other times a full-scale battle is waged throughout the
body. Together, the immune cells work like an internal police
force. When an antigen enters the body, the T cells aided by

*macrophages* (large scavenger cells with insatiable appetites for foreign cells, diseased and run-down red blood cells, and other biological debris) engage in combat with the invader. Meanwhile, the B cells churn out antibodies, which rush to the scene and join in the fray. Also busy at surveillance are natural killer cells that, like the elite forces of a SWAT team, seek out and destroy viruses and cancer cells.

The **lymph nodes,** or glands, are small tissue masses in which some protective cells are stored. If pathogens invade your body, many of them are carried to the lymph nodes to be destroyed. This is why your lymph nodes often feel swollen when you have a cold or the flu.

If the microbes establish a foothold, the blood supply to the area increases, bringing oxygen and nutrients to the fighting cells. Tissue fluids, as well as antibacterial and antitoxic proteins, accumulate. You may develop redness, swelling, local warmth, and pain—the signs of **inflammation.** As more tissue is destroyed, a cavity, or **abscess,** forms, and fills with fluid, battling cells, and dead white blood cells (pus). If the invaders aren't killed or inactivated, the pathogens are able to spread into the bloodstream and cause what is known as **systemic disease.** The toxins released by the pathogens cause fever and the infection becomes more dangerous.

## Immunity and Stress

Whenever we confront a crisis, large or small, our bodies produce powerful hormones that provide extra energy. However, this stress response dampens immunity, reducing the number of some key immune cells and the responsiveness of others.

Stress affects the body's immune system in different ways, depending on two factors: the controllability or uncontrollability of the stressor and the mental effort required to cope with the stress. An uncontrollable stressor that lasts longer than 15 minutes may interfere with cytokine interleukin-6, which plays an essential role in activating the immune defenses. Uncontrollable stressors also produce high levels of the hormone cortisol, which suppress immune system functioning. The mental efforts required to cope with high-level stressors produce only brief immune changes that appear to have little consequence for health. However, stress has been shown to slow pro-inflammatory cytokine production, which is essential for wound healing.

## Immunization: The Key to Prevention

One of the great success stories of American medicine has been the development of vaccines that provide protection against many infectious diseases. Immunization has

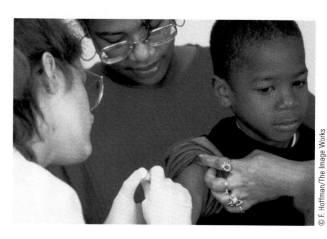

▲ Immunizations are an important protection against childhood diseases. Neighborhood clinics in urban centers offer immunizations to those children at particular risk.

reduced cases of measles, mumps, tetanus, whooping cough, and other life-threatening illnesses by more than 95 percent. Unfortunately, many Americans, including large numbers of children in urban centers and a proportionately high number of African-American youngsters, haven't been properly immunized. About a quarter of children lack complete protection against polio, tetanus, and other illnesses, according to the National Vaccine Advisory Committee. While there has been progress in protecting most American children against diphtheria, whooping cough, tetanus, *Hemophilus influenzae* type B (HIB), polio, and measles, some children are going without the booster shots necessary for complete immunization.[4]

The American Academy of Pediatrics recommends that all children be immunized against hepatitis B, diphtheria, tetanus, whooping cough (pertussis); HIB infection; polio; pneumoccal pneumonia; measles, mumps, German measles (rubella); and chickenpox. Although some vaccines confer lifelong protection, others do not. The protection provided by diphtheria and tetanus vaccinations, for example, diminishes over time, so booster vaccinations are required every ten years.

Table 9-1 shows the recommended immunizations for adults. Health officials also recommend measles booster shots for students entering college, and suggest that people born after 1956 be revaccinated for polio, measles, and other infectious diseases before visiting developing countries. If you're uncertain about your past immunizations, check with family members or your doctor. If you can't find answers, a blood test can show whether you carry antibodies to specific illnesses.

If you're pregnant or planning to get pregnant within the next three months, do not get a measles, mumps, rubella, or oral polio vaccination. If you're allergic to neomycin, consult your doctor before getting a measles, mumps, rubella, or intramuscular polio vaccination. Those with egg allergies should also check with a doctor before

| ▼ Table 9-1 Recommended Immunizations for Adults | | | | | | | | | | | | |
|---|---|---|---|---|---|---|---|---|---|---|---|---|
| Age | 18 | 25 | 30 | 35 | 40 | 45 | 50 | 55 | 60 | 65 | 70 | 75 |
| Hepatitis B | (from age 18–24) | | | | | | | | | | | |
| Influenza | | | | | | | (from age 50 and up) | | | | | |
| Pneumococcus | | | | | | | | | | (from age 65 up) | | |
| Tetanus-Diptheria* | (from age 18 up) | | | | | | | | | | | |

*Get complete TD vaccine series if you have not received primary series; boosters every 10 years or at least at age 50

Source: American Academy of Family Physicians.

getting a measles, mumps, or flu vaccination. Also, never get a vaccination when you have a high fever.

# Infectious Diseases

An estimated 500 microorganisms cause disease; no effective treatment exists for about 200 of these illnesses. Although infections can be unavoidable at times, the more you know about their causes, the more you can do to protect yourself.

## Who Is at Highest Risk of Infectious Diseases?

Like human bullies, the viruses responsible for the most common infectious illnesses tend to pick on those least capable of fighting back. Among the most vulnerable are the following groups:

- **Children and their families.** Youngsters get up to a dozen colds annually; adults average two a year. When a flu epidemic hits a community, about 40 percent of school-age boys and girls get sick, compared with only 5 to 10 percent of adults. But parents get up to six times as many colds as other adults.

- **The elderly.** Statistically, fewer older men and women are likely to catch a cold or flu, yet when they do, they face greater danger than the rest of the population. People over 65 who get the flu have a one in ten chance of being hospitalized for pneumonia or other respiratory problems, and a one in fifty chance of dying from the disease.

- **The chronically ill.** Lifelong diseases, such as diabetes, kidney disease, or sickle-cell anemia, decrease an individual's ability to fend off infections. Individuals taking medications that suppress the immune system, such as steroids, are more vulnerable to infections, as are those with medical conditions that impair immunity, such as infection with HIV.

- **Smokers and those with respiratory problems.** Smokers are a high-risk group for respiratory infections and serious complications, such as pneumonia. Chronic breathing disorders, such as asthma and emphysema, also greatly increase the risk of respiratory infections.

- **Those who live or work in close contact with someone sick.** Health-care workers who treat high-risk patients, nursing home residents, and others living in close quarters—such as students in dormitories—face greater odds of catching others' colds and flus.

- **Residents or workers in poorly ventilated buildings.** Building technology has helped spread certain airborne illnesses, such as tuberculosis, via recirculated air. Indoor air quality can be closely linked with disease transmission in winter, when people spend a great deal of time in tightly sealed rooms.

## Common Cold

There are more than 200 distinct cold viruses, or rhinoviruses. Although in a single season you may develop a temporary immunity to one or two, you may then be hit by a third. Americans come down with 1 billion colds a year. Colds can strike in any season, but different cold viruses are more common at different times of years. Rhinoviruses cause most spring, summer, and early fall colds, and tend to cause more symptoms above the neck (stuffy nose, headache, runny eyes). Adenoviruses, parainfluenza viruses, corona viruses, influenza viruses, and others that strike in the winter are more likely to get into the bronchi and trachea (the breathing passages) and cause more fever and bronchitis.

Cold viruses spread by coughs, sneezes, and touch. Cold-sufferers who sneeze and then touch a doorknob or countertop leave a trail of highly contagious viruses behind them. The best preventive tactics are frequent handwashing, replacing toothbrushes regularly, and avoiding stress overload. High levels of stress increase the risk of becoming infected by respiratory viruses and developing

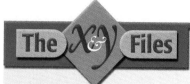

## Gender Differences in Susceptibility

When the flu hits a household, the last one left standing is likely to be Mom. The female immune system responds more vigorously to common infections, offering extra protection against viruses, bacteria, and parasites. But this enhanced immunity doesn't apply to sexually transmitted diseases (STDs). A woman who has unprotected sex with an infected man is more likely to contract an STD than a man who has sex with an infected woman. Symptoms of STDs also tend to be more "silent" in women, so they often go undetected and untreated, leading to potentially serious complications.

The genders also differ in their vulnerability to allergies and **autoimmune disorders.** Although both men and women frequently develop allergies, allergic women are twice as likely to experience potentially fatal anaphylactic shock. A woman's robust immune system also is more likely to overreact and turn on her own organs and tissues. On average, three of four people with autoimmune disorders, such as multiple sclerosis, Hashimoto's thyroiditis, and scleroderma, are women. Of the 8.5 million people in the United States with rheumatoid arthritis, about 6.7 million are women. Another autoimmune disease, lupus, affects nine times as many women as men.

Autoimmune disorders often follow a different course in men and women. Women with multiple sclerosis develop symptoms earlier than men, but the disease tends to progress more quickly and be more severe in men. In lupus, women first show symptoms during their childbearing years, while men develop the illness later in life.

Why are there such large gender differences in susceptibility? Scientists believe that the sex hormones have a great impact on immunity. Through a woman's childbearing years, estrogen, which protects heart, bone, brain, and blood vessels, also bolsters the immune system's response to certain infectious agents. Women produce greater numbers of antibodies when exposed to an antigen; after immunization, they show increased cell-mediated immunity.

In contrast, testosterone may dampen this response—possibly to prevent attacks on sperm cells, which might otherwise be mistaken as alien invaders. When the testes are removed from mice and guinea pigs, their immune systems become more active. Pregnancy dampens a woman's immune response, probably to ensure that her natural protectors don't attack the fetus as a foreign invader. This impact is so great that pregnant women with transplanted kidneys may require lower doses of drugs to prevent organ rejection. Pregnant women with multiple sclerosis and rheumatoid arthritis typically experience decreased symptoms during the nine months of gestation, then return to their prepregnancy state after giving birth. Oral contraceptives also can diminish symptoms of multiple sclerosis and rheumatoid arthritis. Neither pregnancy nor birth control pills has such an impact on lupus.

Other hormones, such as prolactin and growth hormones, may affect autoimmune disease. Women have higher levels of these hormones, which may act directly on immune cells through interactions with receptors on the surface of cells. These hormones also may affect the complex interworkings of the hypothalamus, pituitary, and adrenal glands.

cold symptoms. New research shows that people who feel unable to deal with everyday stresses have an exaggerated immune reaction that may intensify cold or flu symptoms once they've contracted a virus.

Until scientists develop truly effective treatments, experts advise against taking aspirin and acetaminophen (Tylenol), which may suppress the antibodies the body produces to fight cold viruses and increase symptoms such as nasal stuffiness. A better alternative for achiness is ibuprofen (brand names include Motrin, Advil, and Nuprin), which doesn't seem to affect immune response. Children, teenagers, and young adults should never take aspirin for a cold or flu because of the danger of Reye's syndrome, a potentially deadly disorder that can cause convulsions, coma, swelling of the brain, and kidney damage.

The main drawback of antihistamines, the most widely used cold remedy, is drowsiness, which can impair a

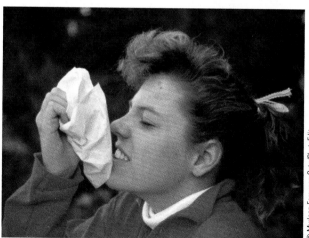

▲ One of the telltale symptoms of a cold is sneezing.

person's ability to safely drive or operate machinery. Another ingredient, pseudoephedrine, can open and drain sinus passages without drowsiness but can speed up heart rate and cause complications for individuals with high blood pressure, diabetes, heart disease, or thyroid disorders. Nasal sprays can clear a stuffy nose, but they invariably cause a rebound effect.

Fluids (especially chicken soup) help, but dairy products contribute to congestion. Mild exercise boosts immunity, but once you're sick, it's better not to work out strenuously. In general, doctors recommend treating specific symptoms—headache, cough, chest congestion, sore throat—rather than taking a multisymptom medication.

For a cough, the ingredient to look for in any suppressant is dextromethrophan, which turns down the brain's cough reflex. In expectorants, the only medicine the FDA has deemed effective is guaifenesin, which helps liquefy secretions so you can bring up mucus from the chest. Unless you're coughing up green or foul yellow mucus (signs of a secondary bacterial infection), antibiotics won't help. They have no effect against viruses and may make your body more resistant to such medications when you develop a bacterial infection in the future.

Many Americans try alternative remedies for colds. One of the most popular herbal remedies is an extract of the echinacea plant, which is widely used in Europe. Although it is not clear how it works, echinacea is believed to increase the number and efficiency of white blood cells, components of the immune system that battle infection. Extensive research has not been done, but some evidence indicates that taking echinacea several times a day at the first sign of sniffles diminishes the symptoms or shortens the duration of an oncoming cold. Most experts recommend only limited use of echinacea, since long-term use can actually suppress the immune system.[5]

Zinc lozenges, another popular alternative treatment in recent years, have not proven to be clearly beneficial. In at least ten studies that have evaluated the benefits of zinc, some have found no benefit, whereas others have found significant reductions in the severity or duration of cold symptoms. Almost all have been criticized for various reasons, such as the size of the sample or the formulation of zinc used. The compound zinc gluconate does seem to have a modest effect in shortening cold symptoms, but zinc acetate has not been shown to have a benefit.[6]

Although sore throats—a frequent cold symptom—are caused by viruses, many people seek treatment with antibiotics, which are effective only against bacteria. An estimated 5 to 17 percent of sore throats in adults are caused by bacteria *(Group A streptococci)*. Yet in one recent survey, primary care physicians prescribed antibiotics for almost three-quarters of patients with sore throats. They were more likely to receive more expensive, broad-spectrum antibiotics rather than the recommended antibiotics for strep (penicillin and erythromycin).[7]

 Colds are common among college students, many of whom do not recognize its signs or respond effectively to its symptoms. In a survey of 425 students at three college campuses in Louisiana and Indiana, 10 percent said they would see a physician for a cold; 41 percent believed that antibiotics were an effective treatment. More students said they would use antibiotics if their symptoms included a fever or discolored nasal discharge.[8]

Your own immune system can do something modern science cannot: cure a cold. All it needs is time, rest, and plenty of fluids. Warmth also is important, because the aptly named "cold" viruses replicate at lower temperatures. Hot soups and drinks (particularly those with a touch of something pungent, like lemon or ginger) raise body temperature and help clear the nose. Even more important is getting off your feet. Taking it easy reduces demands on the body, which helps speed recovery.

## STRATEGIES FOR PREVENTION

### Protecting Yourself from Colds and Flus

▲ Wash your hands frequently with hot water and soap. In a public restroom, use a paper towel to turn off the faucet after you wash your hands, and avoid touching the doorknob.

▲ Wash objects used by someone with a cold.

▲ Take good care of yourself: Make sure you're getting adequate sleep. Eat a balanced diet. Exercise regularly.

▲ Don't share food or drinks.

▲ Spend as little time as possible in crowds, especially in closed places, such as elevators and airplanes. When out, keep your distance from sneezers and coughers.

▲ Don't touch your eyes, mouth, and nose after being with someone who has cold symptoms.

▲ Use tissues rather than cloth handkerchiefs, which may harbor viruses for hours or days.

▲ Try to avoid irritating air pollutants.

▲ Don't smoke, which destroys protective cells in the airways and worsens any cough.

▲ Limit your intake of alcohol, which depresses white blood cells and increases the risk of bacterial pneumonia in flu sufferers.

# Influenza

Although similar to a cold, **influenza**—or the flu—causes more severe symptoms that last longer. Every year an estimated 65 million Americans develop influenza, 30 million seek medical care, 300,000 are hospitalized, and 20,000 die.[9] (See Figure 9-2.)

Flu viruses, transmitted by coughs, sneezes, laughs, and even normal conversation, are extraordinarily contagious, particularly in the first three days of the disease. The usual incubation period is two days, but symptoms can hit hard and fast. Two varieties of viruses—influenza A and influenza B—cause most flus. In recent years, the deadliest flu epidemics have been caused by various forms of influenza A viruses.[10]

A vaccine against the flu is available, but it is not foolproof. "Because the flu virus is constantly changing, you need a new shot every year," explains Edwin Kilbourne, M.D., of New York Medical College, who decides the components of each year's flu vaccine. "And because it takes the body time to manufacture antibodies to the new viruses, you should get a vaccination at least 10 to 14 days before an outbreak hits your area."[11]

Flu shots now are advised for almost everyone. The Center for Infectious Diseases of the CDC recommends a yearly flu shot for people older than age 50, residents of nursing homes and other long-term care facilities, adults and children with chronic illnesses or weakened immune systems, women who will be more than three months pregnant during the flu season, and, when feasible, young, otherwise healthy children between the ages of 6 and 23 months.[12] In older individuals, flu shots may offer significant protection against strokes.[13] The only individuals who should steer clear are those allergic to eggs, since the inactivated flu viruses are grown in chick embryos.

A new alternative to flu shots is an intranasal spray containing a live, attenuated influenza virus (LAIV) vaccine. Researchers have found that the aerosol vaccine significantly reduces flu severity, days lost from work, health-care visits, and the use of over-the-counter medication. The spray represents a particular advantage for children since more than 30 percent of youngsters get the flu, but most don't receive a flu shot. Children who received the vaccine and still got the flu had milder symptoms, were less likely to have a fever, and recovered faster than the children given the placebo.[14]

For those who don't get vaccinated this year, antiviral drugs, such as Relenza (zanamivir) and Tamiflu (oseltamivir), are the next best line of defense.[15] These *neuraminidase inhibitors* are designed to block a protein (neuraminidase) that allows the flu virus to escape from one cell and infect others. A small handheld oral inhaler, used twice a day for five days, delivers Relenza to the surface of the lungs, the primary site of flu infection. Tamiflu, taken twice a day for five days, comes in pill form. These agents act against both influenza A and influenza B viruses and cause few side effects. In research trials, they shortened the duration of flu by up to two days and decreased the likelihood of complications such as bronchitis, sinusitis, and ear infections. However, to be effective treatment with either medication must begin within 36 to 48 hours of the first flu symptom. Although approved only for use as a treatment, antiviral drugs also can prevent flu from spreading through a family, workplace, or school.

# Meningitis

**Meningitis,** or invasive meningococcal disease, attacks the membranes around the brain and spinal cord and can result in hearing loss, kidney failure, and permanent brain damage. An estimated 2,400 to 3,000 cases occur every year; approximately 10 percent are fatal. One of the most common types is caused by the bacterium *Neisseria meningitis,* which is spread through coughing; kissing; sharing drinks, eating utensils, or cigarettes; or prolonged exposure to infected individuals. Viral meningitis is typically less severe.[16]

Most common in the first year of life, the incidence of bacterial meningitis rises in young people between ages 15 and 24.[17] College students are generally not at greater risk, except freshmen living in dormitories (see Table 9-2).

| | |
|---|---|
| Wash hands | 70% |
| Avoid sick people | 52% |
| Get flu shot | 41% |
| Avoid crowds | 24% |

▲ **Figure 9-2**
How Americans Try to Avoid the Flu
Frequent hand washing is the number-one way for most adults. The next most popular technique is avoiding sick people.

Source: Data from Opinion Research Corp. for Kleenex.

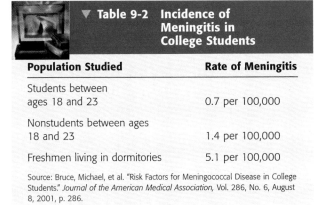

| ▼ Table 9-2 | Incidence of Meningitis in College Students |
|---|---|
| **Population Studied** | **Rate of Meningitis** |
| Students between ages 18 and 23 | 0.7 per 100,000 |
| Nonstudents between ages 18 and 23 | 1.4 per 100,000 |
| Freshmen living in dormitories | 5.1 per 100,000 |

Source: Bruce, Michael, et al. "Risk Factors for Meningococcal Disease in College Students." *Journal of the American Medical Association,* Vol. 286, No. 6, August 8, 2001, p. 286.

In an analysis of data from 50 state health departments and 231 college health centers, CDC researchers found that the risk of meningitis is three times greater for freshmen in dorms than for other college students.[18]

Early symptoms of meningitis include rash, fever, severe headache, nausea, vomiting, and lethargy. A telltale symptom in many, but not all, cases is stiffness of the neck when bending forward. Meningitis progresses rapidly, often in as little time as 12 hours. If untreated, it can lead to permanent hearing loss, brain damage, seizures, or death. If it is caught early and treated with antibiotics, however, it is usually curable.

## Meningitis Vaccination

 The Advisory Committee on Immunization Practices of the CDC and the American Academy of Pediatrics have recommended that all college freshmen be informed that vaccination is effective against 70 percent of the bacterial strains found on campuses. Vaccination could prevent 80 percent or more of cases among undergraduates.[19] Immunization is recommended primarily for freshmen living in dormitories, who make up 4 percent of the total college population but 31 percent of those diagnosed with meningitis.[20] Other factors increasing meningitis risk are smoking and alcohol consumption, especially binge drinking. Smokers, who cough more, and drinkers, who often share glasses, are at higher risk of transmitting and contracting meningitis.[21] Peak incidence for bacterial meningitis is November to March.

Some experts disagree on whether colleges should recommend or require vaccination. According to CDC statistics, only about five deaths as a result of meningitis would be expected annually among the 520,000 freshmen who live in dormitories. By comparison, binge drinking, car accidents, and suicide claim many more lives. Some contend that colleges should devote their limited resources to fighting these threats. Others argue that students should do

everything possible to avoid any potential threat to their health.[22]

At most schools, the cost of vaccination ranges from $50 to $75. Research into the success of meningococcal vaccination programs on college campuses has shown that women are more likely than men to be vaccinated and that vaccination rates for all nonwhite ethnic groups are somewhat lower than rates for whites. Students majoring in science-oriented fields have higher vaccination rates than those majoring in the humanities. More younger students living on campus than older ones get vaccinations, possibly because of greater parental influence or because they see themselves as being at higher risk.[23]

The current vaccine protects against the most common strains for the *N. meningitis* bacterium but does not provide complete protection and remains effective for only about three years. More effective vaccines that confer long-lasting immunity and could be administered with other routine infant immunizations have been developed. Some have been introduced in the United Kingdom and other European countries.[24]

## Hepatitis

An estimated 500,000 Americans contract hepatitis each year. At least five different viruses, referred to as **hepatitis A, B, C, Delta, and E,** can cause this inflammation of the liver. Newly identified viruses also may be responsible for some cases of what is called "non-A, non-B" hepatitis.

All forms of hepatitis target the liver, the body's largest internal organ. Symptoms include headaches, fever, fatigue, stiff or aching joints, nausea, vomiting, and diarrhea. The liver becomes enlarged and tender to the touch; sometimes the yellowish tinge of jaundice develops. Treatment consists of rest, a high-protein diet, and the avoidance of alcohol and drugs that may stress the liver. Alpha interferon, a protein that boosts immunity and prevents viruses from replicating, may be used for some forms.

Most people begin to feel better after two or three weeks of rest, although fatigue and other symptoms can linger. As many as 10 percent of those infected with hepatitis B and up to two-thirds of those with hepatitis C become carriers of the virus for several years or even life. Some have persistent inflammation of the liver, which may cause mild or severe symptoms and increase the risk of liver cancer.

Hepatitis A, a less serious form, is generally transmitted by poor sanitation, primarily fecal contamination of food or water, and is less common in industrialized nations than in developing countries. Among those at highest risk in the United States are children and staff at day-care centers, residents of institutions for the mentally handicapped, sanitation workers, and workers who handle primates such as monkeys. Gamma globulin can provide short-term immunity; vaccines against hepatitis A have been approved by the FDA. The CDC has recommended routine immunization against hepatitis A in 11 Western states with high rates.

Hepatitis B, a potentially fatal disease transmitted through the blood and other bodily fluids, infects an estimated 350,000 people around the world each year. Once spread mainly by contaminated tattoo needles, needles shared by drug users, or transfusions of contaminated blood, hepatitis B is now transmitted mostly through sexual contact. It can cause chronic liver infection, cirrhosis, and liver cancer.

Hepatitis B is a particular threat to young people; 75 percent of new cases are diagnosed in those between ages 15 to 39. They usually contract hepatitis B through high-risk behaviors such as multiple sex partners and use of injected drugs. Individuals who have tattoos or body piercing may also be at risk if procedures are not done under regulated conditions. At highest risk are male homosexuals, heterosexuals with multiple sex partners, health-care workers with frequent contact with blood, injection drug users, and infants born to infected mothers. Vaccination can prevent hepatitis B and is recommended for children, teens, and adults at high risk.

Hepatitis C virus (HCV) is four times as widespread as HIV. However, few of the estimated 3 to 4 million carriers in the U.S. realize they are infected.[25] Without effective prevention strategies, the number of cases is expected to triple in the next decade.[26] Hepatitis C, which can lead to chronic liver disease, cirrhosis, and liver cancer, is the leading reason for liver transplantation in the United States. The CDC estimates that HCV is responsible for 8,000 to 10,000 deaths every year. However, long-term studies have shown that the majority of people infected with HCV do not develop severe liver disease.[27]

## Mononucleosis

You can get **mononucleosis** through kissing—or any other form of close contact. "Mono" is a viral disease that's most common among people 15 to 24 years old; its symptoms include a sore throat, headache, fever, nausea, and prolonged weakness. The spleen is swollen and the lymph nodes are enlarged. You may also develop jaundice or a skin rash similar to German measles.

The major symptoms usually disappear within two to three weeks, but weakness, fatigue, and often depression may linger for at least two more weeks. The greatest danger is from physical activity that might rupture the spleen, resulting in internal bleeding. The liver may also become inflamed. A blood test can determine whether you have mono. However, there's no specific treatment other than rest.[28]

## ???? What Do I Need to Know About Biological Warfare?

Americans have learned firsthand that certain infectious agents can be used as weapons of terrorism and war.[29] Bioterror agents, such as anthrax and, potentially, smallpox or botulism, have been added to the ranks of emerging infectious diseases. Federal and state governments have launched new bioterrorism preparedness programs.

Anthrax, which is found naturally in wild and farm animals, can also be produced in a laboratory. The disease is spread through exposure to anthrax spores, not through exposure to an infected person. Another infectious agent, the smallpox virus, is highly contagious, and could threaten many millions of people because routine inoculations against smallpox stopped in 1972. Those vaccinated before that year may have lost much of their immunity within 10 years. Smallpox was officially eradicated as a disease in 1980, but stores of the virus exist for research purposes. The CDC has developed a response plan, including a large-scale vaccination program, in the event of a smallpox outbreak.[30]

# Reproductive and Urinary Tract Infections

Reproductive and urinary tract infections are very common. Many are not spread exclusively by sexual contact, so they are not classified as sexually transmitted diseases.

## Vaginal Infections

The most common vaginal infections are trichomoniasis, candidiasis, and bacterial vaginosis.

Protozoa (*Trichomonas vaginalis*) that live in the vagina can multiply rapidly, causing itching, burning, and discharge—all symptoms of **trichomoniasis.** Male carriers usually have no symptoms, although some may develop urethritis or an inflammation of the prostate and seminal vesicles. Anyone with this infection should be screened for syphilis, gonorrhea, chlamydia, and HIV. Sexual partners must be treated with oral medication (metronidazole, trade name Flagyl), even if they have no symptoms, to prevent reinfection.

Populations of a yeast called *Candida albicans*—normal inhabitants of the mouth, digestive tract, and vagina—

are usually held in check. Under certain conditions, however (such as poor nutrition, stress, or antibiotic use), the microbes multiply, causing burning, itching, and a whitish discharge, and producing what is commonly known as a yeast infection. Common sites for **candidiasis,** which is also called *moniliasis,* are the vagina, vulva, penis, and mouth. The women most likely to test positive for candidiasis have never been pregnant, use condoms for birth control, have sexual intercourse more than four times a month, and have taken antibiotics in the previous 15 to 30 days. Vaginal medications, such as GyneLotrimin and Monistat, are nonprescription drugs that provide effective treatment. Male sexual partners may be advised to wear condoms during outbreaks of candidiasis. Women should keep the genital area dry and wear cotton underwear.

**Bacterial vaginosis** is characterized by alterations in the microorganisms that live in the vagina, including depletion of certain bacteria and overgrowth of others. It typically causes a white or gray vaginal discharge with a distinctive fishy odor similar to that of trichomoniasis. Its underlying cause is unknown, although it occurs most frequently in women with multiple sex partners. Long-term dangers include pelvic inflammatory disease (PID, discussed later in this chapter) and pregnancy complications. Metronidazole, either in the form of a pill or a vaginal gel, is the primary treatment. According to CDC guidelines, treatment for male sex partners appears to be of little benefit, but some health practitioners recommend treatment for both partners in cases of recurrent infections.

## Urinary Tract Infections

A urinary tract infection (UTI) can be present in any of the three parts of the urinary tract: the urethra, the bladder, or the kidneys. An infection involving the urethra is known as **urethritis.** If the bladder is also infected, it's called **cystitis.** If it reaches the kidneys, it's called **pyelonephritis.**

An estimated 40 percent of women report having had a UTI at some point in their lives. Three times as many women as men develop UTIs, probably for anatomical reasons. A woman's urethra is only 1.5 inches long; a man's is 6 inches. Therefore, bacteria, the major cause of UTIs, have a shorter distance to travel to infect a woman's bladder and kidneys. About one-fourth to one-third of all women between ages 20 and 40 develop UTIs, and 80 percent of those who experience one infection develop recurrences.

Conditions that can set the stage for UTIs include irritation and swelling of the urethra or bladder as a result of pregnancy, bike riding, irritants (such as bubble bath, douches, or a diaphragm), urinary stones, enlargement in men of the prostate gland, vaginitis, and stress. Early diagnosis is critical because infection can spread to the kidneys and, if unchecked, result in kidney failure. Symptoms include frequent burning, painful urination, chills, fever, fatigue, and blood in the urine.

Recurrent UTIs, a frequent problem among young women, have been linked with a genetic predisposition, sexual intercourse, and the use of diaphragms. Postintercourse treatment with antibiotics can lower the risk. Frequent recurrence of symptoms may not be caused by infection but by interstitial cystitis, a little-understood bladder inflammation that afflicts an estimated 450,000 Americans, almost all of them women.

## Sexually Transmitted Diseases

Venereal diseases (from the Latin *venus,* meaning *love* or *lust*) are more accurately called **sexually transmitted diseases (STDs)** or sexually transmitted infections (STIs). Around the world, some 50 million cases of curable STDs occur each year (not including HIV and herpes).[31] Almost 700,000 people are infected every day with one of the over 20 STDs tracked by world health officials. The highest rates of sexually transmitted infections occur among 16- to 24-year-olds, particularly older teenagers.[32] STDs are much more widespread in developing nations because of lack of adequate health standards, prevention practices, and access to treatment.[33]

More Americans are infected with STDs now than at any other time in history. According to the Institute of Medicine, the odds of acquiring an STD during a lifetime are one in four. STDs are among the top ten most frequently reported diseases in the United States, and their annual economic cost is $17 billion. The major cause of preventable sterility in America, STDs have tripled the rate of ectopic (tubal) pregnancies, which can be fatal if not detected early. STD complications, including miscarriage, premature delivery, and uterine infections after delivery, annually affect more than 100,000 women. Moreover, infection with an STD greatly increases the risk of HIV transmission (discussed later in this chapter). The incidence of STDs is highest in young adults and homosexual men. Others affected by STDs include unborn and newborn children who can "catch" potentially life-threatening infections in the womb or during birth.

Although each STD is a distinct disease, all STD pathogens like dark, warm, moist body surfaces, particularly the mucous membranes that line the reproductive organs; they hate light, cold, and dryness. It is possible to catch or have more than one STD at a time. Curing one doesn't necessarily cure another, and treatments don't prevent another bout with the same STD. (See Table 9-3.)

Many STDs, including early HIV infection and gonorrhea in women, may not cause any symptoms. As a result,

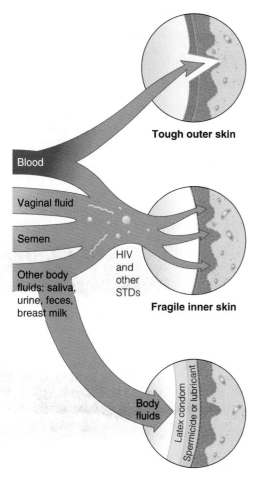

**Tough outer skin** covers the outside of your body, including hands and lips. Viruses and bacteria enter when skin is chapped, or through a hangnail, cut, scrape, sore, or needle puncture.

**Tough outer skin**

Blood

Vaginal fluid

Semen

Other body fluids: saliva, urine, feces, breast milk

HIV and other STDs

**Fragile inner skin** lines the inside of your vagina or penis, anus, and mouth. Viruses and bacteria can enter when skin is torn during sexual contact that involves rubbing, stretching, or not enough lubrication (wetness).

**Fragile inner skin**

Body fluids

Latex condom
Spermicide or lubricant

**Barrier protection** made of latex helps prevent body fluids from entering your body. Latex condoms are recommended for intercourse. Spermicides containing nonoxynol-9 or water-based lubricant help kill many STD microbes. They also reduce friction so latex condoms are less likely to break.

▲ **Figure 9-3** How HIV Infection and Other STDs Are Spread
Most STDs are spread by viruses or bacteria carried in certain body fluids.

infected individuals may continue their usual sexual activity without realizing that they're jeopardizing others' well-being.

## STDs in Adolescents and Young Adults

Nearly two-thirds of the people who acquire STDs in the United States are under age 25. The most common bacterial STD is chlamydia, with two of the highest rates of chlamydia occurring among adolescents in general and among young adult women. Cases of genital herpes among white adolescents have increased five times, and cases among white people in their twenties have doubled over the past few years.

The college years are a prime time for contracting STDs. According to the American College Health Association, chlamydia and HPV have reached epidemic levels at many schools—although many of those infected aren't even aware of it.

In one study of college-age women, cases of human papilloma virus (HPV) infections increased from 26 percent to 43 percent over a three-year period. Contracting STDs may increase the risk of being infected with HIV, and half of new HIV infections occur in people under age 25.[34] Because college students have more opportunities to have different sexual partners and may use drugs and alcohol more often before sex, they are at greater risk. Many college students misjudge the number of people with HIV who live in Africa and who live in the United States.[35] More than half of 13- to 24-year-old women with HIV are infected heterosexually.[36]

Even when high school and college students have generally accurate knowledge about STDs, they don't necessarily practice safe sex. According to research, those students with the greatest number of sexual partners are least likely to use condoms. Other studies have shown that proximity to a high-density AIDS epicenter (such as San Francisco) has no impact on HIV/AIDS knowledge and attitudes, and that religious affiliation does not decrease risky sexual behavior, at least among religious students who are sexually active. While college students admit to engaging in behaviors that put them at risk of HIV and other STDs, they believe that other students do so much more often.[37] (See Student Snapshot: "Perceived and Actual Risky Sexual Behavior" on p. 225.)

According to a survey of 410 students at a public university in the Southeast, students engaged in more unprotected intercourse and oral sex when they were not under the influence of drugs or alcohol—but were more likely to engage in sexual activity with someone they'd just met when drunk or high. However, the undergraduates perceived that the "average" student engaged in risky behaviors more frequently under any circumstance.[38]

Various factors put young people at risk of STDs, including:

✔ **Feelings of invulnerability,** which lead to risk-taking behavior. Even when they are well informed of the risks, adolescents may remain unconvinced that anything bad can or will happen to them.

✔ **Multiple partners.** In surveys of students, a significant minority report having had four or more sexual partners during their lifetime.

▼ **Table 9-3  Common Sexually Transmitted Diseases (STDs):
Mode of Transmission, Symptoms, and Treatment**

| STD | Transmission | Symptoms | Treatment |
|---|---|---|---|
| **Chlamydia** | The *Chlamydia trachomatis* bacterium is transmitted primarily through sexual contact. It can also be spread by fingers from one body site to another. | In women, PID (pelvic inflammatory disease) caused by chlamydia may include disrupted menstrual periods, pelvic pain, elevated temperature, nausea, vomiting, headache, infertility, and ectopic pregnancy. In men, chlamydial infection of the urethra may cause a discharge and burning during urination. Chlamydia-caused epididymitis may produce a sense of heaviness in the affected testicle(s), inflammation of the scrotal skin, and painful swelling at the bottom of the testicle. | Doxycycline, azithromycin, or ofloxacin |
| **Gonorrhea ("clap")** | The *Neisseria gonorrhoeae* bacterium ("gonococcus") is spread through genital, oral-genital, or genital-anal contact. | The most common symptoms in men are a cloudy discharge from the penis and burning sensations during urination. If disease is untreated, complications may include inflammation of scrotal skin and swelling at base of the testicle. In women, some green or yellowish discharge is produced but commonly remains undetected. Later, PID may develop. | Dual therapy of a single dose of ceftriaxone, cefixime, ciprofloxacin, or ofloxacin plus doxycycline for seven days or a single dose of azithromycin |
| **Non-gonococcal urethritis (NGU)** | Primary causes are believed to be the bacteria *Chlamydia trachomatis* and *Ureaplasma urealyticum,* most commonly transmitted through coitus. Some NGU may result from allergic reactions or from *Trichomonas* infection. | Inflammation of the urethral tube. A man has a discharge from the penis and irritation during urination. A woman may have a mild discharge of pus from the vagina but often shows no symptoms. | A single dose of azithromycin or doxycycline for seven days |
| **Syphilis** | The *Treponema pallidum* bacterium ("spirochete") is transmitted from open lesions during genital, oral-genital, or genital-anal contact. | *Primary stage:* A painless chancre appears at the site where the spirochetes entered the body. *Secondary stage:* The chancre disappears and a generalized skin rash develops. *Latent stage:* There may be no visible symptoms. *Tertiary stage:* Heart failure, blindness, mental disturbance, and many other symptoms occur. Death may result. | Benzathine penicillin G, doxycycline, erythromycin, or ceftriaxone |
| **Herpes simplex** | The genital herpes virus (HSV-2) seems to be transmitted primarily by vaginal, anal, or oral-genital intercourse. The oral herpes virus (HSV-1) is transmitted primarily by kissing. | Small, painful red bumps (papules) appear in the genital region (genital herpes) or mouth (oral herpes). The papules become painful blisters that eventually rupture to form wet, open sores. | No known cure. A variety of treatments may reduce symptoms; oral or intravenous acyclovir (Zovirax) promotes healing and suppresses recurrent outbreaks. |
| **Chancroid** | The *Haemophilus ducrevi* bacterium is usually transmitted by sexual interaction. | Small bumps (papules) in genital regions eventually rupture and form painful, soft, crater-like ulcers that emit a foul-smelling discharge. | Single doses of either ceftriaxone or azithromycin, or seven days of erythromycin |
| **Human papilloma virus (HPV) (genital warts)** | The virus is spread primarily through vaginal, anal, or oral-genital sexual interaction. | Hard and yellow-gray on dry skin areas; soft, pinkish-red, and cauliflowerlike on moist areas. | Freezing; application of topical agents like trichloroacetic acid or podofilox; cauterization, surgical removal, or vaporization by carbon dioxide laser |

*(continued)*

▼ **Table 9-3    Common Sexually Transmitted Diseases (STDs):**
**Mode of Transmission, Symptoms, and Treatment (continued)**

| STD | Transmission | Symptoms | Treatment |
|---|---|---|---|
| **Pubic lice ("crabs")** | *Phthirus pubis,* the pubic louse, is spread easily through body contact or through shared clothing or bedding. | Persistent itching. Lice are visible and may often be located in pubic hair or other body hair. | 1% permethrin cream for body areas; 1% Lindane shampoo for hair |
| **Scabies** | *Sarcoptes scabiei* is highly contagious and may be transmitted by close physical contact, sexual and nonsexual. | Small bumps and a red rash that itch intensely, especially at night. | 5% permethrin lotion or cream |
| **Acquired immunodeficiency syndrome (AIDS)** | Blood and semen are the major vehicles for transmitting HIV, which attacks the immune system. It appears to be passed primarily through sexual contact, or needle sharing among injection drug users. | Vary with the type of cancer or opportunistic infections that afflict an infected person. Common symptoms include fevers, night sweats, weight loss, chronic fatigue, swollen lymph nodes, diarrhea and/or bloody stools, atypical bruising or bleeding, skin rashes, headache, chronic cough, and a whitish coating on the tongue or throat. | Commence treatment early after a positive HIV test with a combination of three or more anti-retroviral drugs (HAART) plus other specific treatment(s), if necessary, of opportunistic infections and tumors. |
| **Viral hepatitis** | Hepatitis A seems to be primarily spread via the fecal-oral route, but oral-anal sexual contact is a common mode for sexual transmission. The hepatitis B virus can be transmitted by blood, semen, vaginal secretions, and saliva. Manual, oral, or penile stimulation of the anus are strongly associated with the spread of this virus. | Vary from nonexistent to mild, flulike symptoms to an incapacitating illness characterized by high fever, vomiting, and severe abdominal pain. | No specific therapy for A and B types; treatment generally consists of bed rest and adequate fluid intake. Combination therapy with interferon and ribavarin may be effective for hepatitis C infections. |
| **Bacterial vaginosis** | The most common causative agent, the *Gardnerella vaginalis* bacterium, is sometimes transmitted through coitus. | In women, a fishy- or musty-smelling, thin discharge, like flour paste in consistency and usually gray. Most men are asymptomatic. | Metronidazole (Flagyl) by mouth or intravaginal applications of topical metronidazole gel or clindamycin cream |
| **Candidiasis (yeast infection)** | The *Candida albicans* fungus may accelerate growth when the chemical balance of the vagina is disturbed; it may also be transmitted through sexual interaction. | White, "cheesy" discharge; irritation of vaginal and vulval tissues. | Vaginal suppositories or topical cream, such as clotrimazole and miconazole, or oral fluconazole |
| **Trichomoniasis** | The protozoan parasite *Trichomonas vaginalis* is usually passed through genital sexual contact. | White or yellow vaginal discharge with an unpleasant odor; vulva is sore and irritated. | Metronidazole (Flagyl) for both women and men |

Source: Crooks, Robert L., and Karla Baur. *Our Sexuality,* 8th ed. Pacific Grove, CA: Wadsworth, 2002.

✔ **Failure to use condoms.** Among those who reported having had sexual intercourse in the previous three months, fewer than half reported condom use. Students who'd had four or more sexual partners were significantly less likely to use condoms than those who'd had fewer partners.

✔ **Substance abuse.** Teenagers who drink or use drugs are more likely to engage in sexually risky behaviors, including sex with partners whose health status and history they do not know, and unprotected intercourse.[39]

Although young adulthood is the age of greatest risk for acquiring STDs, the likelihood that men and women will receive information about prevention declines after they graduate from high school. The media, particularly television, is by far the most common source of health information for young men. In a recent survey, about one-third of

## Student Snapshot — Perceived and Actual Risky Sexual Behavior

In a survey of 136 male and 258 female undergraduates, students indicated that they engaged in risky behaviors less frequently than they thought the average student did. The students in the survey ranged in age from 18 to 46 years and attended a public university in the Southeast. For all behaviors, students responded using a 9-point scale:
1 = Never
9 = Everyday

| Type of HIV-risky behavior | Student's personal behavior | Perceived behavior of the "average" student |
|---|---|---|
| **When not drunk or high** | | |
| Genital or anal intercourse without a condom | 3.11 | 4.28 |
| Oral sex | 3.6 | 4.67 |
| Intercourse or oral sex with someone just met | 1.25 | 3.61 |
| **When drunk or high** | | |
| Genital or anal intercourse without a condom | 1.25 | 3.61 |
| Oral sex | 2.14 | 4.5 |
| Intercourse or oral sex with someone just met | 1.32 | 4.18 |

Source: Bon, Rebecca, et al. "Normative Perceptions in Relation to Substance Use and HIV-Risky Sexual Behaviors of College Students." *Journal of Psychology*, Vol. 135, No. 2, March 2001, p. 165.

young adult men said they received no information about AIDS or STDs from any other source.[40] (See also Student Snapshot: "Where Do Young Americans Learn About Relationships and Sexual Health?" in Chapter 7 regarding the Internet as a source of information about STDs.)

 Race and ethnicity also affect risk in the young. Young African-American men, who are more likely to be sexually active and to have more partners than young white men, also have higher STD infection rates. While the chlamydia rate for Hispanics is almost three times that of whites, the rate for blacks is ten times that of whites. The gonorrhea rate for African-American males aged 20 to 24 is 40 times that of whites. Although HIV infection rates have declined for all men, they are falling at a slower rate for African-American men.

Early communication about AIDS and STDs also affects risk later in life. Several studies have shown that discussing sexual risks with parents or counseling by physicians can promote changes in condom use and sexual behavior.[41] Although parents believe that talking to children about sex is important, adolescents say that their parents do not talk to them early enough about sexual issues.

## STRATEGIES FOR CHANGE

### What to Do If You Have an STD

▲ If you suspect that you have an STD, don't feel too embarrassed to get help through a physician's office or a clinic. Treatment relieves discomfort, prevents complications, and halts the spread of the disease.

▲ Following diagnosis, take oral medication (which may be given instead of or in addition to shots) exactly as prescribed.

▲ Try to figure out from whom you got the STD. Be sure to inform that person, who may not be aware of the problem.

▲ If you have an STD, never deceive a prospective partner about it. Tell the truth—simply and clearly. Be sure your partner understands exactly what you have and what the risks are.

## Prevention and Protection

Abstinence is the only guarantee of sexual safety—and an option that more and more young people are choosing. By choosing not to be sexually active with a partner, individuals can safeguard their physical health, their fertility, and their future.

For men and women who are sexually active, a mutually faithful sexual relationship with just one healthy partner is the safest option. For those not in such relationships, safer-sex practices are essential for reducing risks. (See "Safer Sex" in Chapter 7 and Table 8-2 in Chapter 8.) However, no "protection" is 100 percent "safe." For instance, nononxynol-9, the most widely used spermicide in the world, does not protect women from gonorrhea or chlamydia, according to a study of more than 1,200 women being treated for sexually transmitted diseases.[42]

 According to a recent analysis, many factors affect women's decisions about safer sex practices, including race and ethnicity. African-American women were more likely to make contraceptive decisions without the influence of partners and to focus on pregnancy rather than STD prevention. European-American and Hispanic women were more likely to be influenced by their partners in making decisions about safer sex and STD protection. Women who'd had an STD were much more vigilant about using methods to prevent disease and pregnancy.[43] In a survey of 123 sexually experienced African-American undergraduate women, 38 percent reported at least one previous diagnosis of an STD, yet only 24 percent said that they always used condoms. Early age at first intercourse and a greater number of sexual partners increased a woman's likelihood of having an STD.[44]

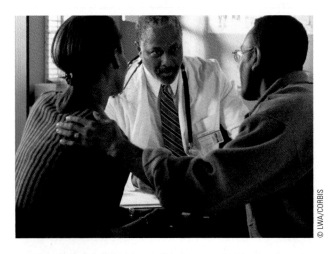

▲ Talking openly about STDs and being tested with your partner will protect your health and foster a sense of trust and commitment.

How can you tell if someone you're dating or hope to date has been exposed to an STD? The bad news is you can't. But the good news is it doesn't matter—as long as you avoid sexual activity that could put you at risk of infection. Ideally, before engaging in any such behavior, both of you should talk about your prior sexual history (including number of partners and sexually transmitted diseases) and other high-risk behavior, such as the use of injection drugs. If you know someone well enough to consider having sex with that person, you should be able to talk about STDs. If the person is unwilling to talk, you shouldn't have sex.

## Chlamydia

The most widespread sexually transmitted bacterium in the United States is *Chlamydia trachomatis,* which causes 3 to 5 million cases of **chlamydia** each year. Chlamydial infections are more common in younger than in older women, in African-American than in white women, and in unmarried than in married pregnant women. They also occur more often in both men and women with gonorrhea.

Those at greatest risk of chlamydial infection are individuals 25 years old or younger who engage in sex with more than one new partner within a two-month period and women who use birth control pills or other nonbarrier contraceptive methods. The U.S. Preventive Services Task Forces recommend regular screening for chlamydia for all sexually active women under age 25 and for older women with multiple sexual partners, a history of STDs, or inconsistent use of condoms.[45]

As many as 75 percent of women and 50 percent of men with chlamydia have no symptoms or symptoms so mild that they don't seek medical attention. Without treatment, up to 40 percent of cases of chlamydia can lead to pelvic inflammatory disease, a serious infection of the woman's fallopian tubes that can also damage the ovaries and uterus. Also, women infected with chlamydia may have three to five times the risk of getting infected with HIV if exposed. Babies exposed to chlamydia in the birth canal during delivery can be born with pneumonia or with an eye infection called conjunctivitis, both of which can be dangerous unless treated early with antibiotics. Symptomless women who are screened and treated for chlamydial infection are almost 60 percent less likely than unscreened women to develop pelvic inflammatory disease.

Traditional methods of screening require a health professional to collect a swab sample of genital secretions. In the past, the sample had to be cultured in a laboratory to look for *C. trachomatis,* and results could take three days or more. Today, a number of tests are available to supplement or sometimes replace the relatively expensive and slow traditional culture. The three major types of nonculture tests are:

✔ Direct fluorescent antibody test (DFA), which uses a scientific method called staining to make chlamydia easier to spot under a microscope. DFA can give quicker results than a culture and can be performed on specimens taken from the eye, cervix, or penis.

✔ Enzyme immunoassays, available in some forms that don't require special lab equipment. Results are more rapid than with culture, and costs can be lower.

✔ Tests to detect the genes of *C. trachomatis* in urine and in genital samples, which can accurately identify even very small numbers of genes in a specimen. While expensive, they are easy to perform and have a high level of accuracy.

According to CDC guidelines, the treatment of choice for uncomplicated chlamydia infections is a seven-day regimen of doxycycline or a single, 1-gram dose of azithromycin (Zithromax). Because chlamydia often occurs along with gonorrhea, some health practitioners prescribe seven days of ofloxacin, a drug effective against both chlamydial and gonorrheal infections. The use of condoms with spermicide can reduce, but not eliminate, the risk of chlamydial infection.[46] Sexual partners should be examined and treated if necessary. The CDC, in its most recent guidelines, recommends that all women with chlamydia be rescreened three to four months after treatment is completed. The reason is that re-infection, which often happens because a patient's sex partners were not treated, increases the risk of pelvic inflammatory disease and other complications.[47]

## Pelvic Inflammatory Disease

Infection of a woman's fallopian tubes or uterus, called **pelvic inflammatory disease (PID),** is not actually an STD, but rather a complication of STDs. About one in every seven women of reproductive age has PID; half of all adult women may have had it. Each year, about 1 million new cases are reported.

Ten to 20 percent of initial episodes of PID lead to scarring and obstruction of the fallopian tubes severe enough to cause infertility. Other long-term complications are ectopic pregnancy and chronic pelvic pain. The risk of these complications rises with subsequent PID episodes, bacterial vaginosis (discussed earlier in this chapter), and use of an IUD. Smoking also may increase the likelihood of PID. Two bacteria—gonococcus (the culprit in gonorrhea) and chlamydia—are responsible for one-half to one-third of all cases of PID. Other organisms are responsible for the remaining cases.

Most cases of PID occur among women under age 25 who are sexually active. Gonococcus-caused cases tend to affect poor women; those caused by chlamydia range across all income levels. One-half to one-third of all cases

are transmitted sexually, and others have been traced to some IUDs that are no longer on the market. Several studies have shown that women with PID are more likely to have used douches than those without the disease. Consistent condom use may decrease PID risk.[48]

PID is a silent disease that, in half of all cases, often produces no noticeable symptoms as it progresses and causes scarring of the fallopian tubes. Experts are encouraging women with mild symptoms, such as abdominal pain or tenderness, to seek medical evaluation, and also encouraging physicians to test these patients for infections. Urine testing is a cost-effective method of detecting gonorrhea and chlamydia in young women and can prevent development of PID. For women with symptoms, magnetic resonance imaging (MRI) is highly accurate in establishing a diagnosis of PID and detecting other diseases that may be responsible for the symptoms.

Women may learn that they have PID only after discovering that they cannot conceive or after they develop an ectopic pregnancy (see Chapter 8). PID causes an estimated 15 to 30 percent of all cases of infertility every year, and about half of all cases of ectopic pregnancy. Most women do not experience any symptoms, but some may develop abdominal pain, tenderness in certain sites during pelvic exams, or vaginal discharge. Treatment may require hospitalization and intensive antibiotics therapy.

## Gonorrhea

**Gonorrhea** (sometimes called "the clap" in street language) is one of the most common STDs in the United States and is increasing in occurrence, reversing a downward trend in the previous two decades.[49] By some estimates, there may be approximately 1 million new cases every year. The incidence is highest among teenagers and young adults. Sexual contact, including oral-genital sex, is the primary means of transmission.

Most men who have gonorrhea know it. Thick, yellow-white pus oozes from the penis and urination causes a burning sensation. These symptoms usually develop two to nine days after the sexual contact that infected them. Men have a good reason to seek help: It hurts too much not to. Women also may experience discharge and burning on urination. However, as many as eight out of ten infected women have no symptoms.

Gonococcus, the bacterium that causes gonorrhea, can live in the vagina, cervix, and fallopian tubes for months, even years, and continue to infect the woman's sexual partners. Approximately 5 percent of sexually active American women have positive gonorrhea cultures but are unaware that they are silent carriers.

If left untreated in men or women, gonorrhea spreads through the urinary-genital tract. In women, the inflammation travels from the vagina and cervix, through

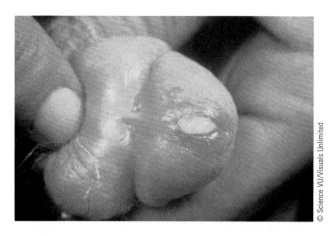

© Science VU/Visuals Unlimited

▲ A cloudy discharge is symptomatic of gonorrhea.

the uterus, to the fallopian tubes and ovaries. The pain and fever are similar to those caused by stomach upset, so a woman may dismiss the symptoms. Eventually these symptoms diminish, even though the disease spreads to the entire pelvis. Pus may ooze from the fallopian tubes or ovaries into the peritoneum (the lining of the abdominal cavity), sometimes causing serious inflammation. However, this, too, can subside in a few weeks. Gonorrhea, the leading cause of sterility in women, can cause PID. In pregnant women, gonorrhea becomes a threat to the newborn. It can infect the infant's external genitals and cause a serious form of conjunctivitis, an inflammation of the eye that may lead to blindness. As a preventive step, newborns may have penicillin dropped into their eyes at birth.

In men, untreated gonorrhea can spread to the prostate gland, testicles, bladder, and kidneys. Among the serious complications are urinary obstruction and sterility caused by blockage of the vas deferens (the excretory duct of the testis). In both sexes, gonorrhea can develop into a serious, even fatal, bloodborne infection that can cause arthritis in the joints, attack the heart muscle and lining, cause meningitis, and attack the skin and other organs.

Although a blood test has been developed for detecting gonorrhea, the tried-and-true method of diagnosis is still a microscopic analysis of cultures from the male's urethra, the female's cervix, and the throat and anus of both sexes.

Because gonorrhea often occurs along with chlamydia, practitioners often prescribe an agent effective against both, such as ofloxacin. In some parts of the United States, gonorrhea has become so resistant to certain antibiotics that they are no longer advised for use in its treatment.[50] Antibiotics taken for other reasons may not affect or cure the gonorrhea because of their dosage or type. And you can't develop immunity to gonorrhea; within days of recovering from one case, you can catch another.

## Nongonococcal Urethritis

The term **nongonococcal urethritis (NGU)** refers to any inflammation of the urethra that is not caused by gonorrhea. NGU is the most common STD in men, accounting for 4 million to 6 million visits to a physician every year. Three microorganisms—*Chlamydia trachomatis, Ureaplasma urealyticum,* and *Mycoplasma genitalium*—are the primary causes; the usual means of transmission is sexual intercourse. Other infectious agents, such as fungi or bacteria, allergic reactions to vaginal secretions, or irritation by soaps or contraceptive foams or gels may also lead to NGU.

In the United States, NGU is more common in men than gonoccocal urethritis. The symptoms in men are similar to those of gonorrhea, including discharge from the penis (usually less than with gonorrhea) and mild burning during urination. Women frequently develop no symptoms or very mild itching, burning during urination, or discharge. Symptoms usually disappear after two or three weeks, but the infection may persist and cause cervicitis or PID in women and, in men, may spread to the prostate, epididymis, or both. Treatment usually consists of doxycycline and should be given to both sexual partners after testing. For men, a single oral dose of azithromycin has proven as effective as a standard seven-day course of doxycycline.

## Syphilis

A corkscrew-shaped, spiral bacterium called *Treponema pallidum* causes **syphilis.** This frail microbe dies in seconds if dried or chilled but grows quickly in the warm, moist tissues of the body, particularly in the mucous membranes of the genital tract. Entering the body through any tiny break in the skin, the germ burrows its way into the bloodstream. Sexual contact, including oral sex or intercourse, is a primary means of transmission. Genital ulcers caused by syphilis may increase the risk of HIV infection, while individuals with HIV may be more likely to develop syphilis.

Public education programs, expanded screening and surveillance, increased tracing of contacts, and condom promotion have helped control the spread of syphilis in some areas. Syphilis rates have fallen to the lowest ever reported in the United States.[51] The decline has been particularly significant in African Americans.

Syphilis has clearly identifiable stages:

✔ **Primary syphilis.** The first sign of syphilis is a lesion, or *chancre* (pronounced "shanker"), an open lump or crater the size of a dime or smaller, teeming with bacteria. The incubation period before its appearance ranges from 10 to 90 days; three to four weeks is average. The chancre appears exactly where the bacteria entered the body: in the mouth, throat, vagina, rectum, or penis. Any contact with the chancre is likely to result in infection.

✔ **Secondary syphilis.** Anywhere from one to twelve months after the chancre's appearance, secondary-stage symptoms may appear. Some people have no symptoms. Others develop a skin rash or a small, flat rash in moist regions on the skin; whitish patches on the mucous membranes of the mouth or throat; temporary baldness; low-grade fever; headache; swollen glands; or large, moist sores around the mouth and genitals. These are loaded with bacteria; contact with them, through kissing or intercourse, may transmit the infection. Symptoms may last for several days or several months. Even without treatment, they eventually disappear as the syphilis microbes go into hiding.

✔ **Latent syphilis.** Although there are no signs or symptoms, no sores or rashes at this stage, the bacteria are invading various organs inside the body, including the heart and brain. For two to four years, there may be recurring infectious and highly contagious lesions of the skin or mucous membranes. However, syphilis loses its infectiousness as it progresses: After the first two years, a person rarely transmits syphilis through intercourse.

After four years, even congenital syphilis is rarely transmitted. Until this stage of the disease, however, a pregnant woman can pass syphilis to her unborn child. If the fetus is infected in its fourth month or earlier, it may be disfigured or even die. If infected late in pregnancy, the child may show no signs of infection for months or years after birth, but may then become disabled with the symptoms of tertiary syphilis.

✔ **Tertiary syphilis.** Ten to twenty years after the beginning of the latent stage, the most serious symptoms of syphilis emerge, generally in the organs in which the bacteria settled during latency. Syphilis that has progressed to this stage has become increasingly rare. Victims of tertiary syphilis may die of a ruptured aorta or of other heart damage, or may have progressive brain or spinal cord damage, eventually leading to blindness, insanity, or paralysis. About a third of those who are not treated during the first three stages of syphilis enter the tertiary stage later in life.

Health experts are urging screening for syphilis for everyone who seeks treatment for an STD, especially adolescents; for everyone using illegal drugs; and for the partners of these two groups. They also recommend that anyone diagnosed with syphilis be screened for other STDs and be counseled about voluntary testing for HIV.

Early diagnosis of syphilis can lead to a complete cure. The most widely used diagnostic techniques are the Venereal Disease Research Laboratory (VDRL) test or the rapid-plasma-reagin (RPR) test. However, these may be positive only during the secondary stage of the disease, when the bacteria have reached the bloodstream. A positive finding always requires additional information, including a physical exam and other laboratory tests, to confirm the diagnosis and plan treatment.

Penicillin is the drug of choice for treating primary, secondary, and latent syphilis. The earlier treatment begins, the more effective it is. Those allergic to penicillin may be treated with doxycycline, ceftriaxone, or erythromycin. An added danger of not getting treatment for syphilis is an increased risk of HIV transmission.

## ???? What Is Herpes?

Herpes (from the Greek word that means *to creep*) collectively describes some of the most common viral infections in humans. Characteristically, **herpes simplex** causes blisters on the skin or mucous membranes. Herpes simplex exists in several varieties. *Herpes simplex virus 1 (HSV-1)* generally causes cold sores and fever blisters around the mouth. *Herpes simplex virus 2 (HSV-2)* may cause blisters on the penis, inside the vagina, on the cervix, in the pubic area, on the buttocks, or on the thighs. With the increase of oral-genital sex, some doctors report finding type 2 herpes lesions in the mouth and throat.

An estimated 135 million Americans age 12 or over carry HSV-1, the most common herpes virus.[52] The prevalence of HSV-2 has increased 30 percent since the late 1970s. According to the CDC, one in five American adolescents and adults is now infected, but 80 to 90 percent of these individuals do not realize they carry the virus because they never develop genital lesions, or they experience only very subtle symptoms. Men and women ages 20 to 29 have higher rates of infection than other age groups.[53]

Recent research with a new, more sensitive test reveals that individuals without any obvious symptoms shed the

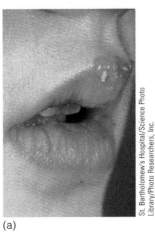
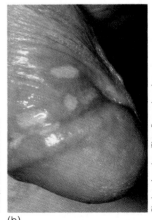

(a)        (b)

St. Bartholomew's Hospital/Science Photo Library/Photo Researchers, Inc.

Biophoto Associates/Photo Researchers, Inc.

▲ (a) Herpes simplex virus (HSV-1) as a mouth sore (b) Herpes simples virus (HSV-2) as a genital sore

virus subclinically, whether or not they have lesions. Most people with herpes contract it from partners who were not aware of any symptoms or of their own contagiousness. Standard methods of diagnosing genital herpes in women, which rely primarily on physical examination and viral cultures, may miss as many as two-thirds of all cases. Newly developed blood tests are more effective in detecting unrecognized and subclinical infections with HSV-2.

A recent study confirmed that people infected with genital herpes can spread it even between flare-ups when they have no symptoms. In the past, patients and most doctors thought people with herpes could safely have unprotected sex when they had no symptoms. Research shows, however, that the herpes virus is present in genital secretions even when patients do not notice any signs of the disease.[54] There is growing evidence that genital herpes promotes the spread of HIV.

HSV transmission occurs through close contact with mucous membranes or abraded skin. Condoms help prevent infection but aren't foolproof. When herpes sores are present, the infected person is highly contagious and should avoid bringing the lesions into contact with someone else's body through touching, sexual interaction, or kissing.

A newborn can be infected with genital herpes while passing through the birth canal, and the frequency of mother-to-infant transmission seems to be increasing. Most infected infants develop typical skin sores, which should be cultured to confirm a herpes diagnosis. Some physicians recommend treatment with acyclovir. Because of the risk of severe damage and possible death, caesarean delivery may be advised for a woman with active herpes lesions.

The virus that causes herpes never entirely goes away; it retreats to nerves near the lower spinal cord, where it remains for the life of the host. Herpes sores can return without warning weeks, months, or even years after their first occurrence, often during menstruation or times of stress, or with sudden changes in body temperature. Of those who experience HSV recurrence, 10 to 35 percent do so frequently—that is, about six or more times a year. In most people, attacks diminish in frequency and severity over time. Herpes, like other STDs, can trigger feelings of shame, guilt, and depression.

Antiviral drugs, such as acyclovir (Zovirax), have proven effective in treating and controlling herpes. Available as an ointment, in capsules, and in injection form, acyclovir relieves the symptoms but doesn't kill the virus. Whereas the ointment works only for the initial bout with herpes, acyclovir in injectable and pill form dramatically reduces the length and severity of herpes outbreaks. Continuing daily oral acyclovir can reduce recurrences by about 80 percent. However, its safety in pregnant women has not been established. Infection with herpes viruses resistant to acyclovir is a growing problem, especially in individuals with immune-suppressing disorders.

Various treatments—compresses made with cold water, skim milk, or warm salt water; ice packs; or a mild anesthetic cream—can relieve discomfort. Herpes sufferers should avoid heat, hot baths, or nylon underwear. In recent years physicians have tried a host of therapies, including topical ointments, various vaccines, exposure to light, and ultrasonic waves—all with little success. Some physicians have used laser therapy to vaporize the lesions. Clinical trials of an experimental vaccine to protect people from herpes infections are underway.[55]

Can stress trigger a flare-up of genital herpes? To test this common assumption, for six months researchers followed 58 women, aged 20 to 44, with a history of herpes; they assessed stress, mood, life changes, and diary reports of herpes recurrences. The researchers found that single stressful events and temporary bad moods were not related to recurrence of the disease, but long-term stresses (lasting more than seven days) were. The more intense the long-term stress, the greater the likelihood of a herpes flare-up.[56]

## Human Papilloma Virus

Infection with **human papilloma virus (HPV),** a pathogen that can cause *genital warts,* is the most common viral STD. By some estimates, 20 million or more women in the United States are infected with HPV, as are three out of four of their male sexual partners. Young women who engage in sexual intercourse at an early age are more likely than those with later sexual debuts to become infected with HPV. Their risk also increases if they have multiple sexual partners or a history of a sexually transmitted disease, use drugs, or have partners with multiple sexual partners.[57]

 College-age women are among those at greatest risk of acquiring HPV infection. In various studies conducted in college health centers, 10 to 46 percent of female students (mean age 20 to 22) had a cervical HPV infection—and increased risk of precancerous cell changes. Risk factors include smoking, use of oral contraceptives, multiple sex partners, anal as well as vaginal intercourse, alcohol consumption at the time of engaging in vaginal intercourse, and sex partners with a history of HPV. Many women erroneously believe they are at low risk for HPV, even if they engage in unprotected sexual activity.

HPV infections in young women tend to be of short duration. In a three-year study, 60 percent of 608 college women became infected with the virus; the average duration of infection was eight months. According to the researchers, many young women who get HPV may not require treatment because the condition often regresses on its own.

HPV is transmitted primarily through vaginal, anal, and oral-genital sex. More than half of HPV-infected individuals do not develop any symptoms. After contact with an infected individual, genital warts may appear from three weeks to eighteen months, with an average period of about three months. The warts are treated by freezing, cauterization, chemicals, or surgical removal. Recurrences are common because the virus remains in the body.

HPV infection may invade the urethra and cause urinary obstruction and bleeding. It greatly increases a woman's risk of developing a precancerous condition called *cervical intraepithelial neoplasia,* which can lead to cervical cancer. There also is a strong association between HPV infections and cancer of the vagina, vulva, urethra, penis, and anus.

HPV may be the single most important risk factor in 95 percent of all cases of cervical cancer. Adolescent girls infected with HPV appear to be particularly vulnerable to developing cervical cancer. It is not known if HPV itself causes cancer or acts in conjunction with cofactors (such as other infections, smoking, or suppressed immunity). HPV transmission may be the reason women are five to eleven times as likely to get cervical cancer if their steady sexual partner has had 20 or more previous partners.

Women who have had an HPV infection should examine their genitals regularly and get an annual Pap smear. However, this standard diagnostic test for cervical cancer doesn't identify HPV infection. A newer, more specific test can recognize HPV soon after it enters the body. Women who test positive should undergo checkups for cervical changes every six to twelve months. If precancerous cells develop, surgery or laser treatment can prevent further growth. Smoking may interact with HPV to increase the risk of cancer.

HPV may also cause genital warts in men and increase the risk of cancer of the penis. HPV-infected men, who may not develop any symptoms, can spread the infection to their partners. People with visible genital warts also may have asymptomatic or subclinical HPV infections that are extremely difficult to treat.

No form of therapy has been shown to completely eradicate HPV, nor has any single treatment been uniformly effective in removing warts or preventing their recurrence. CDC guidelines suggest treatments that focus on the removal of visible warts—cryotherapy (freezing) and topical applications of podofilox, podophyllin, or trichloroacetic acid—and then eradication of the virus. At least 20 to 30 percent of treated individuals experience recurrence. In experimental studies, interferon, a biologic substance produced by virus-infected cells that inhibits viral replication, has proven helpful.

## Chancroid

A **chancroid** is a soft, painful sore or localized infection caused by the bacterium *Haemophilus ducrevi* and usually acquired through sexual contact. Half of the cases heal by themselves. In other cases, the infection may spread to the lymph glands near the chancroid, where large amounts of pus can accumulate and destroy much of the local tissue. The incidence of this STD, widely prevalent in Africa and tropical and semitropical regions, is rapidly increasing in the United States, with outbreaks in several states, including Louisiana, Texas, and New York. Chancroids, which may increase susceptibility to HIV infection, are believed to be a major factor in the heterosexual spread of HIV. This infection is treated with antibiotics (ceftriaxone, azithromycin, or erythromycin) and can be prevented by keeping the genitals clean and washing them with soap and water in case of possible exposure.

## Pubic Lice and Scabies

These infections are sometimes, but not always, transmitted sexually. *Pubic lice* (or "crabs") are usually found in the pubic hair, although they can migrate to any hairy areas of the body. Lice lay eggs called *nits* that attach to the base of the hair shaft. Irritation from the lice may produce intense

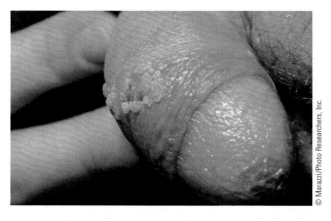

▲ Human papilloma virus, which causes genital warts, is the most common viral STD.

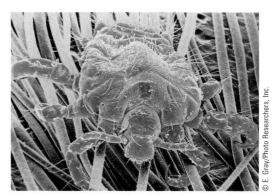

Actual size

▲ A pubic louse, or "crab."

itching. Scratching to relieve the itching can produce sores. *Scabies* is caused by a mite that burrows under the skin, where they lay eggs that hatch and undergo many changes in the course of their life cycle, producing great discomfort, including intense itching.

Lice and scabies are treated with applications of permethrin cream and Lindane shampoo to all the areas of the body where there are concentrations of body hair (genitals, armpits, scalp). You must repeat treatment in seven days to kill any newly developed adults. Wash or dry-clean clothing and bedding.

# HIV

Thirty years ago, no one knew about **human immunodeficiency virus (HIV)**. No one had ever heard of **acquired immune deficiency syndrome (AIDS)**. Once seen as an epidemic affecting primarily gay men and injection drug users, AIDS has taken on a very different form. Today, heterosexuals in developing countries have the highest rates of infection and mortality. And HIV infection continues to spread, doubling at an estimated rate of every ten years. About 40 million people worldwide are infected with HIV; 15,000 more individuals are infected every day.[58]

AIDS has surpassed tuberculosis and malaria as the leading infectious cause of death and has become the fourth-largest killer worldwide. The cumulative death toll for AIDS exceeds 22 million. The region that has been hardest hit is sub-Saharan Africa, the site of seven of every ten of the world's cases of HIV infection and nine of every ten deaths due to AIDS. In the two hardest-hit countries, Zimbabwe and Botswana, one of every four adults is infected, and AIDS has cut the average life expectancy by nearly 20 years.[59] In Asia, the total number of people infected is expanding rapidly, even though the rate of new infection remains relatively low. Russia, China, and India are experiencing dramatic increases in AIDS cases.[60]

In the United States, the CDC estimates that between 800,000 and 900,000 people are living with HIV. The mortality rate for AIDS is declining, but HIV infection rates are increasing in certain groups, including women and racial and ethnic minorities. (See Table 9-4.) Almost two-thirds of new infections occur in blacks and Hispanics, who account for just 24 percent of the population. About 40,000 Americans become infected with HIV every year. HIV infection has continued to climb, but the number of AIDS cases and of deaths has fallen dramatically, thanks to advances in HIVtreatments.[61] However, the rate of decline for both cases and deaths has begun to slow.

There has been progress in lowering the rates of HIV transmission through measures such as reducing the incidence of unprotected intercourse and the number of sex partners, delaying sexual initiation, decreasing the inci-

▼ **Table 9-4  Estimated Annual Rise in New HIV Infections in the United States**

|  | Men | Women |
|---|---|---|
| **Gender** | 70% | 30% |
| **Risk** | | |
| Men who have sex with men | 60% | — |
| Heterosexual sex | 15% | 75% |
| Injection drug use | 25% | 25% |
| **Race** | | |
| Black | 50% | 64% |
| White | 30% | 18% |
| Hispanic | 20% | 18% |

Source: Centers for Disease Control and Prevention.

dence of other STDs, directing injection drug users into drug treatment programs, and reducing needle sharing. Screening the blood supply has reduced the rate of transfusion-associated HIV transmission by 99.9 percent.

Treatment with antiretroviral drugs during pregnancy and birth has reduced transmission by about 90 percent in optimal conditions. Among drug users in some settings, programs that combine addiction treatment and needle exchange reduced the incidence of HIV infection by 30 percent. Even in developing nations, such as Thailand and Uganda, national prevention programs, such as free distribution of condoms and needle-exchange programs, have reduced HIV prevalence by as much as 50 percent.

With the decline in AIDS cases and deaths, there has been an increase in sexually risky behavior.[62] More people at high risk for HIV infection (injection drug users, gay men, heterosexuals diagnosed with STDs) say they are less concerned about HIV/AIDS and more inclined to engage in risky behaviors.[63]

## The Spread of HIV

HIV came to the United States in the late 1970s. Several factors—including frequent sexual activity with multiple, anonymous partners and high-risk sexual practices, such as anal intercourse—may have caused its quick spread through gay communities in the 1980s. As more became known about HIV transmission, many homosexual men adopted safer ways of sexual expression, reduced the number of sexual partners, or entered into monogamous relationships. As a result, the spread of HIV among gay men, especially older men in metropolitan areas, slowed.

In the 1980s, HIV also spread among injection drug users who, by sharing contaminated needles, injected the virus directly into their bloodstream. Injection drug use has been the number-one source of HIV infection in heterosexual men and women in this country. Sex with an infected injection drug user is also a major cause of HIV infection.

The percentage of individuals who acquired HIV through heterosexual contact increased from about 2 percent in 1985 to about 15 percent in 2000. However, many heterosexual adults are not aware of their partners' HIV status and may not see themselves as at risk of HIV infection. According to the CDC, about a third of the HIV-infected individuals in the United States have not been diagnosed.[64]

 Although HIV/AIDS is often seen as a threat to men, 30 percent of new HIV infections in the United States occur among women. About a quarter of Americans living with HIV/AIDS are women. Women of color, particularly African Americans, have been hardest hit. While African-American women make up just 13 percent of the female population of the United States, they account for 63 percent of newly diagnosed cases. HIV/AIDS is most prevalent among women in their childbearing years.[65]

## Reducing the Risk of HIV Transmission

HIV/AIDS can be so frightening that some people have exaggerated its dangers, whereas others understate them. The fact is that although no one is immune to HIV, you can reduce the risk if you abstain from sexual activity, remain in a monogamous relationship with an uninfected partner, and do not inject drugs. If you're not in a long-term monogamous relationship with a partner you're sure is safe, and you're not willing to abstain from sex, there are things you can do to lower your risk of HIV infection. Remember that the risk of HIV transmission depends on sexual behavior, not sexual orientation. Among young men, the prevalence and frequency of sexual risk behaviors are similar regardless of sexual orientation, ethnicity, or age.[66] Homosexual, heterosexual, and bisexual individuals all need to know about the kinds of sexual activity that increase their risk.

Here's what you should know about HIV transmission:

✔ Casual contact does *not* spread HIV infection. You cannot get HIV infection from drinking from a water fountain, contact with a toilet seat, or touching an infected person.[67]

✔ Compared to other viruses, HIV is extremely difficult to get.

✔ HIV can live in blood, semen, vaginal fluids, and breast milk.

✔ Many chemicals, including household bleach, alcohol, and hydrogen peroxide, can inactivate HIV.

✔ In studies of family members sharing dishes, food, clothing, and frequent hugs with people with HIV infection or AIDS, those who have contracted the virus have shared razor blades, toothbrushes, or had other means of blood contact.

✔ You cannot tell visually whether a potential sexual partner has HIV. A blood test is needed to detect the antibodies that the body produces to fight HIV, thus indicating infection.

✔ HIV can be spread in semen and vaginal fluids during a single instance of anal, vaginal, or oral sexual contact between heterosexuals, bisexuals, or homosexuals. The risk increases with the number of sexual encounters with an infected partner.

✔ Teenage girls may be particularly vulnerable to HIV infection because the immature cervix is easily infected.

✔ Anal intercourse is an extremely high-risk behavior because HIV can enter the bloodstream through tiny breaks in the lining of the rectum. HIV transmission is much more likely to occur during unprotected anal intercourse than vaginal intercourse.

✔ Other behaviors that increase the risk of HIV infection include having multiple sexual partners, engaging in sex without condoms or virus-killing spermicides, sexual contact with persons known to be at high risk (for example, prostitutes or injection drug users), and sharing injection equipment for drugs.

✔ Individuals are at greater risk if they have an active sexual infection. Sexually transmitted diseases, such as herpes, gonorrhea, and syphilis, facilitate transmission of HIV during vaginal or rectal intercourse.

✔ No cases of HIV transmission by deep kissing have been reported, but it could happen. Studies have found blood in the saliva of healthy people after kissing; other lab studies have found HIV in saliva. Social (dry) kissing is safe.

✔ Oral sex can lead to HIV transmission. The virus in any semen that enters the mouth could make its way into the bloodstream through tiny nicks or sores in the mouth. A man's risk in performing oral sex on a woman is smaller because an infected woman's genital fluids have much lower concentrations of HIV than does semen.

✔ HIV infection is not widespread among lesbians, although there have been documented cases of possible female-to-female HIV transmission. In each instance, one partner had had sex with a bisexual man or male injection drug user, or had injected drugs herself.

## HIV Infection

HIV infection refers to a spectrum of health problems that results from immunologic abnormalities caused by the virus when it enters the bloodstream. In theory, the body may be able to resist infection by HIV. In reality, in almost all cases, HIV destroys the cell-mediated immune system, particularly the CD4+ T-lymphocytes (also called *T4 helper cells*). The result is greatly increased susceptibility to various cancers and opportunistic infections (infections that take hold because of the reduced effectiveness of the immune system).

Researchers now know that HIV triggers a state of all-out war within the immune system. Almost immediately following infection with HIV, the immune system responds aggressively by manufacturing enormous numbers of CD4+ cells. It eventually is overwhelmed, however, as the viral particles continue to replicate, or multiply. The intense war between HIV and the immune system indicates that the virus itself, not a breakdown in the immune system, is responsible for disease progression.

Shortly after becoming infected with HIV, individuals may experience a few days of flulike symptoms, which most ignore or attribute to other viruses. Some people develop a more severe mononucleosis-type syndrome. After this stage, individuals may not develop any signs or symptoms of disease for a period ranging from weeks to more than 12 years.

HIV symptoms, which tend to increase in severity and number the longer the virus is in the body, may include any of the following:[68]

- Swollen lymph nodes.
- Fever, chills, and night sweats.
- Diarrhea.
- Weight loss.
- Coughing and shortness of breath.
- Persistent tiredness.
- Skin sores.
- Blurred vision and headaches.
- Development of other infections, such as certain kinds of pneumonia.

HIV infection is associated with a variety of HIV-related diseases, including different cancers and dangerous infections. HIV-infected individuals may develop persistent generalized lymphadenopathy, enlargement of the lymph nodes at two or more different sites in the body. This condition typically persists for more than three months without any other illness to explain its occurrence. Diminished mental function may appear before other symptoms. Tests conducted on infected but apparently healthy men have revealed impaired coordination, problems in thinking, or abnormal brain scans.

## HIV Testing

Every year approximately 25 million people in the United States are tested for HIV. About 10,000 facilities provide publicly funded HIV testing and counseling in the United States; approximately 2.6 million tests are performed annually at these sites. Men and women between the ages of 18 and 29 are most likely to report that they've been tested for HIV. The CDC now recommends that all sexually active gay and bisexual men be tested at least once a year for HIV, as well as for chlamydia, syphilis, and gonorrhea.

All HIV tests measure antibodies, cells produced by the body to fight HIV infection. A negative test indicates no exposure to HIV. It can take three to six months for the body to produce the telltale antibodies, however, so a negative result may not be accurate, depending on the timing of the test.

HIV testing can be either confidential or anonymous. In confidential testing, a person's name is recorded along with the test results, which are made available to medical personnel and, in 32 states, the state health department. In anonymous testing, no name is associated with the test results. Anonymous testing is available in 39 states.

 Different groups of individuals at risk prefer different tests. Asian–Pacific Islander and white men who have sex with men are most likely to choose anonymous testing; African-American men who have sex with men are much more likely to choose confidential testing.[69] Consumers must be wary of bogus HIV tests offered via the Internet. (See Savvy Consumer: "Bogus HIV Tests on the Internet.")

The following HIV tests are currently available in the United States:

- **ELISA** (Enzyme-Linked ImmunoSorbent Assay). This is the most commonly used HIV test. A health-care provider draws a blood sample, which is analyzed for antibodies produced to fight against HIV particles. Results are available within a few days to two weeks.
- **Oral HIV tests.** These tests have become available in some doctors' offices and health clinics. A health-care worker swabs a tissue sample from the inside of the mouth. The only oral test approved by the Food and Drug Administration (FDA) is the OraSure.
- **OraQuick Rapid HIV-1 Antibody Test.** This new test approved by the FDA should be available sometime in 2003. OraQuick can be used to detect HIV antibodies in oral mucus and in blood. As its name tells us, the advantage is fast results—in less than an hour.
- **Western blot.** This more accurate and expensive test is used to confirm the results of a positive HIV test.
- **Home Access.** This test—the only home HIV test approved by the FDA—is available in drug stores for $40 to $50. An individual draws a blood sample by pricking a finger and sends it to a laboratory along with a personal identification number. Results are given over the phone by a trained counselor, usually within several days.

Newly developed blood tests can determine how recently a person was infected with HIV and distinguish between long-standing infections and those contracted within the previous four to six months. Health officials recommend HIV testing for the following individuals:

## Savvy Consumer

### Bogus HIV Tests on the Internet

The Internet has been used as a tool for marketing unscientific HIV self-diagnostic tests. The Federal Trade Commission (FTC) has issued a warning that home test kits for HIV that are advertised and sold over the Internet—some of which claim or imply that they are approved by the Food and Drug Administration (FDA) or the World Health Organization—are unreliable. After testing a variety of such kits, the FTC found that in every case, the kits yielded false negatives. In other words, they showed a negative result when they should have shown a positive one. This means that a person who might be infected with HIV would get the false impression that he or she is HIV-negative.

In several court cases, businesspersons have been found guilty of fraud for selling medically useless HIV test kits for home use via the Internet. In one case, the tests were represented as "confidential, safe, accurate, and easy to use," although they lacked any scientific or factual basis. As part of the scheme, the marketer provided bogus test results to purchasers.

The FTC suggests that anyone who has used such a kit be retested for HIV. The only kit approved by the FDA for self-diagnosis is the Home Access Express HIV-1 Test System, which allows a person to collect a blood sample at home and ship it to a laboratory for analysis.

---

- Men who have had sex with other men, regardless of whether they consider themselves homosexual.
- Anyone who uses injection drugs or has shared needles.
- Anyone who has had sex with someone who uses injection drugs or has shared needles.
- Women who have had sex with bisexual men.
- Anyone who has had sex with someone from an area with a high incidence of HIV infection.
- Individuals who have had sex with people they do not know well.
- Anyone who received blood transfusions or blood products between 1978 and 1985, their sexual partners, and, if they are new mothers, their infants.

### AIDS

A diagnosis of AIDS applies to anyone with HIV whose immune system is severely impaired, as indicated by a CD4+ count of less than 200 cells per cubic millimeter of blood, compared to normal CD4+ cell counts in healthy people not infected with HIV of 800 to 1,200 per cubic millimeter of blood. In addition, AIDS is diagnosed in persons with HIV infection who experience recurrent pneumonia, invasive cervical cancer, or pulmonary tuberculosis.

People with AIDS also may experience persistent fever, diarrhea that persists for more than one month, or involuntary weight loss of more than 10 percent of normal body weight. Generalized lymphadenopathy may persist. Neurological disease—including dementia (confusion and impaired thinking) and other problems with thinking, speaking, movement, or sensation—may occur. Secondary infectious diseases that may develop in people with AIDS include *Pneumocystis carinii* pneumonia, tuberculosis, or oral candidiasis (thrush). Secondary cancers associated with HIV infection include Kaposi's sarcoma and cancer of the cervix.

### What Progress Has Been Made in Treating HIV/AIDS?

New forms of therapy have been remarkably effective in boosting levels of protective T cells and reducing *viral load*—the amount of HIV in the bloodstream. People with high viral loads are more likely to progress rapidly to AIDS than people with low levels of the virus.

The current "gold-standard" approach to combating HIV is known as HAART (Highly Active AntiRetroviral Therapies), which dramatically reduces viral load even though it does not eradicate the virus. This complex regimen uses one of 250 different combinations of three or more antiretroviral drugs. Since the development of HAART, the number of deaths among persons with AIDS in the United States has declined substantially, and the number of those living with AIDS has risen. After recent declines, the number of U.S. AIDS cases has remained stable at approximately 10,000 per quarter.[70] An increasing proportion of people living with AIDS in the United States are heterosexual, black or Hispanic, female, and residents of the South.[71]

A year of HAART treatment costs more than $10,000, which is not always covered by health insurance and which has restricted the use of HAART in poor nations. Its success depends on consistent adherence to the drug regimen over a prolonged period of time. However, as many as 30 to 70 percent of patients do not strictly adhere to their schedules.[72] Another drawback is serious side effects, including anemia, mouth ulcers, diarrhea, respiratory difficulties, digestive problems, liver damage, and skin rashes.[73] There also is concern about emerging resistance to some antiretroviral medications.[74] Researchers are continuing to work toward development of more effective and less toxic treatments as well as a vaccine against HIV.[75]

 How large is the threat of emerging or re-emerging infectious diseases?

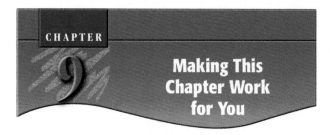

**CHAPTER 9**

## Making This Chapter Work for You

1. Which of the following statements about disease-causing microbes is false?
   a. Helminths cause malaria, one of the major worldwide diseases.
   b. AIDS is caused by a retrovirus.
   c. In the United States, the most common protozoan disease is giardiasis.
   d. Salmonella and botulism are foodborne illnesses caused by bacteria.

2. Which of the following statements about the immune system is false?
   a. The immune system has two types of white blood cells: B cells, which produce antibodies that fight bacteria and viruses, and T cells, which protect against parasites, fungi, and cancer cells.
   b. Immune system structures include the spleen, tonsils, thymus gland, and lymph nodes located throughout the body.
   c. Inoculation with a vaccine confers active immunity.
   d. The effect of stress on the human immune system depends on whether you can control the stressor and on the mental effort required to cope.

3. Adults should receive all of the following immunizations *except*
   a. hepatitis B
   b. influenza

   c. measles
   d. tetanus

4. Which of the following statements about the common cold and influenza is true?
   a. Influenza is just a more severe form of the common cold.
   b. Aspirin should be avoided by children and young adults who have a cold or influenza.
   c. The flu vaccine is also effective against most of the viruses that cause the common cold.
   d. Antibiotics are appropriate treatments for colds but not for influenza.

5. Which of the following statements about specific infectious diseases is false?
   a. Yeast infections can be treated with nonprescription drugs.
   b. Symptoms of UTIs include burning urination, chills, fever, and blood in the urine.
   c. Hepatitis A is usually transmitted through contaminated needles, transfusions, and sexual contact.
   d. College freshmen are at higher risk for contracting meningitis than the general population of young people between the ages of 18 and 23.

6. Sexually transmitted diseases
   a. are the major cause of preventable sterility in the United States.
   b. can result in a severe kidney disease called pylonephritis.
   c. have declined in incidence in developing nations due to improving health standards.
   d. do not increase the risk of being infected with HIV.

7. Bacterial agents cause all of the following STDs except
   a. genital warts
   b. syphilis
   c. chlamydia
   d. gonorrhea

8. Viral agents cause all of the following STDs except
   a. herpes
   b. genital warts
   c. hepatitis B
   d. candidiasis

9. Which of the following statements about HIV transmission is true?
   a. Individuals are not at risk for HIV if they are being treated for chlamydia or gonorrhea.
   b. HIV can be transmitted between lesbians.
   c. Heterosexual men who do not practice safe sex are at less risk for contracting HIV than homosexual men who do practice safe sex.
   d. HIV cannot be spread in a single instance of sexual intercourse.

10. A person with AIDS
    a. has a low viral load and a high number of T4 helper cells.
    b. can no longer pass HIV to a sexual partner.
    c. may suffer from secondary infectious diseases and cancers.
    d. will not respond to treatment.

Answers to these questions can be found on page 415.

## Critical Thinking

1. Before you read this chapter, describe what you did to avoid contracting infectious disease. Now that you have read the chapter, will you be making any changes in your practices? Briefly explain the convenience, advantages, and disadvantages of each practice that you have and/or will be using to prevent infection.

2. The U.S. military and some employers routinely screen personnel for HIV. Some hospitals test patients and note their HIV status on their charts. Some insurance companies test for HIV before selling a policy. Do you believe that an individual has the right to refuse to be tested for HIV? Should a physician be able to order an HIV test without a patient's consent? Can a surgeon refuse to operate on an HIV-infected patient or one who refuses HIV testing? Do patients have the right to know if their doctors, dentists, or nurses are HIV-positive?

3. A man who developed herpes sued his former girlfriend. A woman who became sterile as a result of pelvic inflammatory disease (PID) took her ex-husband to court. A woman who contracted HIV infection from her dentist, who had died of AIDS, filed suit against his estate. Do you think that anyone who knowingly transmits an STD should be held legally responsible? Do you think such an act should be a criminal offense?

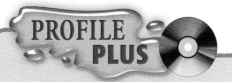

## PROFILE PLUS

Practice self-defense against all forms of infection. Use the following activities from your Profile Plus CD-ROM to assess your risks:

STD Attitude Scale * Self-Quiz on HIV and AIDS

## SITES & BYTES

### Centers for Disease Control and Prevention
**www.cdc.gov**

This comprehensive governmental site sponsored by the U.S. Department of Health and Human Services features information on bioterrorism, travel medicine, infectious diseases, immunization, statistics, and a comprehensive list of health topics.

### Unspeakable: The Naked Truth About STDs
**www.unspeakable.com**

The Risk Profiler on this site can help you determine where your risk of acquiring an STD lies by asking you 13 questions about your age, gender, sexual history, and behavior, and then showing you how these factors play a part in creating your own personal risk profile. In addi-

tion, a 10-question STD Quiz which will test your knowledge of STDs.

### Immunization Action Coalition
**www.immunize.org**

This site features comprehensive vaccination information for children, adolescents, and adults. Vaccine information sheets in English and Spanish are available for measles, rubella, tetanus, hepatitis A & B, influenza, chickenpox, polio, diphtheria, and more.

### InfoTrac College Edition Activity
Bettina M. Beech, Leann Myers, and Derrick J. Beech. "Hepatitis B and C Infections Among Homeless Adolescents." *Family and Community Health*, July 2002, Vol. 25, No. 2, p. 28.

1. Why are homeless adolescents considered to have a higher risk of acquiring hepatitis infections than other adolescents?

2. What are the similarities between hepatitis B and hepatitis C regarding mode of transmission and risk factors?

3. According to the study's results, what are the strongest predictors of positive hepatitis status?

You can find additional readings related to infectious diseases with InfoTrac College Edition, an online library of more than 900 journals and publications. Follow the instructions for accessing InfoTrac that were packaged with your textbook; then search for articles using a keyword search.

For additional links, resources, and suggested readings on InfoTrac, visit our Health & Wellness Resource Center at http://health.wadsworth.com.

## Key Terms

The terms listed here are used within the chapter on the page indicated. Definitions of the terms are in the Glossary at the end of this book.

abscess 214
acquired immune deficiency
  syndrome (AIDS) 232
antibiotics 210
antiviral drug 210
autoimmune disorders 216
bacteria 210
bacterial vaginosis 221
candidiasis 221
cell-mediated immunity 212
chanchroid 231
chlamydia 226

cystitis 221
fungi 210
gamma globulin 212
gonorrhea 227
helminth 211
hepatitis 219
herpes simplex 229
host 210
human immunodeficiency
  virus (HIV) 232
human papilloma virus
  (HPV) 230

humoral immunity 212
immunity 212
incubation period 212
inflammation 214
influenza 218
lymph nodes 214
meningitis 218
mononucleosis 220
nongonococcal urethritis
  (NGU) 228
pathogen 210

pelvic inflammatory disease
  (PID) 227
protozoa 210
pyelonephritis 221
sexually transmitted
  diseases (STDs) 221
syphilis 228
systemic disease 214
trichomoniasis 220
urethritis 221
vector 210
virus 210

## References

1. Centers for Disease Control and Prevention.
2. Centers for Disease Control and Prevention, www.cdc.gov. "West Nile Virus Activity." *Morbidity and Mortality Weekly Report,* Vol. 51, No. 32, August 16, 2002, p. 708.
3. "West Nile Virus Becoming Endemic in the United States." *British Medical Journal,* Vol. 325, No. 7360, August 17, 2002, p. 354.
4. "One More Visit Could Close Demographic Gaps in Infant Immunization Efforts." Media Release, National Center for HIV, STD, and TB Prevention, Office of Communication, April 20, 2001.
5. "Cold-Fighting Echinacea." *Psychology Today,* March 2000, p. 40.
6. Kirchner, Jeffrey. "A Final Look at Oral Zinc for the Common Cold." *American Family Physician,* Vol. 63, No. 9, May 1, 2001, p. 1851.
7. Linder, Jeffrey, and Randall Stafford. "Antibiotic Treatment of Adults with Sore Throat by Community Primary Care Physicians." *Journal of the American Medical Association,* Vol. 286, No. 10, September 12, 2001, p. 1181.
8. Zoorob, Roger, et al. "Use and Perceptions of Antibiotics for Upper Respiratory Infections Among College Students." *Journal of Family Practice,* Vol. 50, No. 1, January 2001, p. 32.
9. "WHO Plans New Fight Against Flu." *Medical Letter on the CDC & FDA,* August 26, 2001.
10. "Flu Season 2000–01." Centers for Disease Control and Prevention, Division of Media Relations, June 22, 2000.
11. Kilbourne, Edwin. Personal Interview.
12. "Prevention and Control of Influenza, Recommendations of the Advisory Committee on Immunization Practices (ACIP)." *Morbidity and Mortality Weekly Report,* Vol. 51, No. RR-3, April 12, 2002, p. 1.
13. Stephenson, Joan. "Flu Shots for Stroke Prevention?" *Journal of the American Medical Association,* Vol. 287, No. 10, March 13, 2002, p. 1255.
14. Luce, Bryan, et al. "Cost-Effectiveness Analysis of an Intranasal Influenza Vaccine for the Prevention of Influenza in Healthy Children." *Pediatrics,* Vol. 108, No. 2, August 2001, p. 456.
15. "Flu Drugs (Antiviral)." Centers for Disease Control and Prevention, Division of Media Relations, June 22, 2000.
16. Myers, Frank. "Meningitis: The Fears, the Facts." *RN,* Vol. 63, No. 11, November 2000.
17. Harrison, Lee, and Margaret Pass. "Invasive Meningococcal Disease in Adolescents and Young Adults." *Journal of the American Medical Association,* Vol. 286, No. 6, August 8, 2001.
18. Bruce, Michael, et al. "Risk Factors for Meningococcal Disease in College Students." *Journal of the American Medical Association,* Vol. 286, No. 6, August 8, 2001, p. 286.
19. "Parents Urged to Learn About Campus Meningitis Risk." *TB & Outbreaks Week,* September 17, 2002, p. 15.
20. Wenger, Jay. "Toward Control of Meningococcal Disease: Reducing Risk in College Students." *Journal of the American Medical Association,* Vol. 286, No. 6, August 8, 2001.
21. Brody, Jane. "Lowering the Risk of Bacterial Meningitis." *New York Times,* September 4, 2001, p. D8.
22. Nice, Ruth. "Meningitis, Life and Death, and Why We Do What We Do." *Journal of American College Health,* Vol. 50, No. 6, May 2002, p. 313.
23. Paneth, Nigel, et al. "Predictors of Vaccination Rates During a Mass Meningococcal Vaccination Program on a College Campus." *Journal of American College Health,* Vol. 49, No. 1, July 2000.

24. Wenger, "Toward Control of Meningococcal Disease."

25. "Hepatitis C Fact Sheet." www.cdc.gov/hepatitis.

26. Dougherty, Augustine, and Heyward Dreher. "Hepatitis C: Current Treatment Strategies for an Emerging Epidemic." *MedSurg Nursing,* Vol. 10, No. 1, February 2001, p. 9.

27. Bren, Linda. "Hepatitis C." *FDA Consumer,* Vol. 35, No. 4, July 2001, p. 24.

28. Riccio, Nina. "When Mono Strikes." *Current Health 2,* Vol. 26, No. 7, March 2000, p. 16.

29. Perkins, Bradley, et al. "Bioterrorism-Related Anthrax: Public Health in the Time of Bioterrorism." *Emerging Infectious Diseases,* Vol. 8, No. 10, October 2002, p. 1015.

30. Centers for Disease Control and Prevention. "Smallpox Response Plan and Guidelines." September 23, 2002, www.bt.cdc.gov/agent/ smallpox/response-plan/index.asp.

31. Panchaud, Christine, et al. "Sexually Transmitted Diseases Among Adolescents in Developed Countries." *Family Planning Perspectives,* Vol. 32, No. 1, January 2000.

32. Catchpole, Mike. "Sexually Transmitted Infections: Control Strategies." *British Medical Journal,* Vol. 322, No. 7295, May 12, 2001, p. 1135.

33. Celentano, David, et al. "Preventive Intervention to Reduce Sexually Transmitted Infections." *Archives of Internal Medicine,* Vol. 160, No. 4, February 28, 2000.

34. Stephenson, Joan. "Youth Ignorance of HIV/AIDS." *Journal of the American Medical Association,* Vol. 288, No. 6, August 14, 2002, p. 689.

35. Dowd, Timothy. "College Students Perceptions of the HIV Epidemic." Presentation, American Psychological Society, New Orleans, July 2002.

36. Bon, Rebecca, et al. "Normative Perceptions in Relation to Substance Use and HIV-Risky Sexual Behaviors of College Students." *Journal of Psychology,* Vol. 135, No. 2, March 2001, p. 165.

37. Buunk, Bram, et al. "The Double-Edge Sword of Providing Information About Safer Sex." *Journal of Applied Social Psychology,* Vol. 32, No. 4, April 2002, p. 684.

38. Bon et al., "Normative Perceptions."

39. O'Connor, M. L. "Social Factors Play Major Role in Making Young People Sexual Risk-Takers." *Family Planning Perspectives,* Vol. 32, No. 1, January 2000.

40. Bradner, Carolyn, et al. "Older, But Not Wiser: How Men Get Information about AIDS and Sexually Transmitted Diseases After High School." *Family Planning Perspectives,* Vol. 32, No. 1, January 2000.

41. "Counseling Can Help Correct Misconceptions About Sexually Transmitted Diseases." *Medical Letter on the CDC & FDA,* October 8, 2000.

42. "Nonoxynol-9 Found Ineffective Against STDs." *Contemporary OB/GYN,* Vol. 47, No. 7, July, 2002, p. 33.

43. Wyatt, Gail. "Factors Affecting HIV Contraceptive Decision-Making Among Women." *Sex Roles: A Journal of Research,* April 2000.

44. Lewis, Lisa, et al. "Factors Influencing Condom Use and STD Acquisition Among African-American College Women." *Journal of American College Health,* Vol. 49, No. 1, July 2000.

45. "Chlamydia Screening for Young Women." *American Journal of Preventive Medicine,* Vol. 20, April 2001, p. 90.

46. Roddy, Ronald, et al. "Effect of Nonoxynol-9 Gel on Urogenital Gonorrhea and Chlamydial Infection." *Journal of the American Medical Association,* Vol. 287, No. 9, March 6, 2002, p. 1117.

47. Centers for Disease Control and Prevention. "New CDC Treatment Guidelines Critical to Preventing Health Consequences of Sexually Transmitted Diseases." May 9, 2002.

48. Ross, Jonathan. "Pelvic Inflammatory Disease." *British Medical Journal,* Vol. 322, No. 7287, March 17, 2001, p. 658.

49. Altman, Lawrence. "Rates of Gonorrhea Rise After a Long Decline." *New York Times,* December 6, 2000.

50. "CDC Issues New STD Screening, Treatment Guidelines." *Clinical Infectious Diseases,* Vol. 35, No. 1, July 1, 2002, p. i.

51. Mitka, Mike. "U.S. Effort to Eliminate Syphilis Moving Forward." *Journal of the American Medical Association,* Vol. 283, No. 12, March 22/29, 2000.

52. "Taming Herpes." Mayo Clinic Women's HealthSource, September 2001.

53. Armstrong, Gregory, et al. "Herpes." *American Journal of Epidemiology,* Vol. 153, May 2001, p. 912.

54. Wald, Ann, et al. "Reactivation of Genital Herpes Simplex Virus Type 2 Infection in Asymptomatic Seropositive Persons." *New England Journal of Medicine,* Vol. 343, No. 12, March 23, 2000.

55. Drake, Susan, et al. "Improving the Care of Patients with Genital Herpes." *British Medical Journal,* Vol. 321, No. 7261, September 9, 2000.

56. Cohen, Frances. "Persistent Stress As a Predictor of Genital Herpes Recurrence." *Archives of Internal Medicine,* Vol. 282, No. 11, March 15, 2000.

57. Rosenberg, J. "Age at First Sex and Human Papillomavirus Infection Linked Through Behavioral Factors and Partner's Traits." *Perspectives on Sexual and Reproductive Health,* Vol. 34, No. 3, May–June 2002, p. 171.

58. "Update: AIDS—United States, 2000." *Journal of the American Medical Association,* Vol. 288, No. 6, August 14, 2002, p. 691.

59. "The 20th Year of AIDS: A Time to Re-energize Prevention." *Morbidity and Mortality Weekly Report,* Vol. 50, No. 21, June 1, 2001, p. 444.

60. Stephenson, Joan. "At International HIV/AIDS Conference, Daunting Challenges Mixed with Hope." *Journal of the American Medical Association,* Vol. 288, No. 6, August 14, 2002.

61. "HIV and AIDS—United States, 1981–2000." *Morbidity and Mortality Weekly Report,* Vol. 50, No. 21, June 1, 2001, p. 444.

62. "The 20th Year of AIDS: A Time to Re-energize Prevention."

63. Scheer, Susan, et al. "Effects of Highly Active Antiretroviral Therapy on Diagnosis of Sexually Transmitted Disease in People with AIDS." *Lancet,* Vol. 357, No. 9254, February 10, 2001, p. 432.

64. Klevens, R. Monina, et al. "Many Heterosexuals Unaware of their HIV Risk." *American Journal of Preventive Medicine,* April 2001.

65. "Women and HIV/AIDS Fact Sheet." Menlo Park, CA: Henry J. Kaiser Family Foundation, May 2001.

66. Rotheram-Borus, Mary Jane, et al. "HIV Risk Among Homosexual, Bisexual, and Heterosexual Male and Female Youths." *Archives of Sexual Behavior,* Vol. 28, No. 2, April 1999.

67. Stevens, Lisa. "HIV Infection: The Basics." *Journal of the American Medical Association,* Vol. 288, No. 2, July 10, 2002, p. 268.

68. Ibid.

69. Centers for Disease Control and Prevention. "Anonymous or Confidential HIV Counseling and Voluntary Testing in Federally Funded Testing Sites." *Journal of the American Medical Association,* Vol. 282, No. 4, July 28, 1999.

70. "Number of U.S. AIDS Cases Remains Stable After Recent Declines." Office of Communications, National Center for HIV, STD, and TB Prevention, Centers for Disease Control and Prevention, July 7, 2002.

71. "Update: AIDS—United States, 2000."

72. Murphy, Debra, et al. "Barriers to Antiretroviral Adherence Among HIV-Infected Adults." *AIDS Patient Care and STDs,* Vol. 14, No. 1, 2000, p. 47.

73. Barreiro, P., et al. "Risks and Benefits of Replacing Protease Inhibitors by Nevirapine in HIV-infected Subjects Under Long-Term Successful Triple Combination Therapy." *AIDS 2000,* No. 4, p. 807.

74. Trachtenberg, Joel, and Merle Sande. "Emerging Resistance to Nonnucleoside Reverse Transcriptase Inhibitors: A Warning and a Challenge." *Journal of the American Medical Association,* Vol. 288, No. 2, July 10, 2002, p. 239.

75. Baltimore, David. "Steering a Course to an AIDS Vaccine." *Science,* Vol. 296, June 28, 2002, p. 2297.

# Lowering Your Risk
# of Major Diseases

**W**hether or not you will get a serious disease at some time in your life may seem to be a matter of odds. Genetic tendencies, environmental factors, and luck affect your chances of having to face many health threats. However, you do have some control over such risks, and even if a major illness may be inevitable, you can often prevent or delay it for years, even decades.

Cardiovascular disease—the term for all disorders of the heart and blood vessels—is an excellent example. Although cardiovascular disease—the term for all disorders of the heart and blood vessels—remains the nation's top killer, death rates have dropped by 60 percent since 1950. Much of the credit goes to lifestyle changes, such as quitting smoking and making dietary changes that lower blood pressure and cholesterol levels. Overall cancer death rates in the United States also are coming down. Some experts predict that within 20 years, cancer deaths could be cut an additional 25 percent.

Start protecting your health now. People mistakenly think of heart disease, cancer, and other disorders as illnesses of middle and old age. But, the events leading up to these diseases often begin in childhood, develop in adolescence, and become a health threat to men in their thirties and forties and to women in their forties and fifties. This chapter provides the information about the risk factors, silent dangers, and medical advances that can improve your chances of a healthier, longer life.

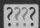

# How the Heart Works

The heart is a hollow, muscular organ with four chambers that serve as two pumps (see Figure 10-1). It is about the size of a clenched fist. Each pump consists of a pair of chambers formed of muscles. The upper two—each called an **atrium**—receive blood, which then flows through valves into the lower two chambers, the **ventricles,** which contract to pump blood out into the arteries through a second set of valves. A thick wall divides the right side of the heart from the left side; even though the two sides are separated, they contract at almost the same time. Contraction of the ventricles is called **systole;** the period of relaxation between contractions is called **diastole.** The heart valves, located at the entrance and exit of the ventricular chambers, have flaps that open and close to allow blood to flow through the chambers of the heart.

The *myocardium* (heart muscle) consists of branching fibers that enable the heart to contract or beat between 60 and 80 times per minute, or about 100,000 times a day. With each beat, the heart pumps about 2 ounces of blood. This may not sound like much, but it adds up to nearly 5 quarts of blood pumped by the heart in one minute, or about 75 gallons per hour.

The heart is surrounded by the *pericardium,* which consists of two layers of a tough membrane. The space between the two contains a lubricating fluid that allows the heart muscle to move freely. The *endocardium* is a smooth membrane lining the inside of the heart and its valves.

Blood circulates through the body by means of the pumping action of the heart, as shown in Figure 10-2. The right ventricle (on your own right side) pumps blood, via the *pulmonary arteries,* to the lungs, where it picks up oxygen (a gas essential to the body's cells) and gives off carbon dioxide (a waste product of metabolism). The blood returns from the lungs via the *pulmonary veins* to the left side of the heart, which pumps it, via the **aorta,** to the arteries in the rest of the body.

The arteries divide into smaller and smaller branches, and finally into **capillaries,** the smallest blood vessels of all (only slightly larger in diameter than a single red blood cell). The blood within the capillaries supplies oxygen and nutrients to the cells of the tissues, and takes up vari-

ous waste products. Blood returns to the heart via the veins: The blood from the upper body (except the lungs) drains into the heart through the *superior vena cava,* while blood from the lower body returns via the *inferior vena cava.*

The workings of this remarkable pump affect your entire body. If the flow of blood to or through the heart or to the rest of the body is reduced, or if a disturbance occurs in the small bundle of highly specialized cells in the heart that generate electrical impulses to control heartbeats, the result may at first be too subtle to notice. However, without diagnosis and treatment, these changes could develop into a life-threatening problem.

Perhaps the biggest breakthrough in the field of cardiology has been not a test or a treatment, but a realization: Heart disease is not inevitable. We can keep our hearts healthy for as long as we live, but the process of doing so must start early and continue throughout life.

# Preventing Heart Problems

Risk factors related to lifestyle—smoking, physical inactivity, a high-fat diet, raised blood pressure—account for at least three in every four new cases of cardiovascular disease.[1] The best way to protect your heart is by making positive changes in your lifestyle, such as not smoking, exercising, controlling your weight, and limiting fat in your diet.[2]

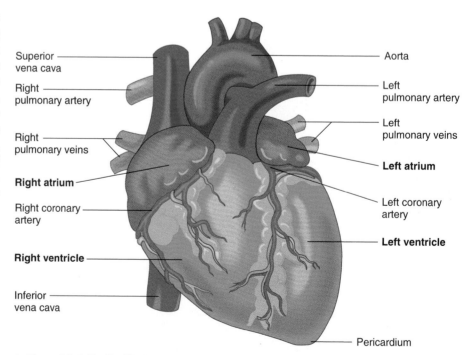

▲ **Figure 10-1** The Healthy Heart
The heart muscle is nourished by blood from the coronary arteries, which arise from the aorta. The pericardium is the outer covering of the heart.

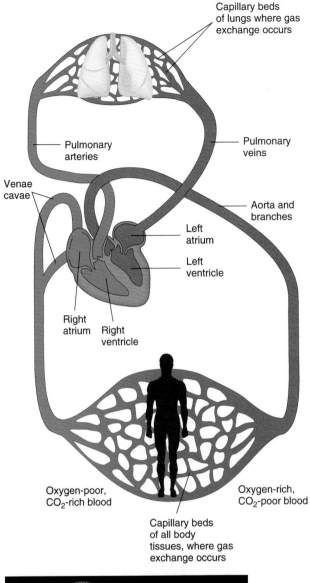

Capillary beds of lungs where gas exchange occurs

Pulmonary arteries

Pulmonary veins

Venae cavae

Aorta and branches

Left atrium

Left ventricle

Right atrium

Right ventricle

Oxygen-poor, $CO_2$-rich blood

Oxygen-rich, $CO_2$-poor blood

Capillary beds of all body tissues, where gas exchange occurs

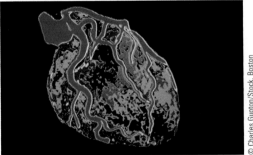

© Charles Gupton/Stock, Boston

▲ **Figure 10-2** The Path of Blood Flow
Blood is pumped from the right ventricle into the pulmonary arteries, which lead to the lungs, where gas exchange (oxygen for carbon dioxide) occurs. Oxygenated blood returning from the lungs drains into the left atrium and is then pumped into the left ventricle, which sends the blood into the aorta and its branches. The oxygenated blood flows through the arteries, which extend to all parts of the body. Again, gas exchange occurs in the body tissues; this time oxygen is "dropped off" and carbon dioxide "picked up." The photo depicts a computer-enhanced image of a healthy heart.

# Physical Activity

For years we've known that regular exercise reduces the risk of heart attack, helps maintain a healthy body weight, lowers blood pressure, and improves metabolism. If rigorous and frequent enough, it also may increase longevity. But you don't have to head to a gym or hit the bike path to keep your heart healthy. As recent studies have confirmed, lifestyle activities, such as walking, housecleaning, and gardening, are as effective as a structured exercise program in improving heart function, lowering blood pressure, and maintaining or losing weight.[3] (See Chapter 4 for a complete discussion of physical activity.)

The federal government recommends that adults try to get 60 minutes of moderate-intensity physical activity every day of the week.[4] While moderate exercise is beneficial, vigorous exercise is more clearly associated with longer life. In a study that followed Harvard alumni for several decades, those who participated in activities such as jogging and swimming lived, on average, a year and a half longer than those who engaged in less intense activities.[5]

## ???? What Kind of Diet Is Best for a Healthy Heart?

A balanced, low-fat diet is the best recipe for a healthy heart. Fruits and vegetables, in particular, are associated with a reduced risk of cardiovascular disease, including lower blood pressure.[6] Saturated fat is the number-one dietary villain in the development of heart disease. However, debate continues over the role of other foods and nutrients in threatening or protecting our hearts. Among the heart-healthy foods are fruits, vegetables, whole grain cereals, fish and fish oils, unsalted nuts, soy products, low-fat dairy products, and alcohol (in moderate amounts).[7]

Fish, as confirmed in several large studies, improves cardiovascular health in several ways. Eating fish instead of red meat reduces the amount of saturated fat in the diet. The omega-3 fatty acids in fish may prevent erratic heart rhythms, a common cause of sudden cardiac death. Fish oils also keep blood clots from forming by making platelets less sticky and less likely to clump, just as aspirin does. They may also improve blood vessel function and ease inflammation, a recently identified threat to the heart. People who regularly eat fish may also tend to do other healthy things, such as exercise, not smoke, or eat more fruits and vegetables. The American Heart Association recommends eating fish twice a week. Walnuts, soybeans, flaxseeds, and oils made from all three also provide omega-3 fatty acids.[8]

## Risk Factors for Cardiovascular Disease

Many people don't realize that they're at risk of heart disease; one-quarter of heart attack victims have no prior symptoms.[9] The best way of identifying individuals in potential danger is by looking for risk factors. About 35 percent of adults over age 25 have no elevated risk factors and can be categorized as low risk. Roughly 40 percent with one or more elevated risk factors are at intermediate risk. They should undergo regular testing by a physician. Approximately 25 percent of adults have multiple risk factors, some form of heart disease, or type 2 diabetes. They are considered at high risk and should work with their physicians on specific strategies to protect their hearts.

### ???? Why Should I Worry About Heart Disease?

Although many people think of it as a threat to older individuals, heart disease is the third leading cause of death among adults aged 25 to 44. Many behaviors that endanger a heart's health begin in adolescence and early adulthood, including tobacco use, high-fat diets, sedentary lifestyles, and high stress.

 Even college students who indicate that they're aware of cardiovascular risks often behave in ways that do not reflect their knowledge. In one recent study of 226 students at a New Jersey college, half or more ate a high-fat diet or reported moderate to severe stress. Many did not exercise frequently; some already had high cholesterol or high blood pressure.[10] (See Student Snapshot: "Heart Disease Risk Factors on Campus.")

### Risk Factors You Can Control

The choices individuals make and the habits they follow can have a significant impact on whether or not their hearts remain healthy. You can choose to avoid the following potential risks for the sake of your heart's health.

---

## Student Snapshot ❯ Heart Disease Risk Factors on Campus

| Risk Factor | Percentages of Students* |
|---|---|
| Moderate to extreme stress | 54 |
| Diet high in saturated fat | 52 |
| Diet with high cholesterol or high blood pressure | 50 |
| Exercise fewer than two times a week | 36 |
| Undesirable total cholesterol levels | 29 |
| Current smoker | 14 |
| High diastolic blood pressure | 11 |
| High systolic blood pressure | 10 |
| High cholesterol | 10 |

*Percentages are based on a study of 226 college students, ages 18 to 26.
Source: Data from Spencer, Leslie. "Results of a Heart Disease Risk-Factor Screening Among Traditional College Students." *Journal of American College Health,* Vol. 50, No. 6, p. 291, May 2002.

## Physical Inactivity

Most Americans get too little physical activity. About one-quarter of U.S. adults are sedentary and another third are not active enough to reach a healthy level of fitness. People who are not even somewhat physically active face a much greater risk of fatal heart attack than those who engage in some form of exercise or activity. Women who are active have lower coronary heart disease rates than those who are inactive. According to a recent study, even walking for a minimum of half an hour a day reduces women's risk of coronary heart disease.[11] However, in men, more rigorous exercise produced greater protection against heart disease. Those who ran for an hour or more per week reduced their risk of heart disease by 42 percent, compared with an 18 percent reduction for those who walked briskly for a half-hour per day or more. With walking, pace, not duration, was linked with lower danger of heart disease.[12]

## Tobacco Smoke

Each year smoking causes more than 250,000 deaths from cardiovascular disease—far more than it causes from cancer and lung disease. Smokers who have heart attacks are more likely to die from them than are nonsmokers. Smoking is the major risk factor for *peripheral vascular disease,* in which the vessels that carry blood to the leg and arm muscles become hardened and clogged.

Cigar smoking causes a moderate, but significant increase in an individual's risk for coronary artery disease, as well as for cancers of the upper digestive tract and chronic obstructive pulmonary disease. Men who smoke five or more cigars per day have the highest risk, compared with those who do not smoke cigars at all.[13]

Both active and passive smoking accelerate the process by which arteries become clogged and increase the risk of heart attacks and strokes. The American Heart Association estimates that 37,000 to 40,000 nonsmokers die each year from cardiovascular diseases as a result of exposure to environmental tobacco smoke. Overall, nonsmokers exposed to environmental tobacco smoke are at a 25 percent higher relative risk of developing coronary heart disease than nonsmokers not exposed to environmental tobacco smoke.

Cigarette smoking and secondhand smoke can damage the heart in several ways:

✔ The nicotine may repeatedly overstimulate the heart.
✔ Carbon monoxide may take the place of some of the oxygen in the blood, which reduces the oxygen supply to the heart muscle.
✔ Tars and other smoke residues may damage the lining of the coronary arteries, making it easier for cholesterol to build up and narrow the passageways.
✔ Smoking increases blood clotting, leading to a higher incidence of clotting in the coronary arteries and subsequent heart attack. Clotting in the peripheral arter-

ies is also increased, which can cause leg pain with walking and, ultimately, stroke.
✔ Even ex-smokers may have irreversible damage to their arteries.

## High Blood Pressure (Hypertension)

Blood pressure is a result of the contractions of the heart muscle, which pumps blood through your body, and the resistance of the walls of the vessels through which the blood flows. Each time your heart beats, your blood pressure goes up and down within a certain range. It's highest when the heart contracts; this is called *systolic blood pressure.* It's lowest between contractions; this is called *diastolic blood pressure.* A blood pressure reading consists of the systolic measurement "over" the diastolic measurement, recorded in millimeters of mercury (mmHg) by a sphygmomanometer (see Figure 10-3).

High blood pressure, or **hypertension,** occurs when the artery walls become constricted so that the force exerted as the blood flows through them is greater than it should be. Physicians see blood pressure as a continuum: the higher the reading, the greater the risk of stroke and heart disease. (See the discussion of high blood pressure later in this chapter.)

As a result of the increased work in pumping blood, the heart muscle of a person with hypertension can become stronger and also stiffer. This stiffness increases resistance to filling up with blood between beats, which can cause shortness of breath with exertion. Hypertension can also act on the kidney arteries, which can lead to kidney failure in some cases. In addition, hypertension accelerates the development of plaque buildup within the arteries. Especially when combined with obesity, smoking, high cholesterol levels, or diabetes, hypertension increases the risks of cardiovascular problems several times. However, you can control high blood pressure through diet, exercise, and medication (if necessary).

## Blood Fats

**Cholesterol** is a fatty substance found in certain foods and also manufactured by the body. The measurement of cholesterol in the blood is one of the most reliable indicators of the formation of plaque, the sludgelike substance that builds up on the inner walls of arteries. You can lower blood cholesterol levels by cutting back on high-fat foods and exercising more, thereby reducing the risk of a heart attack. According to the National Heart, Lung, and Blood Institute (NHLBI), for every 1 percent drop in blood cholesterol, studies show a 2 percent decrease in the likelihood of a heart attack.[14]

**Lipoproteins** are compounds in the blood that are made up of proteins and fat. The different types are classified by their size or density. The heaviest are *high-density lipoproteins,* or HDLs, which have the highest portion of protein. These "good guys," as some cardiologists refer to them, pick up excess cholesterol in the blood and carry it

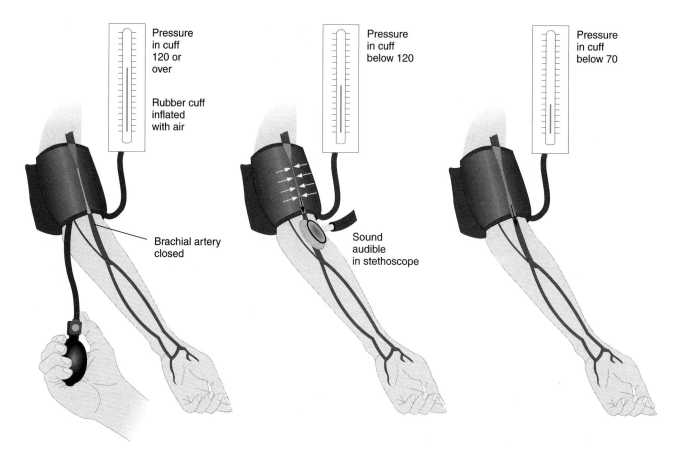

1. The cuff of the sphygmomanometer (blood pressure cuff) is wrapped snugly around the arm just above the elbow and inflated until the blood flow into the brachial artery is stopped. This stoppage is detected with a stethoscope.

2. The cuff is gradually loosened while the examiner listens carefully for pulse sounds with the stethoscope. The pressure reading as the first soft tapping sounds are heard (as a small amount of blood spurts through the constricted artery) is the systolic pressure.

3. As the cuff is loosened still farther, the pulse sounds become louder and more distinct. When the artery is no longer constricted and blood flows freely, however, the pulse sounds can no longer be heard. The reading at which the sounds disappear is recorded as the diastolic pressure.

▲ **Figure 10-3** Measurement of Blood Pressure
The three steps in measuring the blood pressure in a young, healthy individual, with a result of 120/70 (120 systolic, 70 diastolic).

back to the liver for removal from the body. An HDL level of 40 mg/dL or lower substantially increases the risk of heart disease. (Cholesterol levels are measured in milligrams of cholesterol per deciliter of blood—mg/dL.) The average HDL for men is about 45 mg/dL; for women, it is about 55 mg/dL. *Low-density lipoproteins*, or LDLs, and very low-density lipoproteins (VLDLs) carry more cholesterol than HDLs and deposit it on the walls of arteries—they're the "bad guys." The higher your LDL cholesterol, the greater your risk for heart disease. If you are at high risk of heart disease, any level of LDL higher than 100 mg/dL may increase your danger. (See "Your Lipoprotein Profile" later in this chapter.)

**Triglycerides** are fats that flow through the blood after meals and have been linked to increased risk of coronary artery disease, especially in women. Triglyceride levels tend to be highest in those whose diets are high in calories, sugar, alcohol, and refined starches. High levels of these fats may increase the risk of obesity, and cutting back on these foods can reduce high triglyceride levels.

## Metabolic Syndrome

**Metabolic syndrome,** also known as Syndrome X or insulin-resistant syndrome, is a cluster of medical abnormalities that increases the risk of heart disease and diabetes. Genetics, lack of exercise, and overeating are its probable causes. According to the National Institutes of Health, three or more of the following symptoms indicate metabolic syndrome:

✓ Waist measurement of 40 inches or more in men and 35 inches or more in women. (In one recent study, waist circumference proved the best indicator of increased heart risk.)[15]
✓ Levels of triglycerides of 150 mg/dL or more.
✓ Levels of high-density lipoprotein—"good" cholesterol—of less than 40 mg/dL in men or 50 mg/dL in women.
✓ Blood pressure of 130 mm/Hg systole over 85 mmHg diastole (130/85), or higher.
✓ Fasting blood sugar of 110 mg/dL or higher.[16]

## Diabetes Mellitus

**Diabetes mellitus,** a disorder of the endocrine system, increases the likelihood of hypertension and atherosclerosis, thereby increasing the risk of heart attack and stroke.[17] A physician can detect diabetes and prescribe a diet, exercise program, and, if necessary, medication to keep it in check. Even before developing diabetes, individuals at high risk for this disease—those who are overweight, have a family history of the disease, have mildly elevated blood pressure and blood sugar levels, and above-ideal levels of harmful blood fats—may already be at increased risk of heart disease. Up to one-half of diabetics also have hypertension, another risk factor. Diabetics who develop heart disease are more likely to die if they suffer a heart attack or develop heart failure.[18] Two-thirds of people with diabetes die from cardiovascular disease.[19]

## Weight

According to the NHLBI, losing weight at any age can help reduce the risk of heart problems. For women, obesity is as great a cause of death and disability from heart disease as smoking and heavy drinking. Even mild to moderately obese women are more likely to suffer chest pain or a heart attack than thinner women. Weight loss significantly reduces high blood pressure, another risk factor for heart disease. (See Chapter 6 for a discussion of weight control.)

## Psychosocial Factors

How we respond to everyday sources of stress can affect our hearts as well as our overall health. While we may not be able to control the sources of stress, we can change how we habitually respond to it. Various psychological and social influences may affect vulnerability to heart disease. The most widely studied are Type A traits, particularly anger and hostility, depression and anxiety, work characteristics, and social supports. These factors may act alone or combine and exert different effects at different ages and stages of life. They may influence behaviors such as smoking, diet, alcohol consumption, and physical activity, and they also may directly cause changes in physiology.

Although Type A behavior—especially anger—has long been linked with heart disease, a recent review of all prospective studies of its effects found no increased risk for Type A patients with coronary heart disease. However, women who bottle up their anger may be more likely to have a heart attack by age 60 than other women. According to a ten-year study of 200 women, those who conceal their anger or are concerned about their public appearance may have rising heart rates, elevated stress hormones, and high blood pressure—all associated with thickening of the carotid arteries.

Depression itself can be a risk factor for heart disease. Individuals who become depressed after a heart attack are significantly more likely to die or suffer a subsequent heart attack. Regardless of whether it's mild or severe, depression decreases the ability to function on a daily basis by amplifying heart disease symptoms and reducing patients' interest in daily activities. Research from the University of Michigan School of Public Health shows a link between feelings of hopelessness—a sense of futility and negative expectations for the future—and the development of hypertension.[20]

Some psychological factors take a long-term toll. In a 20-year study of more than 2,000 Californians, women who were depressed and felt socially alienated and men who felt inadequate in their jobs were more likely than their peers to develop high blood pressure decades later. In women, much of the association between psychosocial factors and high blood pressure was the result of unhealthy lifestyle habits, such as smoking, obesity, and a sedentary lifestyle.[21]

Job stress also can be hard on the heart, particularly for employees who have little control over their work. A lack of social supports also seems to increase risk, possibly because intimate, caring relationships may buffer the effect of other stressors in life.

# Risk Factors You Can't Control

## Heredity

Anyone whose parents, siblings, or other close relatives suffered heart attacks before age 50 is at increased risk of developing heart disease. Certain risk factors, such as abnormally high blood levels of lipids, can be passed down from generation to generation. Although you can't rewrite your family history, individuals with an inherited vulnerability to cardiovascular disease can lower the danger by changing the risk factors within their control. Your heart's health depends to a great extent on your behavior, including the decisions you make about the foods you eat or the decision not to smoke. As an added preventive step, cardiologists may prescribe a small daily dose of aspirin to individuals with a history of coronary artery disease who are at risk of forming clots that could block blood supplies to the heart, brain, and other organs. (Note: Daily aspirin is not advised for individuals who are not at risk because of their age or health history.)

## Race and Ethnicity

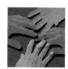 African Americans are twice as likely to develop high blood pressure as whites. African Americans also suffer strokes at an earlier age and of greater severity. Poverty may be an unrecognized risk factor for members of this minority group, who are less likely to receive medical treatments or undergo corrective surgery. Family history, lifestyle, diet, and stress may also play a role, starting early in life. However, researchers have found no single explanation for why African-American youngsters, like their parents, tend to have higher blood pressure than white children.

## Age

Almost four out of five people who die of a heart attack are over age 65. Heart disease accounts for more than 40 percent of deaths among people between 65 and 74, and almost 60 percent at age 85 and above. However, the risk factors that are likely to cause heart disease later in life, including high blood pressure and high levels of "bad" cholesterol, may begin to develop in childhood. Nevertheless, although cardiovascular function declines with age, heart disease is not an inevitable consequence of aging. Many 80- and 90-year-olds have strong, healthy hearts.

## Gender

Men have a higher incidence of cardiovascular problems than women, particularly before age 40. The incidence of coronary artery disease in women remains lower than in men until the sixth and seventh decades of life, but heart disease often takes a greater toll on women.[22] The major risk factors for heart disease in women are diabetes and menopause; intermediate risk factors are hypertension, smoking, and abnormal blood fats (lipids); and relatively minor risk factors are sedentary lifestyle, obesity, age, and family history.[23]

The heart attack rate for women increased by 36 percent during the 1980s and 1990s, a time when heart attacks among men were declining by 8 percent, according to a Mayo Clinic study.[24] Women report poorer physical and psychological functioning than men immediately after hospital treatment and for a year following a heart attack.

Heart disease is the fourth leading cause of death among women aged 30 to 34, third among women aged 35 to 39, second among women aged 40 to 64, and first among women over age 65. Although heart disease causes greater disability in women, it is routinely treated less aggressively than in men.[25]

Researchers long believed that postmenopausal hormone replacement therapy (HRT) protected women from heart disease. However, recent studies have shown this not to be true. A major long-term study, the Women's Health Initiative, has shown that women on HRT actually have an increased risk of heart attack and stroke.[26] (See The X & Y Files: "Gender Differences in Disease" on p. 267.)

## Male Pattern Baldness

**Male pattern baldness** (the loss of hair at the vertex, or top, of the head) is associated with increased risk of heart attack in men under age 55. A study of 1,437 men showed a "modest" increased risk for those men who'd lost hair at the top of their heads but not for those with receding hairlines. The speed at which men lose their hair also may be an indicator of risk. Scientists speculate that men with male pattern baldness who lose their hair quickly may metabolize male sex hormones differently than others, thereby increasing the likelihood of heart disease.[27] Although it's premature to say that baldness is definitely bad news for the heart, health experts advise bald men to follow basic guidelines, such as not smoking and controlling their cholesterol levels, to lower any possible risk.

# Your Lipoprotein Profile

Medical science has changed the way it views and targets the blood fats that endanger the healthy heart. In the past, the focus was primarily on total cholesterol in the blood. The higher this number was, the greater the risk of heart disease. In 2001, the NHLBI's National Cholesterol Education Program revised federal guidelines and recommended more comprehensive testing, called a *lipoprotein profile,* for all individuals age 20 or older.[28] (See Savvy Consumer: "What You Need to Know About Testing Lipoproteins.")

This blood test, which should be performed after a 9- to 12-hour fast and repeated at least once every five years, provides readings of:

✔ Total cholesterol.
✔ LDL (bad) cholesterol, the main culprit in the buildup of plaque within the arteries.
✔ HDL (good) cholesterol, which helps prevent cholesterol buildup.
✔ Triglycerides, which are blood fats released into the bloodstream after a meal.

## *Savvy Consumer*

### What You Need to Know About Testing Lipoproteins

- Go to your primary health-care provider to get a lipoprotein profile. Although cholesterol tests at shopping malls or health fairs can help identify people at risk, the analyzers are often not certified technicians, and the readings may occasionally be inaccurate. In addition, without a health expert to counsel them, some people may be unnecessarily frightened by a high reading—or falsely reassured by a low one.

- Ask about accuracy. Even at first-rate laboratories, cholesterol readings are often inaccurate. Find out if the lab is using the National Institutes of Health standards, and ask about the lab's margin for error (which should be less than 5 percent).

- Fast beforehand. Lipoprotein tests are most accurate after a 9- to 14-hour fast. Schedule the test before breakfast if you can. Women may not want to get tested at the end of their menstrual cycles, when minor elevations in cholesterol levels occur because of lower estrogen levels. Cholesterol levels can also rise 5 to 10 percent during periods of stress. Reschedule the test if you come down with an intestinal flu because the viral infection could interfere with the absorption of food and thus with cholesterol levels. Let your doctor know if you're taking any drugs. Common medications, including birth control pills and hypertension drugs, can affect cholesterol levels.

- Sit down before allowing blood to be drawn or your finger to be pricked; fluids pool differently in the body when you're standing than when you're sitting. Don't let a technician squeeze blood from your finger, which forces fluid from cells, diluting the blood sample and possibly leading to a falsely low reading.

- Get real numbers. Don't settle for "normal" or "high" because laboratories can inaccurately label results. Find out exactly what your reading is. Find out your HDL/ LDL ratio, and HDL and LDL levels.

- Some physicians advise getting two tests in the same month and averaging the result. A person's cholesterol levels vary so much from day to day that a single measurement may not be significant.

### What Is a Healthy Cholesterol Reading?

The answer to this question has become more complex. In general, a total cholesterol reading of less than 200 mg/dL is considered healthy. However, one single cholesterol count no longer applies to everyone. (See Table 10-1.)

The greatest threat to your heart's health is LDL cholesterol. The degree of danger of a higher reading depends, not just on the number itself, but on whether or not you have other risk factors for heart disease. These include age (over 45 in men, over 55 in women), smoking, high blood pressure, high blood sugar, diabetes, abdominal obesity ("belly" fat), and a family history of heart disease. Depending on your individual risk, your doctor may recommend lifestyle changes or medications that lower cholesterol.

An optimal LDL reading of less than 100 mg/dL should be the goal of those at highest risk of heart disease. Those at moderate risk should keep their LDL level under 130 mg/dL; those at low risk should keep their LDL level at or below 160 mg/dL.[29]

HDL, good cholesterol, also is important, particularly in women. Federal guidelines define an HDL reading of less than 40 mg/dL as a major risk factor for developing heart disease. HDL levels of 60 mg/dL or more are protective and lower the risk of heart disease.

A lipoprotein profile also measures triglycerides, the free-floating molecules that transport fats in the bloodstream. Ideally this should be below 150 mg/dL. Individuals with readings of 150 to 199 mg/dL, considered borderline, as well as those with higher readings, may benefit from weight control, physical activity, and, if necessary, medication.

The National Heart, Lung, and Blood Institute (NHLBI) has developed an easy-to-use interactive website that weighs your risk factors, assesses your lipoprotein profile, and calculates how likely you are to have a heart attack in the next ten years. You can perform these calculations by clicking on www.nhlbi.nih.gov. Some doctors may recommend additional tests, such as measurements of homocysteine (hs-CRP) or of the size and density of cholesterol particles. In general, small, dense particles of LDL cholesterol seem more dangerous.

## ▼ Table 10-1 What Do Your Cholesterol Numbers Mean?*

| Total Cholesterol Level | Category |
|---|---|
| Less than 200 mg/dL | Desirable |
| 200–238 mg/dL | Borderline high |
| 240 mg/dL and above | High |

| LDL ("Bad") Cholesterol | Category |
|---|---|
| Less than 100 mg/dL | Optimal |
| 100–129 mg/dL | Near optimal/above optimal |
| 130–159 mg/dL | Borderline high |
| 160–189 mg/dL | High |
| 190 mg/dL and above | Very high |

**HDL ("Good") Cholesterol**

For HDL, higher numbers are better. A level less than 40 mg/dL is considered a major risk factor because it increases your risk for developing heart disease. An HDL level of 60 mg/dL or more helps lower your risk for heart disease.

**Triglycerides**

Triglycerides can also raise heart disease risk. Levels that are borderline high (150–199 mg/dL) or high (200 mg/dL or more) may need treatment in some people.

*Cholesterol levels are measured in milligrams (mg) of cholesterol per deciliter (dL) of blood.
Source: "High Blood Cholesterol: What You Need to Know." National Cholesterol Education Program, 2001.

## Lowering Cholesterol

According to federal guidelines, about one in five Americans may require treatment to lower their cholesterol level and the risk of dying from heart disease.[30] The National Cholesterol Education Program (NCEP) estimates that some 36 million Americans should be watching their diet and exercising more. Another 65 million should be taking cholesterol-lowering drugs. Depending on your lipoprotein profile and an assessment of other risk factors, your physician may recommend that you take steps to lower your LDL cholesterol. For some people, therapeutic life changes can make a difference. Simply eating more often may have an effect on cholesterol. According to several small studies, "grazers" who eat small meals six or more times a day tend to have lower cholesterol levels than "gorgers" who eat three times a day.[31]

## The Silent Killers

The two most common forms of cardiovascular disease in this country are high blood pressure (hypertension) and coronary artery disease, the gradual narrowing of the blood vessels of the heart. Often these two problems go together.

## High Blood Pressure

Hypertension forces the heart to pump harder than is healthy. Because the heart must force blood into arteries that are offering increased resistance to blood flow, the left side of the heart often becomes enlarged. The term *essential hypertension* indicates that the cause is unknown, as is usually the case. Occasionally, abnormalities of the kidneys or the blood vessels feeding them, or certain substances in the bloodstream, are identified as the culprits. Whatever its cause, hypertension is dangerous because excessive pressure can wear out arteries, leading to serious cardiovascular diseases, vision problems, and kidney disease. (See Figure 10-4.)

About 50 million Americans—one in four adults—have high blood pressure that requires monitoring or treatment. (See Table 10-2.) Hypertension has become increasingly common among people in their twenties and thirties. High blood pressure is more prevalent among southerners than among people of other regions of the same age and gender.[32] The absolute risk of heart disease related to elevated blood pressure varies in different geographic locations.[33] Physicians urge all adults to have their blood pressure checked at least once a year.

A blood pressure reading that's slightly above normal isn't necessarily proof of a blood pressure problem. Due to nervousness, blood pressure may shoot up when anxious individuals enter a medical office, causing what's known as *white coat hypertension*. Other factors, such as warm weather or variations in how health-care practitioners do the test, also can cause elevated readings. It can help to take blood pressure readings at home and compare them with your physician's readings. (Equipment for measuring blood pressure is sold at most pharmacies.)

### ????  What Is a Healthy Blood Pressure?

Ideal blood pressure is 120/80 mmHg (120 systolic pressure, 80 diastolic pressure). Hypertension is diagnosed when blood pressure rises above 140/90 mmHg. (See Table 10-3.) In the past, physicians relied mainly on the diastolic read-

## ▼ Table 10-2 Heart Disease Deaths Per 100,000 People

| | Men | Women |
|---|---|---|
| **African American** | 841 | 553 |
| **White** | 666 | 388 |
| **Native American** | 465 | 259 |
| **Hispanic** | 432 | 265 |
| **Asian** | 372 | 221 |

Source: Centers for Disease Control and Prevention.

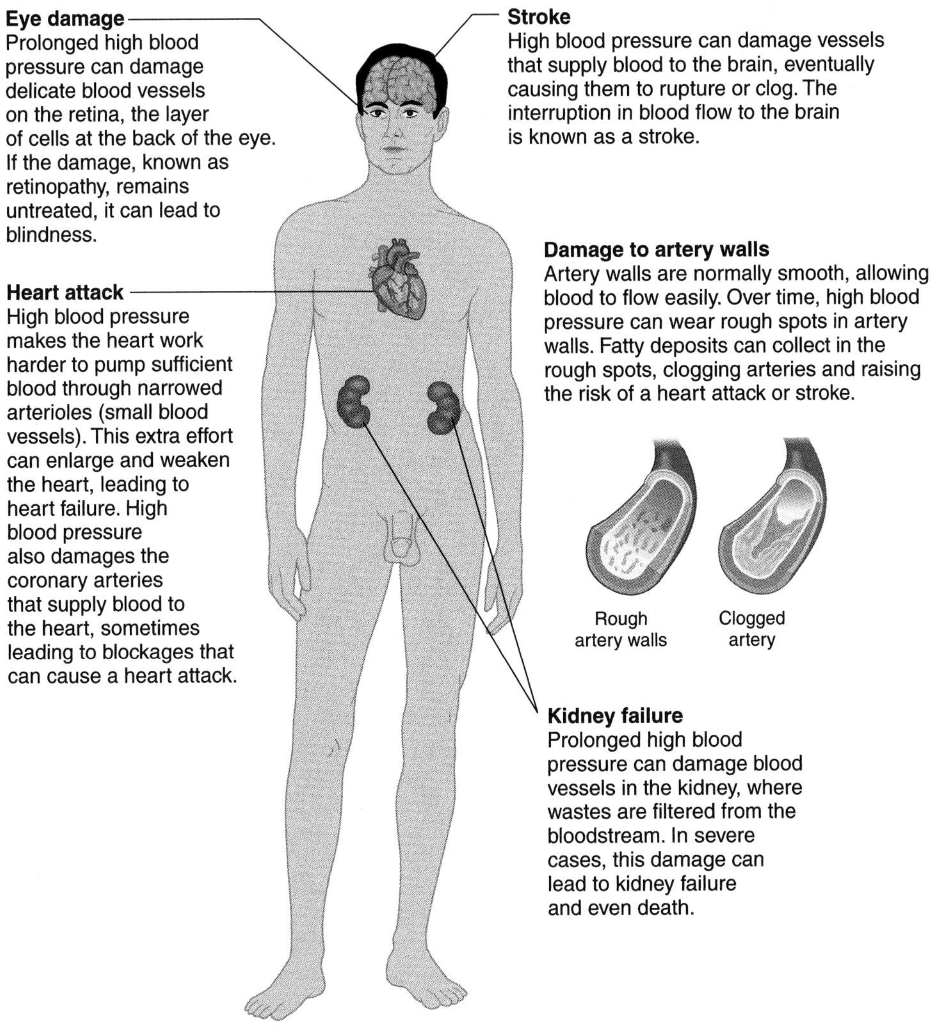

**Eye damage**
Prolonged high blood pressure can damage delicate blood vessels on the retina, the layer of cells at the back of the eye. If the damage, known as retinopathy, remains untreated, it can lead to blindness.

**Heart attack**
High blood pressure makes the heart work harder to pump sufficient blood through narrowed arterioles (small blood vessels). This extra effort can enlarge and weaken the heart, leading to heart failure. High blood pressure also damages the coronary arteries that supply blood to the heart, sometimes leading to blockages that can cause a heart attack.

**Stroke**
High blood pressure can damage vessels that supply blood to the brain, eventually causing them to rupture or clog. The interruption in blood flow to the brain is known as a stroke.

**Damage to artery walls**
Artery walls are normally smooth, allowing blood to flow easily. Over time, high blood pressure can wear rough spots in artery walls. Fatty deposits can collect in the rough spots, clogging arteries and raising the risk of a heart attack or stroke.

Rough artery walls

Clogged artery

**Kidney failure**
Prolonged high blood pressure can damage blood vessels in the kidney, where wastes are filtered from the bloodstream. In severe cases, this damage can lead to kidney failure and even death.

▲ **Figure 10-4** Consequences of High Blood Pressure
If left untreated, elevated blood pressure can damage blood vessels in several areas of the body and lead to serious health problems.

▼ **Table 10-3 What the Blood Pressure Numbers Mean**

Blood pressure on arteries, measured in millimeters of mercury, has two components. The harder it is for blood to flow, the higher both readings are.

| Rating | First Number: Systolic — Pressure When Heart Beats | Second Number: Diastolic — Pressure Between Heartbeats |
|---|---|---|
| High | 140 and up | 90 and up |
| High Normal | 130–139 | 85–89 |
| Normal | Less than 130 | Less than 85 |
| Optimal | Less than 120 | Less than 80 |

Source: *American Heart Association.*

ing—the second and lower of the two blood pressure numbers—in diagnosing hypertension. In young people, diastolic pressure, a reflection of the constriction of the small blood vessels, continues to be a good indicator of cardiovascular risk. However, a rise in systolic blood pressure—the first and higher of the numbers in a blood pressure reading also can be dangerous.

Systolic hypertension, a reading of 140 mmHg or higher, reflects stiffening or hardening of the large arteries and is the most common blood pressure problem in the United States. (See Figure 10-5.)[34] "The traditional belief was that a systolic blood pressure of 100 plus your age is okay, but this is simply not true," says Joseph Izzo, M.D., an adviser to the NHLBI. "Research data have convinced us that it's time to blow the whistle about the danger of systolic hypertension."[35] A reduction as small as 2 mmHg in the average American's systolic blood pressure could save more than 70,000 lives per year.[36]

Systolic blood pressure typically rises with age and poses the greatest risk for those middle-aged and older.[37] However, the ideal time to start caring about blood pressure is in your twenties and thirties. In a young person, even mild hypertension can cause organs such as the heart, brain, and kidneys to start to deteriorate. By age 50 or 60, the damage may be irreversible.

## Know Your Numbers

"Everyone, regardless of age, should know his or her blood pressure—the actual numbers, not just that it's 'fine' or 'normal,'" says Claude Lenfant, M.D., director of the NHLBI. "If your reading is higher than 140 over 80 mmHg, ask your doctor why and find out what you can do about it."[38]

Although anyone can develop high blood pressure, some groups are at greater risk. In any decade of life, African Americans have higher blood pressure levels and

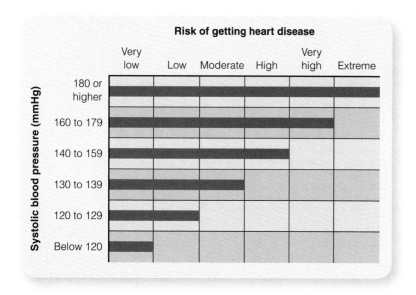

**Risk of getting heart disease**

| Systolic blood pressure (mmHg) | Very low | Low | Moderate | High | Very high | Extreme |
|---|---|---|---|---|---|---|
| 180 or higher | | | | | | |
| 160 to 179 | | | | | | |
| 140 to 159 | | | | | | |
| 130 to 139 | | | | | | |
| 120 to 129 | | | | | | |
| Below 120 | | | | | | |

▲ **Figure 10-5** Dangers of Systolic Hypertension
As systolic blood pressure (the top number) rises, so does the risk of getting heart disease. If your systolic is too high—140 or above—see your doctor.

Source: Framingham Heart Study, National Heart, Lung, and Blood Institute, National Institutes of Health.

suffer more consequences of high blood pressure. An African American with the same elevated blood pressure reading as a Caucasian faces a greater risk of stroke, heart disease, and kidney problems. No one knows why African Americans are more vulnerable, although some speculate that overweight or dietary factors may contribute.

Family history also plays a role. "If you study healthy college students with normal blood pressures, those who have one parent with hypertension will have blood pressure that's a little higher than average," notes Rose Marie Robertson, M.D., of the American Heart Association. "If two parents have high blood pressure, their levels will be a little higher, and they're destined to go higher still. If your parents have high blood pressure, have yours checked regularly."[39]

In a study that followed more than 10,000 healthy men for 25 years, those with high blood pressure in young adulthood were at higher risk for eventually dying from heart disease.[40] Men and women are equally likely to develop hypertension, but in women, blood pressure tends to rise around the time of menopause. Half of all women over age 45 have hypertension. For individuals who smoke, are overweight, don't exercise, or have high cholesterol levels, hypertension multiplies the risk of heart disease and stroke. At ultrahigh risk are people with diabetes or kidney disease.[41]

## Preventing Hypertension

Prevention pays off when it comes to high blood pressure. The most effective preventive measures involve lifestyle changes. Losing weight is the best approach for individuals

with high normal values. Exercise may be effective in lowering mildly elevated blood pressure. Among the approaches that have not proven effective are dietary supplements, such as calcium, magnesium, potassium, and fish oil.

The National Heart, Lung, and Blood Institute has developed what is known as the DASH diet. Following DASH, which stands for Dietary Approaches to Stop Hypertension, has proven as effective as drug therapy in lowering blood pressure.[42] An additional benefit: The DASH diet also lowers harmful blood fats, including cholesterol and low-density lipoprotein, and the amino acid homocysteine (one of the new suspects in heart disease risk).[43]

Restriction of sodium intake also helps. Most Americans consume more salt than they need. The current federal recommendation is to limit sodium to less than 2.4 grams (2,400 milligrams) a day. That equals 6 grams (about a teaspoon) of salt a day, including salt used in cooking and at the table. Doctors may advise those with high blood pressure to eat less salt. According to recent research, diets of less than 1,500 milligrams of sodium produce even greater benefits and help blood pressure medicines work better.

The lower the amount of sodium in the diet, the lower the blood pressure for both those with and those without hypertension, and for both genders and all racial and ethnic groups. However, reducing dietary sodium has an even greater effect on blood pressure in blacks than whites, in women than men, and in individuals with hypertension.[44]

The most recent federal recommendations for preventing hypertension emphasize six approaches:[45]

- ✔ Engage in moderate physical activity.
- ✔ Maintain normal body weight.
- ✔ Limit alcohol consumption.
- ✔ Reduce sodium intake.
- ✔ Maintain adequate intake of potassium.
- ✔ Consume a diet rich in fruits, vegetables, and low-fat dairy products, and reduced in saturated and total fat.

Researchers caution that fish oil (omega-3 polyunsaturated fatty acids) and calcium supplements lower blood pressure only slightly in individuals with hypertension. In addition, the ability of herbal and botanical supplements to lower blood pressure is unproven.[46]

## Treating Hypertension

For some people, particularly those with mild hypertension, lifestyle changes alone can bring blood pressure down. "The most important thing is to be active—not just sit in front of the TV," says Dr. Lenfant. "Control your weight, watch what you eat, limit alcohol. Some people are more sensitive to salt than others and have to be especially careful, but everyone should monitor their salt intake."[47]

For other people, diet and exercise are not enough. "The good news is that today we can treat high blood pressure with medications that don't make people feel bad," says Dr. Robertson. "In the past, blood pressure medicines often caused so many side effects that people didn't take them. Now there are multiple classes of drugs, and many drugs in every class. With good communication between patient and doctor, virtually every case can be successfully treated with medications that are effective and don't cause side effects."[48]

Medications called beta-blockers and diuretics are recommended as the first-line treatment for hypertension, but newer drugs such as angiotensin-converting enzyme (ACE) inhibitors and calcium channel blockers are becoming increasingly popular. They account for 55 percent of prescriptions of antihypertensives in the United States. Nevertheless, there is no conclusive evidence that they are more effective and better tolerated. No single drug works well in everyone, so physicians have to rely on clinical judgment and trial-and-error to find the best possible medication for an individual patient.[49]

## Coronary Artery Disease

The general term for any impairment of blood flow through the blood vessels, often referred to as "hardening

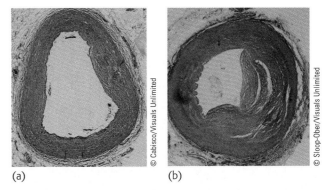

(a)                    (b)

▲ (a) A healthy coronary artery. (b) An artery partially blocked by the buildup of atherosclerotic plaque.

of the arteries," is **arteriosclerosis.** The most common form is **atherosclerosis,** a disease of the lining of the arteries in which **plaque**—deposits of fat, fibrin (a clotting material), cholesterol, other cell parts, and calcium—narrows the artery channels. (See photos above.)

## ???? What Happens During a Heart Attack?

Each year an estimated 1 million Americans suffer a heart attack; nearly half of them die. The medical name for a heart attack, or coronary, is **myocardial infarction (MI).** The *myocardium* is the cardiac muscle layer of the wall of the heart. It receives its blood supply, and thus its oxygen

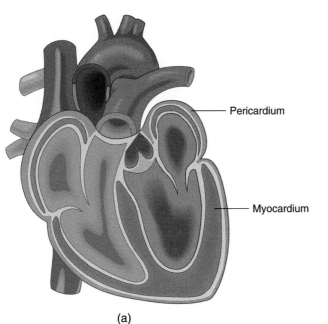

(a)

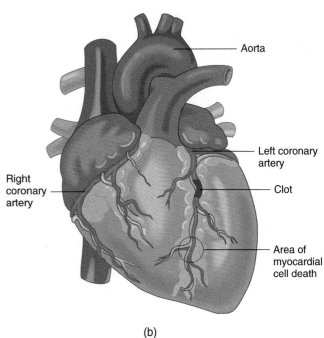

(b)

▲ **Figure 10-6** The Making of a Heart Attack
(a) The bulk of the heart is composed mainly of the myocardium, the muscle layer that contracts. (b) A clot in one of the arteries that feeds into the myocardium can cut off the blood supply to part of the myocardium, causing cells in that area to die. This is called a myocardial infarction, or heart attack.

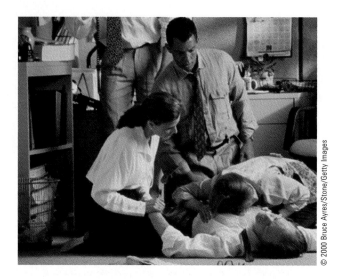

▲ If you witness someone who appears to be experiencing a heart attack, the best thing you can do is immediately call for emergency help. Only after medical emergency personnel are called should you begin any CPR efforts.

and other nutrients, from the coronary arteries. If an artery is blocked by a clot or plaque, or by a spasm, the myocardial cells do not get sufficient oxygen, and the portion of the myocardium deprived of its blood supply begins to die. (See Figure 10-6.) Although such an attack may seem sudden, usually it has been building up for years, particularly if the person has ignored risk factors and early warning signs.

Individuals should seek immediate medical care if they experience the following symptoms:

✔ A tight ache, heavy, squeezing pain, or discomfort in the center of the chest, which may last for 30 minutes or more and is not relieved by rest.

✔ Chest pain that radiates to the shoulder, arm, neck, back, or jaw.

✔ Anxiety.

✔ Sweating or cold, clammy skin.

✔ Nausea and vomiting.

✔ Shortness of breath.

✔ Dizziness, fainting, or loss of consciousness.

The two hours immediately following the onset of such symptoms are the most crucial. About 40 percent of those who suffer an MI die within this time. According to the American Heart Association, most patients wait three hours after the initial symptoms begin before seeking help. By that time, half of the affected heart muscle may already be lost.

Heart attacks in the United States may be becoming less severe, as measured by the average size of myocardial infarcts. Prompt treatment may be one reason. However, this is not true for women.

Women's heart attacks are more likely to be fatal than men's. Heart attacks are twice as likely to kill women under age 50 than men in the same age range. A review of the records of 384,878 heart attack victims found that 17 percent of female heart attack victims die while still in the hospital, compared with 12 percent of males. The difference results entirely from a much higher death rate among the younger victims.[50]

Women wait hours longer after a heart attack before going to the hospital, then are treated less aggressively than men. This delay, which allows further damage to the oxygen-starved heart, results partly because women tend to experience less painful heart attack symptoms. Sometimes they feel only pressure or a burning feeling, not crushing pain. Younger female victims are more likely than men to have other health problems, such as diabetes, high blood pressure, and heart failure.[51]

In another study of 12,142 men and women who had bad heart attacks, milder ones, or severe chest pain, women were up to twice as likely to suffer serious complications. Among those who had heart attacks, the women were 50 percent more likely to die within 30 days.

More doctors' offices, airlines, and public meeting places, such as casinos, are purchasing heart defibrillators. This life-saving equipment may seem expensive, at an estimated $3,500, but the cost of defibrillators and training teams of nurses in their use comes to only about a nickel per paying patient. State-of the-art treatments for heart attacks include clot-dissolving drugs, early administration of medications to thin the blood, intravenous nitroglycerin, and, in some cases, a beta-blocker (which blocks many of the effects of adrenaline in the body, particularly its stimulating impact on the heart).

Clot-dissolving drugs called thrombolytic agents are the treatment of choice for acute myocardial infarction in most clinical settings. Administered through a *catheter* (flexible tube) threaded through the arteries to the site of the blockage (the more effective method of delivery) or injected intravenously (the faster, cheaper method of delivery), these agents can save lives and dissolve clots, but don't remove the underlying atherosclerotic plaque.

Two clot-thinning drugs may be better than one for treating heart attacks. One drug, called a thrombolytic, dissolves blood clots. The second drug, a platelet receptor blocker, keeps platelets from clumping and forming the blood clots that can obstruct blood flow and thereby trigger a heart attack or stroke. The platelet blockers, sometimes called "super aspirin," are more potent than aspirin. They are also administered through an intravenous drip or infusion. Patients receiving such therapy may require further procedures, such as bypass surgery or angioplasty, which can reduce their risk of another heart attack or death. In a coronary bypass, an artery from the patient's leg or chest wall is grafted onto a coronary artery to detour blood around the blocked area.

Emergency balloon **angioplasty** has shown greater effectiveness than clot-dissolving medication in restoring blood flow in arteries immediately after an attack. With this approach, arteries are less likely to close down again and patients have shorter hospital stays and fewer hospital readmissions. Angioplasty patients also are less likely to die of the heart attack or to experience repeat attacks. However, most American hospitals do not perform angioplasty, and not all can do it on an emergency basis.

## Stroke

When the blood supply to a portion of the brain is blocked, a cerebrovascular accident, or **stroke,** occurs. Someone in the United States suffers a stroke every 53 seconds; more than a quarter are under age 65. An estimated 20 percent of stroke victims die within three months; 50 to 60 percent are disabled. About half of those who have a stroke are partially paralyzed on one side of their body; between a quarter and a half are partially or completely dependent on others for daily living; a third become depressed; a fifth cannot walk.[52]

Strokes rank third, after heart disease and cancer, as a cause of death in this country.[53] After decades of steady decline, the number of strokes per year has begun to rise.[54] The main reasons seem to be that more people in the United States are living longer, advanced medical care is allowing more people to survive heart disease, and doctors are better able to diagnose and detect strokes. Yet 80 percent of strokes are preventable, and key risk factors can be modified through either lifestyle changes or drugs. The most important steps are treating hypertension, not smoking, managing diabetes, lowering cholesterol, and taking aspirin.

Strokes continue to occur 40 percent more often in the Southeast (the so-called Stroke Belt) than in other regions of the United States. However, stroke rates have fallen in Mississippi and Alabama while they've increased in Oregon, Washington, and Arkansas. The decline in deaths among stroke victims has been greatest in white men and smallest among black men.[55]

### What Causes a Stroke?

There are two types of stroke: *ischemic stroke,* which is the result of a blockage that disrupts blood flow to the brain, and *hemorrhagic stroke,* which occurs when blood vessels rupture. One of the most common causes of ischemic stroke is the blockage of a brain artery by a thrombus, or blood clot—a *cerebral thrombosis.* Clots generally form around deposits sticking out from the arterial wall. Sometimes a wandering blood clot (embolus), carried in the bloodstream, becomes wedged in one of the cerebral arteries. This is called a *cerebral embolism,* and it can completely plug up a cerebral artery.

In hemorrhagic stroke, a diseased artery in the brain floods the surrounding tissue with blood. The cells nourished by the artery are deprived of blood and can't function, and the blood from the artery forms a clot that may interfere with brain function. This is most likely to occur if the patient suffers from a combination of hypertension and atherosclerosis.

Hemorrhage (bleeding) may also be caused by a head injury or by the bursting of an aneurysm, a blood-filled pouch that balloons out from a weak spot in the wall of an artery.

Brain tissue, like heart muscle, begins to die if deprived of oxygen, which may then cause difficulty speaking and walking, and loss of memory. These effects may be slight or severe, temporary or permanent, depending on how widespread the damage and whether other areas of the brain can take over the function of the damaged area. About 30 percent of stroke survivors develop dementia, a disorder that robs a person of memory and other intellectual abilities.

The following symptoms should alert you to the possibility that you or someone with you has suffered a stroke:

- ✔ Sudden weakness or loss of strength.
- ✔ Numbness of face, arm, or leg.
- ✔ Loss of speech, or difficulty speaking or understanding speech.
- ✔ Dimness or loss of vision, particularly double vision in one eye.
- ✔ Unexplained dizziness.
- ✔ Change in personality.
- ✔ Change in pattern of headaches.

## Risk Factors for Strokes

People who've experienced Transient Ischemic Attacks (TIAs) are at the highest risk for stroke. Other risk factors, like those for heart disease, include some that can't be changed (such as gender and race) and some that can be controlled:[56]

### STRATEGIES FOR PREVENTION

#### How to Prevent a Stroke

▲ Quit smoking. Smokers have twice the risk of stroke that nonsmokers have. When they quit, their risk drops 50 percent in two years. Five years after quitting, their risk is nearly the same as nonsmokers.

▲ Keep blood pressure under control. Treating hypertension with medication can lead to a 40 percent reduction in fatal and nonfatal strokes.

▲ Eat a low-fat, low-cholesterol diet, which reduces your risk of fatty buildup in blood vessels.

▲ Avoid obesity, which burdens the blood vessels as well as the heart.

▲ Exercise. Moderate amounts of exercise improve circulation and may help dissolve deposits in the blood vessels that can lead to stroke.

✔ **Gender.** Men have a greater risk of stroke than women. However, women are at increased risk at times of marked hormonal changes, particularly pregnancy and childbirth. Past studies have shown an association between oral contraceptive use and stroke, particularly in women over age 35 who smoke. The newer low-dose oral contraceptives have not shown an increased stroke risk among women ages 18 to 44. A woman's stroke risk may increase markedly at menopause. (See the X & Y Files: "Gender Differences in Disease" on p. 267.)

✔ **Race.** African Americans have a much greater risk of stroke than whites. Hispanics also are more likely to develop hemorrhagic strokes than whites.

✔ **Age.** A person's risk of stroke more than doubles every decade after age 55.

✔ **Hypertension.** Detection and treatment of high blood pressure are the best means of stroke prevention.

✔ **High red blood cell count.** A moderate to marked increase in the number of a person's red blood cells increases the risk of stroke.

✔ **Heart disease.** Heart problems can interfere with the flow of blood to the brain; clots that form in the heart can travel to the brain, where they may clog an artery.

✔ **Blood fats.** Although the standard advice from cardiologists is to lower harmful LDL levels, what may be more important for stroke risk is a drop in the levels of protective HDL.

✔ **Diabetes mellitus.** Diabetics have a higher incidence of stroke than nondiabetics.

# Understanding Cancer

The uncontrolled growth and spread of abnormal cells causes cancer. Normal cells follow the code of instructions embedded in DNA (the body's genetic material); cancer cells do not. Think of the DNA within the nucleus of a cell as a computer program that controls the cell's functioning, including its ability to grow and reproduce itself. If this program or its operation is altered, the cell goes out of control. The nucleus no longer regulates growth. The abnormal cell divides to create other abnormal cells, which again divide, eventually forming **neoplasms** (new formations), or tumors.

Tumors can be either *benign* (slightly abnormal,

not considered life-threatening) or *malignant* (cancerous). The only way to determine whether a tumor is benign is by microscopic examination of its cells. Cancer cells have larger nuclei than the cells in benign tumors, they vary more in shape and size, and they divide more often.

At one time cancer was thought to be a single disease that attacked different parts of the body. Now scientists believe that cancer comes in countless forms, each with a genetically determined molecular "fingerprint" that indicates how deadly it is. With this understanding, doctors can identify how aggressively a tumor should be treated.

Without treatment, cancer cells continue to grow, crowding out and replacing healthy cells. This process is called **infiltration,** or invasion. Cancer cells may also **metastasize,** or spread to other parts of the body via the bloodstream or lymphatic system (see Figure 10-7). For many cancers, as many as 60 percent of patients may have metastases (which may be too small to be felt or seen without a microscope) at the time of diagnosis.

Although all cancers have similar characteristics, each is distinct. Some cancers are relatively simple to cure, whereas others are more threatening and mysterious. The earlier any cancer is found, the easier it is to treat and the better the patient's chances of survival.

Cancers are classified according to the type of cell and the organ in which they originate, such as the following:

✔ *Carcinoma,* the most common kind, which starts in the epithelium, the layers of cells that cover the body's surface or line internal organs and glands.

✔ *Sarcoma,* which forms in the supporting, or connective, tissues of the body: bones, muscles, blood vessels.

✔ *Leukemia,* which begins in the blood-forming tissues (bone marrow, lymph nodes, and the spleen).

✔ *Lymphoma,* which arises in the cells of the lymph system, the network that filters out impurities.

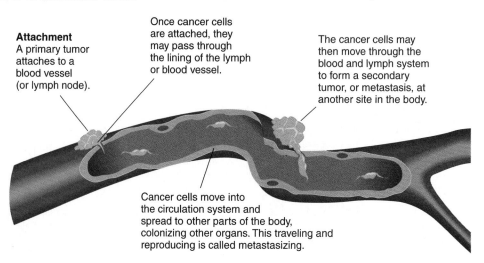

**Attachment**
A primary tumor attaches to a blood vessel (or lymph node).

Once cancer cells are attached, they may pass through the lining of the lymph or blood vessel.

The cancer cells may then move through the blood and lymph system to form a secondary tumor, or metastasis, at another site in the body.

Cancer cells move into the circulation system and spread to other parts of the body, colonizing other organs. This traveling and reproducing is called metastasizing.

▲ **Figure 10-7** Metastasis, or Spread of Cancer
Cancer cells can travel through the blood vessels to spread to other organs, or through the lymphatic system to form secondary tumors.

## ????  Who Is at Risk for Developing Cancer?

Everyone and anyone can develop cancer. However, since the occurrence of cancer increases over time, most cases affect adults who are middle-aged or older (see Table 10-4). In the United States, men have a one in two lifetime risk of developing cancer; for women, the risk is one in three.[57] (See The X & Y Files: "Gender Differences in Cancer.")

The term **relative risk** compares the risk of developing cancer in people with a certain exposure or trait to the risk

### ▼ Table 10-4 Age and the Risk of Cancer (All Sites)

|  | Men | Women |
|---|---|---|
| Birth to age 39 | 1 in 64 | 1 in 51 |
| Ages 40 to 59 | 1 in 12 | 1 in 11 |
| Ages 60 to 79 | 1 in 3 | 1 in 4 |
| Birth to death | 1 in 2 | 1 in 3 |

Source: *Cancer Facts & Figures 2001.* Atlanta, GA: American Cancer Society, 2001.

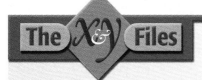 The X & Y Files

## Gender Differences in Cancer*

| Cancer Cases by Site and Sex per Year | | Cancer Deaths by Site and Sex per Year | |
|---|---|---|---|
| **Male** | **Female** | **Male** | **Female** |
| Prostate 189,000 (30%) | Breast 203,500 (31%) | Lung and bronchus 89,200 (31%) | Lung and bronchus 65,700 (25%) |
| Lung and bronchus 90,200 (14%) | Lung and bronchus 79,200 (12%) | Prostate 30,200 (11%) | Breast 39,600 (15%) |
| Colon and rectum 72,600 (11%) | Colon and rectum 75,700 (12%) | Colon and rectum 27,800 (10%) | Colon and rectum 28,800 (11%) |
| Urinary bladder 41,500 (7%) | Uterine Corpus 39,300 (6%) | Pancreas 14,500 (5%) | Pancreas 15,200 (6%) |
| Melanoma of the skin 30,100 (5%) | Non-Hodgkin's lymphoma 25,700 (4%) | Non-Hodgkin's lymphoma 12,700 (5%) | Ovary 13,900 (5%) |
| Non-Hodgkin's lymphoma 28,200 (4%) | Melanoma of the skin 23,500 (4%) | Leukemia 12,100 (4%) | Non-Hodgkin's lymphoma 11,700 (4%) |
| Kidney 19,100 (3%) | Ovary 23,300 (4%) | Esophagus 9,600 (3%) | Leukemia 9,600 (4%) |
| Oral Cavity 18,900 (3%) | Thyroid 15,800 (2%) | Liver 8,900 (3%) | Uterine Corpus 6,600 (2%) |
| Leukemia 17,600 (3%) | Pancreas 15,600 (2%) | Urinary bladder 8,600 (3%) | Brain 5,900 (2%) |
| Pancreas 14,700 (2%) | Urinary bladder 15,000 (2%) | Kidney 7,200 (3%) | Multiple myeloma 5,300 (2%) |
| All sites 637,500 | All sites 647,400 | All sites 288,200 | All sites 267,300 |

▲ **Figure 10-8**
Gender Differences in Cancer Sites and Deaths.

*Excludes basal and squamous cell skin cancers and in situ carcinoma except urinary bladder. Percentages may not total 100% due to rounding.
Source: Surveillance Research, American Cancer Society, Inc., 2002.

in those who do not have this exposure or trait. Smokers, for instance, have a ten-times-greater relative risk of developing lung cancer than nonsmokers. Most relative risks are smaller. For example, women who have a first-degree (mother, sister, or daughter) family history of breast cancer have about a twofold increased risk of developing breast cancer compared with women who do not have a family history of the disease. This means that they are about twice as likely to develop breast cancer.

## Heredity

An estimated 13 to 14 million Americans may be at risk of a hereditary cancer. In hereditary cancers, such as retinoblastoma (an eye cancer that strikes young children) or certain colon cancers, a specific cancer-causing gene is passed down from generation to generation. The odds of any child with one affected parent inheriting this gene and developing the cancer are fifty-fifty. In familial cancers, close relatives develop the same types of cancer, but no one knows exactly how the disease is transmitted. Genetic tests can identify some individuals who are born with an increased susceptibility. Tracing cancers through a family tree is one simple way of checking your own risk.

The most likely sites for inherited cancers to develop are the breast, brain, blood, muscles, bones, and adrenal glands. The telltale signs of inherited cancers include:

✔ **Early development.** Genetic forms of certain diseases strike earlier than noninherited cancers. For example, the average age of women diagnosed with breast cancer is 62. But if breast cancer is inherited, the average age at diagnosis is 44, an 18-year difference.

✔ **Family history.** Anyone with a close relative (mother, father, sibling, child) with cancer has about three times the usual chance of getting the same type of cancer.

✔ **Multiple targets.** The same type of hereditary cancer often strikes more than once—in both breasts or both kidneys, for instance, or in two separate parts of the same organ.

✔ **Unusual gender pattern.** Genes may be responsible for cancers that generally don't strike a certain gender—for example, breast cancer in a man.

✔ **Cancer family syndrome.** Some families, with unusually large numbers of relatives affected by cancer, seem clearly cancer-prone. For instance, in Lynch syndrome (a form of colon cancer), more than 20 percent of the family members in at least two generations develop cancer of both the colon and the endometrium.

## Racial and Ethnic Groups

The American Cancer Society estimates 1,284,900 cases of cancer are diagnosed each year, with more cases in black

Americans than in any other racial or ethnic group.[58] Blacks are about 33 percent more likely to die of cancer than whites. African-American women have the highest incidence of colorectal and lung cancers of any ethnic group, while black men have the highest rates of prostate, colorectal, and lung cancer. African Americans also have higher rates of incidence and deaths from other cancers, including those of the mouth, throat, esophagus, stomach, pancreas, and larynx. The National Cancer Institute (NCI) has launched the Southern Community Cohort Study to determine why African Americans are more likely to develop and die from cancer.[59]

Cancer rates also vary in other racial and ethnic groups. Hispanics have six times lower risk of developing melanoma than Caucasians, yet tend to have a worse prognosis than Caucasians when they do develop this skin cancer. The incidence of female breast cancer is highest among white women and lowest among Native American women.[60]

## Viruses

Researchers have long known that viruses can cause tumors in animals, but only recently have they shown a connection between several different viruses and cancer in humans. Viruses have been implicated in certain leukemias (cancers of the blood system) and lymphomas (cancers of the lymphatic system), cancers of the nose and pharynx, liver cancer, and cervical cancer. Human immune deficiency virus (HIV) can lead to certain lymphomas and leukemias and to a type of cancer called Kaposi's sarcoma. Human papilloma virus (HPV) has been linked to an increased risk of cervical cancer and cancer of the penis.[61]

## ????  How Can I Reduce My Cancer Risk?

Environmental factors may cause between 80 and 90 percent of cancers. At least in theory, these cancers can be prevented by avoiding cancer-causing substances (such as tobacco and sunlight) or using substances that protect against cancer-causing factors (such as antioxidants and vitamin D). How do you start protecting yourself? Simple changes in lifestyle—smart eating, not smoking, protecting yourself from the sun, exercising regularly—are essential.

## Cancer-Smart Nutrition

Diets high in antioxidant-rich fruits and vegetables have long been linked with lower rates of esophageal, lung, colon, and stomach cancer. At least in theory, antioxidants—substances that prevent the damaging effects of oxidation in cells—can block genetic damage induced by free radicals that could lead to some cancers. However, scientific studies have not proven conclusively that any specific antioxidant, particularly in supplement form, can prevent cancer.

In studies of beta-carotene (found in dark green and dark yellow fruits and vegetables), this carotenoid did not reduce overall cancer rates or mortality. In two studies of smokers, beta-carotene actually was associated with increased mortality from lung cancer. Researchers are continuing to investigate a variety of antioxidants that have shown promise as cancer-fighters. The mineral selenium, which promotes antioxidant activity, may protect against prostate cancer and possibly also lower the risk of cancer of the lung, colon, and esophagus. Diets rich in vitamin C and folate also may have some specific benefits against breast cancer.

Eating as many different types of fruits and vegetables as possible—for a total of five to nine servings a day—remains a standard recommendation. However, a low-fat diet rich in fruit, vegetables, and fiber did not influence the risk of recurrence of colorectal polyps.[62] Some studies have found a correlation between very high consumption of fruits and vegetables and lower risk of breast cancer, but the overall findings have been inconclusive.[63]

Another way to lower your cancer risk is to reduce the fat in your diet. There is solid evidence that cutting back on fat can lower the risks of colon, ovarian, and pancreatic cancer.

It's also important to pay attention to food processing and preparation. Whenever possible, select foods close to their natural state, grown locally and without pesticides. Avoid cured, pickled, or smoked meats. When cooking, try not to fry or barbecue often; these cooking methods can produce mutagens that induce cancer in animals. The process of smoking or charcoal-grilling releases carcino-genic tar that may increase the risk of cancer of the stomach and esophagus.

## Tobacco Smoke

Cigarette smoking is the single most devastating and preventable cause of cancer deaths in the United States. People who smoke two or more packs of cigarettes a day are 15 to 25 times more likely to die of cancer than nonsmokers. Cigarettes cause most cases of lung cancer and increase the risk of cancer of the mouth, pharynx, larynx, esophagus, pancreas, and bladder. Pipes, cigars, and smokeless tobacco also increase the danger of cancers of the mouth and throat.

Environmental tobacco smoke can increase the risk of cancer even among those who've never smoked. For example, researchers have found that exposure to others' tobacco smoke for as little as three hours a day can increase the risk of developing cancer threefold. (See the discussion of environmental tobacco smoke in Chapter 12.)

## Possible Carcinogens

Although it may not be possible to avoid all possible **carcinogens** (cancer-causing chemicals), you can take steps to minimize your danger. Many chemicals used in industry, including nickel, chromate, asbestos, and vinyl chloride, are carcinogens; employees as well as people living near a factory that creates smoke, dust, or gases are at risk. If your job involves their use, follow safety precautions at work. If you are concerned about possible hazards in your community, check with local environmental protection officials.

Women and men who frequently dye their hair, particularly with very dark shades of permanent coloring, may be at increased risk for leukemia (cancer of blood-forming cells), non-Hodgkin's lymphoma (cancer of the lymph system), multiple myeloma (cancer of the bone marrow), and, in women, ovarian cancer. Lighter shades and less permanent tints do not seem to be a danger.

## Early Detection

Cancers that can be detected by screening account for approximately half of all new cancer cases. Screening examinations, conducted regularly by a health-care professional, can lead to early diagnosis of cancers of the breast, colon, rectum, cervix, prostate, testicles, and oral cavity, and can improve the odds of successful treatment. (See Table 10-5.) Self-examinations for cancers of the breast, testicles, and skin may also result in detection of tumors at earlier stages. The five-year relative survival rate for all these cancers is about 81 percent. If all Americans participated in regular cancer screenings, this rate could increase to more than 95 percent.[64]

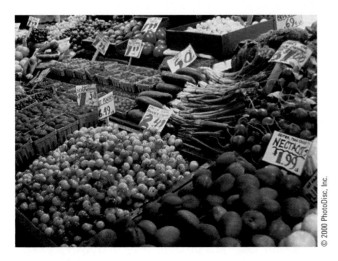

© 2000 PhotoDisc, Inc.

▲ Eating at least five servings of fruits and vegetables a day can help reduce your cancer risk.

▼ **Table 10-5 American Cancer Society Recommendations for the Early Detection of Cancer in Asymptomatic People**

| Cancer Type | Recommended Screening |
|---|---|
| **General cancer prevention** | A cancer-related checkup is recommended every 3 years for people aged 20–40 and every year for people age 40 and older. The exam should include health counseling and depending on a person's age might include examinations for cancers of the thyroid, oral cavity, skin, lymph nodes, testes, and ovaries, as well as some nonmalignant diseases. |
| **Breast** | Women 40 and older should have an annual mammogram and an annual clinical breast examination (CBE) by a health-care professional. The CBE should be conducted close to and preferably before the scheduled mammogram. Women aged 20–39 should have a CBE by a health-care professional every 3 years. |
| **Colon and rectum** | Beginning at age 50, men and women at average risk should follow one of the examination schedules below: <br>• Fecal occult blood test (FOBT) every year<br>• Flexible sigmoidoscopy every 5 years*<br>• Double-contrast barium enema every 5 years*<br>• Colonoscopy every 10 years* |
| **Prostate** | Beginning at age 50, the prostate-specific antigen (PSA) test and the digital rectal exam should be offered annually to men who have a life expectancy of at least 10 years. Men at high risk (African-American men and men who have a first-degree relative who was diagnosed with prostate cancer at a young age) should begin testing at age 45. Patients should be given information about the benefits and limitations of tests so they can make an informed decision. |
| **Uterus** | **Cervix:** All women who are or have been sexually active or who are 18 and older should have an annual Pap test and pelvic examination. After three or more consecutive satisfactory examinations with normal findings, the Pap test may be performed less frequently. Discuss the matter with your physician. <br><br>**Endometrium:** Beginning at age 35, women with or at risk for hereditary non-polyposis colon cancer should have an endometrial biopsy annually to screen for endometrial cancer. |

*A digital rectal exam should be done at the same time. People at increased or high risk for colorectal cancer should talk with a doctor about a different testing schedule.

Source: *Cancer Facts and Figures—2002,* Reprinted by permission American Cancer Society, Inc.

© Corbis Images
© Bill Crump/Brand X Pictures/PictureQuest
© 2001 PhotoDisc, Inc.
© Corbis Images
© 2001 PhotoDisc, Inc.

# Common Types of Cancer

Cancer refers to a group of more than a hundred diseases characterized by abnormal cell growth. The most common are discussed in the following sections.

## Skin Cancer

Sunlight is the primary culprit in the 1 million new cases of skin cancer that develop every year. Once scientists thought exposure to the B range of ultraviolet light (UVB), the wavelength of light responsible for sunburn, posed the greatest danger. However, longer-wavelength UVA, which penetrates deeper into the skin, also plays a major role in skin cancers.[65] An estimated 80 percent of total lifetime sun exposure occurs during childhood, so sun protection is especially important in youngsters. Tanning salons and sunlamps also increase the risk of skin cancer because they produce ultraviolet radiation. A half-hour dose of radiation from a sunlamp can be equivalent to the amount you'd get from an entire day in the sun.

The most common skin cancers are *basal-cell* (involving the base of the epidermis, the top level of the skin) and *squamous-cell* (involving cells in the epidermis). Every year more than 5 million Americans develop skin lesions known as actinic keratoses (AKs), rough red or brown scaly patches that develop in the upper layer of the skin, usually on the face, lower lip, bald scalp, neck, and back of the hands and forearms. Forty percent of squamous cell carcinomas, the second leading cause of skin cancer deaths, begin as AKs. Treatments include surgical removal, cryosurgery (freezing the skin), electrodesiccation (heat generated by an electric current), topical chemotherapy, and removal with lasers, chemical peels, or dermabrasion.

Smoking and exposure to certain hydrocarbons in asphalt, coal tar, and pitch may increase the risk of squamous-cell skin cancer. Other risk factors include occupational exposure to carcinogens and inherited skin disorders, such as xeroderma pigmentosum and familial atypical multiple-mole melanoma.

Malignant *melanoma,* the deadliest type of skin cancer, causes 1 to 2 percent of all cancer deaths.[66] During the 1930s, the lifetime risk of melanoma was about 1 in 1,500. Today it is 1 in 75. This increase in risk is due mostly to overexposure to UV radiation. The use of a tanning bed ten times or more a year doubles the risk for individuals over age 30. For those younger than 30, this type of exposure increases the risk by a factor of 7.7.[67]

Melanoma occurs more often among people over 40 but is increasing in younger people, particularly those who had severe sunburns in childhood.[68] The rate of increase in melanoma also has risen more in men (4.6 percent a year) than for women (3.2 percent). Men are more likely than women to be diagnosed with melanoma after age 40.[69]

Individuals with any of the following characteristics are at increased risk:

✔ Fair skin, light eyes, or fair hair.
✔ A tendency to develop freckles and to burn instead of tan.
✔ A history of childhood sunburn or intermittent, intense sun exposure.
✔ A personal or family history of melanoma.
✔ A large number of *nevi,* or moles (200 or more, or 50 or more if under age 20), or dysplastic (atypical) moles.[70]

## Detection

The most common predictor for melanoma is a change in an existing mole or development of a new and changing pigmented mole. The most important early indicators are change in color, an increase in diameter, and changes in the borders of a mole. (See Figure 10-9.) An increase in height signals a corresponding growth in depth under the skin. Itching in a new or long-standing mole also should not be ignored.[71]

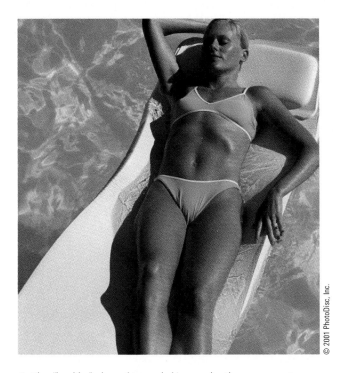

▲ The "healthy" glow of tanned skin may be the precursor to a severe, even fatal, case of skin cancer.

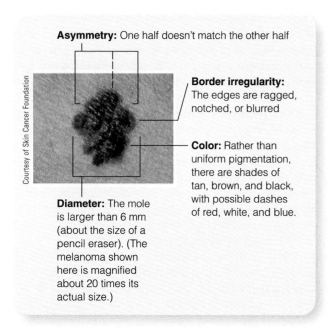

**Asymmetry:** One half doesn't match the other half

**Border irregularity:** The edges are ragged, notched, or blurred

**Color:** Rather than uniform pigmentation, there are shades of tan, brown, and black, with possible dashes of red, white, and blue.

**Diameter:** The mole is larger than 6 mm (about the size of a pencil eraser). (The melanoma shown here is magnified about 20 times its actual size.)

*Courtesy of Skin Cancer Foundation*

▲ **Figure 10-9** ABCD: The Warning Signs of Melanoma
An estimated 95 percent of cases of melanoma arise from an existing mole. A normal mole is usually round or oval, less than 6 millimeters (about 1/4 inch) in diameter, and evenly colored (black, brown, or tan). Seek prompt evaluation of any moles that change in ways shown in the photo.

## Treatment

If caught early, melanoma is highly curable, usually with surgery alone. Once it has spread, chemotherapy with a single drug or a combination can temporarily shrink tumors in some people. However, the five-year survival rate for metastatic melanoma is less than 10 percent.

## Breast Cancer

Every 3 minutes a woman in the United States learns that she has breast cancer. Every 12 minutes a woman dies of breast cancer. Many women misjudge their own likelihood of developing breast cancer, either overestimating or underestimating their susceptibility. In a national poll, one in every ten surveyed considered herself at no risk at all. This is never the case. "Every woman is at risk for breast cancer simply because she's female," says Leslie Ford, M.D., associate director for early detection at the National Cancer Institute (NCI).[72]

However, not all women's risks are equal. NCI has developed a computerized Breast Cancer Risk Assessment Tool, based on data from more than 280,000 women, that allows a woman to sit down with her doctor and discuss her own odds of developing breast cancer within the next five years and over her entire lifetime. These calculations include a variety of risk factors, including the following:

✔ **Age.** As shown in Figure 10-10, at 25, a woman's chance of developing breast cancer is 1 in 19,608; at 45, 1 in 93; at 65, 1 in 17; at 85, 1 in 9. By age 90 to 95, 1 in 8 women will have developed breast cancer. The mean age at which women are diagnosed is 63.

✔ **Family history.** The overwhelming majority of breast cancers—90 to 95 percent—are not due to strong genetic factors. However, having a first-degree relative—mother, sister or daughter—with breast cancer does increase risk, and if the relative developed breast cancer before menopause, the cancer is more likely to be hereditary. Genetic testing, controversial but sometimes recommended for women in cancer-prone families, can identify these defects. However, it's not yet clear how many women with a defective gene actually will develop breast cancer; estimates range from 50 to 80 percent, or higher in families with many affected members.[73]

✔ **Age at menarche.** Women who had their first period before age 12 are at greater risk than women who began menstruating later. The reason is that the more menstrual cycles a woman has, the longer her exposure to estrogen, a hormone known to increase breast cancer danger. For similar reasons, childless women, who menstruate continuously for several decades, are also at greater risk.

✔ **Age at birth of first child.** An early pregnancy—in a woman's teens or twenties—changes the actual maturation of breast cells and decreases risk. But if a woman has her first child in her forties, precancerous cells may actually flourish with the high hormone levels of the pregnancy.

✔ **Breast biopsies.** Even if laboratory analysis finds no precancerous abnormalities, women who require such tests are more likely to develop breast cancer. Fibrocystic breast disease, a term often used for "lumpy" breasts, is not a risk factor.

 ✔ **Race.** Breast cancer rates are lower in Hispanic and Asian populations than in whites, but higher in African-American women up to age 50. In post-

| By age 25 | 1 in 19,608 | By age 60 | 1 in 24 |
|---|---|---|---|
| By age 30 | 1 in 2,525 | By age 65 | 1 in 17 |
| By age 35 | 1 in 622 | By age 70 | 1 in 14 |
| By age 40 | 1 in 217 | By age 75 | 1 in 11 |
| By age 45 | 1 in 93 | By age 80 | 1 in 10 |
| By age 50 | 1 in 50 | By age 85 | 1 in 9 |
| By age 55 | 1 in 33 | Ever | 1 in 8 |

▲ **Figure 10-10** A Woman's Risk of Developing Breast Cancer
Source: Surveillance Program, National Cancer Institute.

menopausal African-American women, rates are lower. Nonetheless, African-American women are still more likely to die of breast cancer than whites. Scientists don't know if that's because they don't have equal access to care, if they don't get optimal care, or if the disease itself is more aggressive in black women.

✔ **Occupation.** Based on two decades of following more than a million women, Swedish researchers have developed a list of jobs linked with a high risk of breast cancer. These include pharmacists, certain types of teachers, schoolmasters, systems analysts and programmers, telephone operators, telegraph and radio operators, metal platers and coaters, and beauticians.

✔ **Estrogen.** The role of estrogen replacement as a cancer risk factor remains controversial. Some studies have documented an increase in certain types of breast cancer in women who have used hormone replacement therapy (HRT) for more than five years. Some experts believe that the failure of well-designed epidemiological studies conducted over the last 25 years to confirm a risk indicates that the dangers, if they exist, are not great.

## Detection

In the past, women were advised to perform monthly breast self-exams seven to ten days after their periods. According to a recent study, breast self-examination (BSE) does *not* appear to decrease the number of deaths from breast cancer. Highly motivated women practicing BSE, the researchers found, are more likely to find benign tumors and undergo expensive and unnecessary testing.[74] Based on the new findings, rather than spending time teaching BSE, physicians have been urged to educate women about breast cancer symptoms and spend a little longer on the clinical breast exam.[75]

The best tool for early detection is the diagnostic X-ray exam called **mammography.** Overall, screening mammograms could reduce breast cancer deaths by 25 percent. Mammograms can detect a tumor two to three years before it can be detected by manual exam (see Figure 10-11). According to a recent report, annual mammography for women in their forties is more cost-effective than Pap smear tests for cervical cancer and installation of airbags and seat belts in vehicles. The American Cancer Society, the American Medical Association, and the National Cancer Society recommend that all women begin routine mammographic screening by age 40.

Recent reviews of mammography's impact on breast cancer mortality have triggered disagreements about the benefits of routine mammograms.[76] Some experts have concluded there isn't enough evidence to support the claim that routine mammography lessens deaths from breast cancer.[77] Others, including the American Cancer Society,

continue to recommend regular screening for women age 40 and older, not just women 50 and older.

Mammography is more likely to detect early-stage disease in white than black and Hispanic women, possibly because of lack of insurance coverage for the screening tests.[78] Hispanic women undergo these potentially live-saving tests less often than white and African-American women and appear less likely than other women to seek follow-up mammograms in the recommended time frame.[79]

## Treatment

Breast cancer can be treated with surgery, radiation, and drugs (chemotherapy and hormonal therapy). Doctors may use one of these options or a combination, depending on the type and location of the cancer and whether the disease has spread.

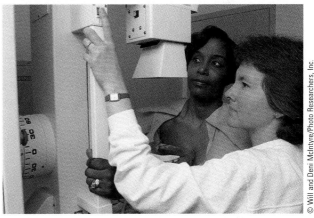

© Will and Deni McIntyre/Photo Researchers, Inc.

Cancer calcifications of this size and smaller can be seen on mammograms.

Average-size lump found by mammogram.

Average-size lump found by women practicing frequent breast self-exam.

Smallest-size cancer that can be felt by physician's palpation exam.

Average-size lump found by women practicing occasional breast self-exam.

▲ **Figure 10-11** Cancer Sizes Found by Breast-Cancer Detection Methods
Mammography is able to detect a lump much smaller than a woman can find with regular breast self-exams.

Most women undergo some type of surgery. **Lumpectomy** or breast-conserving surgery removes only the cancerous tissue and a surrounding margin of normal tissue. A modified radical **mastectomy** includes the entire breast and some of the underarm lymph nodes. Radical mastectomy, in which the breast, lymph nodes, and chest wall muscles under the breast are removed, is rarely performed today because modified radical mastectomy has proven just as effective. Removing underarm lymph nodes is important to determine if the cancer has spread, but a new method, sentinel node biopsy, allows physicians to pinpoint the first lymph node into which a tumor drains (the sentinel node), and remove only the nodes most likely to contain cancer cells.

Radiation therapy is treatment with high-energy rays or particles to destroy cancer. In almost all cases, lumpectomy is followed by six to seven weeks of radiation. Chemotherapy is used to reach cancer cells that may have spread beyond the breast—in many cases even if no cancer is detected in the lymph nodes after surgery.

The use of the drugs paclitaxe (Taxol) or docetaxel (Taxotere), which inhibit cell division, in addition to standard chemotherapy, can significantly lower the risk of recurrence.[80] A new biotherapy—a monoclonal antibody that zeros in on cancer cells like a miniature guided missile—also has shown promise against some aggressive breast tumors. The drug Herceptin targets a defective growth-promoting gene (HER-2/neu) found in about 30 percent of women with breast cancer. The combination of Herceptin and standard chemotherapy has significantly improved survival rates in women with this gene.

## Cervical Cancer

 An estimated 12,900 cases of invasive cervical cancer are diagnosed in the United States every year, with about 4,400 annual deaths from this disease. The highest incidence rate occurs among Vietnamese women; Alaskan Native, Korean, and Hispanic women also have higher rates than the national average. The mortality rate for African-American women is more than twice that of whites, largely because of a high number of deaths among older black women.

The primary risk factor for cervical cancer is infection with certain types of the human papilloma virus (HPV), discussed in Chapter 9. However, not every HPV infection becomes cervical cancer, and while HPV infection is very common, cervical cancer is not. Other risk factors for cervical cancer include early age of first intercourse, multiple sex partners, genital herpes, and significant exposure to passive smoking.

The standard screening test for cervical cancer is the Pap smear. Each year this test detects about 1.2 million cases of abnormal cell growth.

## Ovarian Cancer

Ovarian cancer is the leading cause of death from gynecological cancers, with 23,400 new cases diagnosed and 13,900 deaths each year. Risk factors include a family history of ovarian cancer; personal history of breast cancer; obesity; infertility (because the abnormality that interferes with conception may also play a role in cancer development); and low levels of transferase, an enzyme involved in the metabolism of dairy foods. Often women develop no obvious symptoms until the advanced stages, although they may experience painless swelling of the abdomen, irregular bleeding, lower abdominal pain, digestive and urinary abnormalities, fatigue, backache, bloating, and weight gain.

## Colon and Rectal Cancer

Colon and rectal, or colorectal, cancer accounts for 10 percent of cancer deaths. Most cases occur after age 50. Both age and gender influence the risk of colon cancer. Older individuals and men are more likely to develop *polyps* (nonmalignant growths that may turn cancerous at some point) and tumors in the colon than young people and women. Men are 52 percent more likely to have polyps and 43 percent more likely to have cancer of the colon than women. When women do develop tumors, they are more likely to occur in the right side of the colon and are more responsive to chemotherapy.[81]

Risk factors include a personal or family history of colon and rectal cancer, polyps in the colon or rectum, and ulcerative colitis. Early signs of colorectal cancer are bleeding from the rectum, blood in the stool, or a change in bowel habits.

Sixty percent of eligible people in the United States have never been screened for colorectal cancer.[82] The simplest test for this common cancer, the fecal occult blood test, detects blood in a person's stool.

Treatment may involve surgery, radiation therapy, or chemotherapy. Regular exercise can lower the risk of colon and rectal cancer in both men and women. Hormone replacement after menopause may significantly reduce women's risk of colon cancer.

## Prostate Cancer

After skin cancer, prostate cancer is the most common form of cancer in American men, according to National Cancer Institute statistics. More than a quarter of men diagnosed with cancer have prostate cancer. The disease strikes black men more often than white; Asian and American Indian men are affected less often.[83]

The risk of prostate cancer increases with age, family history, exposure to the heavy metal cadmium, high number of sexual partners, and history of frequent sexually transmitted diseases. An inherited predisposition may account for 5 to 10 percent of cases. A purported link between vasectomy and prostate cancer has been disproven.[84]

The development of a simple screening test that measures levels of a protein called prostate-specific antigen (PSA) in the blood has revolutionized the diagnosis of prostate cancer.

## Testicular Cancer

In the last 20 years the incidence of testicular cancer has risen 51 percent in the United States—from 3.61 to 5.44 per 100,000. It is not clear why testicular cancer is on the rise, although researchers speculate that changing environmental or socioeconomic risk factors could have a role. Testicular cancer occurs mostly among young men between the ages of 18 and 35, who are not normally at risk of cancer. At highest risk are men with an undescended testicle (a condition that is almost always corrected in childhood to prevent this danger). To detect possibly cancerous growths, men should perform monthly testicular self-exams, as shown in Figure 10-12.

 Although college-age men are among those at highest risk of testicular cancer, three in four do not know how to perform a testicular self-examination. Only 8 to 14 percent examine their testicles regularly.[85]

Often the first sign of this cancer is a slight enlargement of one testicle. There also may be a change in the way it feels when touched. Sometimes men with testicular cancer report a dull ache in the lower abdomen or groin, along with a sense of heaviness or sluggishness. Lumps on the testicles also may indicate cancer.

A man who notices any abnormality should consult a physician. If a lump is indeed present, a surgical biopsy is necessary to find out if it is cancerous. If the biopsy is positive, a series of tests generally is needed to determine whether the disease has spread.

Treatment for testicular cancer generally involves surgical removal of the diseased testis, sometimes along with radiation therapy, chemotherapy, and the removal of nearby lymph nodes. The remaining testicle is capable of maintaining a man's sexual potency and fertility. Only in rare cases is removal of both testicles necessary. Testosterone injections following such surgery can maintain potency. The chance for a cure is very high if testicular cancer is spotted early.

## Diabetes Mellitus

About 100 million people around the world, including nearly 16 million people in the United States, have diabetes mellitus, a disease in which the body doesn't produce or respond properly to insulin, a hormone essential for daily life. In those who have diabetes, the pancreas, which produces insulin (the hormone that regulates carbohydrate and fat metabolism) doesn't function as it should. When the pancreas either stops producing insulin (type 1 or *insulin-dependent diabetes*) or doesn't produce sufficient insulin to meet the body's needs (type 2 or *non-insulin-dependent diabetes*), almost every body system can be damaged.

### ???? Who Is at Risk for Developing Diabetes?

One in three Americans with diabetes is not aware of having an illness that increases the risk of blindness, kidney failure, cardiovascular disease, and premature death.[86] The incidence of this potential killer, which jumped about a third in the last decade, is growing so fast that Dr. Allen Spiegel, director of the National Institute of Diabetes and Digestive and Kidney Diseases (NIDDK), describes it as "a definite epidemic."[87] There has been a particularly dramatic rise in type 2 diabetes in children and adolescents, especially among minority populations.[88] "The fact that kids just past puberty are getting type 2 diabetes blows us out of the water compared to what we were taught in medical school, which was that type 2 diabetes was a disease of aging," says Dr. Spiegel.

Uncontrolled glucose levels slowly damage blood vessels throughout the body, thus individuals who become

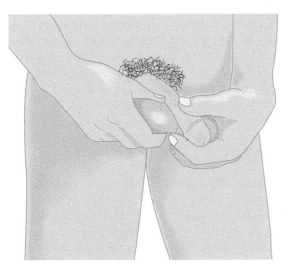

▲ **Figure 10-12** Testicular Self-Exam
The best time to examine your testicles is after a hot bath or shower, when the scrotum is most relaxed. Place your index and middle fingers under each testicle and the thumb on top, and roll the testicle between the thumb and fingers. If you feel a small, hard, usually painless lump or swelling, or anything unusual, consult a urologist.

diabetic early in life may face devastating complications even before they reach middle age. "Diabetes is already the number one cause of blindness, nontraumatic amputations, and kidney failure, and diabetes increases by two or three times the risk of heart attack or stroke," says Dr. Robert Sherwin of Yale University, president of the American Diabetes Association, who estimates that the disease may affect 22 million Americans within the next two decades.[89]

Lifestyle factors, especially a lack of physical activity, greatly increase the risk for type 2 diabetes.[90] Television watching, more than other sedentary activities such as sewing, reading, writing, and driving, is strongly associated with weight and obesity, a risk factor for diabetes in both children and adults. In a ten-year study of 1,058 individuals with type 2 diabetes, watching television for 2 to 10 hours a week increased the risk of diabetes 66 percent; 21 to 40 hours per week more than doubled the risk; more than 40 hours a week nearly tripled the risk.[91]

To identify individuals with this disease as early as possible, the American Diabetes Association now recommends screening every three years for all men and women beginning at age 45. Those at highest risk include relatives of diabetics (whose risk is two and a half times that of others), obese persons (85 percent of diabetics are or were obese), older persons (four out of five diabetics are over age 45), and mothers of large babies (an indication of maternal prediabetes). A child of two parents with type 2 diabetes faces an 80 percent likelihood of also becoming diabetic.

The early signs of diabetes are frequent urination, excessive thirst, a craving for sweets and starches, and weakness. Diagnosis is based on tests of the sugar level in the blood. Researchers are working to develop a test that would help identify telltale antibodies in the blood; this could indicate that pancreas cells are being destroyed years before the first signs of diabetes.

## Dangers of Diabetes

Before the development of insulin injections, diabetes was a fatal illness. Today diabetics can have normal life spans. However, both types of diabetes can lead to devastating complications, including increased risk of heart attack or stroke, kidney failure, blindness, and loss of circulation to the extremities. Although few people realize it, diabetes claims more than 100,000 women's lives a year—more than the number who succumb to breast cancer.

Diabetic women who become pregnant face higher risks of miscarriage and babies with serious birth defects; however, precise control of blood sugar levels before conception and in early pregnancy can lower the likelihood of these problems. The development of diabetes during pregnancy, called *gestational diabetes,* may pose potentially serious health threats to mother and child years later. Women who develop gestational diabetes are more than three times

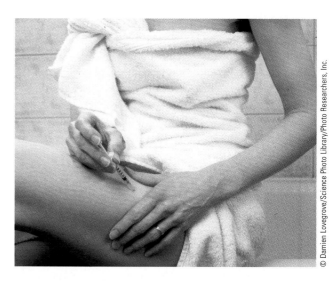

▲ Individuals with type 1 or insulin-dependent diabetes control their disease by injecting themselves with insulin.

as likely to develop type 2 diabetes if they have a second pregnancy; their infants may be at increased risk of cardiovascular disease later in life.

## Diabetes and Ethnic Minorities

 Several minority groups, especially African Americans, Native Americans, and Hispanics, are at high risk of developing diabetes. One in every ten African Americans and Hispanics has this disease. The members of some Native American tribes are 300 percent more likely to develop diabetes than the general population. For many, obesity and unhealthy food choices increase the risk. Researchers now believe that the interaction of environmental factors and genes varies among different racial and ethnic groups.

## Treatment

There's no cure for diabetes at this time. The best treatment option is to keep blood sugar levels as stable as possible to prevent complications, such as kidney damage. Home glucose monitoring allows diabetics to check their blood sugar levels as many times a day as necessary and to adjust their diet or insulin doses as appropriate.

Those with type 1 diabetes require daily doses of insulin via injections, an insulin infusion pump, or oral medication. Those with type 2 diabetes can control their disease through a well-balanced diet, exercise, and weight management. However, insulin therapy may be needed to keep blood glucose levels near normal or normal, thereby reducing the risk of damage to the eyes, nerves, and kidneys.

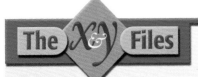

## Gender Differences in Disease

isease doesn't discriminate. In general, men and women are vulnerable to the same illnesses, but there are differences in the diseases that strike each gender. Women are more prone to arthritis, osteoporosis, and joint problems, while more men are felled by heart attacks and cancer. Of the top ten causes of death in the United States—including heart disease, lung cancer, cirrhosis of the liver, and homicide—every single one kills roughly twice as many men as women.

Half of all men, compared to a third of women, develop cancer. Smoking, which for many years was much more prevalent among men, accounts for some of this difference. As more women became smokers in the last 30 years, lung cancer rates in women have doubled.

In some cancers, estrogen may somehow protect against distant metastases. This protection may be why women have a 12 percent lower death rate from cancer of the stomach and lung than men and a 33 percent greater chance of surviving malignant melanoma. Men account for two of every three melanoma deaths. (See The X & Y Files: "Gender Differences in Cancer" for differences in cancer sites and deaths in men and women.)

Some diseases, such as diabetes, afflict more women than men and pose a graver threat to their health. While more men develop ulcers and hernias, women are three to four times more likely to get gallbladder disease. Irritable bowel syndrome (IBS), one of the most common digestive disorders, causes such varied symptoms in the genders that some gastroenterologists think of it as a completely different disease in men and women. IBS affects women three times as often as men, and white women five times more often than African Americans. The incidence of diabetes, hypertension, stroke, lupus, and other serious illnesses is higher in African-American women than in other racial groups.

---

Medical advances hold out bright hopes for diabetics. Laser surgery, for instance, is saving eyesight. Bypass operations are helping restore blood flow to the heart and feet. Dialysis machines and kidney and pancreas transplants save many lives. Researchers are exploring various approaches to prevention, including early low-dose insulin therapy, oral insulin to correct immune intolerance, and immunosuppressive drugs. Still on the horizon is the promise of a true cure through transplanting insulin-producing cells from healthy pancreases. In preliminary trials, this procedure has helped patients become insulin-independent.[92]

 What are the greatest risk factors for heart disease?

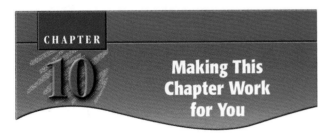

CHAPTER
10

**Making This Chapter Work for You**

1. The heart
   a. has four chambers, which are responsible for pumping blood into the veins for circulation through the body.
   b. pumps blood first to the lungs where it picks up oxygen and discards carbon dioxide.
   c. beats about 10,000 times and pumps about 75 gallons of blood per day.
   d. has specialized cells that generate electrical signals to control the amount of blood that circulates through the body.

2. Risk factors for heart disease that cannot be controlled include
   a. male pattern baldness
   b. diabetes mellitus
   c. sedentary lifestyle
   d. blood fat cells

3. Your lipoprotein profile
   a. provides a breakdown of the different types and levels of blood fats circulating in your body.
   b. is best obtained at a health fair where the results are uniformly accurate.
   c. will give a total cholesterol level, which is the amount of triglycerides and LDL cholesterol levels added together.
   d. should be evaluated after eating a full meal.

4. Hypertension
   a. is diagnosed when blood pressure is consistently less than 130/85 mmHg.
   b. may be treated with dietary changes, which include eating low-fat foods and avoiding sodium.
   c. can cause fatty deposits to collect on the artery walls.

d. usually does not respond to medication, especially in severe cases.

5. A heart attack
   a. occurs when the myocardium receives an excessive amount of blood from the coronary arteries.
   b. is typically suffered by individuals who have irregular episodes of atherosclerosis.
   c. can be treated successfully up to four hours after the event.
   d. occurs when the myocardial cells are deprived of oxygen-carrying blood, causing them to die.

6. You can protect yourself from certain types of cancer by
   a. eating a diet rich in antioxidants.
   b. avoiding people who have had cancer.
   c. wearing sunscreen with an SPF of less than 15.
   d. using condoms during sexual intercourse.

7. Which of the following statements about skin cancer is true?
   a. Individuals with a large number of moles are at decreased risk for melanoma.
   b. The most serious type of skin cancer is squamous-cell carcinoma.
   c. The safest way to get a tan and avoid skin cancer is to use tanning salons and sunlamps instead of sunbathing in direct sunlight.
   d. Individuals with a history of childhood sunburn are at increased risk for melanoma.

8. A woman's risk of developing breast cancer increases if
   a. she is African American under the age of 50.
   b. she had her first child when in her teens or twenties.
   c. her husband's mother had breast cancer.
   d. she began menstruating when she was 15 or 16.

9. Prostate cancer
   a. occurs mostly among men between the ages of 18 and 35.
   b. is usually more aggressive in men older than 70.
   c. may be treated by implanting radioactive iodine in the prostate.
   d. can be detected through a screening test that measures the levels of prostate-serum antibody in the blood.

10. Which of the following statements about diabetes mellitus is false?
   a. The two types of diabetes are insulin-dependent and non–insulin-dependent.
   b. The incidence of diabetes has decreased in the last decade, especially among African Americans, Native Americans, and Latinos.
   c. Individuals with diabetes must measure the levels of glucose in their blood to ensure that it does not rise to unsafe levels.
   d. Untreated or uncontrolled diabetes can lead to coma and eventual death.

Answers to these questions can be found on page 415.

## Critical Thinking

1. Have you had a lipoprotein profile lately? Do you think it's necessary for you to obtain one? If your reading was/is borderline or high, what lifestyle changes can you make to help control your cholesterol level?

2. The costs for a heart transplant are over $100,000. The annual price tag for a year's worth of cyclosporine, the drug that prevents rejection and must be taken for the rest of a transplant recipient's life, is about $5,000. The total medical bill can come to hundreds of thousands of dollars—enough to fund programs to improve the nutrition of poor pregnant women, to treat alcoholism, or to provide regular preventive care. Does treatment of any single individual justify such huge costs? Should our society try to balance the costs versus the benefits of such heroic measures as heart transplants? How would you go about making such decisions?

3. Do you have family members who have had cancer? Were these individuals at risk for cancer because of specific environmental factors, such as long-term exposure to tobacco smoke? If no particular cause was identified, what other factors could have triggered their diseases? Are you concerned that you might have inherited a genetic predisposition to any particular type of cancer because of your family history?

4. A friend of yours, Karen, discovered a small lump in her breast during a routine self-examination. When she mentions it, you ask if she has seen a doctor. She tells you that she hasn't had time to schedule an appointment; besides, she says she's not sure it's really the kind of lump one has to worry about. It's clear to you that Karen is in denial and procrastinating about seeing a doctor. What advice would you give her?

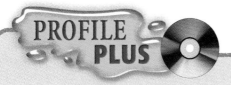

Assess your risks for cardiovascular disease and different types of cancer with the following activities on your Profile Plus CD-ROM:

Cardiovascular Risk * Cancer Risk

## SITES & BYTES

### American Heart Association
www.americanheart.org

This comprehensive site features a searchable database of all major cardiovascular diseases, plus information on healthy lifestyles, current research, CPR, cardiac warning signs, risk awareness, low-cholesterol diets, and family health. The interactive Heart Profiler provides personalized information about treatment options for common cardiovascular conditions such as hypertension, heart failure, and cholesterol.

### American Cancer Society
www.cancer.org

The site features comprehensive information about different kinds of cancer: statistics, early detection, prevention, treatment options, alternative treatments, and coping strategies for families. In addition, you can type in your zip code and find local resources or order books from the online bookstore.

### American Diabetes Association
www.diabetes.org

Here you will find the latest information on both type 1 and type 2 diabetes mellitus, including suggestions regarding diet and exercise. The online bookstore features meal planning guides, cookbooks, and self-care guides. Type in your zip code to find community resources.

Please note that links are subject to change. If you find a broken link, use a search engine such as www.yahoo.com and search for the website by typing in keywords.

**InfoTrac College Edition Activity** Julia Hippisley-Cox, et al. "Married Couples' Risk of Same Disease: Cross Sectional Study." *British Medical Journal*, Vol. 325, No. 7365, September 21, 2002, p. 636.

1. Married partners of people with which types of chronic diseases are at increased risk of developing the same disease themselves?

2. What factors could explain this finding?

3. According to this study, there was a lack of adequate evidence for spouse concordance for which types of chronic diseases?

You can find additional readings relating to major diseases with InfoTrac College Edition, an online library of more than 900 journals and publications. Follow the instructions for accessing InfoTrac College Edition that were packaged with your textbook; then search for articles using a keyword search.

For additional links, resources, and suggested readings on InfoTrac College Edition, visit our Health & Wellness Resource Center at http://health.wadsworth.com.

## Key Terms

The terms listed here are used within the chapter on the page indicated. Definitions of the terms are in the Glossary at the end of the book.

| | | | |
|---|---|---|---|
| angioplasty 254 | atrium 242 | diabetes mellitus 247 | lipoproteins 245 |
| aorta 242 | capillary 242 | diastole 242 | lumpectomy 264 |
| arteriosclerosis 253 | carcinogen 259 | hypertension 245 | male pattern baldness 248 |
| atherosclerosis 253 | cholesterol 245 | infiltration 256 | mammography 263 |

*continued*

## References

1. Beaglehole, Robert. "Global Cardiovascular Disease Prevention: Time to Get Serious." *Lancet,* Vol. 358, No. 9282, August 25, 2001, p. 661.

2. Edwards, Thomas. "Lifestyle Influences and Coronary Artery Disease Prevention." *Physician Assistant,* Vol. 25, No. 8, August 2001, p. 19.

3. Lenfant, Claude. "Benefits of Exercise and Lifestyle Modification." National Heart, Lung, and Blood Institute, August 23, 2000.

4. "Exercise Standards Testing and Training." *Circulation,* October 2001.

5. Leiter, Lorene. "Study Finds Vigorous Exercise May Be Best." *Focus: News from Harvard Medical, Dental and Public Health Schools,* March 10, 2000.

6. John J. H., et al. "Effects of Fruit and Vegetable Consumption on Plasma Antioxidant Concentrations and Blood Pressure: A Randomised Controlled Trial." *Lancet,* Vol. 359, No. 9322, June 8, 2002, p. 1969.

7. Mann, J. I., "Diet and Risk of Coronary Heart Disease and Type 2 Diabetes." *Lancet,* Sept 7, 2002, p. 783.

8. "Angling for a Healthier Heart." *Harvard Heart Letter,* Vol. 12, No. 11, July 2002.

9. "A Few Minutes of Risk Assessment Could Mean More of Life." News Release, American Heart Association, October 8, 2001.

10. Spencer, Leslie. "Results of a Heart Disease Risk-Factor Screening Among Traditional College Students." *Journal of American College Health,* Vol. 50, No. 6, p. 291, May 2002.

11. Weemering, Mary Lynne. "Physical Activity and Coronary Heart Disease in Women: Is "No Pain, No Gain" Passé?" *Association of Perioperative Registered Nurses Journal,* Vol. 76, No. 2, August, 2002, p. 331.

12. Tanasescu, Mihaela, et al. "Exercise Type and Intensity in Relation to Coronary Heart Disease in Men." *Journal of the American Medical Association,* Vol. 288, No. 16, October 23, 2002, p. 1994.

13. Iribarren, Carlos. "The Effect of Cigar Smoking on the Risk of Cardiovascular Disease, Chronic Obstructive Pulmonary Disease, and Cancer in Men." *New England Journal of Medicine,* Vol. 342, No. 12, March 23, 2000.

14. National Cholesterol Education Program Expert Panel on Detection, Evaluation, and Treatment of High Blood Cholesterol in Adults. "Prevalence of Metabolic Syndrome Based on Results of NHANES III." *Nutrition Research Newsletter,* Vol. 21, No. 2, February 2002, p. 7.

15. Siani, Alfonso, et al. "The Relationship of Waist Circumference to Blood Pressure: The Olivetti Heart Study." *American Journal of Hypertension,* Vol. 15, No. 9, September 2002, p. 780.

16. National Cholesterol Education Program Expert Panel on Detection, Evaluation, and Treatment of High Blood Cholesterol in Adults. "Prevalence of Metabolic Syndrome Based on Results of NHANES III."

17. "Diabetes and Heart Disease: More Closely Linked Than Most Think." *Tufts University Health & Nutrition Letter,* Vol. 19, No. 5, July 2001, p. 2.

18. American Diabetes Association. www.diabetes.org.

19. "One for 2001: Take Lifestyle to Heart." *Harvard Women's Health Watch,* Vol. 8, No. 5, January 2001.

20. Reyes, Amy. "Link Between Hopelessness and Hypertension." University of Michigan News Service, February 18, 2000.

21. Levenstein, Susan, et al. "Psychosocial Predictors of Hypertension in Men and Women." *Archives of Internal Medicine,* Vol. 161, No. 10, May 28, 2001.

22. Anderson, Judith, and Cathy Kessenich. "Women and Coronary Heart Disease." *Nurse Practitioner,* Vol. 26, No. 8, August 2001, p. 12.

23. Hu, Frank, et al. "The Impact of Diabetes Mellitus on Mortality from All Causes and Coronary Heart Disease in Women: 20 Years of Follow-Up." *Archives of Internal Medicine,* Vol. 161, No. 14, July 23, 2001, p. 1717.

24. "Men and Women Are Different." *Mayo Clinic Women's HealthSource,* September 2002.

25. Roger, Veronique, et al. "Sex Differences in Evaluation and Outcome of Unstable Angina." *Journal of the American Medical Association,* Vol. 263, No. 5, February 2, 2000.

26. Writing Group for the Women's Health Initiative Investigators. "Risks and Benefits of Estrogen Plus Progestin Healthy Postmenopausal Women: Principal Results from the Women's Health Initiative Randomized Controlled Trial." *Journal of the American Medical Association,* Vol. 288, No. 3, p. 321.

27. Lotufo, Paolo, et al. "Male Pattern Baldness and Coronary Heart Disease." *Journal of the American Medical Association,* Vol. 160, No. 2, January 24, 2000.

28. Expert Panel on Detection, Evaluation, and Treatment of High Blood Cholesterol in Adults. "Executive Summary of the Third Report of the National Cholesterol Education Program (NCEP) Expert Panel on Detection, Evaluation, and Treatment of High Blood Cholesterol in Adults." *Journal of the American Medical Association,* Vol. 285, No. 19, May 16, 2001, p. 2486.

29. "Cholesterol: Highlight of the New Guidelines." *Harvard Health Letter,* Vol. 26, No. 9, July 2001.

30. Expert Panel on Detection, Evaluation, and Treatment of High Blood Cholesterol in Adults. "Executive Summary of the Third Report."

31. "Heartbeats: Graze Your Way to Lower Cholesterol." *Havard Heart Letter,* Vol. 12, No. 9, May 2002.

32. Bullock, Carole. "Southerners At Risk for High Blood Pressure." American Heart Association, January 7, 2000.

33. Van den Hoogen, Peggy, et al. "The Relation Between Blood Pressure and Mortality Due to Coronary Heart Disease Among Men in Different Parts of the World." *New England Journal of Medicine,* Vol. 342, No. 1, January 6, 2000.

34. National Heart, Lung, and Blood Institute. "Clinical Advisory on Systolic Blood Pressure." May 4, 2000, available at www.nhlbi.nih.gov.

35. Izzo, Joseph. Personal interview.

36. Sagusti, Susan. "New Recommendations to Prevent High Blood Pressure Issued." National Heart, Blood, and Lung Institute Media Office, October 15, 2002.

37. Baker, C., et al. "Hypertension." *Heart,* Vol. 86, No. 3, September 2001, p. 251.

38. Lenfant, Claude. Personal interview.

39. Robertson, Rose Marie. Personal interview.

40. Miura, Katsuyuki, and Martha Daviglus. "Relationship of Blood Pressure to 25-Year Mortality Due to Coronary Heart Disease,

Cardiovascular Diseases, and All Causes in Young Adult Men." *Archives of Internal Medicine,* Vol. 161, No. 12, June 2001, p. 1501.

41. Hales, Dianne. "The Stealth Killer." *Parade,* June 25, 2000.

42. Greenland, Philip. "Beating High Blood Pressure with Low-Sodium DASH." *New England Journal of Medicine,* Vol. 344, No. 1, January 4, 2001.

43. "DASH Hypertension Diet Also Lowers Cholesterol." NIH News Release, June 21, 2001.

44. Greenland, "Beating High Blood Pressure with Low-Sodium DASH."

45. Whelton, Paul, et al. "Primary Prevention of Hypertension: Clinical and Public Health Advisory from the National High Blood Pressure Education Program." *Journal of the American Medical Association,* Vol. 288, No. 15, October 16, 2002, p. 1882.

46. John et al., "Effects of Fruit and Vegetable Consumption on Plasma Antioxidant Concentrations and Blood Pressure."

47. Lenfant, Claude. Personal interview.

48. Hales, "The Stealth Killer."

49. Malik, Iqbal, et al. "Easier to Take a Pill Than Change the Lifestyle, But Not As Effective As the Combination." *Heart,* Vol. 87, No. 5, May 2002, p. 494.

50. Legato, Marianne. "Gender and the Heart: Sex-Specific Differences in Normal Anatomy and Physiology." *Journal of Gender-Specific Medicine,* Vol. 3, No. 7, October 2000.

51. Mark, Daniel. "Sex Bias in Cardiovascular Care: Should Women Be Treated More Like Men?" *Journal of the American Medical Association,* Vol. 263, No. 5, February 2, 2000.

52. Liebman, Bonnie. "Brain Attack." *Nutrition Action Newsletter,* Vol. 28, No. 7, September 2001, p. 1.

53. "More People Are Hospitalized for Stroke, But Fewer Strokes Are Fatal. News release, American Heart Association, October 4, 2001.

54. "Strokes and Mini-Strokes on the Rise: Total May Exceed 1.2 Million." American Heart Association News Media Relations, February 10, 2000.

55. "Stroke Mortality Varies by Race and Region." News release, American Heart Association, October 4, 2001.

56. Chatfield, Joanne. "American Heart Association Scientific Statement on the Primary Prevention of Ischemic Stroke." *American Family Physician,* Vol. 64, No. 3, August 1, 2001, p. 513.

57. Wizeman, Theresa, and Mary-Lou Pardue. *Exploring the Biological Contributions to Human Health: Does Sex Matter?* Washington, DC: National Academy Press, 2001.

58. *Cancer Prevention & Early Detection.* Atlanta: American Cancer Society. 2002.

59. "Why Blacks Get, Die from Cancer More." Press release, National Cancer Institute, October 18, 2001.

60. *Cancer Facts & Figures 2002.* Atlanta: American Cancer Society. 2002.

61. Zenilman, Jonathan. "Chlamydia and Cervical Cancer." *Journal of the American Medical Association,* Vol. 285, No. 1, January 3, 2001.

62. Velie, E.M., et al. "A Prospective Study of Dietary Patterns and Colorectal Cancer." *American Journal of Epidemiology,* Vol. 153, No. 11, June 1, 2001, p. S194.

63. Slattery, Martha. "Can an Apple a Day Keep Breast Cancer Away? *Journal of the American Medical Association,* Vol. 285, No. 6, February 14, 2001.

64. Zoorob, Roger, et al. "Cancer Screening Guidelines." *American Family Physician,* Vol. 63, No. 6, March 15, 2001, p. 1101.

65. Goldstein, Beth, and Adam Goldstein. "Diagnosis and Management of Malignant Melanoma." *American Family Physician,* Vol. 63, No. 7, April 1, 2001, p. 1101.

66. Ibid.

67. Ibid.

68. "Skin Cancer: Shedding Light on Melanoma." *Harvard Women's Health Watch,* Vol. 9, No. 1, September 2001.

69. Beddingfield, Frederick. "Melanoma Strikes Men and Women Differently." Presentation, Society for Investigative Dermatory, Annual Meeting, Washington, DC, May 12, 2001.

70. "Skin Cancer: Shedding Light on Melanoma."

71. Goldstein and Goldstein, "Diagnosis and Management of Malignant Melanoma."

72. Ford, Leslie. Personal interview.

73. Iversen, Edwin, Jr., et al. "Genetic Susceptibility and Survival: Application to Breast Cancer." *Journal of the American Statistical Association,* Vol. 95, No. 449, March 2000.

74. Thomas, David B., et al. "Randomized Trial of Breast Self-Examination in Shanghai: Final Results." *Journal of National Cancer Institute,* Vol. 94, No. 19, October 2, 2002, p. 1445.

75. Harris, Russell, and Linda Kinsinger. "Routinely Teaching Breast Self-Examination Is Dead. What Does This Mean?" *Journal of National Cancer Institute,* Vol. 94, No. 19, October 2, 2002, p. 1420.

76. Christensen, Damaris. "A Decades-Old Debate: Do Mammograms Save Lives?" *Consumers Research Magazine,* Vol. 85, No. 7, July, 2002, p. 26.

77. Duffy, Stephen, et al. "The Impact of Organized Mammography Service Screening on Breast Carcinoma Mortality in Seven Swedish Counties." *Cancer,* Vol. 95, No. 3, August 1, 2002, p. 458.

78. Jacobellis, Jillian, and Gary Cutter. "Mammography Screening and Differences in Stage of Disease by Race/Ethnicity." *American Journal of Public Health,* Vol. 92, No. 7, July 2002, p. 1144.

79. Stidley, Christine, et al. "Mammography Utilization After a Benign Breast Biopsy Among Hispanic and Non-Hispanic Women." *Cancer,* Vol. 91, No. 9, May 1, 2001, p. 1716.

80. Hellekson, Karen. "NIH Statement on Adjuvant Therapy for Breast Cancer." *American Family Physician,* May 1, 2001.

81. McCashland, Timothy, et al. "Age and Gender Influence Colon Cancer Risk." *American Journal of Gastroenterology,* Vol. 96, April 2001, p. 882.

82. Woolf, Steven. "The Best Screening Test for Colorectal Cancer: A Personal Choice." *New England Journal of Medicine,* Vol. 343, No. 22, November 30, 2000.

83. "Prostate Cancer: New Test Identifies Aggressive and Less Aggressive Forms." *Cancer Weekly,* July 9, 2002, p. 25.

84. Strayer, Scott. "Vasectomy Not a Risk Factor for Prostate Cancer." *Journal of Family Practice,* Vol. 51, No. 9, September 2002, p. 791.

85. Courtenay, Will. "Behavioral Factors Associated with Disease, Injury, and Death Among Men: Evidence and Implications for Prevention." *Journal of Men's Studies,* Vol. 9, No. 1, Fall 2000, p. 81.

86. Hales, Dianne. "Should You Be Tested for Diabetes?" *Parade,* February 4, 2001.

87. Spiegel, Allen. Personal interview.

88. Levetan, Claresa. "Into the Mouth of Babes: The Diabetes Epidemic in Children." *Clinical Diabetes,* Vol. 19, No. 3, Summer 2001, p. 102.

89. Sherwin, Robert. Personal interview.

90. Hu, Frank, et al. "Diet, Lifestyle, and the Risk of Type 2 Diabetes Mellitus in Women." *New England Journal of Medicine,* Vol. 345, No. 11, September 13, 2001, p. 790.

91. Ibid.

92. Hales, "Should You be Tested for Diabetes?"

# Drug Use, Misuse, and Abuse

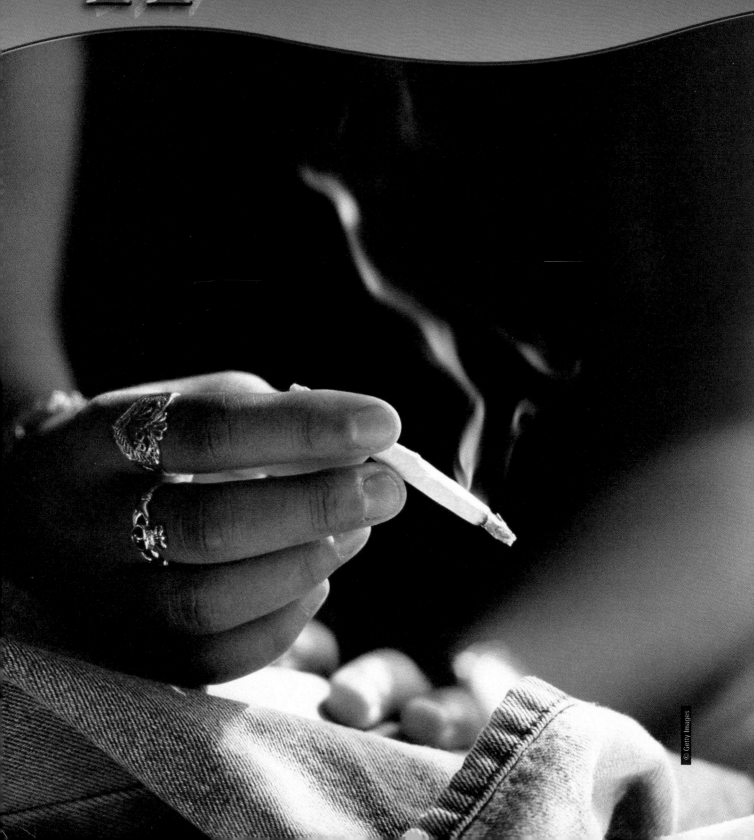

After studying the material in this chapter, you should be able to:

- **Describe** the factors affecting individuals' response to drugs.
- **Give examples** of appropriate and inappropriate use of over-the-counter and prescription medications.
- **Discuss** the factors affecting drug dependence.
- **Describe** the methods of use and the effects of common drugs of abuse.
- **Describe** the treatment methods available for drug dependence.

People who try illegal drugs don't think they'll ever lose control. Even regular drug users are convinced that they are smart enough, strong enough, lucky enough not to get caught and not to get hooked. But with continued use, drugs produce changes in an individual's body, mind, and behavior. In time, a person's need for a drug can outweigh everything else, including the values, people, and relationships he or she once held dearest.

After years of decline, illegal drug use may be on the rise. As many as one in five young adults—almost 16 million Americans—report current drug use. According to the National Household Survey on Drug Abuse, the percentage of young adults between the ages of 18 and 25 who use drugs has increased to 18.8 percent, up from 15.9 percent in 2000.[1] However, other studies have reported a decline in drug, alcohol, and cigarette use among sixth- to twelfth-graders.[2] About half of American adults surveyed report having used an illicit drug at some time in their lives.

This chapter provides information on the nature and effects of drugs, the impact of drugs on individuals and society, and the drugs Americans most commonly use, misuse, and abuse.

 **FREQUENTLY ASKED QUESTIONS**

**FAQ: What should I know about buying over-the-counter drugs? p. 275**

**FAQ: What causes drug dependence and abuse? p. 280**

**FAQ: How common is drug use on campus? p. 282**

# Understanding Drugs and Their Effects

A **drug** is a chemical substance that affects the way you feel and function. In some circumstances, taking a drug can help the body heal or relieve physical and mental distress. In other circumstances, taking a drug can distort reality, undermine well-being, and threaten survival. No drug is completely safe; all drugs have multiple effects that vary greatly in different people at different times. Knowing how drugs affect the brain, body, and behavior is crucial to understanding their impact and making responsible decisions about their use.

**Drug misuse** is the taking of a drug for a purpose or by a person other than that for which it was medically intended. Borrowing a friend's prescription for penicillin when your throat feels scratchy is an example of drug misuse. The World Health Organization defines **drug abuse** as excessive drug use that's inconsistent with accepted medical practice. Taking prescription painkillers to get high is an example of drug abuse.

Risks are involved with all forms of drug use. Even medications that help cure illnesses or soothe symptoms have side effects and can be misused. Some substances that millions of people use every day, such as caffeine, pose some health risks. Others—like the most commonly used drugs in our society, alcohol and tobacco—can lead to potentially life-threatening problems. With some illicit drugs, any form of use can be dangerous.

Many factors determine the effects a drug has on an individual. These include how the drug enters the body, the dosage, the drug action, and the presence of other drugs in the body—as well as the physical and psychological makeup of the person taking the drug and the setting in which the drug is used.

## Routes of Administration

Drugs can enter the body in a number of ways (see Figure 11-1). The most common way of taking a drug is by swallowing a tablet, capsule, or liquid. However, drugs taken orally don't reach the bloodstream as quickly as drugs introduced into the body by other means. A drug taken orally may not have any effect for 30 minutes or more.

Drugs can enter the body through the lungs either by inhaling smoke, for example, from marijuana, or by inhaling gases, aerosol sprays, or fumes from solvents or other compounds that evaporate quickly. Young users of such inhalants, discussed later in this chapter, often soak a rag with fluid and press it over their nose. Or they may place inhalants in a plastic bag, put the bag over their nose and mouth, and take deep breaths—a practice called *huffing* and one that can produce serious, even fatal consequences.

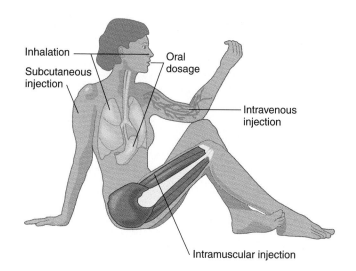

▲ **Figure 11-1** Routes of Administration of Drugs

Drugs can also be injected with a syringe subcutaneously (beneath the skin), intramuscularly (into muscle tissue, which is richly supplied with blood vessels), or intravenously (directly into a vein). **Intravenous** (IV) injection gets the drug into the bloodstream immediately (within seconds in most cases); **intramuscular** injection, moderately fast (within a few minutes); and **subcutaneous** injection, more slowly (within ten minutes).

Approximately 1.5 million Americans use illegal injected drugs. This practice is extremely dangerous because many diseases, including hepatitis and infection with human immune deficiency virus (HIV), can be transmitted by sharing contaminated needles. Injection-drug users who are HIV-positive are the chief source of transmission of HIV among heterosexuals. (See Chapter 9 for more on HIV infection and AIDS.)

## Dosage and Toxicity

The effects of any drug depend on the amount an individual takes. Increasing the dose usually intensifies the effects produced by smaller doses. Also, the kind of effect may change at different dose levels. For example, low doses of barbiturates may relieve anxiety, while higher doses can induce sleep, loss of sensation, even coma and death.

The dosage level at which a drug becomes poisonous to the body, causing either temporary or permanent damage, is called its **toxicity**. In most cases, drugs are eventually broken down in the liver by special body chemicals called *detoxification enzymes*.

## Individual Differences

Each person responds differently to different drugs, depending on circumstances or setting. The enzymes in the body reduce the levels of drugs in the bloodstream; because there can be 80 variants of each enzyme, every person's body may react differently.

Often drugs intensify the emotional state of a person. If you're feeling depressed, a drug may make you feel more depressed. A generalized physical problem, such as having the flu, may make your body more vulnerable to the effects of a drug. Genetic differences among individuals may account for varying reactions.

Personality and psychological attitude also play a role in drug effects, so that one person may have a frighteningly bad trip on the same LSD dosage on which another person has a positive experience. To a certain extent, this depends on each user's *mind-set*—his or her expectations or preconceptions about using the drug. Someone who snorts cocaine to enhance sexual pleasure may feel more stimulated simply because that's what he or she expects.

# Medications

Many of the medications and pharmaceutical products available in this country do indeed relieve symptoms and help cure various illnesses. However, improper use of medications leads to more than 170,000 hospitalizations and costs of about $750 million every year. Because drugs are powerful, it's important to know how to use them appropriately.

### ???? What Should I Know About Buying Over-the-Counter Drugs?

More than half a million health products—remedies for everything from bad breath to bunions—are readily available without a doctor's prescription. This doesn't mean that they're necessarily safe or effective. Indeed, many widely used **over-the-counter (OTC) drugs** pose unsuspected hazards.

Among the most potentially dangerous is aspirin, the "wonder drug" in practically everyone's home pharmacy. When taken by someone who's been drinking (often to prevent or relieve hangover symptoms), for instance, aspirin increases blood-alcohol concentrations (see Chapter 12). Along with other nonsteroidal anti-inflammatory drugs, such as ibuprofen (brand names include Advil and Nuprin), aspirin can damage the lining of the stomach and lead to ulcers in those who take large daily doses for arthritis or other problems. Kidney problems have also been traced to some pain relievers including acetaminophen (Tylenol). Some health products that aren't even considered true drugs can also cause problems. Many Americans take food supplements, even though the Food

and Drug Administration (FDA) has never approved their use for any medical disorder.

A growing number of drugs that once were available only with a doctor's prescription can now be bought over the counter. These include Gyne-Lotrimin and Monistat, which combat vaginal yeast infections, and famotidine (sold as Pepcid AC) and cimetidine (sold as Tagamet), which offer an alternative to antacids for people suffering from heartburn and acid indigestion. For consumers, the advantages of this greater availability include lower prices and fewer visits to the doctor. The disadvantages, however, are the risks of misdiagnosing a problem and misusing or overusing medications.

Like other drugs, OTC medications can be used improperly, often simply because of a lack of education about proper use. Among those most often misused are the following:

✔ **Nasal sprays.** Nasal sprays relieve congestion by shrinking blood vessels in the nose. If they are used too often or for too many days in a row, however, the blood vessels widen instead of contracting, and the surrounding tissues become swollen, causing more congestion. To make the vessels shrink again, many people use more spray more often. The result can be permanent damage to nasal membranes, bleeding, infection, and partial or complete loss of smell.

✔ **Laxatives.** Believing that they must have one bowel movement a day (a common misconception), many people rely on laxatives. Brands that contain phenolphthalein irritate the lining of the intestines and cause muscles to contract or tighten, often making constipation worse rather than better. Bulk laxatives are less dangerous, but regular use is not advised. A high-fiber diet and more exercise are safer and more effective remedies for constipation.

✔ **Eye drops.** Eye drops make the blood vessels of the eye contract. However, as in the case of nasal sprays, with overuse (several times a day for several weeks), the blood vessels expand, making the eye look redder than before.

✔ **Sleep aids.** Although over-the-counter sleeping pills are widely used, there has been little research on their use and possible risks.

✔ **Cough syrup.** Chugging cough syrup (also called *roboing,* after the over-the-counter medication Robitussin) is a growing problem, in part because young people think of dextromethorphan (DXM), a common ingredient in cough medicine, as a "poor man's version" of the popular drug ecstasy.[3]

## Prescription Drugs

Medications are a big business in this country. However, the latest, most expensive drugs aren't necessarily the best. Each year the FDA approves about 20 new drugs, yet no more than 4 are rated as truly meaningful advances. The others often are no better or worse than what's already on the market. (For tips on using prescription drugs, see Savvy Consumer: "Getting the Most Out of Medications.")

 College students, like other consumers, often take medicines, particularly nonprescription pain pills, without discussing them with their physician. Both doctors and patients make mistakes when it comes to prescription drugs. The most frequent mistakes doctors make are over- or under-dosing, omitting information from prescriptions, ordering the wrong dosage form (a pill instead of a liquid, for example), and not recognizing a patient's allergy to a drug.

## Nonadherence

Many prescribed medications aren't taken the way they should be; millions simply aren't taken at all. As many as 70 percent of adults have trouble understanding dosage information and 30 percent can't read standard labels, according to the FDA, which has called for larger, clearer drug labeling. The dangers of nonadherence (not properly taking prescription drugs) include recurrent infections, serious medical complications, and emergency hospital treatment. The drugs most likely to be taken incorrectly are those that treat problems with no obvious symptoms (such as high blood pressure), that require complex dosage schedules, that treat psychiatric disorders, or that have unpleasant side effects.

Some people skip prescribed doses or stop taking medications because they fear that any drug can cause tolerance and eventual dependence. Others fail to let doctors know about side effects. For instance, patients may stop taking anti-inflammatory drugs because they irritate their stomach. However, taking the drugs with food can eliminate this problem. The side effects of other drugs may disappear as the person's body becomes accustomed to the drug.

## Physical Side Effects

Most medications, taken correctly, cause only minor complications. However, no drug is entirely without side effects for all individuals taking it. Serious complications that may occur include heart failure, heart attack, seizures, kidney and liver failure, severe blood disorders, birth defects, blindness, memory problems, and allergic reactions.

Allergic reactions to drugs are common. The drugs that most often provoke allergic responses are penicillin and other antibiotics (drugs used to treat infection). Aspirin, sulfa drugs, barbiturates, anticonvulsants, insulin, and local anesthetics can also provoke allergic responses. Allergic reactions range from mild rashes or hives to anaphylaxis—a life-threatening constriction of the airways and sudden drop of blood pressure that causes rapid pulse, weakness, paleness, confusion, nausea, vomiting, unconsciousness, and collapse. This extreme response, which is rare, requires immediate treatment with an injection of

## *Savvy* Consumer

### Getting the Most Out of Medications

Before you leave with a prescription, be sure to ask the following questions:

- What is the name of the drug?
- What's it supposed to do?
- How and when do I take it? For how long?
- What foods, drinks, other medications, or activities should I avoid while taking this drug?
- Are there any side effects? What do I do if they occur?
- What written information is available on this drug?
- How should I store my prescriptions? (A hot, damp bathroom medicine chest is often the worst place.)
- Are there other, possibly cheaper alternatives? Why do you recommend this particular drug?

- Are there nondrug alternatives, such as using a vaporizer, gargling with salt water, and drinking plenty of liquids for a viral infection; or losing weight and exercising to lower blood pressure?

If you're taking a medication, tell your doctor if you plan to change your diet significantly—cutting calories or fat, stopping or starting vitamin supplements, or changing the amount of fiber you consume.

Don't keep old medications (discard after the expiration date). Don't take drugs prescribed for someone else unless your doctor tells you to. Keep medications out of the reach of small children.

Have all prescriptions filled at the same pharmacy, and ask your pharmacist to keep a record of your medications to avoid hazardous interactions.

epinephrine (adrenaline) to open the airways and blood vessels.

## Psychological Side Effects

Dozens of drugs—both over-the-counter and prescription—can cause changes in the way people think, feel, and behave. Unfortunately, neither patients nor their physicians usually connect such symptoms with medications. Doctors may not even mention potential mental and emotional problems because they don't want to scare patients away from what otherwise may be a very effective treatment. What you don't know about a drug's effects on your mind *can* hurt you.

Among the medications most likely to cause psychiatric side effects are drugs for high blood pressure, heart disease, asthma, epilepsy, arthritis, Parkinson's disease, anxiety, insomnia, and depression. Some drugs—such as the powerful hormones called *corticosteroids,* used for asthma, autoimmune diseases, and cancer—can cause different psychiatric symptoms, depending on dosage and other factors. Other drugs, such as ulcer medications, can cause delirium and disorientation, especially when given in high doses or to elderly patients. More subtle problems, such as forgetfulness or irritability, are common reactions to many drugs that are likely to be ignored or dismissed. The older you are, the sicker you are, and the more medications you're taking, the greater your risk of developing some psychiatric side effects. Even medications that don't usually cause problems, such as antibiotics, can cause psychiatric side effects in some individuals.

Any medication that slows down bodily systems, as many high blood pressure and cardiac drugs do, can cause depressive symptoms. Estrogen in birth control pills can cause mood changes. As many as 15 percent of women using oral contraceptives have reported feeling depressed or moody. For many people, switching to another medication quickly lifts a drug-induced depression.

All drugs that stimulate or speed up the central nervous system can cause agitation and anxiety—including the almost 200 allergy, cold, and congestion remedies containing pseudoephedrine hydrochloride (Sudafed). Other common culprits in inducing anxiety are caffeine and theophylline, a chemical relative of caffeine found in many medications for asthma and other respiratory problems. These drugs act like mild amphetamines in the body, making people feel hyper and restless.

## Drug Interactions

OTC and prescription drugs can interact in a variety of ways. For example, mixing some cold medications with tranquilizers can cause drowsiness and coordination problems, thus making driving dangerous. Moreover, what you eat or drink can impair or completely wipe out the effectiveness of drugs or lead to unexpected effects on the body. For instance, aspirin takes five to ten times as long to be absorbed when taken with food or shortly after a meal than when taken on an empty stomach. If tetracyclines encounter calcium in the stomach, they bind together and cancel each other out.

To avoid potentially dangerous interactions, check the label(s) for any instructions on how or when to take a medication, such as "with a meal." If the directions say that you should take a drug on an empty stomach, take it at least one hour before eating or two or three hours after eating. Don't drink a hot beverage with a medication; the temperature may interfere with the effectiveness of the drug. Don't open, crush, or dissolve tablets or capsules without checking first with your physician or pharmacist.

Whenever you take a drug, be especially careful of your intake of alcohol, which can change the rate of metabolism and the effects of many different drugs. Because it dilates the blood vessels, alcohol can add to the dizziness sometimes caused by drugs for high blood pressure, angina, or depression. Also, its irritating effects on the stomach can worsen stomach upset from aspirin, ibuprofen, and other anti-inflammatory drugs.

## Caffeine Use and Misuse

Caffeine, which has been drunk, chewed, and swallowed since the Stone Age, is the most widely used **psychotropic** (mind-affecting) drug in the world. Eighty percent of Americans drink coffee, our principal caffeine source—an average of 3.5 cups a day. Coffee contains 100 to 150 milligrams of caffeine per cup; tea, 40 to 100 milligrams; cola, about 45 milligrams. Most medications that contain caffeine are one-third to one-half the strength of a cup of coffee. However, some, such as Excedrin, are very high in caffeine. (See Table 11-1.)

The effects of caffeine vary. As a **stimulant,** it relieves drowsiness, helps in the performance of repetitive tasks, and improves the capacity for work. Some athletes feel that caffeine gives them an extra boost that allows them to go farther and longer in endurance events. Consumption of high doses of caffeine can lead to dependence, anxiety, insomnia, rapid breathing, upset stomach and bowels, and dizziness.

In a study of college men and women who normally consumed fewer than three caffeinated beverages per day, caffeine boosted anxiety but did not significantly affect performance on various low-intensity tasks, except for hand-eye coordination, which improved.[4]

Although there is no conclusive proof that caffeine causes birth defects, it does cross the placenta into the tissues of a growing fetus. Because of an increased risk of

| ▼ Table 11-1 Caffeine Counts | |
|---|---|
| Substance (typical serving) | Caffeine (milligrams) |
| No Doz, one pill | 200 |
| Coffee (drip), one 5-ounce cup | 130 |
| Excedrin, two pills | 130 |
| Espresso, one 2-ounce cup | 100 |
| Instant coffee, one 5-ounce cup | 74 |
| Coca-Cola, 12 ounces | 46 |
| Tea, one 5-ounce cup | 40 |
| Dark chocolate, 1 ounce | 20 |
| Milk chocolate, 1 ounce | 6 |
| Cocoa, 5 ounces | 4 |
| Decaffeinated coffee, one 5-ounce cup | 3 |

miscarriage, the U.S. surgeon general has recommended that pregnant women avoid or restrict their caffeine intake. Some fertility specialists also have urged couples trying to conceive to reduce caffeine to increase their chance of success. Women who are heavy caffeine users tend to have shorter menstrual cycles than nonusers. A recent analysis drawing upon data from the ongoing Nurses Health Study found that moderate amounts of coffee may protect women from Parkinson's disease.[5]

# Substance Use Disorders

People have been using **psychoactive** (mood-altering) chemicals for centuries. Citizens of ancient Mesopotamia

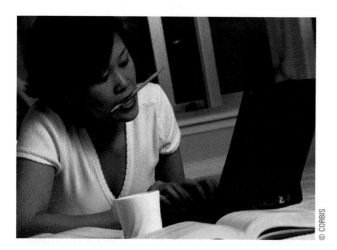

▲ Coffee and work often go hand in hand, but too much caffeine can lead to dependence, anxiety, and other problems.

© CORBIS

and Egypt used opium. More than 3,000 years ago, Hindus included cannabis in religious ceremonies. For centuries the Inca in South America have chewed the leaves of the coca bush. Although drugs existed in most ancient societies, their use was usually limited to small groups. Today millions of people regularly turn to drugs to pick them up, bring them down, alter perceptions, or ease psychological pain.

Both men and women are vulnerable to substance use disorders, although they tend to have different patterns of drug use. (See The X & Y Files: "Men, Women, and Drugs.") The 1960s ushered in an explosive increase in drug use and in the number of drug users in our society. Marijuana use soared in the 1960s and 1970s; cocaine, in the 1980s. In 1986, crack—a cheap, smokeable form of cocaine—hit the streets of the United States, and the number of regular cocaine users zoomed. By the twenty-first century, club drugs, such as ecstasy (MDMA), were growing in popularity.[6]

The word **addiction,** as used by the general population, refers to the compulsive use of a substance, loss of control, negative consequences, and denial. Mental health professionals describe drug-related problems in terms of *dependence* and *abuse.*

## Dependence

Individuals may develop **psychological dependence** and feel a strong craving for a drug because it produces pleasurable feelings or relieves stress and anxiety. **Physical dependence** occurs when a person develops *tolerance* to the effects of a drug and needs larger and larger doses to achieve intoxication or another desired effect. Individuals who are physically dependent and have a high tolerance to a drug may take amounts many times those that would produce intoxication or an overdose in someone who was not a regular user.

Men and women with a substance dependence disorder may use a drug to avoid or relieve withdrawal symptoms, or they may consume larger amounts of a drug or use it over a longer period than they'd originally intended. They may repeatedly try to cut down or control drug use without success; spend a great deal of time obtaining or using drugs or recovering from their effects; give up or reduce important social, occupational, or recreational activities because of their drug use; or continue to use a drug despite knowledge that the drug is likely to cause or worsen a persistent or recurring physical or psychological problem.

Specific symptoms of dependence vary with particular drugs. Some drugs, such as marijuana, hallucinogens, and phencyclidine, do not cause withdrawal symptoms. The degree of dependence also varies. In mild cases, a person may function normally most of the time. In severe cases,

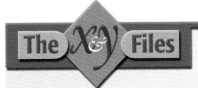

## Men, Women, and Drugs

Beginning at a very early age, males and females show different patterns in drug use. Among 12-year-olds who have been offered drugs, boys are more likely to have received those offers from other males or their parents. Girls are most likely to have been offered drugs by a female friend or family member. The social setting and nature of drug offers also differ by gender. Boys are more likely to receive offers in a public setting, such as on the street or in a park, and the offers typically emphasize "benefits," such as improved status or self-image. Girls are more likely to receive a straightforward "do you want some?" offer or one that minimizes the risks of drug use. For girls, these offers are usually made in a private setting such as a friend's home.

Later in life men generally encounter more opportunities to use drugs than women, but given an opportunity to use drugs for the first time, both genders are equally likely to do so and to progress from initial use to dependence. Vulnerability to some drugs varies with gender. Both are equally likely to become addicted to or dependent on cocaine, heroin, hallucinogens, tobacco, and inhalants. Women are more likely than men to become addicted to or dependent on sedatives and drugs designed to treat anxiety or sleeplessness, and less likely than men to abuse alcohol and marijuana.

Males and females may differ in their biological responses to drugs. In studies of animals given the opportunity to self-administer intravenous doses of cocaine or heroin, females began self-administration sooner than males and administered larger amounts of the drugs. Women may be more sensitive than men to the cardiovascular effects of cocaine. In human studies, women and men given equal doses of cocaine experienced the same cardiovascular response despite the fact that blood concentrations of cocaine did not rise as high in women as in men. Male and female long-term cocaine users showed similar impairment in tests of concentration, memory, and academic achievement following sustained abstinence, even though women in the study had substantially greater exposure to cocaine. Women cocaine users also were less likely than men to exhibit abnormalities of blood flow in the brain's frontal lobes. These findings suggest a gender-related mechanism that may protect women from some of the damage cocaine inflicts on the brain. However, women are more vulnerable to poor nutrition and below-average weight, depression, physical abuse, and if pregnant, preterm labor or early delivery.

Substance abuse compounds the risk of AIDS for women, who may become infected with HIV by sharing needles with other injection-drug users and by engaging in unprotected sex. In all, drug abuse is nearly twice as likely to be directly or indirectly associated with AIDS in women (66 percent) as in men (34 percent).

There are also differences between men and women who seek treatment for drug abuse. Women in treatment programs are less likely than men to have graduated from high school and to be employed, and are more likely than men to have other health problems, to have sought previous drug treatment, to have attempted suicide, and to have suffered sexual abuse or other physical abuse. Traditional drug treatment programs, created for men, have proven to be less effective for women than programs that provide more comprehensive services, including child care, assertiveness training, and parenting training.

---

the person's entire life may revolve around obtaining, using, and recuperating from the effects of a drug.

Individuals with drug dependence become intoxicated or high on a regular basis—whether every day, every weekend, or several binges a year. They may try repeatedly to stop using a drug and yet fail, even though they realize their drug use is interfering with their health, family life, relationships, and work.

## Abuse

Some drug users do not develop the symptoms of tolerance and withdrawal that characterize dependence, yet they use drugs in ways that clearly have a harmful effect on them. These individuals are diagnosed as having a *psychoactive*

*substance abuse disorder.* They continue to use drugs despite their awareness of persistent or repeated social, occupational, psychological, or physical problems related to drug use, or they use drugs in dangerous ways or situations (before driving, for instance).

## Intoxication and Withdrawal

**Intoxication** refers to maladaptive behavioral, psychological, and physiologic changes that occur as a result of substance use. **Withdrawal** is the development of symptoms that cause significant psychological and physical distress when an individual reduces or stops drug use. (Intoxication and withdrawal from specific drugs are discussed later in this chapter.)

## Polyabuse

Most users prefer a certain type of drug but also use several others; this behavior is called **polyabuse.** The average user who enters treatment is on five different drugs. The more drugs anyone uses, the greater the chance of side effects, complications, and possibly life-threatening interactions.

## Coexisting Conditions

Mental disorders and substance abuse disorders have a great deal of overlap. "A little more than a third of those with a psychiatric disorder also have a chemical dependency problem, and a little more than a third of those with a chemical dependency problem have a psychiatric disorder," notes psychiatrist Richard Frances, M.D., founding president of the American Association of Addiction Psychiatry.[7] Individuals with such *dual diagnoses* require careful evaluation and appropriate treatment for the complete range of complex and chronic difficulties they face.

## What Causes Drug Dependence and Abuse?

No one fully understands why some people develop drug dependence or abuse disorders, whereas others, who may experiment briefly with drugs, do not. Inherited body chemistry, genetic factors, and sensitivity to drugs may make some individuals more susceptible. These disorders may stem from many complex causes.

## Biology of Dependence

Scientists now view drug dependence as a brain disease triggered by frequent use of drugs that change the biochemistry and anatomy of neurons and alter the way they work.[8] A major breakthrough in understanding dependence has been the discovery that certain mood-altering substances and experiences—a puff of marijuana, a slug of whiskey, a snort of cocaine, a big win at blackjack—trigger a rise in a brain chemical called *dopamine,* which is associated with feelings of satisfaction and euphoria. This brain chemical or neurotransmitter, one of the crucial messengers that links nerve cells in the brain, rises during any pleasurable experience, whether it be a loving hug or a taste of chocolate.

Addictive drugs have such a powerful impact on dopamine and its receptors (its connecting cells) that they change the pathways within the brain's pleasure centers. (See Figure 11-2.) Various psychoactive chemicals create a craving for more of the same. According to this hypothesis, addicts do not specifically yearn for heroin, cocaine, or nico-

### STRATEGIES FOR PREVENTION

#### Saying No to Drugs

If people offer you a drug, here are some ways to say no:

▲ Let them know you're not interested. Change the subject. If the pressure seems threatening, just walk away.

▲ Have something else to do: "No, I'm going for a walk now."

▲ Be prepared for different types of pressure. If your friends tease you, tease them back.

▲ Keep it simple. "No, thanks," "No," or "No way" all get the point across.

▲ Hang out with people who won't offer you drugs.

tine but for the rush of dopamine that these drugs produce. Other brain chemicals, including glutamate, GABA (gamma-aminobutyric acid) and possibly norepinephrine, may also be involved. Some individuals, born with low levels of dopamine, may be particularly susceptible to addiction.

## Other Routes of Addiction

Although scientists do not believe there is an addictive personality, certain individuals are at greater risk of drug dependence because of psychological factors, including difficulty controlling impulses, a lack of values that might constrain drug use (whether based in religion, family, or society), low self-esteem, feelings of powerlessness, and depression. The one psychological trait most often linked with drug use is denial. Young people in particular are absolutely convinced that they will never lose control or suffer in any way as a result of drug use.

Many diagnosed drug users have at least one mental disorder, particularly depression or anxiety. Disorders that emerge in adolescence, such as bipolar disorder, may increase the risk of substance abuse. Many people with psychiatric disorders abuse drugs. Individuals may self-administer drugs to treat psychiatric symptoms; for example, they may take sedating drugs to suppress a panic attack.

Individuals who are isolated from friends and family, or who live in communities where drugs are widely used (such as poor inner-city areas), have higher rates of drug abuse. Young people from lower socioeconomic back-

**NORMAL STATE**

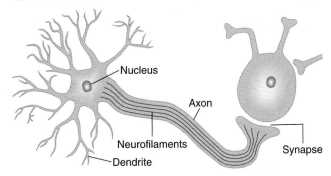

**DRUG-DEPENDENT STATE**

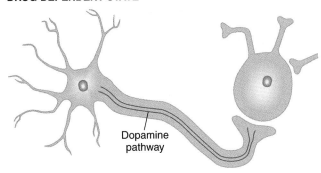

**AFFECTED AREAS
OF THE BRAIN**

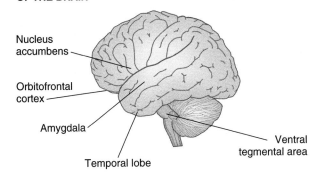

▲ **Figure 11-2** The Nervous System on Drugs
Repeated drug doses overload normal neurotransmitter systems in nerve cells. The cells compensate by becoming smaller, thereby making dopamine less effective. When doses stop, craving ensues.

Source: *The Neuroscientist.*

grounds are more likely to use drugs than their more affluent peers, possibly because of economic disadvantage; family instability; a lack of realistic, rewarding alternatives and role models; and increased hopelessness.

Those whose companions are substance abusers are far more likely to use drugs. Peer pressure to use drugs can be a powerful factor for adolescents and young adults. The likelihood of drug abuse is also related to family instability, parental rejection, and divorce.

When researchers followed families for a decade and a half and interviewed both children and their mothers, they found that youngsters who felt attached to their parents and showed greater responsibility and less rebelliousness were less likely to use drugs. Their attitudes and behaviors insulated them from socializing with drug-using peers, resulting in less drug use in their early and late twenties.[9] Clear rules and expectations from parents also can go a long way toward preventing or delaying alcohol and marijuana use in children, even if there is tension in the parent-child relationship.[10]

Parents' own attitudes and drug-use history affect their children's likelihood of using marijuana, according to the Substance Abuse and Mental Health Services Administration. Parents who perceived little risk associated with marijuana use had children with similar attitudes, and the children of parents who had used marijuana were about three times more likely to try the drug than children whose parents had never used the drug.[11]

Drugs like crack cocaine that produce an intense, brief high lead to dependence more quickly than slower-acting agents like cocaine powder. Drugs that cause uncomfortable withdrawal symptoms, such as barbiturates, may lead to continued use to avoid such discomfort.

Drug use involves certain behaviors, situations, and settings that users may, in time, associate with getting high. Even after long periods of abstinence, some former drug users find that they crave drugs when they return to a site of drug use or meet people with whom they used drugs. Former cocaine users report that the sight of white powder alone can serve as a cue that triggers a craving.

Most individuals who use drugs first try them as adolescents. Teens are likely to begin experimenting with tobacco, beer, wine, or hard liquor, then smoke marijuana or sniff inhalants. Teens who smoke cigarettes are more likely to use drugs and to drink heavily than nonsmoking youths. Some then go on to try sedative-hypnotics, stimulants (including cocaine), and hallucinogens such as LSD. A much smaller percentage of teens try the opioids. Over time some individuals give up certain drugs, such as hallucinogens, and return to old favorites, such as alcohol and marijuana. A smaller number continues using several drugs.

## The Toll of Drugs

Drugs affect a person's physical, psychological, and social health. The effects of drugs can be *acute* (resulting from a single dose or series of doses) or *chronic* (resulting from long-term use). Acute effects vary with different drugs. Stimulants may trigger unpredictable rage; an overdose of heroin may lead to respiratory depression, a breathing impairment that can be fatal.

Over time, chronic drug users may feel fatigued, cough constantly, lose weight, become malnourished, and ache from head to toe. They may suffer blackouts, flashbacks, and episodes of increasingly bizarre behavior, often triggered by escalating paranoia. Their risk of overdose rises steadily, and they must live with constant stress: the fear of getting busted for possession or of losing a job if they test positive for drugs, the worry of getting enough money for their next fix, the dangers of associating with dealers and other users.

The toll of drug use can be especially great on the young because it disrupts many critical developmental tasks of adolescence and young adulthood. Early use of drugs can lead to drug-related crime (including stealing), poor achievement in high school or college, and job instability.

## How Common Is Drug Use on Campus?

Alcohol is the number-one drug of abuse on college campuses. Marijuana remains the most commonly used illegal drug.[12] (See Student Snapshot: "Illegal Drug Use by Undergraduates.") However, there is a large gap between actual drug use on campus and how prevalent students believe drug use to be. When researchers compared students' self-reports of frequency of drug use with what students perceived to be the frequency of drug use by "the average student," they found that students greatly overestimate the use of a variety of drugs.[13]

Various factors influence which students use drugs, including the following:

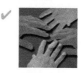

✔ **Race/ethnicity.** In general, white students have higher levels of alcohol and drug use than African-American students. In a comparison of African-American students at predominantly white and predominantly black colleges, those at historically black colleges had lower rates of alcohol and drug use than either white or African-American students at white schools. The reason, according to the researchers, may be that these colleges provide a greater sense of self-esteem, which helps prevent alcohol and drug use.

✔ **Perception of risk.** Students seem most likely to try substances they perceive as being safe or low risk. Of these, the top three are caffeine, alcohol, and tobacco;

### Student Snapshot — Illegal Drug Use by Undergraduates

| Drug | Undergraduates reporting current use | Undergraduates reporting lifetime use |
|---|---|---|
| Marijuana | 17% | 43% |
| Cocaine | 1% | 7% |
| Other illegal drugs (ecstasy, LSD, PCP, etc.) | 3% | 16% |

Source: Jones, Sherry, et al. "Binge Drinking Among Undergraduate College Students in the United States: Implications for Other Substance Use." *Journal of American College Health*, Vol. 50, No. 1, July 2001, p. 33.

marijuana is listed fourth in terms of perceived safety. Other agents—barbiturates, heroin, cocaine, PCP, speed, LSD, crack, and inhalants—are viewed as about equally risky and are used much less often.

✔ **Alcohol use.** Individuals often engage in more than one risk behavior, and researchers have documented correlations among smoking, drinking, and drug use. Among college students, those who report binge drinking (discussed in depth in Chapter 12) are much more likely than other students to report current or past use of marijuana, cocaine, or other illegal drugs.[14]

✔ **Environment.** As with alcohol use, students are influenced by their friends, their residence, the general public's attitude toward drug use, and even the Internet. Increasingly, college health officials are realizing that, rather than simply trying to change students' substance abuse, they also must change the environment to promote healthier lifestyle choices. One successful innovation is substance-free dorms.[15]

## Drugs and Driving

One important impact of drugs is their effect on driving ability. Alcohol and drug use are equally common in drivers injured in traffic accidents. Often drivers using alcohol also test positive for other drugs. Different drugs affect driving ability in different ways. Here are the facts from the National Institute on Drug Abuse:

✔ Alcohol affects perception, coordination, and judgment, and increases the sedative effects of tranquilizers and barbiturates.

✔ Marijuana affects a wide range of driving skills—including the ability to track (stay in the lane) through curves, brake quickly, and maintain speed and a safe distance between cars—and slows thinking and reflexes. Normal driving skills remain impaired for four to six hours after smoking a single joint.

✔ Sedatives, hypnotics, and antianxiety agents slow reaction time, and interfere with hand–eye coordination and judgment. The greatest impairment is in the first hour after taking the drug. The effects depend on the particular drug: Some build up in the body and can impair driving skills the morning after use; others make drivers very sleepy and, therefore, incapable of driving safely.

✔ Amphetamines, after repeated use, impair coordination. They can also make a driver more edgy and less coordinated, and thus more likely to be involved in an accident.

✔ Hallucinogens distort judgment and reality, and cause confusion and panic, thus making driving extremely dangerous.

# Common Drugs of Abuse

The psychoactive substances most often associated with both abuse and dependence include alcohol (discussed in Chapter 12), amphetamines, cannabis (marijuana), cocaine, club drugs, hallucinogens, inhalants, opioids, phencyclidine (PCP), and sedative-hypnotic drugs. Table 11-2 groups the common drugs of abuse by their effect on the mind.

## Amphetamines

**Amphetamines,** stimulants that were once widely prescribed for weight control because they suppress appetite, have emerged as a global danger. They trigger the release of epinephrine (adrenaline), which stimulates the central nervous system. Amphetamines are sold under a variety of names: amphetamine (brand name Benzedrine, street-name bennies), dextroamphetamine (Dexedrine, dex), methamphetamine (Methedrine, meth, speed), and Desoxyn (copilots). Related *uppers* include the prescription drugs methylphenidate (Ritalin), pemoline (Cylert), and phenmetrazine (Preludin).

Amphetamines are available in tablet or capsule form. Abusers may grind and sniff the capsules, or make a solution and inject the drug. *Ice* is a smokeable form of methamphetamine that is highly addictive and produces an intense physical and psychological high that can last from four to fourteen hours. *Crank* is the street term for another central nervous system stimulant, propylexedrine, which is less potent than amphetamine. Abusers often extract the drug from the cotton plug of decongestant inhalants and inject it intravenously.

### How Users Feel

Amphetamines produce a state of hyper-alertness and energy. Users feel confident in their ability to think clearly and to perform any task exceptionally well—although amphetamines do not, in fact, significantly boost performance or thinking. Higher doses make users feel *wired:* talkative, excited, restless, irritable, anxious, moody.

If taken intravenously, amphetamines produce a characteristic rush of elation and confidence, as well as adverse effects, including confusion, rambling or incoherent speech, anxiety, headache, and palpitations. Individuals may become paranoid; be convinced they are having profound thoughts; feel increased sexual interest; and experience unusual perceptions, such as ringing in the ears, a sensation of insects crawling on their skin, or hearing their name called. Crank users may feel high and sleepy or may hallucinate and lose contact with reality. Methamphetamine,

▼ **Table 11-2 Common Drugs of Abuse**

| Type of Drug | Drug Name | Street Name | Description | How It's Used | Related Paraphernalia | Signs and Symptoms of Use |
|---|---|---|---|---|---|---|
| **Cannabis** | **Marijuana** | Pot, grass, reefer, weed, Colombian hash, sinsemilla, joint, blunts, Acapulco gold, Thai sticks | Like dried oregano leaves, dark green or brown | Usually smoked in hand-rolled cigarettes, pipes, or thin cigars, or eaten | Rolling papers, pipes, bongs, baggies, roach clips | Sweet burnt odor, neglect of appearance, loss of motivation, slow reactions, red eyes, memory lapses |
| **Depressants** (Depress the nervous system) | **Alcohol** | Booze, hooch, juice, brew, alcopops (hard lemonade or fruit juices) | Clear or amber-colored liquid; sweet, fruit-flavored malt-based drinks | Swallowed in liquid form | Flask, bottles, cans, use of food color to disguise it; colorful and innocent-looking labels | Impaired judgment, poor muscle coordination, lowered inhibitions |
| | **Barbiturates** Amyl, Seconal, Nembutal, Butisol, Tuinal | Barbs, downers, yellow jackets, red devils, blue devils | Variety of tablets, capsules, powder | Swallowed in pill form or injected into the veins | Syringe, needles | Drowsiness, confusion, impaired judgment, slurred speech, needle marks, staggering gait |
| | **Tranquilizers/ Benzodiazepines** Valium, Librium, Miltown, Xanax | V's, blues, downers, candy | Variety of tablets | Swallowed in pill form or injected | Syringe, pill bottles, needles | Drowsiness, faulty judgment, disorientation |
| | **Narcotics/ Opioids** heroin, morphine | Dreamer, junk, smack, horse | White or brown powders, tablets, capsules, liquid | Injected, smoked, may be blended with marijuana | Syringes, spoon, lighter, needles, medicine dropper | Lethargy, loss of skin color, needle marks, constricted pupils, decreased coordination |
| **Stimulants** (Stimulate the nervous system) | **Amphetamines** amphetamine, dextroamphetamine methamphetamine | Speed, uppers, pep pill, bennies, dexies, meth, crank, crystal, black beauties, white crosses | Variety of tablets, capsules, and crystal-like rock salt | Swallowed in pill or capsule form, or injected | Syringe, needles | Excess activity, irritability, nervousness, mood swings, needle marks, dilated pupils, talkativeness then depression |
| | **Methylphenidate** | Ritalin, MDMA (ecstasy) | Tablets, imprinted logos | Crushed and sniffed | Razor blade, straws, glass surfaces | Increased alertness, excitation, insomnia, loss of appetite |
| | **Cocaine** | Coke, snow, toot, white lady | White odorless powder | Usually inhaled; can be injected, swallowed, or smoked | Razor blade, straws, glass surfaces | Restlessness, dilated pupils, oily skin, talkativeness; euphoric short-term high, followed by depression |
| | **Tobacco/ Nicotine** | Smokes, butts, cigs, cancer sticks, snuff, dip, chew, plug | Dried brown organic material, bidis flavored with mint or chocolate; smokeless is moist | Burned and inhaled as cigarettes, pipes, cigars, cigarillos; chewed; or inhaled through the nose as snuff. | Rolling papers, pipes, spit cups, cigar cutters, lighters, matches | Shortness of breath, respiratory illnesses; oral, lung, and other cancers |

## ▼ Table 11-2 Common Drugs of Abuse

| Type of Drug | Drug Name | Street Name | Description | How It's Used | Related Paraphernalia | Signs and Symptoms of Use |
|---|---|---|---|---|---|---|
| **Hallucinogens** (Alter perceptions of reality) | **PCP** (Phencyclidine) | Angel dust, killer weed, supergrass, hog, peace pill | White powder or tablet | Usually smoked, can be inhaled (snorted), injected, or swallowed in tablets | Tinfoil | Slurred speech, blurred vision, lack of coordination, confusion, agitation, violence, unpredictability, "bad trips" |
| | **LSD** (Lysergic Acid Diethylamide) | Acid, cubes, purple haze, white lightning | Odorless, colorless, tasteless powder | Injected, or swallowed in tablets or capsules | Blotter papers, tinfoil | Dilated pupils, illusions, hallucinations, disorientation, mood swings, nausea, flashbacks |
| | **Mescaline** caps, psilocybin, psilocin, mushrooms | Mesc, cactus, caps, magic mushroom, shrooms | Capsules, tablets, mushrooms | Ingested in its natural form, smoked, or brewed as tea | Dried mushrooms | Same as LSD above |
| **Inhalants** (Substances abused by sniffing) | **Solvents, aerosols** airplane glue, gasoline, dry cleaning solution, correction fluid | | Chemicals that produce mind-altering vapors | Inhaled or sniffed, often with the use of paper or plastic bags | Cleaning rags, empty spray cans, tubes of glue, baggies | Poor motor coordination; bad breath; impaired vision, memory and thoughts; violent behavior |
| | **Nitrates** Amyl & Butyl | Poppers, locker room, rush, snappers | Clear yellowish liquid | Inhaled or sniffed from gauze or single-dose glass vials | Cloth-covered bulb that pops when broken, small bottles | Slowed thought, headache |
| | **Nitrous oxide** | Laughing gas, whippets | Colorless gas with sweet taste and smell | Inhaled or sniffed by mask or cone | Aerosol cans such as whipped cream, small canisters | Light-headed, loss of motor control |
| **Club Drugs/ Designer Drugs** (Stimulants, depressants, and/or hallucinogens) | **MDMA, MDA, MDEA** | Ecstasy, XTC, X, Adam, Clarity | Tablet or capsule; colorless, tasteless, and odorless | Swallowed, can be added to beverages by individuals who want to intoxicate others | Pacifiers, glow sticks (used at all-night dance parties, raves, or trances) | Agitated state, confusion, sleep problems, paranoia |
| | **Date-rape drug** Rohypnol | Roofies, roche, love drug, forget-me pill | Tasteless, odorless, dissolves easily in all beverages | Swallowed, can be added to beverages by individuals who want to sedate others | Drinks, soda cans | 1 milligram can impair a victim for 8 to 12 hours, can cause amnesia, decreased blood pressure, urinary retention |
| | **GHB** | Liquid Ecstasy, Grievous Bodily Harm, G | Clear liquid, tablet, capsule | Swallowed, dissolved in drinks | Drinks, soda cans | Can relax or sedate |

Source: "A Parent's Guide for the Prevention of Alcohol, Tobacco and Other Drug Use." Copyright © 2000 Lowe Family Foundation, Inc., Revised 2001. (Lowe Family Foundation, 3339 Stuyvesant Pl. NW, Washington DC, 20015, 202-362-4883.) Used with permission.

which produces a rapid high when inhaled, produces exceptionally long-lasting toxic effects, including psychosis, violence, seizures, and cardiovascular abnormalities. Brain-imaging studies show changes in heavy users' brains that may affect learning and memory for as long as a year.[16]

## Risks

Dependence on amphetamines can develop with episodic or daily use. Users typically take amphetamines in large doses to prevent crashing. Bingeing—taking high doses over a period of several days—can lead to an extremely intense and unpleasant crash characterized by a craving for the drug, shakiness, irritability, anxiety, and depression. Two or more days are required for recuperation.

Amphetamine intoxication may cause the following symptoms:

✔ Feelings of grandiosity, anxiety, tension, hypervigilance, anger, social hypersensitivity, fighting, jitteriness or agitation, paranoia, and impaired judgment in social or occupational functioning.

✔ Increased heart rate, dilated pupils, elevated blood pressure, perspiration or chills, and nausea or vomiting.

✔ Less frequent effects such as speeding up or slowing down of physical movement; muscular weakness; impaired breathing, chest pain, heart arrhythmia; confusion, seizures, impaired movements or muscle tone; or even coma.

✔ In high doses, a rapid or irregular heartbeat, tremors, loss of coordination, and collapse.

Smokeable methamphetamine, or ice, also increases heart rate and blood pressure; high doses can cause permanent damage to blood vessels in the brain. Other physical effects of methamphetamine include dilated pupils, blurred vision, dry mouth, and increased breathing rate. Prolonged use can cause fatal lung and kidney disorders. Injecting propylexedrine can lead to convulsions, strokes, and respiratory and kidney failure. Abusers also may develop infected veins, and if they share needles, they risk HIV infection.

The long-term effects of amphetamine abuse include malnutrition, skin disorders, ulcers, insomnia, depression, vitamin deficiencies, and, in some cases, brain damage that results in speech and thought disturbances. Sexual dysfunction and impaired concentration or memory also may occur.

## Withdrawal

When the immediate effects of amphetamines wear off, users experience a *crash*—they crave the drug and become shaky, irritable, anxious, and depressed. Amphetamine withdrawal usually persists for more than 24 hours after cessation of prolonged, heavy use. Its characteristic features include fatigue, disturbing dreams, much more or less than usual sleep, increased appetite, and speeding up or slowing down of physical movements. Those who are unable to sleep despite their exhaustion often take sedative-hypnotics (discussed later in this chapter) to help them rest, and may then become dependent on them as well as amphetamines. Symptoms usually reach a peak in two to four days, although depression and irritability may persist for months. Suicide is a major risk.

## Cannabis

**Marijuana** (pot) and **hashish** (hash)—the most widely used illegal drugs—are derived from the cannabis plant. The major psychoactive ingredient in both is *THC (delta-9-tetrahydrocannabinol)*. Nearly one of every three people in the United States over age 12 has tried marijuana at least once. After a decline in teen marijuana use in the late 1990s, surveys indicate a moderate increase in the years since.[17] Some 12 million Americans use cannabis; more than 1 million cannot control this use.

THC triggers a series of reactions in the brain that ultimately lead to the high that users experience when they smoke marijuana. Heredity influences an individual's response to marijuana. Identical male twins, who share all their genes, are more likely than fraternal male twins, who share only about half their genes, to report similar responses to marijuana use, indicating a genetic basis for their response.

Different types of marijuana have different percentages of THC. Because of careful cultivation, the strength of today's marijuana is much greater than that used in the 1970s; the physical and mental effects are therefore greater. Usually, marijuana is smoked in a joint (hand-rolled cigarette) or pipe; it may also be eaten as an ingredient in other foods (as when baked in brownies), though with a less predictable effect. The drug high is enhanced by holding the marijuana smoke in the lungs, and experienced smokers learn to hold the smoke for longer periods to increase the amount of drug diffused into the bloodstream. The circumstances in which marijuana is smoked, the communal aspects of its use, and the user's experience all can affect the way a marijuana-induced high feels.

Marijuana has been used therapeutically, primarily to ease the nausea of chemotherapy. A report from the Institute of Medicine (IOM) found "strong scientific evidence" that the active ingredients in marijuana (cannabinoids) are potentially effective in treating pain, nausea, and the severe weight loss associated with AIDS. Other studies have found that cannabinoids are more effective than conventional drugs in treating chemotherapy-related sickness, but there is no substantial proof of its effectiveness in easing pain.[18] The American Medical Association has rejected a proposal to endorse the medical use of marijuana under controlled circumstances.[19] Some jurisdictions, such as San Francisco, have legalized marijuana use for medical purposes.

## How Users Feel

In low to moderate doses, marijuana typically creates a mild sense of euphoria, a sense of slowed time (five minutes may feel like an hour), a dreamy sort of self-absorption, and some impairment in thinking and communicating. Users report heightened sensations of color, sound, and other stimuli, relaxation, and increased confidence. The sense of being *stoned* peaks within half an hour and usually lasts about three hours. Even when alterations in perception seem slight, as noted earlier, it is not safe to drive a car for

as long as four to six hours after smoking a single joint. Some users—particularly those smoking marijuana for the first time or taking a high dose in an unpleasant or unfamiliar setting—experience acute anxiety, which may be accompanied by a panicky fear of losing control. They may believe that their companions are ridiculing or threatening them and experience a panic attack, a state of intense terror.

The immediate physical effects of marijuana include increased pulse rate, bloodshot eyes, dry mouth and throat, slowed reaction times, impaired motor skills, increased appetite, and diminished short-term memory. (See Figure 11-3.) High doses reduce the ability to perceive and to react; all the reactions experienced with low doses are intensified, leading to sensory distortion and, in the case of hashish, vivid hallucinations and LSD-like psychedelic reactions. The drug remains in the body's fat cells 50 hours or more after use, so people may experience psychoactive

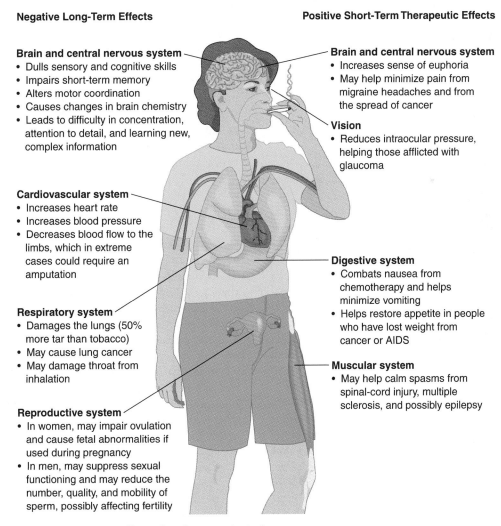

**Negative Long-Term Effects**

**Brain and central nervous system**
- Dulls sensory and cognitive skills
- Impairs short-term memory
- Alters motor coordination
- Causes changes in brain chemistry
- Leads to difficulty in concentration, attention to detail, and learning new, complex information

**Cardiovascular system**
- Increases heart rate
- Increases blood pressure
- Decreases blood flow to the limbs, which in extreme cases could require an amputation

**Respiratory system**
- Damages the lungs (50% more tar than tobacco)
- May cause lung cancer
- May damage throat from inhalation

**Reproductive system**
- In women, may impair ovulation and cause fetal abnormalities if used during pregnancy
- In men, may suppress sexual functioning and may reduce the number, quality, and mobility of sperm, possibly affecting fertility

**Positive Short-Term Therapeutic Effects**

**Brain and central nervous system**
- Increases sense of euphoria
- May help minimize pain from migraine headaches and from the spread of cancer

**Vision**
- Reduces intraocular pressure, helping those afflicted with glaucoma

**Digestive system**
- Combats nausea from chemotherapy and helps minimize vomiting
- Helps restore appetite in people who have lost weight from cancer or AIDS

**Muscular system**
- May help calm spasms from spinal-cord injury, multiple sclerosis, and possibly epilepsy

▲ **Figure 11-3** Some Effects of Marijuana on the Body
Some negative long-term effects and positive short-term therapeutic effects of marijuana use.

Source: *Time,* November 4, 2002.

effects for several days after use. Drug tests may produce positive results for days or weeks after last use.

## Risks

Marijuana produces a range of effects in different bodily systems, such as diminished immune responses and impaired fertility in men. Other risks include damage to the brain, lungs, and heart, and to babies born to mothers who use marijuana during pregnancy or while nursing. (See Figure 11-3.)

**Brain** THC produces changes in the brain that affect learning, memory, and the way the brain integrates sensory experiences with emotions and motivations. Short-term effects include problems with memory and learning; distorted perceptions; difficulty thinking and problem-solving; loss of coordination; increased anxiety; and panic attacks. Long-term use produces changes in the brain similar to those seen with other major drugs of abuse.[20]

 According to a study of college students, heavy marijuana use impairs critical skills related to attention, memory, and learning, even 24 hours after its use. Heavy users who smoked marijuana almost every day showed significant difficulty sustaining attention, shifting attention to meet the demands of changes in the environment, and registering, processing, and using information.[21]

Teenagers below college age who use marijuana have lower achievement than nonusers, more acceptance of illegal or socially deviant behavior, more aggression, greater rebelliousness, poorer relationships with parents, and more delinquent and drug-using friends. Those who regularly smoke marijuana often lose interest in school and do not remember what they learned when they were high. Some long-term regular users may experience *burnout,* a dulling of their senses and responses termed *amotivational syndrome.*

Over time, continued heavy marijuana use can interfere with students' ability to learn and perform well in school and in challenging careers. Marijuana contributes significantly to accidental death and injury among adolescents, especially through motor vehicle crashes.

**Lungs** Regular marijuana smokers have many of the same respiratory problems as tobacco smokers, including daily cough and phlegm, chronic bronchitis, and more frequent chest colds. The amount of tar inhaled by marijuana smokers and the level of carbon monoxide absorbed are three to five times greater than among tobacco smokers. The reasons may be that marijuana users inhale more deeply, hold the smoke in the lungs longer, and do not use filters. Chronic use can lead to bronchitis, emphysema, and lung cancer. Smoking a single joint can be as damaging to the lungs as smoking five tobacco cigarettes.

**Heart** Otherwise healthy people have suffered heart attacks shortly after smoking marijuana. Experiments have also linked marijuana use to elevated blood pressure and decreased oxygen supply to the heart muscle. According to recent estimates, the risk of heart attack triples within an hour of smoking pot.[22] Smoking marijuana while shooting cocaine can potentially cause deadly increases in heart rate and blood pressure.[23]

**Pregnancy** Babies born to mothers who use marijuana during pregnancy are smaller than those born to mothers who did not use the drug, and the babies are more likely to develop health problems.[24] A nursing mother who uses marijuana passes some of the THC to the baby in her breast milk. This may impair the infant's motor development (control of muscle movement).

## Withdrawal

Marijuana users can develop a compulsive, often uncontrollable craving for the drug. More than 120,000 people enter treatment every year for marijuana addiction. In addition, animal studies suggest that marijuana causes physical dependence. Stopping after long-term marijuana use can produce *marijuana withdrawal syndrome,* which is characterized by insomnia, restlessness, loss of appetite, and irritability. People who smoked marijuana daily for many years may become aggressive after they stop using it and may relapse to prevent aggression and other symptoms.

## Cocaine

**Cocaine** (coke, snow, lady) is a white crystalline powder extracted from the leaves of the South American coca plant. Usually mixed with various sugars and local anesthetics like lidocaine and procaine, cocaine powder is generally inhaled. When sniffed or snorted, cocaine anesthetizes the nerve endings in the nose and relaxes the lung's bronchial muscles.

Cocaine can be dissolved in water and injected intravenously. The drug is rapidly metabolized by the liver, so the high is relatively brief, typically lasting only about 20 minutes. This means that users will commonly inject the drug repeatedly, increasing the risk of infection and damage to their veins. Many intravenous cocaine users prefer the practice of *speedballing,* the intravenous administration of a combination of cocaine and heroin.

Cocaine alkaloid, or *freebase,* is obtained by removing the hydrochloride salt from cocaine powder. *Freebasing* is smoking the fumes of the alkaloid form of cocaine. *Crack,* pharmacologically identical to freebase, is a cheap, easy-to-use, widely available, smokeable, and potent form of cocaine named for the popping sound it makes when burned. Because it is absorbed rapidly into the bloodstream and large doses reach the brain very quickly, it is particularly dangerous. However, its low price and easy availability have made it a common drug of abuse in poor urban areas.

## How Users Feel

A powerful stimulant to the central nervous system, cocaine targets several chemical sites in the brain, producing feelings of soaring well-being and boundless energy. Users feel they have enormous physical and mental ability, yet are also restless and anxious. After a brief period of euphoria, users slump into a depression. They often go on cocaine binges, lasting from a few hours to several days, and consume large quantities of cocaine.

With crack, dependence develops quickly. As soon as crack users come down from one high, they want more crack. Whereas heroin addicts may shoot up several times a day, crack addicts need another hit within minutes. Thus, a crack habit can quickly become more expensive than heroin addiction. Some *crackheads* have $1,000-a-day habits. Police in big cities have traced many brutal crimes and murders to young crack addicts, who often are extremely paranoid and dangerous. Smoking crack doused with liquid PCP, a practice known as *space-basing,* has especially frightening effects on behavior.

With continuing use, cocaine users experience less pleasure and more unpleasant effects. Eventually they may reach a point at which they no longer experience euphoric effects and crave the drug simply to alleviate their persistent hunger for it. They constantly think about it, dream about it, spend all their money on it, and borrow, steal, or deal to pay for it. They cannot concentrate on work; they become increasingly irritable and confused. They may also become dependent on alcohol, sedatives, or opioids, which they use to calm down from cocaine's aftereffects.

## Risks

Cocaine dependence is an easy habit to acquire. With repeated use, the brain becomes tolerant of the drug's stimulant effects, and users must take more of it to get high. Its grip is strong. Those who smoke or inject cocaine can develop dependence within weeks. Those who sniff cocaine may not become dependent on the drug for months or years. It is thought that 5 to 20 percent of all coke users—a group as large as the estimated total number of heroin addicts—are dependent on the drug.

The physical effects of acute cocaine intoxication include dilated pupils, elevated or lowered blood pressure, perspiration or chills, nausea or vomiting, speeding up or slowing down of physical activity, muscular weakness, impaired breathing, chest pain, and impaired movements

or muscle tone. Prolonged cocaine snorting can result in ulceration of the mucous membrane of the nose and damage to the nasal septum (the membrane between the nostrils) severe enough to cause it to collapse.

Although some users initially try cocaine as a sexual stimulant, it does not enhance sexual performance. At low doses, it may delay orgasm and cause heightened sensory awareness, but men who use cocaine regularly have problems maintaining erections and ejaculating. They also tend to have low sperm counts, less active sperm, and more abnormal sperm than nonusers. Both male and female chronic cocaine users tend to lose interest in sex and have difficulty reaching orgasm.

Cocaine use can cause blood vessels in the brain to clamp shut and can trigger a stroke, bleeding in the brain, and potentially fatal brain seizures. Cocaine users can also develop psychiatric or neurological complications. (See Figure 11-4.) Repeated or high doses of cocaine can lead to impaired judgment, hyperactivity, nonstop babbling, feelings of suspicion and paranoia, and violent behavior. The brain never learns to tolerate cocaine's negative effects; users may become incoherent and paranoid, and may experience unusual sensations, such as ringing in their ears, feeling insects crawling on the skin, or hearing their name called.

Cocaine can damage the liver and cause lung damage in freebasers. Smoking crack causes bronchitis as well as lung damage, and may promote the transmission of HIV through burned and bleeding lips. Some smokers have died

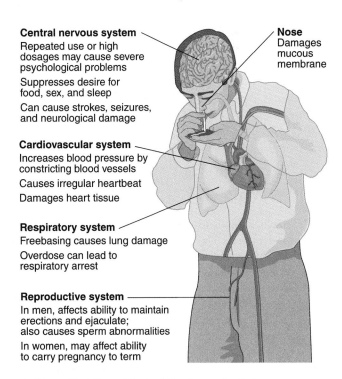

**Central nervous system**
Repeated use or high dosages may cause severe psychological problems
Suppresses desire for food, sex, and sleep
Can cause strokes, seizures, and neurological damage

**Nose**
Damages mucous membrane

**Cardiovascular system**
Increases blood pressure by constricting blood vessels
Causes irregular heartbeat
Damages heart tissue

**Respiratory system**
Freebasing causes lung damage
Overdose can lead to respiratory arrest

**Reproductive system**
In men, affects ability to maintain erections and ejaculate; also causes sperm abnormalities
In women, may affect ability to carry pregnancy to term

▲ **Figure 11-4** Some Effects of Cocaine on the Body

of respiratory complications, such as pulmonary edema (the buildup of fluid in the lungs).

Cocaine causes the heart rate to speed up and blood pressure to rise suddenly. Its use is associated with many cardiac complications, including arrhythmia (disruption of heart rhythm), angina (chest pain), and acute myocardial infarction (heart attack). These cardiac complications can lead to sudden death.[25] The most common ways of dying from cocaine use are persistent seizures that result in respiratory collapse, cardiac arrest from arrhythmias, myocardial infarction, and intracranial hemorrhage or stroke. Cocaine-induced elevations in blood pressure can lead to kidney failure.

Cocaine users who inject the drug and share needles put themselves at risk for another potentially lethal problem: HIV infection. Other complications of injecting cocaine include skin infections, hepatitis, inflammation of the arteries, and infection of the lining of the heart.

The combination of alcohol and cocaine is particularly lethal. Alcohol and cocaine together are second only to the combination of heroin and alcohol in causing deaths related to substance abuse. When people mix cocaine and alcohol, they compound the danger each drug poses. The liver combines the two agents and manufactures cocaethylene, which intensifies cocaine's euphoric effects, while possibly increasing the risk of sudden death.[26]

Cocaine is dangerous for pregnant women and their babies, causing miscarriages, developmental disorders, and life-threatening complications during birth. Women who use the drug while pregnant are more likely to miscarry in the first three months of pregnancy than women who do not use drugs or who use heroin and other opioids. Cocaine can reduce the fetal oxygen supply, possibly interfering with the development of the fetus's nervous system. Infants born to cocaine and crack users can suffer withdrawal and may have major complications or permanent disabilities. Cocaine babies have higher-than-normal rates of respiratory and kidney troubles, visual problems, and developmental retardation, and they may be at greater risk of sudden infant death syndrome.

### Withdrawal

When addicted individuals stop using cocaine, they often become depressed. This may lead to further cocaine use to alleviate depression. Other symptoms of cocaine withdrawal include fatigue, vivid and disturbing dreams, excessive or too little sleep, irritability, increased appetite, and physical slowing down or speeding up. This initial crash may last one to three days after cutting down or stopping the heavy use of cocaine. Some individuals become violent, paranoid, and suicidal.

Symptoms usually reach a peak in two to four days, although depression, anxiety, irritability, lack of pleasure in usual activities, and low-level cravings may continue for weeks. As memories of the crash fade, the desire for cocaine intensifies. For many weeks after stopping, individuals may feel an intense craving for the drug. Experimental medical approaches for treating cocaine dependence include antidepressant drugs, anticonvulsant drugs, and the naturally occurring amino acids tryptophan and tyrosine. However, these have only limited benefit, and much more research into medical treatments is needed. Recent research has found that, depending on personal characteristics such as abstract reasoning ability and religious motivation, some cocaine abusers fare better with cognitive-behavioral therapy (discussed in Chapter 3); others, with 12-step programs (discussed later in this chapter).[27]

## Club Drugs

**Club drugs** include MDMA (ecstasy), GHB, GBL, ketamine (Special-K), fentanyl, Rohypnol, amphetamines, methamphetamine, and LSD. (See Table 11-2.) Their primary users are teens and young adults at nightclubs, bars, and raves or trance events, night-long dances often held in warehouses. They try these low-cost drugs to increase their stamina and experience a high that supposedly deepens the rave or trance experience.

Some club drugs are legal and have legitimate medical uses. They include gamma hydroxybutyrate (GHB), a depressant with potential benefits for people with narcolepsy, and Rohypnol, a tranquilizer used overseas that also can be slipped into someone's drink to knock them out and cause short-term amnesia. (See Chapter 14 for a discussion of date-rape drugs.) Since Rohypnol is odorless and tasteless, victims have no way of knowing whether

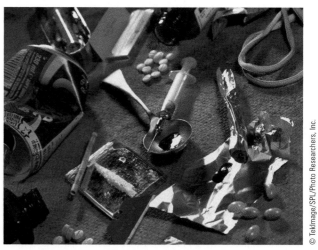

© Tekimage/SPL/Photo Researchers, Inc.

▲ Club drugs, made in a laboratory and sold on the street, aren't subject to quality controls and don't always contain what the buyer expects.

their drink has been tampered with; the subsequent loss of memory leaves them with no explanation for where they've been or what's happened in the hours before they regain consciousness.

Although users may think of ecstasy and other club drugs as harmless and fun, they can produce a range of unwanted effects, including hallucinations, paranoia, amnesia, and, in some cases, death. When used with alcohol, these drugs can be even more harmful because they involve the same brain mechanism. Also, there are great differences in how individuals react to club drugs. Some people have been known to have extreme, even fatal, reactions the first time they use club drugs. Club drugs found in party settings are often adulterated or impure and thus even more dangerous.[28]

## Ecstasy

**Ecstasy** is the most common street name for methylenedioxymethamphetamine (MDMA), a synthetic compound with both stimulant and mildly hallucinogenic properties. Ecstasy use has been increasing substantially, particularly among young people.

 Some 8.1 million Americans have tried ecstasy, according to the National Household Survey on Drug Abuse.[29] Nearly 5 percent of college students have tried the drug. Ecstasy users are more likely to spend a lot of time socializing, attend a residential college, and belong to a fraternity or sorority. However, they do not differ from other students in grade point average, nor in the emphasis they place on community service and the arts.[30]

### How It Feels

Although it can be smoked, inhaled (snorted), or injected, ecstasy is almost always taken as a pill or tablet. Its effects begin in 45 minutes and last for two to four hours.

MDMA belongs to a family of drugs called *enactogens,* which literally means "touching within." As a mood elevator, it produces a relaxed, euphoric state but does not produce hallucinations. Users of ecstasy often say they feel at peace with themselves and at ease and empathic with others. In some settings, they reveal intimate details of their lives (which they may later regret); in other settings, they join in collective rejoicing. Like hallucinogenic drugs, MDMA can enhance sensory experience, but it rarely causes visual distortions, sudden mood changes, or psychotic reactions. Regular users may experience depression and anxiety the week after taking MDMA.

Psychologists have experimented with MDMA as a way to enhance self-revelation, self-criticism, and self-exploration, and to boost trust between a patient and a therapist. Most clinicians are highly skeptical of its benefits, and there has been no officially sanctioned research on its therapeutic benefits.[31]

## Risks

Ecstasy poses risks similar to those of cocaine and amphetamines. These include psychological difficulties (confusion, depression, sleep problems, drug craving, severe anxiety, and paranoia) and physical symptoms (muscle tension, involuntary teeth clenching, nausea, blurred vision, rapid eye movement, faintness, chills, sweating, and increases in heart rate and blood pressure that pose a special risk for people with circulatory or heart disease).[32]

Continued use of ecstasy can lead to psychological dependence because users seek to recreate the exhilarating high and avoid the plunge into unhappiness and emptiness that comes after use. Because ecstasy is *neurotoxic* (damaging to brain cells), it depletes the brain of serotonin, a messenger chemical involved with mood, sleep, and appetite, and can lead to depression, anxiety, and impaired thinking and memory.[33]

According to brain-imaging studies, users, although as mentally alert as nonusers, fared far worse on measures of memory, learning, and general intelligence. The more frequently they took ecstasy, the worse they did, probably because ecstasy alters neuronal function in a brain structure called the hippocampus, which helps create short-term memory.[34] (See Figure 11-5.) Other experiments have shown increased impulsiveness and attention deficits in MDMA users.

MDMA can produce nausea, vomiting, and dizziness. When combined with extended physical exertion like dancing, club drugs can lead to hyperthermia (severe overheating), severe dehydration, serious increases in blood pressure, stroke, and heart attack. Without sufficient water, dancers at raves may suffer dehydration and heat stroke, which can be fatal. Individuals with high blood pressure, heart trouble, or liver or kidney disease are in the greatest danger.[35] Several deaths have occurred in teens who suffered brain damage by drinking large amounts of water to counteract the raised body temperature induced by the drug.

MDMA has been implicated in some cases of acute hepatitis, which can lead to liver failure. Even after liver transplantation, the mortality rate for individuals with this condition is 50 percent.[36] Another danger comes from the practice of taking Prozac, a drug that modulates the mood-altering brain chemical serotonin, before ecstasy. This can cause jaw clenching, nausea, tremors, and, in extreme cases, potentially fatal elevations in body temperature.

Although not a sexual stimulant (if anything, MDMA has the opposite effect), ecstasy fosters strong feelings of intimacy that may lead to risky sexual behavior. The psychological effects of ecstasy become less intriguing with

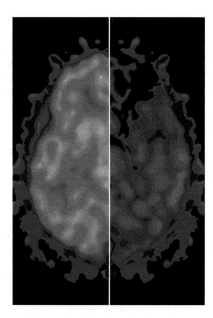

▲ **Figure 11-5** Effects of Ecstasy on the Brain
These brain scans show the sharp difference in human brain function for an individual who has never used drugs (left) and one who used the club drug ecstasy many times but had not used any drugs for at least three weeks before the scan (right). In the left scan, the bright reddish color shows active serotonin sites in the brain. Serotonin is a critical neurochemical that regulates mood, emotion, learning, memory, sleep, and pain. In the right scan, the dark sections indicate areas where serotonin is not present even after three weeks without any drugs.

Source: National Institute on Drug Abuse, www.clubdrugs.org.

repeated use, and the physical side effects become more uncomfortable. Ecstasy poses risks to a developing fetus, including a greater likelihood of heart and skeletal abnormalities and long-term learning and memory impairments in children born to women who used MDMA during pregnancy.[37]

Herbal ecstasy, also known as Herbal Bliss, Cloud 9, and Herbal X, is a mixture of stimulants such as ephedrine, pseudoephedrine, and caffeine. Sold in tablet form as a "natural" alternative to ecstasy, its ingredients vary greatly. Reactions have included seizures, heart attacks, and stroke.[38]

# Hallucinogens

The drugs known as **hallucinogens** produce vivid and unusual changes in thought, feeling, and perception. The most widely used in the United States is *LSD (lysergic acid diethylamide,* acid), which was initially developed as a tool to explore mental illness. It became popular in the 1960s and resurfaced among teenagers in the 1990s. LSD is taken orally, either blotted onto pieces of paper that are held in the mouth or chewed along with another substance, such as a sugar cube. Much less commonly used in this country is *peyote* (whose active ingredient is *mescaline*).

## How Users Feel

LSD produces hallucinations, including bright colors and altered perceptions of reality. Effects from a single dose begin within 30 to 60 minutes and last 10 to 12 hours. During this time, there are slight increases in body temperature, heart rate, and blood pressure. Sweating, chills, and goose pimples may appear. Some users develop headache and nausea. Mescaline produces vivid hallucinations—including brightly colored lights, animals, and geometric designs—within 30 to 90 minutes of consumption. These effects may persist for 12 hours.

The effects of hallucinogens depend greatly on the dose, the individual's expectations and personality, and the setting for drug use. Many users report religious or mystical imagery and thoughts; some feel they are experiencing profound insights. Usually the user realizes that perceptual changes are caused by the hallucinogen, but some become convinced that they have lost their minds. Drugs sold as hallucinogens are frequently mixed with other drugs, such as PCP and amphetamines, combinations that can produce unexpected and frightening effects.

Hallucinogens do not produce dependence in the same way as cocaine or heroin. Individuals who have an unpleasant experience after trying a hallucinogen may stop using the drug completely without suffering withdrawal symptoms. Others continue regular or occasional use because they enjoy the effects.

## Risks

Physical symptoms include dilated pupils, rapid heart rate, sweating, heart palpitations, blurring of vision, tremors, and poor coordination. These effects may last 8 to 12 hours. Hallucinogen intoxication also produces changes in emotions and mood, such as anxiety, depression, fear of losing one's mind, and impaired judgment.

LSD can trigger irrational acts. LSD users have injured or killed themselves by jumping out of windows, swimming out to sea, or throwing themselves in front of cars. Some individuals develop a delusional disorder in which they become convinced that their distorted perceptions and thoughts are real. They may experience *flashbacks* (re-experiencing symptoms felt while intoxicated), which include geometric hallucinations, flashes of color, halos around objects, and other perceptual changes.

Individuals having a *bad trip* may blame themselves and feel excessively guilty, tense, and so agitated that they cannot stop talking and have trouble sleeping. They may fear that they have destroyed their brains and will never return to normal. Someone who already is depressed may take a hallucinogen to lift his or her spirits, only to become more depressed. Suicide is a real danger.

## Inhalants

**Inhalants** or **deleriants** are chemicals that produce vapors with psychoactive effects. The most commonly abused inhalants are solvents, aerosols, model-airplane glue, cleaning fluids, and petroleum products like kerosene and butane. Some anesthetics and nitrous oxide (laughing gas) are also abused. Almost 21 percent of eighth graders surveyed have used household products, such as glue, solvents, and aerosols, to get high.[39]

### How Users Feel

Inhalants very rapidly reach the lungs, bloodstream, and other parts of the body. At low doses, users may feel slightly stimulated; at higher doses, they may feel less inhibited. Intoxication often occurs within five minutes and can last more than an hour. Inhalant users do not report the intense rush associated with other drugs, nor do they experience the perceptual changes associated with LSD. However, inhalants interfere with thinking and impulse control, so users may act in dangerous or destructive ways.

Often there are visible external signs of use: a rash around the nose and mouth; breath odors; residue on face, hands, and clothing; redness, swelling, and tearing of the eyes; and irritation of throat, lungs, and nose that leads to coughing and gagging. Nausea and headache also may occur.

### Risks

Regular use of inhalants leads to tolerance, so the sniffer needs more and more to attain the desired effects. Younger children who use inhalants several times a week may develop dependence. Older users who become dependent may use the drugs many times a day. They are likely to have used many different substances as adolescents, and to have gradually turned to inhalants as their preferred substance.

Although some young people believe inhalants are safe, this is far from true. Inhalation of butane from cigarette lighters displaces oxygen in the lungs, causing suffocation. Users also can suffocate while covering their heads with a plastic bag to inhale the substance, or from inhaling vomit into their lungs while high. According to the International Institute on Inhalant Abuse, the effects of inhalants are unpredictable, and even a single episode can trigger asphyxiation or cardiac arrhythmia, leading to disability or death. Abusers also can develop difficulties with memory and abstract reasoning, problems with coordination, and uncontrollable movements of the extremities.[40]

## Opioids

The **opioids** include *opium* and its derivatives (*morphine, codeine,* and *heroin*) and nonopioid synthetic drugs that have similar sleep-inducing and pain-relieving properties. The opioids come from a resin taken from the seedpod of the Asian poppy. **Nonopioids,** such as *meperidine* (Demerol), *methadone,* and *propoxyphene* (Darvon), are chemically synthesized. Whether natural or synthetic, these drugs are powerful *narcotics,* or painkillers.

Heroin (also known as horse, junk, smack, or downtown), the most widely abused opioid, is illegal in this country. In other nations it is used as a potent painkiller for conditions such as terminal cancer. There are an estimated 600,000 heroin addicts in the United States, with men outnumbering women addicts by three to one. The number of young adults who use heroin is growing in suburban and rural areas, according to the Centers for Disease Control and Prevention (CDC). Among people aged 18 to 25, the percentage of heroin users who inject the drug has doubled in the last decade. While the number of young heroin users in major cities has dropped by 50 percent, their numbers almost tripled in suburban and rural areas.[41]

Heroin users typically inject the drug into their veins. However, individuals who experiment with recreational drugs often prefer *skin-popping* (subcutaneous injection) rather than *mainlining* (intravenous injection); they also may snort heroin as a powder, or dissolve it and inhale the vapors. To try to avoid addiction, some users begin by *chipping,* taking small or intermittent doses. Regardless of the method of administration, tolerance can develop rapidly.

Morphine, used as a painkiller and anesthetic, acts primarily on the central nervous system, eyes, and digestive tract. By producing mental clouding, drowsiness, and euphoria, it does not decrease the physical sensation of

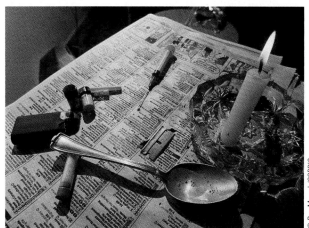

▲ Opioid drugs, made from the Asian poppy, come in both legal and illegal forms. In any form, these substances can readily become addictive.

pain as much as it alters a person's awareness of the pain; in effect, he or she no longer cares about it.

Two semisynthetic derivatives of morphine are *hydromorphone* (trade name Dilaudid, little D), with two to eight times the painkilling effect of morphine, and *oxycodone* (Oxycontin, Percocet, Percodan, perkies), similar to codeine but more potent. The synthetic narcotic *meperidine* (Demerol, demies) is now probably second only to morphine for use in relieving pain. It is also used by addicts as a substitute for morphine or heroin.

Codeine, a weaker painkiller than morphine, is an ingredient in liquid products prescribed for relieving coughs and in tablet and injectable form for relieving pain. The synthetic narcotic *propoxyphene* (Darvon), a somewhat less potent painkiller than codeine, is no more effective than aspirin in usual doses. It has been one of the most widely prescribed drugs for headaches, dental pain, and menstrual cramps. At higher doses, Darvon produces a euphoric high, which may lead to misuse.

Prescription opioids are taken orally in pill form but can also be injected intravenously. Some individuals first take a medically prescribed opioid for pain relief or cough suppression, then gradually increase the dose and frequency of use on their own, often justifying this because of their symptoms rather than for the sensations the drug induces. They expend increasing efforts to obtain the drug, frequently seeking out several doctors to write prescriptions.

## How Users Feel

All opioids relax the user. When injected, they can produce an immediate *rush* (high) that lasts 10 to 30 minutes. For two to six hours thereafter, users may feel indifferent, lethargic, and drowsy; they may slur their words and have problems paying attention, remembering, and going about their normal routine. The primary attractions of heroin are the euphoria and pain relief it produces. However, some people experience very unpleasant feelings, such as anxiety and fear. Other effects include a sensation of warmth or heaviness, dry mouth, facial flushing, and nausea and vomiting (particularly in first-time users).

Some addicts report a rush when heroin is injected directly into their veins. Since the effects of heroin do not last long—usually only two to four hours—addicts have to "shoot up" two to five times a day. With large doses, the pupils become smaller; and the skin becomes cold, moist, and bluish. Breathing slows down; the user cannot be awakened and may stop breathing completely.

## Risks

Addiction is common. Almost all regular users of opioids rapidly develop drug dependence, which can lead to lethargy, weight loss, loss of sex drive, and the continual effort to avoid withdrawal symptoms through repeated drug administration. In addition, they experience anxiety, insomnia, restlessness, and craving for the drug. Users continue taking opioids as much to avoid the discomfort of withdrawal, a classic sign of opioid addiction, as to experience pleasure.

Opioid intoxication is characterized by changes in mood and behavior, such as initial euphoria followed by apathy or discontent and impaired judgment. Physical symptoms include constricted pupils (although pupils may dilate from a severe overdose), drowsiness, slurred speech, and impaired attention or memory. Morphine affects blood pressure, heart rate, and blood circulation in the brain. Both morphine and heroin slow down the respiratory system; overdoses can cause fatal respiratory arrest.

Opioid poisoning or overdose causes shock, coma, and depressed respiration and can be fatal. Emergency medical treatment is critical, often with drugs called *narcotic antagonists* that rapidly reverse the effects of opioids when administered intravenously.

Over time, users who inject opioids may develop infections of the heart lining and valves, skin abscesses, and lung congestion. Infections from unsterile solutions, syringes, and shared needles can lead to hepatitis, tetanus, liver disease, and HIV transmission. Depression is common, and may be both an antecedent and a risk factor for needle-sharing.

## Withdrawal

If a regular user stops taking an opioid, withdrawal begins within 6 to 12 hours. The intensity of the symptoms depends on the degree of the addiction; they may grow stronger for 24 to 72 hours and gradually subside over a period of 7 to 14 days, though some symptoms, such as insomnia, may persist for several months. Individuals may develop craving for an opioid, irritability, nausea or vomiting, muscle aches, runny nose or eyes, dilated pupils, sweating, diarrhea, yawning, fever, and insomnia. Desperately craving the drug, users may plead, demand, or manipulate others to obtain more. Opioid withdrawal usually is not life-threatening.

## Methadone Maintenance

Opioid dependence is a very difficult addiction to overcome. Studies demonstrate that only 10 to 30 percent of heroin users are able to maintain abstinence. This fact contributed to the development of a unique, yet still controversial, treatment for opioid dependence: the use of methadone, a long-acting opioid that users can substitute for heroin or other opioids.[42]

Methadone is used in two basic ways to treat opioid dependence: as an opioid substitute for detoxification, usually with a gradual tapering of methadone over a period of 21 to 180 days, and as a maintenance treatment. Methadone maintenance has been criticized by some as

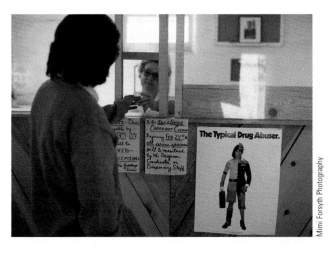

▲ Methadone has been criticized as a treatment for opioid addiction, but research clearly demonstrates positive benefits. Those who participate in long-term methadone maintenance programs usually move out of the drug culture and are candidates for eventually leaving methadone dependence behind them.

*Mimi Forsyth Photography*

nothing more than the substitution of a legal opioid, methadone, for an illegal opioid, heroin.

Methadone maintenance may be the most thoroughly studied drug treatment. Research has clearly documented several important positive benefits, including decreased use of illicit opioids; decreased criminal behavior; decreased risk of contracting HIV infection (through sharing of infected needles); and improvements in physical health, employment, and other lifestyle factors. Individuals who have been on methadone maintenance for a long time (often years), have stable relationships and employment, have assimilated themselves into the nondrug culture, and are highly motivated to get off methadone have the best chance for successful detoxification from methadone.

## Phencyclidine (PCP)

**PCP** (phencyclidine, brand name Sernyl; street names angel dust, peace pill, lovely, and green) is an illicit drug manufactured as a tablet, capsule, liquid, flake, spray, or crystal-like white powder that can be swallowed, smoked, sniffed, or injected. Sometimes it is sprinkled on crack, marijuana, tobacco, or parsley, and smoked. A fine-powdered form of PCP can be snorted or injected. Once PCP was thought to have medicinal value as an anesthetic, but its side effects, including delirium and hallucinations, now make it unacceptable for medical use.

PCP use peaked in the 1970s, but it remains a popular drug of abuse in both inner-city ghettos and suburban high schools. Users often think that the PCP they take together with another illegal psychoactive substance, such as amphetamines, coke, or hallucinogens, is responsible for the highs they feel, so they seek it out specifically.

## How Users Feel

The effects of PCP are utterly unpredictable. It may trigger violent behavior or irreversible psychosis the first time it is used, or the twentieth time, or never. In low doses, PCP produces changes—from hallucinations or euphoria to feelings of emptiness or numbness—similar to those produced by other psychoactive drugs. Higher doses may produce a stupor that lasts several days, increased heart rate and blood pressure, flushing, sweating, dizziness, and numbness.

The behavioral changes associated with PCP intoxication, which can develop within minutes, include belligerence, aggressiveness, impulsiveness, unpredictability, agitation, poor judgment, and impaired functioning at work or in social situations. The physical symptoms of PCP intoxication include involuntary eye movements, increased blood pressure or heart rate, numbness or diminished responsiveness to pain, impaired coordination and speech, muscle rigidity, seizures, and a painful sensitivity to sound. Some people experience repetitive motor movements (such as facial grimacing), hallucinations, and paranoia. Suicide is a definite risk. Intoxication typically lasts four to six hours, but some effects can linger for several days. Delirium may occur within 24 hours of taking PCP or after recovery from an overdose and can last as much as a week.

## Sedative-Hypnotic Drugs

**Sedative-hypnotics,** also known as anxiolytic or antianxiety drugs, depress the central nervous system, reduce activity, and induce relaxation, drowsiness, or sleep. They include the benzodiazepines and the barbiturates.

The **benzodiazepines**—the most widely used drugs in this category—are commonly prescribed for tension, muscular strain, sleep problems, anxiety, panic attacks, anesthesia, and in the treatment of alcohol withdrawal. They include such drugs as *chlordiazepoxide* (Librium), *diazepam* (Valium), *oxazepam* (Serax), *lorazepam* (Ativan), *flurazepam* (Dalmane), and *alprazolam* (Xanax). They differ widely in their mechanism of action, absorption rate, and metabolism, but all produce similar intoxication and withdrawal symptoms.

Benzodiazepine sleeping pills have largely replaced the **barbiturates,** which were used medically in the past for inducing relaxation and sleep, relieving tension, and treating epileptic seizures. These drugs are usually taken by mouth in tablet, capsule, or liquid form. When used as a general anesthetic, they are administered intravenously. Barbiturates such as *pentobarbital* (Nembutal, yellow jackets), *secobarbital* (Seconal, reds), and *thiopental* (Pentothal) are short-acting and rapidly absorbed into the brain. The longer-acting barbiturates, such as *amobarbital* (Amytal, blues, downers) and *phenobarbital* (Luminal, phennies), are usually taken orally and absorbed slowly into the bloodstream, taking a while to reach the brain and having an effect for several days.

## How Users Feel

Low doses of these drugs may reduce or relieve tension, but increasing doses can cause a loosening of sexual or aggressive inhibitions. Individuals using this class of drugs may experience rapid mood changes, impaired judgment, and impaired social or occupational functioning. High doses produce slurred speech, drowsiness, and stupor.

Young people in their teens or early twenties who have used many illegal substances typically take sedative-hypnotics to obtain a high or a state of euphoria. Some use them in combination with other drugs. Less commonly, individuals may first obtain sedatives, hypnotics, or antianxiety medications by prescription from a physician for insomnia or anxiety, and then gradually increase the dose or frequency of use on their own, often by seeking prescriptions from several physicians. While they justify this continued use because of their symptoms, the fact is that they reach a state in which they cannot function normally without the drug.

## Risks

All sedative-hypnotic drugs can produce physical and psychological dependence within two to four weeks. A complication specific to sedatives is *cross-tolerance* (cross-addiction), which occurs when users develop tolerance for one sedative or become dependent on it and develop tolerance for other sedatives as well.

Intoxication with these drugs can produce changes in mood or behavior, such as inappropriate sexual or aggressive acts, mood swings, and impaired judgment. Physical signs include slurred speech, poor coordination, unsteady gait, involuntary eye movements, impaired attention or memory, and stupor or coma.

Taken in combination with alcohol, these drugs have a synergistic effect that can be dangerous or even lethal. For example, an individual's driving ability, already impaired by alcohol, will be made even worse, increasing the risk of an accident. Alcohol in combination with sedative-hypnotics leads to respiratory depression and may result in respiratory arrest and death. Regular users of any of these drugs who become physically dependent should not try to cut down or quit on their own. If they try to quit suddenly, they run the risk of seizures, coma, and death.

## Withdrawal

Withdrawal from sedative-hypnotic drugs may range from relatively mild discomfort to a severe syndrome with grand mal seizures, depending on the degree of dependence. Withdrawal symptoms include malaise or weakness, sweating, rapid pulse, coarse tremors (of the hands, tongue, or eyelids), insomnia, nausea or vomiting, temporary hallucinations or illusions, physical restlessness, anxiety or irritability, and grand mal seizures. Withdrawal may begin within two to three days after stopping drug use, and symptoms may persist for many weeks.

## Treating Drug Dependence and Abuse

An estimated 6.1 million Americans are in need of drug treatment, but the vast majority—some 5 million—never get treatment.[43] The most difficult step for a drug user is to admit that he or she *is* in fact an addict. If drug abusers are not forced to deal with their problem through some unexpected trauma, such as being fired or going bankrupt, those who care—family, friends, coworkers, doctors—may have to confront them and insist that they do something about their addiction. Often this *intervention* can be the turning point for addicts and their families. Treatment has proven equally successful for young people and for older adults.[44]

Treatment may take place in an outpatient setting, a residential facility, or a hospital. Increasingly, treatment thereafter is tailored to address coexisting or dual diagnoses. A personal treatment plan may consist of individual psychotherapy, marital and family therapy, medication, and behavior therapy. Once an individual has made the decision to seek help for substance abuse, the first step usually is detoxification, which involves clearing the drug from the body. An exception is methadone maintenance, discussed earlier in this chapter, which does not rely on complete detoxification.

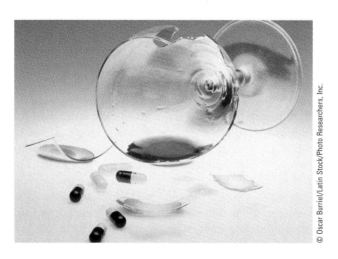

▲ Benzodiazepines and barbiturates react dangerously with alcohol.

© Oscar Burriel/Latin Stock/Photo Researchers, Inc.

Controlled and supervised withdrawal within a medical or psychiatric hospital may be recommended if an individual has not been able to stop using drugs as an outpatient or in a residential treatment program. Detoxification is most likely to be complicated in a polysubstance abuser, who may require close monitoring and treatment of potentially fatal withdrawal symptoms. Other reasons for inpatient treatment include lack of psychosocial support for maintaining abstinence and the absence of a drug-free living environment. Restrictions on insurance coverage may limit the number of days of inpatient care. Increasingly, once individuals complete detoxification, they continue treatment in residential programs or as outpatients.

Medications are used in detoxification to alleviate withdrawal symptoms and prevent medical and psychiatric complications.[45] Once withdrawal is complete, these medications are discontinued, so the individual is in a drug-free state. However, individuals with mental disorders may require appropriate psychiatric medication to manage their symptoms and reduce the risk of relapse. For example, a person suffering from major depression or panic disorder may require ongoing treatment with antidepressant medication.

The aim of chemical dependence treatment is to help individuals establish and maintain their recovery from alcohol and drugs of abuse. Recovery is a dynamic process of personal growth and healing in which the drug user makes the transition from a lifestyle of active substance use to a drug-free lifestyle.

Whatever their setting, chemical dependence treatment programs initially involve some period of intensive treatment followed by one or two years of continuing aftercare. Most freestanding programs (those not affiliated with a hospital) follow what is known as the *Minnesota model*, a treatment approach developed at Hazelden Recovery Center in Center City, Minnesota, more than 30 years ago. Its key principles include a focus on drug use as the primary problem, not as a symptom of underlying emotional problems; a multidisciplinary approach that addresses the physical, emotional, spiritual, family, and social aspects of the individual; a supportive community; and a goal of abstinence and health.

Outpatient programs for substance abuse, offered by freestanding centers, hospitals, and community mental health centers, often run four or five nights a week for four to eight weeks, or in daily eight-hour sessions for seven to eight days, followed by weekly group therapy. These outpatient programs allow recovering drug users to go on with their daily lives and learn to deal with day-to-day work and family stresses. Mental health professionals in private practice also offer individually structured outpatient treatment.

Therapy groups provide an opportunity for individuals who have often been isolated by their drug use to participate in normal social settings. Small groups with other former drug users can be especially valuable because they all share the experience of drug use. Group members can confront one another with frankness and cut through lies and rationalizations. A professional therapist keeps members of the group from ganging up on one person. After their discharge from inpatient treatment, individuals who became involved in self-help groups are less likely to use drugs, cope better with stress, and develop richer friendship networks.

## 12-Step Programs

Since its founding in 1935, Alcoholics Anonymous (AA)—the oldest, largest, and most successful self-help program in the world—has spawned a worldwide movement. As many as 200 different recovery programs are based on the spiritual **12-step program** of AA. Participation in 12-step programs for drug abusers, such as Substance Anonymous, Narcotics Anonymous, and Cocaine Anonymous, is of fundamental importance in promoting and maintaining long-term abstinence.

The basic precept of 12-step programs is that members have been powerless when it comes to controlling their addictive behavior on their own. These programs don't recruit members. The desire to stop must come from the individual, who can call the number of a 12-step program, listed in the telephone book, and find out when and where the next nearby meeting will be held. A representative may offer to send someone to the caller's house to talk about the problem and to escort him or her to the next meeting.

Meetings of various 12-step programs are held daily in almost every city in the country. (Some chapters, whose members often include the disabled or those in remote areas, meet via Internet chat rooms or electronic bulletin boards.) There are no dues or fees for membership. Many individuals belong to several programs because they have several problems, such as alcoholism, substance abuse, and pathological gambling. All have only one requirement for membership: a desire to stop an addictive behavior.

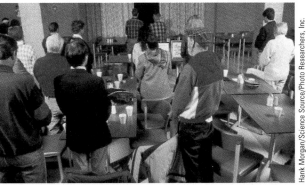

Hank Morgan/Science Source/Photo Researchers, Inc.

▲ Based on the Alcoholics Anonymous model, 12-step programs have helped many people overcome addictions. The one requirement for membership is a desire to stop following a pattern of addictive behavior.

To get the most out of a 12-step program:

✔ Try out different groups until you find one you like and in which you feel comfortable.

✔ Once you find a group in which you feel comfortable, go back several times (some recommend a minimum of six meetings) before making a final decision on whether to continue.

✔ Keep an open mind. Listen to other people's stories and ask yourself if you've had similar feelings or experiences.

✔ Accept whatever feels right to you and ignore the rest. One common saying in 12-step programs is "Take what you like and leave the rest."

## Relapse Prevention

The most common clinical course for substance abuse disorders involves a pattern of multiple relapses over the course of a lifespan. It is important for individuals with these problems and their families to recognize this fact. When relapses do occur, they should be viewed as neither a mark of defeat nor evidence of moral weakness. While painful, they do not erase the progress that has been achieved and ultimately may strengthen self-understanding. They can serve as reminders of potential pitfalls to avoid in the future.

One key to preventing relapse is learning to avoid obvious cues and associations that can set off intense cravings. This means staying away from the people and places linked with past drug use. Some therapists use conditioning techniques to give former users some sense of control over their urge to use the drug. The theory behind this approach, which is called *extinction* of conditioned behavior, is that with repeated exposure—for example, to videotapes of dealers selling crack cocaine—the arousal and craving will diminish. While this technique by itself cannot ward off relapses, it does seem to enhance the overall effectiveness of other therapies.

Another important lesson that therapists emphasize is that every lapse does not have to lead to a full-blown relapse. Users can turn to the skills acquired in treatment—calling people for support or going to meetings—to avoid a major relapse. Ultimately, users must learn much more than how to avoid temptation; they must examine their entire view of the world and learn new ways to live in it without turning to drugs. This is the underlying goal of the recovery process.

 Why is there a growing trend in ritalin abuse among college students?

### STRATEGIES FOR PREVENTION

**Relapse-Prevention Planning**

The following steps, from Terence Gorski and Merlene Miller's *Staying Sober: A Guide for Relapse Prevention,* can lower the likelihood of relapses:

1. *Stabilization and self-assessment.* Get control of yourself. Find out what's going on in your head, heart, and life.

2. *Education.* Learn about relapse and what to do to prevent it.

3. *Warning-sign identification and management.* Make a list of your personal relapse warning signs. Learn how to interrupt them before you lose control.

4. *Inventory training.* Learn how to become consciously aware of warning signs as they develop.

5. *Review of the recovery program.* Make sure your recovery program is able to help you manage your warning signs of relapse.

6. *Involvement of significant others.* Teach them how to help you avoid relapses.

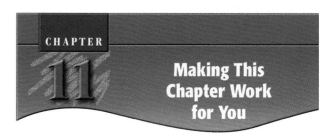

CHAPTER

**Making This Chapter Work for You**

1. Which of the following statements about drugs is false?
   a. Toxicity is the dosage level of a prescription.
   b. Drugs can be injected into the body intravenously, intramuscularly, or subcutaneously.
   c. Drug misuse is the taking of a drug for a purpose other than that for which it was medically intended.
   d. An individual's response to a drug can be affected by the setting in which the drug is used.

2. To help ensure that an over-the-counter or prescription drug is safe and effective,
   a. take smaller dosages than indicated in the instructions.
   b. test your response to the drug by borrowing a similar medication from a friend.

c. ask your doctor or pharmacist about possible interactions with other medications.

d. buy all of your medications online.

3. Which of the following drugs does not cause withdrawal symptoms?
   a. caffeine
   b. marijuana
   c. heroin
   d. aspirin

4. Individuals with substance use disorders
   a. are usually not physically dependent on their drug of choice.
   b. have a compulsion to use one or more addictive substances.
   c. require less and less of the preferred drug to achieve the desired effect.
   d. suffer withdrawal symptoms when they use the drug regularly.

5. Amphetamine is very similar to which of the following in its effects on the central nervous system?
   a. marijuana
   b. heroin
   c. cocaine
   d. alcohol

6. Which of the following statements about marijuana is false?
   a. People who have used marijuana may experience psychoactive effects for several days after use.
   b. Marijuana has shown some effectiveness in treating chemotherapy-related nausea.
   c. Unlike long-term use of alcohol, regular use of marijuana does not have any long-lasting health consequences.
   d. Depending on the amount of marijuana used, its effects can range from a mild sense of euphoria to extreme panic.

7. Cocaine dependence can result in all of the following *except*
   a. stroke.

b. paranoia and violent behavior.
c. heart failure.
d. enhanced sexual performance.

8. Which of the following statements about club drugs is true?
   a. Club drugs can produce many unwanted effects, including hallucinations and paranoia.
   b. Most club drugs do not pose the same health dangers as "hard" drugs such as heroin.
   c. MDMA is the street name for ecstasy.
   d. When combined with extended physical exertion, club drugs can lead to hypothermia (lowered body temperature).

9. The opioids
   a. are not addictive if used in a prescription form such as codeine or Demerol.
   b. produce an immediate but short-lasting high and feeling of euphoria.
   c. include morphine, which is typically used for cough suppression.
   d. are illegal in the United States, although they are allowed in other countries to help control severe pain.

10. Which of the following statements about drug dependence treatment is false?
    a. Chemical dependence treatment programs usually involve medications to alleviate withdrawal symptoms.
    b. Detoxification is usually the first step in a drug treatment program.
    c. Relapses are not uncommon for a person who has undergone drug treatment.
    d. The 12-step recovery program modeled after Alcoholics Anonymous has been shown to be ineffective with individuals with drug dependence disorders.

Answers to these questions can be found on p. 415.

## Critical Thinking

1. Some argue that marijuana should be a legal drug like alcohol and tobacco. What is your opinion on this issue? Defend your position.

2. Suppose a close friend is using amphetamines to keep her energy levels high so that she can continue to attend school full-time and hold down a job to pay her school expenses. You fear that she is developing a substance abuse disorder. What can you do to help her realize the dangers of her behavior? What resources are available at your school or in your community to help her deal with both her drug problem and her financial needs?

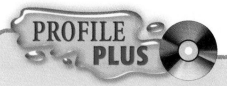

Drug dependency robs you of enjoying a full, happy life. Are you concerned about your drug use? Begin the process of change with this activity on your Profile Plus CD-ROM:

Is it a substance abuse problem?

## SITES & BYTES

### Partnership for a Drug-Free America
www.drugfreeamerica.org

This comprehensive site features current resources and photographs on a variety of drugs, including a special section on ecstasy and club drugs. This site also includes resources, several video clips, and true-life stories revealing the consequences of drug use.

### American Council for Drug Education
www.acde.org

This site features current news topics and general information on a variety of drugs, with special sections for college students, parents, youth, and health professionals.

### National Institute on Drug Abuse
www.nida.nih.gov

This government site—a virtual clearinghouse of information for students, parents, teachers, researchers, and health professionals—features current treatment and research, as well as a comprehensive database on common drugs of abuse.

**InfoTrac College Edition Activity** "Report Finds Link Between Early Marijuana Use and Adult Drug Dependence." *Alcoholism & Drug Abuse Weekly,* Vol. 14, No. 34, September 9, 2002, p. 1.

1. What is the relationship between age of first use of marijuana and the subsequent use of other drugs as adults?

2. According to the study, the prior use of which two other types of drugs is highly correlated with becoming a new marijuana user?

3. What are the physical and mental health risks of early marijuana use?

You can find additional readings related to drug abuse with InfoTrac College Edition, an online library of more than 900 journals and publications. Follow the instructions for accessing InfoTrac that were packaged with your textbook; then search for articles using a keyword search.

For additional links, resources, and suggested readings on InfoTrac, visit our Health & Wellness Resource Center at http://health.wadsworth.com.

## Key Terms

The terms listed here are used within the chapter on the page indicated. Definitions of terms are in the Glossary at the end of the book.

addiction 278
amphetamine 283
barbiturates 295
benzodiazepines 295
club drugs 290
cocaine 288
deleriants 293
drug 274
drug abuse 274

drug misuse 274
ecstasy (MDMA) 291
hallucinogen 292
hashish 286
inhalants 293
intoxication 279
intramuscular 274
intravenous 274
marijuana 286

nonopioids 293
opioids 293
over-the-counter (OTC) drugs 275
PCP(phencyclidine) 295
physical dependence 278
polyabuse 280
psychoactive 278

psychological dependence 278
psychotropic 277
sedative-hypnotics 295
stimulant 277
subcutaneous 274
toxicity 274
12-step program 297
withdrawal 279

# References

1. National Institute on Drug Abuse, www.drugabuse.gov.
2. "Teenage Drug Use Drops to an 8-Year Low." *New York Times,* July 18, 2002.
3. "A Cough Syrup Ingredient Is a Popular Drug." *Pediatrics,* Vol. 106, No. 5, November 2000, p. 1125.
4. Scott, William H., Jr., et al. "Effects of Caffeine on Performance of Low Intensity Tasks." *Perceptual and Motor Skills,* Vol. 94, No. 2, April 2002, p. 521.
5. Cerrato, Paul. "Caffeine May Protect Women from Parkinson's." *Contemporary OB/GYN,* Vol. 47, No. 5, May 2002, p. 168. "Too Much Caffeine May Be Detrimental for People with Glaucoma and Ocular Hypertension." *Environmental Nutrition,* Vol. 25, No. 9, September 2002, p. 3.
6. "Ecstasy Use Up Sharply; Use of Other Illegal Drugs Steady, or Declining." *Medical Letter on the CDC & FDA,* January 14, 2001.
7. Frances, Richard. Personal interview.
8. "Report Makes Case for Addiction As Chronic Disease." *Alcoholism & Drug Abuse Weekly,* Vol. 12, No. 43, November 6, 2000, p. 3.
9. Brook, Judith, et al. "Longitudinally Foretelling Drug Use in the Late Twenties: Adolescent Personality and Social-Environment Antecedents." *Journal of Genetic Psychology,* Vol. 161, No. 1, March 2000, p. 37.
10. "Parental Ground Rules Work in Prevention." *Alcoholism & Drug Abuse Weekly,* Vol. 12, No. 30, July 31, 2000, p. 7.
11. "Parental Attitudes, History Affect Children's Drug Use." *Alcoholism & Drug Abuse Weekly,* Vol. 13, No. 32, August 20, 2001, p. 7.
12. Jones, Sherry, et al. "Binge Drinking Among Undergraduate College Students in the United States: Implications for Other Substance Use." *Journal of American College Health,* Vol. 50, No. 1, July 2001, p. 33.
13. Bon, Rebecca, et al. "Normative Perceptions in Relation to Substance Use and HIV-Risky Sexual Behaviors of College Students." *Journal of Psychology,* Vol. 135, No. 2, March 2001, p. 165.
14. Jones et al., "Binge Drinking Among Undergraduate College Students in the United States."
15. Wechsler, Henry, et al. "Drinking Levels, Alcohol Problems and Secondhand Effects in Substance-Free College Residences: Results of a National Study." *Journal of Studies on Alcohol,* Vol. 62, No. 1, January 2001, p. 23.
16. Volkow, Nora, et al. "Higher Cortical and Lower Subcortical Metabolism in Detoxified Methamphetamine Abusers." *American Journal of Psychiatry,* Vol. 158, March 2001, p. 383.
17. *Substance Use and Risky Sexual Behavior: Attitudes and Practices Among Adolescents and Young Adults.* Menlo Park, CA: Henry J. Kaiser Family Foundation, February 2002.
18. "Research Casts Doubt on Marijuana for Pain." *Alcoholism & Drug Abuse Weekly,* Vol. 13, No. 27, July 16, 2001, p. 8.
19. "Doctors Reject Proposal Backing Medical Marijuana." *Alcoholism & Drug Abuse Weekly,* Vol. 13, No. 26, July 2, 2001, p. 8.
20. National Institute on Drug Abuse, www.nida.nih.gov.
21. Ibid.
22. Mittleman, Murray. "Triggering Myocardial Infarction by Marijuana." *Journal of the American Medical Association,* Vol. 286, No. 6, August 8, 2001, p. 655.
23. "Marijuana May Boost Heart Attack Risk." *Alcoholism & Drug Abuse Weekly,* Vol. 13, No. 37, October 1, 2001, p. 7.
24. Walling, Anne. "Marijuana Use During Pregnancy." *American Family Physician,* Vol. 63, No. 12, June 15, 2001, p. 2463.
25. Swift, Pauline, and Donald Singer. "Cocaine Use and Acute Left Ventricular Dysfunction." *Lancet,* Vol. 357, No. 9268, May 19, 2001, p. 1586.
26. National Institute on Drug Abuse, www.nida.nih.gov.
27. Shine, Barbara. "Some Cocaine Abusers Fare Better with Cognitive-Behavioral Therapy, Others with 12-Step Programs." *National Institute on Drug Abuse, NIDA Notes,* Vol. 15, No. 1, March 2000.
28. "Officials Should Monitor Drugs Collected at Clubs." *Alcoholism & Drug Abuse Weekly,* Vol. 13, No. 36, September 24, 2001, p. 8.
29. National Institute on Drug Abuse, www.drugabuse.gov.
30. Strote, Jared, et al. "Increasing MDMA Use Among College Students: Results of a National Survey." *Journal of Adolescent Health,* Vol. 30, No. 1, January 2002, p. 64.
31. "MDMA (Ecstasy)." *Harvard Mental Health Letter,* Vol. 18, No. 1, July 2001.
32. National Institute on Drug Abuse, www.nida.nih.gov.
33. "Ecstasy." *Psychiatric Services,* Vol. 53, No. 6, June 2002, p. 667.
34. "Long-Term Ecstasy Use Impairs Memory." *Science News,* Vol. 159, No. 18, May 5, 2001, p. 280.
35. "From MDMA to Ecstasy." *Brown University Digest of Addiction Theory and Application,* Vol. 20, No. 6, June 2001, p. 4.
36. Hilliard, Malaika. "Ecstasy, Liver Failure, and Death in a Young Adult." Press release, American College of Gastroenterology, October 22, 2001.
37. "Can Ecstasy's Effects Be Passed on to Offspring?" *Brown University Child and Adolescent Behavior Letter,* Vol. 17, No. 8, August 2001, p. 1.
38. National Institute on Drug Abuse, www.clubdrugs.org.
39. National Institute on Drug Abuse, www.nida.nih.gov/ ResearchReports/Inhalants/Inhalants.html.
40. "Getting High with Inhalants." *State Legislatures,* Vol. 41, No. 7, July 2001, p. 14.
41. "Heroin." National Institute on Drug Abuse, www.nida.nih.gov.
42. Stancliff, Sharon, et al. "Methadone Maintenance." *American Family Physician,* Vol. 63, No. 12, June 15, 2001, p. 2335.
43. National Institute on Drug Abuse, www.drugabuse.gov.
44. "Youth Treatment Study Shows Good Results, Parallels Findings for Adult Outcomes." *Alcoholism & Drug Abuse Weekly,* Vol. 13, No. 27, July 16, 2001, p. 1.
45. Sloves, Harold. "Drug Treatment for Drug Addiction: Surmounting the Barriers." *Behavioral Health Management,* Vol. 20, No. 4, July 2000, p. 42.

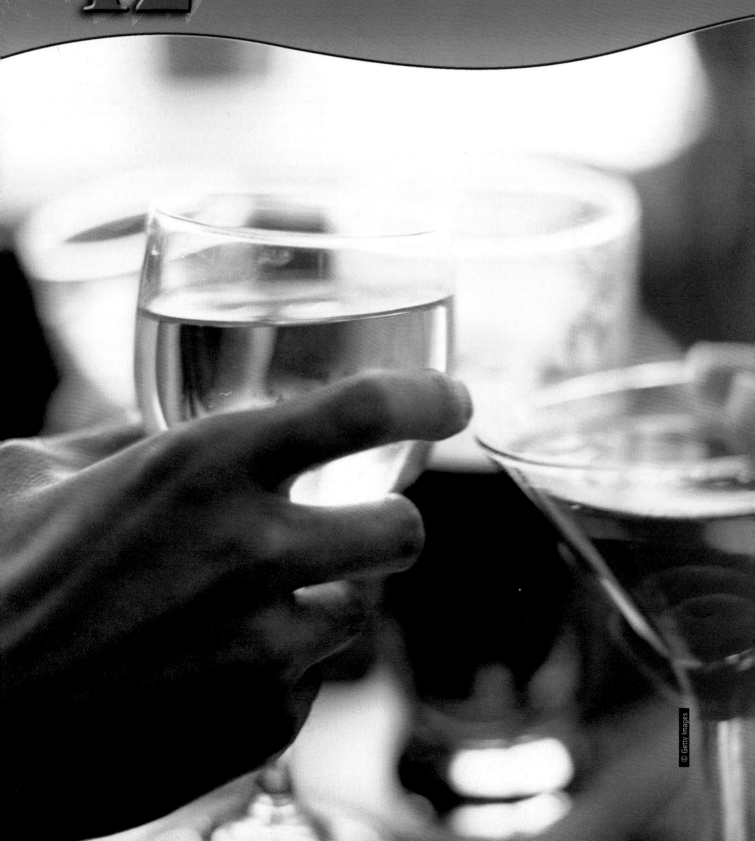

# Alcohol and Tobacco Use, Misuse, and Abuse

Alcohol and tobacco are the most widely used mind-altering substances in the world. College campuses are no exception. About eight in ten college students drink, at least occasionally. An increasing number—about two in five—engage in the dangerous practice of binge drinking.[1] There also has been an increase in tobacco use by students. Almost half report using tobacco in the last year, including cigarettes, cigars, smokeless tobacco, or a combination of these products.[2]

These trends are worrisome. Tobacco use remains the single leading preventable cause of death in the world. According to World Health Organization statistics, tobacco products annually cause 2 million deaths in developed countries and 1 million in developing countries. The death toll is expected to rise to 10 million a year by the 2020s, with 70 percent of these deaths in developed countries.

Each dangerous in itself, drinking and smoking tend to go together. Heavy drinking is more common among current smokers than former or nonsmokers. The more individuals smoke and drink, the less likely they are to eat a nutritious diet and follow a healthy lifestyle. Even if you never drink to excess and don't smoke, you live with the consequences of others' drinking and smoking. That's why it's important for everyone to know about these harmful habits. This chapter provides information that can help you understand, avoid, and change behaviors that could destroy your health, happiness, and life.

**After studying the material in this chapter, you should be able to:**

- **Describe** the effects of alcohol on the body, behavior, and thought.
- **Define** alcohol abuse, dependence, and alcoholism, and **list** their symptoms.
- **List** the negative consequences to individuals and to our society from alcohol abuse.
- **List** the health effects of smoking tobacco or using smokeless tobacco.
- **Describe** the social impact of tobacco use.
- **List** the health effects of environmental tobacco smoke.

# Alcohol and Its Effects

Pure alcohol is a colorless liquid obtained through the fermentation of a liquid containing sugar. **Ethyl alcohol,** or *ethanol,* is the type of alcohol in alcoholic beverages. Another type—methyl, or wood, alcohol—is a poison that should never be drunk. Any liquid containing 0.5 to 80 percent ethyl alcohol by volume is an alcoholic beverage. However, different drinks contain different amounts of alcohol (see Figure 12-1).

One drink can be any of the following:

✔ One bottle or can (12 ounces) of beer, which is 5 percent alcohol.

✔ One glass (4 ounces) of table wine, such as burgundy, which is 12 percent alcohol.

✔ One small glass (2½ ounces) of fortified wine, which is 20 percent alcohol.

✔ One shot (1 ounce) of distilled spirits (such as whiskey, vodka, or rum), which is 50 percent alcohol.

All of these drinks contain close to the same amount of alcohol—that is, if the number of ounces in each drink is multiplied by the percentage of alcohol, each drink contains the equivalent of approximately ½ ounce of 100 percent ethyl alcohol. With distilled spirits (such as bourbon, scotch, vodka, gin, and rum), alcohol content is expressed in terms of **proof,** a number that is *twice* the percentage of alcohol: 100-proof bourbon is 50 percent alcohol; 80-proof gin is 40 percent alcohol.

But the words *bottle* and *glass* can be deceiving in this context. Drinking a 16-ounce bottle of malt liquor, which is 6.4 percent alcohol, is not the same as drinking a 12-ounce glass of 3.2 percent beer. Two bottles of high-alcohol wines (such as Cisco), packaged to resemble much less powerful wine coolers, can lead to alcohol poisoning, especially in those who weigh less than 150 pounds. This is one reason alcoholic drinks are a serious danger for young people.

## ????  How Much Alcohol Can I Drink?

The best way to figure how much you can drink safely is to determine the amount of alcohol in your blood at any given time, or your **blood-alcohol concentration (BAC).** BAC is expressed in terms of the percentage of alcohol in the blood and is often measured from breath or urine samples. Law enforcement officers use BAC to determine whether a driver is legally drunk. The federal Department of Transportation has called on states to set 0.08 percent—the BAC that a 150-pound man would have after consuming about three mixed drinks within an hour—as the threshold at which a person can be cited for drunk driving. In the past, 0.1 percent was often the legal limit. (See Figure 12-2.) According to the National Institute on Alcohol Abuse and Alcoholism, lowering the BAC can lead to a significant drop in fatal car crashes related to alcohol.[3]

A BAC of 0.05 percent indicates approximately 5 parts alcohol to 10,000 parts other blood components. Most people reach this level after consuming one or two drinks and experience all the positive sensations of drinking—relaxation, euphoria, and well-being—without feeling intoxicated. If they continue to drink past the 0.05 percent BAC level, they start feeling worse rather than better, gradually losing control of speech, balance, and emotions. At a BAC of 0.2 percent, they may pass out. At a BAC of 0.3 percent, they could lapse into a coma; at 0.4 percent, they could die.

For some people, even very low blood alcohol concentrations can cause a headache, upset stomach, or dizziness. These reactions often are inborn. People who have suffered brain damage, often as a result of head trauma or encephalitis, may lose all tolerance for alcohol, either temporarily or permanently, and behave abnormally after drinking small amounts. The elderly, as well as those who are unusually fatigued or have a debilitating physical illness, may also have a low tolerance for alcohol and respond inappropriately to a small amount.

## ????  How Much Alcohol Is Too Much?

Federal health authorities at the National Institute of Alcohol Abuse and Alcoholism recommend that men have no more than two drinks a day and women, no more than one. The American Heart Association advises that alcohol account for no more than 15 percent of the total calories

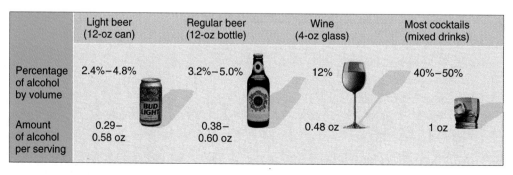

| | | Light beer (12-oz can) | Regular beer (12-oz bottle) | Wine (4-oz glass) | Most cocktails (mixed drinks) |
|---|---|---|---|---|---|
| Percentage of alcohol by volume | | 2.4%–4.8% | 3.2%–5.0% | 12% | 40%–50% |
| Amount of alcohol per serving | | 0.29–0.58 oz | 0.38–0.60 oz | 0.48 oz | 1 oz |

▲ **Figure 12-1** The Alcohol Content of Different Drinks

| Men | Approximate blood alcohol percentage | | | | | | | | |
|---|---|---|---|---|---|---|---|---|---|
| | Body weight in pounds | | | | | | | | |
| Drinks | 100 | 120 | 140 | 160 | 180 | 200 | 220 | 240 | |
| 0 | .00 | .00 | .00 | .00 | .00 | .00 | .00 | .00 | Only safe driving limit |
| 1 | .04 | .03 | .03 | .02 | .02 | .02 | .02 | .02 | Impairment begins |
| 2 | .08 | .06 | .05 | .05 | .04 | .04 | .03 | .03 | |
| 3 | .11 | .09 | .08 | .07 | .06 | .06 | .05 | .05 | Driving skills significantly affected |
| 4 | .15 | .12 | .11 | .09 | .08 | .08 | .07 | .06 | |
| 5 | .19 | .16 | .13 | .12 | .11 | .09 | .09 | .08 | Possible criminal penalties |
| 6 | .23 | .19 | .16 | .14 | .13 | .11 | .10 | .09 | |
| 7 | .26 | .22 | .19 | .16 | .15 | .13 | .12 | .11 | |
| 8 | .30 | .25 | .21 | .19 | .17 | .15 | .14 | .13 | Legally intoxicated |
| 9 | .34 | .28 | .24 | .21 | .19 | .17 | .15 | .14 | Criminal penalties |
| 10 | .38 | .31 | .27 | .23 | .21 | .19 | .17 | .16 | |

Subtract .01% for each 40 minutes of drinking.
One drink is 1.25 oz. of 80 proof liquor, 12 oz. of beer, or 5 oz. of table wine.

| Women | Approximate blood alcohol percentage | | | | | | | | | |
|---|---|---|---|---|---|---|---|---|---|---|
| | Body weight in pounds | | | | | | | | | |
| Drinks | 90 | 100 | 120 | 140 | 160 | 180 | 200 | 220 | 240 | |
| 0 | .00 | .00 | .00 | .00 | .00 | .00 | .00 | .00 | .00 | Only safe driving limit |
| 1 | .05 | .05 | .04 | .03 | .03 | .03 | .02 | .02 | .02 | Impairment begins |
| 2 | .10 | .09 | .08 | .07 | .06 | .05 | .05 | .04 | .04 | Driving skills significantly affected |
| 3 | .15 | .14 | .11 | .10 | .09 | .08 | .07 | .06 | .06 | |
| 4 | .20 | .18 | .15 | .13 | .11 | .10 | .09 | .08 | .08 | Possible criminal penalties |
| 5 | .25 | .23 | .19 | .16 | .14 | .13 | .11 | .10 | .09 | |
| 6 | .30 | .27 | .23 | .19 | .17 | .15 | .14 | .12 | .11 | |
| 7 | .35 | .32 | .27 | .23 | .20 | .18 | .16 | .14 | .13 | |
| 8 | .40 | .36 | .30 | .26 | .23 | .20 | .18 | .17 | .15 | Legally intoxicated |
| 9 | .45 | .41 | .34 | .29 | .26 | .23 | .20 | .19 | .17 | Criminal penalties |
| 10 | .51 | .45 | .38 | .32 | .28 | .25 | .23 | .21 | .19 | |

Subtract .01% for each 40 minutes of drinking.
One drink is 1.25 oz. of 80 proof liquor, 12 oz. of beer, or 5 oz. of table wine.

▲ **Figure 12-2** Alcohol Impairment Charts

Source: Data supplied by the Pennsylvania Liquor Control Board.

The dangers of alcohol increase along with the amount you drink. Heavy drinking destroys the liver, weakens the heart, elevates blood pressure, damages the brain, and increases the risk of cancer. Individuals who drink heavily have a higher mortality rate than those who have two or fewer drinks a day. However, the boundary between safe and dangerous drinking isn't the same for everyone. For some people, the upper limit of safety is zero: Once they start, they can't stop.

## Intoxication

If you drink too much, the immediate consequence is that you get drunk—or, more precisely, intoxicated. According to the American Psychiatric Association's definition, **intoxication** consists of "clinically significant maladaptive behavioral or psychological changes," such as inappropriate sexual or aggressive behavior, mood changes, impaired judgment, and impaired social and occupational functioning. Alcohol intoxication, which can range from mild inebriation to loss of consciousness, is characterized by at least one of the following signs: slurred speech, poor coordination, unsteady gait, abnormal eye movements, impaired attention or memory, stupor, or coma. Medical risks of intoxication include falls, hypothermia in cold climates, and increased risk of infections because of suppressed immune function.

Time and a protective environment are the recommended treatments for alcohol intoxication. Anyone who passes out after drinking heavily should be monitored regularly to ensure that vomiting (the result of excess alcohol irritating the stomach) doesn't block the breathing airway. Always make sure that an unconscious drinker is lying on his or her side, with the head lower than the body.

consumed by an individual every day, up to an absolute maximum of 1.75 ounces of alcohol a day—the equivalent of three beers, two mixed drinks, or three and a half glasses of wine. Your own limit may well be less, depending on your gender, size, and weight. Some people—such as women who are pregnant or trying to conceive; individuals with problems, such as ulcers, that might be aggravated by alcohol; those taking medications such as sleeping pills or antidepressants; and those driving or operating any motorized equipment—shouldn't drink at all.

Intoxicated drinkers can slip into shock, a potentially life-threatening condition characterized by a weak pulse, irregular breathing, and skin-color changes. This is an emergency, and professional medical care should be sought immediately.

## Impact of Alcohol

Unlike drugs in tablet form or food, alcohol is directly and quickly absorbed into the bloodstream through the stomach walls and upper intestine. The alcohol in a typical drink reaches the bloodstream in 15 minutes and rises to its peak concentration in about an hour. The bloodstream carries the alcohol to the liver, heart, and brain. (See Figure 12-3.)

Alcohol is a *diuretic,* a drug that speeds up the elimination of fluid from the body. Most of the alcohol you drink can leave your body only after metabolism by the liver, which converts about 95 percent of the alcohol to carbon dioxide and water. The other 5 percent is excreted unchanged, mainly through urination, respiration, and perspiration. Alcohol lowers body temperature, so you should never drink to get or stay warm. Alcohol affects the major organ systems of the body, and its effects are cumulative.

## Digestive System

Alcohol reaches the stomach first, where it is partially broken down. The remaining alcohol is absorbed easily through the stomach tissue into the bloodstream. In the stomach, alcohol triggers the secretion of acids, which irritate the stomach lining. Excessive drinking at one sitting may result in nausea; chronic drinking may result in peptic ulcers (breaks in the stomach lining) and bleeding from the stomach lining.

The alcohol in the bloodstream eventually reaches the liver. The liver, which bears the major responsibility of fat metabolism in the body, converts this alcohol to fat. After a

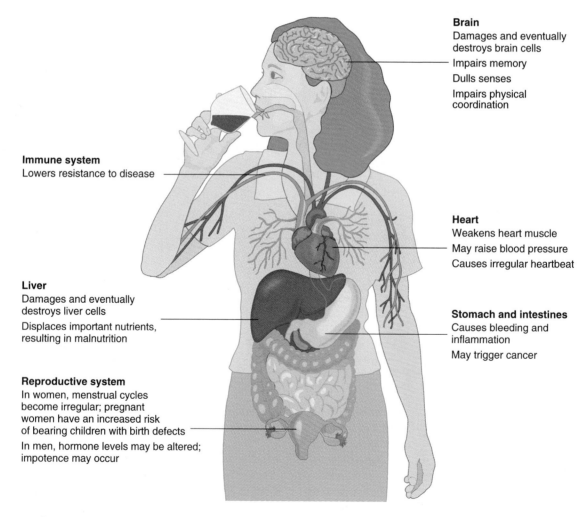

**Brain**
Damages and eventually destroys brain cells
Impairs memory
Dulls senses
Impairs physical coordination

**Immune system**
Lowers resistance to disease

**Liver**
Damages and eventually destroys liver cells
Displaces important nutrients, resulting in malnutrition

**Reproductive system**
In women, menstrual cycles become irregular; pregnant women have an increased risk of bearing children with birth defects
In men, hormone levels may be altered; impotence may occur

**Heart**
Weakens heart muscle
May raise blood pressure
Causes irregular heartbeat

**Stomach and intestines**
Causes bleeding and inflammation
May trigger cancer

▲ **Figure 12-3** The Effects of Alcohol Abuse on the Body

few weeks of four or five drinks a day, liver cells start to accumulate fat. Alcohol also stimulates liver cells to attract white blood cells, which normally travel throughout the bloodstream engulfing harmful substances and wastes. If white blood cells begin to invade body tissue, such as the liver, they can cause irreversible damage.

## Cardiovascular System

Alcohol gets mixed reviews regarding its effects on the cardiovascular system. People who drink moderate amounts of alcohol have lower mortality rates after a heart attack, as well as a lower risk of heart attack, compared to abstainers and heavy drinkers.[4] Moderate drinkers also have less buildup of cholesterol in their arteries, and are less likely to die of heart disease than heavy drinkers or teetotalers. French researchers have associated moderate drinking of only wine with lower mortality, although drinking both wine and beer reduced the risk of cardiovascular death.

However, heavier drinking triggers the release of harmful oxygen molecules called free radicals, which can increase the risk of heart disease, stroke, and cirrhosis of the liver. Alcohol can weaken the heart muscle, causing a disorder called *cardiomyopathy*. The combined use of alcohol and other drugs, including tobacco and cocaine, greatly increases the likelihood of damage to the heart.

## Immune System

Chronic alcohol use can inhibit the production of both white blood cells, which fight off infections, and red blood cells, which carry oxygen to all the organs and tissues of the body. Alcohol may increase the risk of HIV infection by altering the judgment of users so that they more readily engage in activities, such as unsafe sexual practices, that put them in danger. If you drink when you have a cold or the flu, alcohol interferes with the body's ability to recover. It also increases the chance of bacterial pneumonia in flu sufferers.

## Brain and Behavior

At first, when you drink, you feel up. In low dosages, alcohol affects the regions of the brain that inhibit or control behavior, so you feel looser and act in ways you might not otherwise. However, you also experience losses of concentration, memory, judgment, and fine motor control; and you have mood swings and emotional outbursts. Moderate and heavy drinkers show signs of impaired intelligence, slowed-down reflexes, and difficulty remembering. Research has shown that heavy drinking also depletes the brain's supplies of crucial chemicals, including dopamine, gamma aminobutyric acid, opioid peptides, and serotonin, that are responsible for our feelings of pleasure and well-being. At the same time, alcohol promotes the release of stress chemicals, such as corticotropin releasing factor (CRF), that create tension and depression.

Heavy alcohol use may pose special dangers to the brains of drinkers at both ends of the age spectrum. Adolescents who drink regularly show impairments in their neurological and cognitive functioning.[5] Elderly people who drink heavily appear to have more brain shrinkage, or atrophy, than those who drink lightly or not at all. In general, moderate drinkers have healthier brains than those who don't drink and those who drink to excess.[6]

Because alcohol is a central nervous system depressant, it slows down the activity of the neurons in the brain, gradually dulling the responses of the brain and nervous system. One or two drinks act as a tranquilizer or relaxant. Additional drinks result in a progressive reduction in central nervous system activity, leading to sleep, general anesthesia, coma, and even death. Moderate amounts of alcohol can have disturbing effects on perception and judgment, including the following:

- **Impaired perceptions.** You're less able to adjust your eyes to bright lights because glare bothers you more. Although you can still hear sounds, you can't distinguish between them or accurately determine their source.
- **Dulled smell and taste.** Alcohol itself may cause some vitamin deficiencies, and the poor eating habits of heavy drinkers result in further nutrition problems.
- **Diminished sensation.** On a freezing winter night, you may walk outside without a coat and not feel the cold.
- **Altered sense of space.** You may not realize, for instance, that you have been in one place for several hours.
- **Impaired motor skills.** Writing, typing, driving, and other tasks involving your muscles are impaired. This is why law enforcement officers sometimes ask suspected drunk drivers to touch their nose with a finger or to walk a straight line. Drinking large amounts of alcohol impairs reaction time, speed, accuracy, and consistency, as well as judgment.
- **Impaired sexual performance.** While drinking may increase your interest in sex, it may also impair sexual response, especially a man's ability to achieve or maintain an erection. As Shakespeare wrote, "It provokes the desire, but it takes away the performance."

## Increased Risk of Dying

Alcohol kills. Alcohol is responsible for 100,000 deaths each year and is the third leading cause of death after tobacco and improper diet and lack of exercise.[7] The leading alcohol-related cause of death is injury. Alcohol plays a role in at least half of all traffic fatalities, half of all homicides, and a quarter of all suicides. The second leading cause of alcohol-related deaths is cirrhosis of the liver, a chronic disease that causes extensive scarring and irreversible damage. In addition, as many as half of patients admitted to hospitals and 15 percent of those making office visits seek or need medical care because of the direct or indirect effects of alcohol.

Young drinkers—teens and those in their early twenties—are at highest risk of dying from injuries, mostly car accidents. Older drinkers over age 50 face the greatest danger of premature death from cirrhosis of the liver, hepatitis, and other alcohol-linked illnesses. Light alcohol intake (no more than one drink a day for women and two for men) is associated with lower mortality than abstinence, but mortality rates increase with the amount of alcohol consumed. The mortality rate for alcoholics is two and a half times higher than for nonalcoholics of the same age.

## Interaction with Other Drugs

Alcohol can interact with other drugs—prescription and nonprescription, legal and illegal. Of the 100 most frequently prescribed drugs, more than half contain at least one ingredient that interacts adversely with alcohol. Because alcohol and other psychoactive drugs may work on the same areas of the brain, their combination can produce an effect much greater than that expected of either drug by itself. The consequences of this synergistic interaction can be fatal. (See Savvy Consumer: "Alcohol and Drug Interactions.") Alcohol is particularly dangerous when combined with depressants and antianxiety medications.

Aspirin, long used to prevent or counter alcohol's effects, may actually enhance its impact by significantly lowering the body's ability to break down alcohol in the stomach. In a study of healthy men between the ages of 30 and 45, volunteers who took two extra-strength aspirin tablets an hour before drinking a glass and a half of wine had a 30 percent higher BAC than when they drank alcohol alone. This increase could make a difference in impairment for individuals driving cars or operating machinery.

If you want to drink while taking medication, be sure you read the warnings on nonprescription-drug labels or prescription-drug containers; ask your doctor about possible alcohol–drug interactions; and check with your phar-

## Savvy Consumer

## Alcohol and Drug Interactions

| Drug | Possible Effects of Interaction |
|---|---|
| Analgesics (painkillers) | |
|    Narcotic (Codeine, Demerol, Percodan) | Increase in central nervous system depression, possibly leading to respiratory failure and death. |
|    Nonnarcotic (aspirin, acetaminophen) | Irritation of stomach resulting in bleeding and increased susceptibility to liver damage. |
| Antabuse | Nausea, vomiting, headache, high blood pressure, and erratic heartbeat. |
| Antianxiety drugs (Valium, Librium) | Increase in central nervous system depression; decreased alertness and impaired judgment. |
| Antidepressants | Increase in central nervous system depression; certain antidepressants in combination with red wine could cause a sudden increase in blood pressure. |
| Antihistamines (Actifed, Dimetap, and other cold medications) | Increase in drowsiness; driving more dangerous. |
| Antibiotics | Nausea, vomiting, headache; some medications rendered less effective. |
| Central nervous system stimulants (caffeine, Dexedrine, Ritalin) | Stimulant effects of these drugs may reverse depressant effect of alcohol but do not decrease its intoxicating effects. |
| Diuretics (Diuril, Lasix) | Reduction in blood pressure resulting in dizziness upon rising. |
| Sedatives (Dalmane, Nembutal, Quaalude) | Increase in central nervous system depression, possibly leading to coma, respiratory failure, and death. |

macist if you have any questions about your medications, especially over-the-counter (OTC) products.

## Drinking in America

According to the most recent statistics available from the National Institute on Alcohol Abuse and Alcoholism, about 60 percent of American adults use alcohol, although they vary in how much and how often they drink. Whites are more likely to be daily or near-daily drinkers than nonwhites. Men tend to drink more and more often than women. Young people between the ages of 21 and 34 are most likely to drink, and alcohol use typically declines with age.

## Why People Drink

The most common reason people drink alcohol is to relax. Because it depresses the central nervous system, alcohol can make people feel less tense. Other motivations for drinking include the following:

✓ **Celebration.** Unless alcohol use violates family, ethnic, or religious values, people raise their glasses together on life's important occasions—births, graduations, weddings, promotions.

✓ **Friendship.** When friends visit, they may have a drink, or they may meet somewhere "for a drink." Young people are much more likely to experiment with alcohol if their friends drink.

✓ **Social ease.** When people use alcohol, they may seem bolder, wittier, sexier. At the same time, they become more relaxed and seem to enjoy each other's company

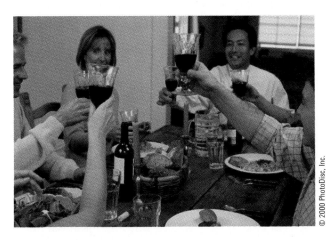

▲ Alcohol can be part of many enjoyable social situations, as long as individuals know when to say "no more." Many people are increasingly substituting nonalcoholic drinks.

more. Because alcohol lowers inhibitions, some people see it as a prelude to seduction.

✓ **Self-medication.** Like other drugs, alcohol may be the means some people use to treat—or escape from—painful feelings or bad moods.

✓ **Role models.** Athletes, some of the most admired celebrities in our country, have a long history of appearing in commercials for alcohol. Many advertisements feature glamorous women holding or sipping alcoholic beverages.

✓ **Advertising.** Brewers and beer distributors spend $15 to $20 million a year promoting the message: If you want to have fun, have a drink. Adolescents may be especially responsive to such sales pitches. Nearly two dozen national groups, including the American Medical Association, have petitioned the Federal Trade Commission to ban alcohol advertisements that link drinking to risky activities (such as driving, water skiing, and skydiving) and that target youth.

##  How Common Is Drinking on College Campuses?

Drinking has long been part of the college experience. For the majority of students, alcohol usually does not interfere with their school and work responsibilities. However, alcohol use can—and too often does—become problematic and even tragic. A single episode, combined with poor judgment or bad luck, can lead to life-altering and sometimes life-threatening consequences.[8]

In the last decade, patterns in college drinking have changed in some ways, but not in others. (See Student Snapshot: "Drinking on Campus.") More students abstain—19.3 percent, up from 16.4 percent in 1993.[9] However, more students now say that they drink primarily for the purpose of getting drunk. While fewer students attend or drink heavily at fraternity and sorority parties than a decade ago, more are drinking heavily at off-campus parties. College women are as likely to drink, but men drink more heavily. About half of college men and a third of college women report drinking to excess.

Fewer underage students (77.4 percent) drink than 21- to 23-year-olds (85.6 percent). They also drink less frequently and are less likely to binge. However, increased numbers of underage students report being drunk three or more times in the past 30 days. Students under age 21 in states with tough laws against underage drinking are less likely to drink than those in states with fewer restrictions. When they drink, underage students are more likely to drink to excess than older ones—possibly because they feel greater pressure to drink quickly before some authority cuts off their alcohol supply or they get caught.[10]

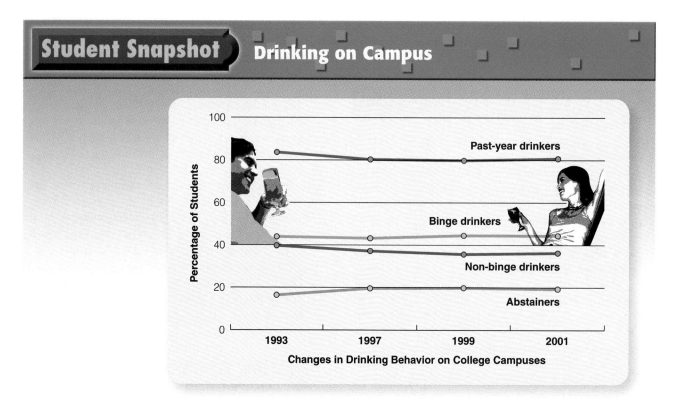

**Student Snapshot** **Drinking on Campus**

Percentage of Students

Past-year drinkers

Binge drinkers

Non-binge drinkers

Abstainers

1993  1997  1999  2001

**Changes in Drinking Behavior on College Campuses**

Source: Data from Wechsler, Henry, et al. "Trend in College Binge Drinking During a Period of Increased Prevention Efforts." *Journal of American College Health,* Vol. 50, No. 5, March 2002, p. 203.

Two in five students, 44 percent, report at least occasional **binge drinking,** which generally means at least five drinks for men and four for women. Schools with large fraternity systems and rural colleges typically report more heavy drinking, while Christian and women's colleges have less drinking. However, heavy drinking has become more prevalent on most campuses.[11] An estimated 10 percent of college students drink more than 15 alcoholic beverages per week.[12]

Every year students spend $5.5 billion on alcohol, mostly beer—more than they spend on books, soda pop, coffee, juice, and milk combined. The total amount of alcohol consumed by college students each year is 430 million gallons, enough for every college and university in the United States to fill an Olympic-size swimming pool.

Virtually all colleges provide alcohol education programs. Many universities prohibit delivery of beer kegs to dormitories, fraternity houses, and sorority houses.[13] Some schools are studying whether they're scheduling too few classes on Fridays, which might spur Thursday-night partying. Other colleges are trying a social-norms approach, spreading the message to students that their peers drink less than they think, in an attempt to make heavy drinking less socially acceptable.[14] Some have developed programs that extend beyond the campus to reach families or high school students.

The U.S. Department of Education has begun highlighting innovative antidrinking practices on campus; Mothers Against Drunk Driving (MADD) is planning to rank colleges based on how well they curb student drinking. There has been an increase in on-campus chapters of national support groups such as AA, Al-Anon, Adult Children of Alcoholics, and a peer-education program called BACCHUS: Boost Alcohol Consciousness Concerning the Health of University Students.

## Why College Students Drink

Most college students drink for the same reasons undergraduates have always turned to alcohol: Away from home, often for the first time, many are excited by and apprehensive about their newfound independence. When new pressures seem overwhelming, when they feel awkward or insecure, when they just want to let loose and have a good time, they reach for a drink.

Freshmen may be especially vulnerable to dangerous drinking as they struggle to adapt to an often bewildering new world. In a study of freshmen at a medium-sized state university and at a small, predominantly African-American university who were nondrinkers as high school seniors, almost half (46.5 percent) started to drink in college. They were less likely to do so if they had friends who discouraged them from drinking.

Other studies have also linked alcohol consumption with where students live on campus and what they perceive as the norm for acceptable drinking.[15] Stress-related drinking is common. Students in competitive academic environments may turn to alcohol to reduce their anxiety and the pressure to perform. Athletes have higher drinking rates than nonathletes.[16] Members of sororities and fraternities rated all drinking norms as more extreme and perceived fraternity drinking as particularly heavy. Fraternity leaders are among the heaviest drinkers and the most out-of-control partygoers, with the highest incidence of heavy drinking and bingeing.

The most dramatic increases in college drinking have been among women: Eight in ten female undergraduates say they drink; one in four get drunk three or more times in a month. (See The X & Y Files: "Alcohol, Tobacco, and Gender.")

Among both men and women, those with alcoholic parents and dysfunctional families are at greater risk of substance abuse. By some estimates, one of five college students comes from an alcoholic home and may be at increased risk of developing a drinking problem. More than two of every five students report at least one symptom of alcohol abuse or dependence (discussed later in this chapter) and are at increased risk of developing a true alcohol disorder.[17]

## Binge Drinking

Binge drinking—defined as the consumption of five or more alcoholic drinks in a row by men and four or more by women—is the leading cause of preventable death among undergraduates and the most serious threat to their intellectual, physical, and psychological development.[18] In recent years, several students have died after consuming numerous drinks in a short period of time, sometimes as part of hazing rituals.

According to the most recent findings of the Harvard School of Public Health's College Alcohol Study, which has

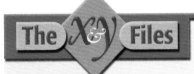

## Alcohol, Tobacco, and Gender

According to conventional gender stereotypes, drinking is a symbol of manliness. In the past, far more men than women drank. In the United States today, both genders are likely to consume alcohol. However, there are well-documented differences in how often and how much men and women drink. In general, men drink more frequently, consume a larger quantity of alcohol per drinking occasion, and report more problems related to drinking.

Women are at greater risk of organ damage from heavy alcohol use and have higher rates of liver cirrhosis. One reason is that females do not respond to long-term heavy use of alcohol with the same protective physiological mechanisms as men. As a result, drinking the same amount of alcohol causes more damage to the female liver. Women drinkers also are at greater risk of heart disease, osteoporosis, and breast cancer.

In recent years, researchers have been comparing and contrasting the reasons why men and women drink. Undergraduate women and men are equally likely to drink for stress-related reasons; both perceive alcohol as a means of tension relaxation. Some psychologists theorize that men engage in *confirmatory drinking,* that is, they drink to reinforce the image of masculinity associated with alcohol consumption. Both genders may engage in *compensatory drinking,* consuming alcohol to

heighten their sense of masculinity or femininity.

According to the Centers for Disease Control and Prevention, 28 percent of men and 22 percent of women are smokers. Among teens, more girls than boys smoke.

Male and female smokers share certain characteristics: Most start smoking as teenagers; the lower their educational level, the more likely they are to smoke. But there are gender differences in tobacco use. In the last decade, smoking rates among adult women stopped their previous decline and have risen sharply among teenage girls. Men of all ages are more likely than women to use other forms of tobacco, such as cigars and chewing tobacco.

The genders smoke for different reasons. Men smoke to decrease boredom and fatigue and to increase arousal and concentration. Women smoke to control their weight and to decrease stress, anger, and other negative feelings.

Women tend to be less successful than men in quitting smoking. Possible reasons include gender differences in the effectiveness of therapies, a greater fear of weight gain among women, the inability to take certain antismoking drugs while pregnant, and the menstrual cycle's effect on withdrawal symptoms. Women drop out at higher rates from traditional stop-smoking programs and are less responsive to nicotine replacement therapies. The approaches that work best for them combine medication and behavioral treatments, including support groups.

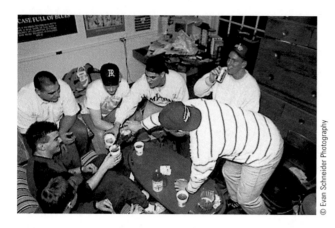

▲ Binge drinkers can get into—and cause—trouble. Dangerously large amounts of alcohol can cause death, and heavy party drinking often results in violence.

conducted four national surveys of students at 119 colleges, 40 to 45 percent of college students report binge drinking. This percentage has remained stable in the last decade—despite greater awareness, more efforts at prevention, and demands for greater accountability.[19]

The number of frequent binge drinkers has increased somewhat in the last decade, even though fewer undergraduates say they were binge drinkers in high school.[20] Frequent binge drinkers account for almost 70 percent of all alcohol consumed by college students.[21] Students in four-year colleges are more likely to binge than those in two-year colleges. Many more of those living in fraternity or sorority houses (65.9 percent) report bingeing than stu-  dents living elsewhere (38.1 percent).[22] The students least likely to binge drink were African American or Asian, aged 24 years or older, married, and had not been binge drinkers in high school.[23]

More women now binge. At coed schools, 41.2 percent report at least one binge within the previous two weeks; 17.4 percent are frequent bingers. At all-female colleges, binge drinking has jumped 125 percent, from 24.5 percent in 1993 to 32.1 percent in 2001.[24] Unplanned sexual activities, date rape, and sexual assault are 150 percent more likely among women who drink than among those who do not. Sophomore, junior, and senior women are much less likely to engage in heavy episodic drinking than freshman women.[25]

Why do students binge? Some educators view bingeing as a product of the college environment.[26] More students binge drink at the beginning of the school year and then cut back as the semester progresses and academic demands increase. Binge drinking also peaks following exam times, during home football weekends, and during spring break. Many new students engage in binge drinking for the first

time very soon after they arrive on campus. Binges become less common in their subsequent years at school and almost always end with education. Real life, one educator notes, is "a strong disincentive" to this type of drinking.[27]

Fewer than 10 percent of frequent binge drinkers experience any disciplinary action as a result of their drinking.[28] Support for tougher campus restrictions has grown among students, particularly those who do not binge drink and who have experienced the negative consequences of others' drinking, such as violence and vandalism.[29] According to studies of schools that have lowered binge drinking rates, a combination of social and environmental approaches has the greatest impact on reducing binge drinking. Key elements are involvement of students and development of alternatives, such as alcohol-free parties and events.[30]

Despite their heavy drinking as undergraduates, within three years of graduation, students who had been members of fraternities and sororities drink no more than students who did not join Greek houses. Heavy drinking may be the result of students' perceptions that excessive alcohol use is normal in Greek houses, along with the encouragement of peers.[31]

Surveys consistently show that students who engage in binge drinking, particularly those who do so more than once a week, experience a far higher rate of problems than other students. Frequent binge drinkers are likely to miss classes, vandalize property, and drive after drinking. Frequent binge drinkers are also more likely to experience five or more different alcohol-related problems and to use other substances, including nicotine, marijuana, cocaine, and LSD.[32]

Students on campuses with many binge drinkers report higher rates of secondhand problems caused by others' alcohol use, compared with students on campuses with lower rates of binge drinking. These problems include loss of sleep, interruption of studies, assaults, vandalism, and unwanted sexual advances. Students living on campuses with high rates of binge drinking are two or more times as likely to experience these secondhand effects as those living on campuses with low rates.[33]

## The Toll of College Drinking

More than 1,400 students die from alcohol-related accidents every year. More than 500,000 students experience drinking-related injuries; more than 600,000 are hit or assaulted by another student who has been drinking.[34] Of the 8 million college students in the United States, 2 million have driven under the influence of alcohol; more than 3 million have ridden with a drinking driver.[35] More than a third of students surveyed reported doing some-

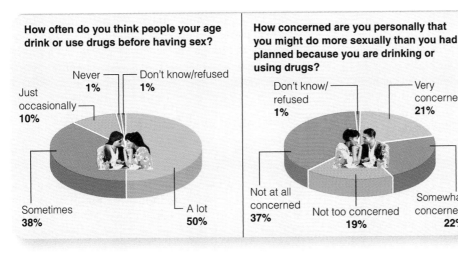

**How often do you think people your age drink or use drugs before having sex?**

Never 1%
Don't know/refused 1%
Just occasionally 10%
Sometimes 38%
A lot 50%

**How concerned are you personally that you might do more sexually than you had planned because you are drinking or using drugs?**

Don't know/refused 1%
Very concerned 21%
Not at all concerned 37%
Not too concerned 19%
Somewhat concerned 22%

▲ **Figure 12-4** Substance Abuse and Risky Sexual Behavior

Source: Henry J. Kaiser Family Foundation

thing they regretted while under the influence of alcohol.[36] See Table 12-1.

According to the Commission on Substance Abuse at Colleges and Universities, alcohol is involved in two-thirds

▼ **Table 12-1 Alcohol-Related Problems Among Students Who Drink Alcohol**

| Alcohol-Related Problem | Percentage of Students Reporting the Problem |
| --- | --- |
| Miss a class | 29.5 |
| Get behind in school work | 21.6 |
| Do something you regret | 35.0 |
| Forget where you were or what you did | 26.8 |
| Argue with friends | 22.9 |
| Engage in unplanned sexual activities | 21.3 |
| Not use protection when you had sex | 10.4 |
| Damage property | 10.7 |
| Get into trouble with the campus or local police | 6.5 |
| Get hurt or injured | 12.8 |
| Require medical treatment for an overdose | 0.8 |
| Drive after drinking | 29.0 |

Source: Wechsler, Henry, et al. "Trends in College Binge Drinking During a Period of Increased Prevention Efforts." *Journal of American College Health*, Vol. 50, No. 5, March 2002, p. 203.

of college student suicides, nine of ten rapes, and 95 percent of violent crimes on campus.[37] According to a national survey released by the Higher Education Center for Alcohol and Other Drug Prevention, 75 to 90 percent of all violence on college campuses is alcohol-related. About 300,000 of today's college students will eventually die from alcohol-related causes, including drunk-driving accidents, cirrhosis of the liver, various cancers, and heart disease, estimates the Core Institute, an organization that studies college drinking.

Drinking also increases sexual risks for college students. (See Figure 12-4). Heavy drinking has been correlated with increased casual sex without condoms, an increased number of sex partners, and sexual attacks on women. According to a 2002 survey, half of 15- to 24-year-olds mix alcohol, drugs, and sex "a lot." Alcohol and drug use can lead to earlier sexual initiation, unprotected sexual intercourse, multiple sex partners, and increased risk of sexually transmitted diseases.[38]

The impact of student drinking spills beyond campus borders. Neighbors living within a mile of a college are much more likely to experience disturbances such as vandalism, assault, noise, litter, and drunkenness than those living farther away.[39] Support for tougher restrictions on alcohol has grown on some campuses. Laws restricting underage drinking or governing the volume of sales and consumption of alcohol are associated with less drinking among underage students.[40]

## Drinking and Race

Experts in alcohol treatment are increasingly recognizing racial and ethnic differences in risk factors for drinking problems, patterns of drinking, and most effective types of treatment. Increases in drinking have been traced to stresses related to immigration, acculturation, poverty, racial discrimination, and powerlessness. Environmental factors, such as aggressive marketing and advertising of alcoholic beverages in minority neighbor-

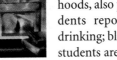

hoods, also play a role. On campus white students report the highest rates of heavy drinking; black students, the lowest. Hispanic students are intermediate.[41]

## African-American Community

Overall, African Americans consume less alcohol per person than whites, yet twice as many blacks die of cirrhosis of the liver each year. In some cities, the rate of cirrhosis is ten times higher among African-American than white men. Alcohol also contributes to high rates of hypertension, esophageal cancer, and homicide among African-American men.

The makers of alcoholic beverages aggressively market their products to African Americans, and there are many more liquor stores (per capita) in many African-American neighborhoods than in white communities. Peer pressure to drink, the easy accessibility of alcohol, and socioeconomic frustrations increase the likelihood of alcohol problems among African Americans. Moreover, recovery can be especially difficult because of the lack of treatment programs and role models in the African-American community and ongoing pressures to resume drinking.

## Hispanic Community

The various Hispanic cultures tend to discourage any drinking by women but encourage heavy drinking by men as part of machismo, or feelings of manhood. According to the Department of Health and Human Services, Hispanic men have higher rates of alcohol use and abuse than the general population and suffer a high rate of cirrhosis. Moreover, American-born Hispanic men drink more than those born in other countries.

Few Hispanics enter treatment, partly because of a lack of information, language barriers, and poor community-

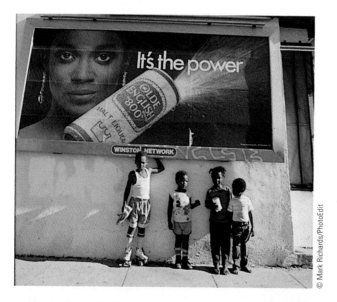

▲ The makers of alcoholic beverages aggressively market their products in poor urban neighborhoods, where liquor stores and bars are common.

based services. Hispanic families generally try to resolve problems themselves, and their cultural values discourage the sharing of intimate personal stories, which characterizes Alcoholics Anonymous and other support groups. Churches often provide the most effective forms of help.

## Native American Community

European settlers introduced alcohol to Native Americans. Because of the societal and physical problems resulting from excessive drinking, at the request of tribal leaders, the U.S. Congress in 1832 prohibited the use of alcohol by Native Americans. Many reservations still ban alcohol use, so Native Americans who want to drink may have to travel long distances to obtain alcohol, which may contribute to the high death rate from hypothermia and pedestrian and motor-vehicle accidents among Native Americans. (Injuries are the leading cause of death among this group.)

Certainly, not all Native Americans drink, and not all who drink do so to excess. However, they have three times the general population's rate of alcohol-related injury and illness. Cirrhosis of the liver is the fourth-leading cause of death among this cultural group. While many Native American women don't drink, those who do have high rates of alcohol-related problems, which affect both them and their children. Their rate of cirrhosis of the liver is 36 times that of white women. In some tribes, 10.5 out of every 1,000 newborns have fetal alcohol syndrome, compared with 1 to 3 out of 1,000 in the general population. (See the discussion on fetal alcohol syndrome in the next section.)

Both a biological predisposition and socioeconomic conditions may contribute to alcohol abuse by Native Americans. In addition, alcoholism is not a physical disease according to their cultural beliefs, but a spiritual disorder, making it less likely that they'll seek appropriate treatment.

## Asian-American Community

Asian Americans tend to drink very little or not at all, in part because of an inborn physiological reaction to alcohol that causes facial flushing, rapid heart rate, lowered blood pressure, nausea, vomiting, and other symptoms. A very high percentage of women of all Asian-American nationalities abstain completely. Some sociologists have expressed concern, however, that as Asian Americans become more assimilated into American culture, they'll drink more—and possibly suffer very adverse effects from alcohol.

## Women and Alcohol

More than half of women drink: Of these, 45 percent are light drinkers; 3 percent, moderate drinkers; 2 percent, heavy drinkers; and 21 percent, binge drinkers. According to the National Institute of Alcohol Abuse and Alcoholism, almost 4 million women suffer from alcohol abuse or dependence. But women who drink have different risk factors, potential dangers, and drinking patterns than men.[42]

## Why Women Drink

In the past, most people, including physicians and therapists, assumed that women who drank heavily did so primarily for social and psychological reasons—because they were lonely, isolated, brokenhearted. Many of these assumptions have proven to be false. The following are more likely to lead to drinking problems in women.

✓ **Inherited susceptibility.** In women, as in men, genetics accounts for 50 to 60 percent of a person's vulnerability to a serious drinking problem. Although heredity increases the risk of alcoholism, life circumstances also play an important role in determining whether young women will have a drinking problem. Female alcoholics are more likely than males to have a parent who abused drugs or alcohol, who had psychiatric problems, or who attempted suicide.

✓ **Childhood traumas.** Female alcoholics often report that they were physically or sexually abused as children or suffered great distress because of poverty or a parent's death.

✓ **Depression.** Women are more likely than men to be depressed prior to drinking and to suffer from both depression and a drinking problem at the same time. Even after women enter and complete treatment for their alcohol problems, depressive symptoms may persist.[43]

✓ **Relationship issues.** Single, separated, or divorced women drink more and more often than married women; women with live-in male partners have the highest rates of drinking problems. "Functioning

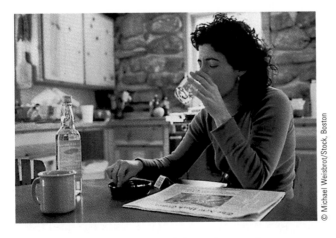

▲ Genetics, childhood trauma, and depression contribute to a woman's vulnerability to heavy drinking and alcohol dependence.

women alcoholics may be very successful in other areas of their lives but have problems in their relationships," says Sharon Wilsnack, Ph.D., a professor at the University of North Dakota School of Medicine who studied the drinking habits of more than 1,100 women over ten years.[44]

✓ **Psychological factors.** Like men, women may drink to compensate for feelings of inadequacy. Women who tend to ruminate or mull over bad feelings may find that alcohol increases this tendency and makes them feel more distressed. Women involved with heavy drinkers are at risk of drinking heavily themselves, at least as long as the relationship continues.

✓ **Employment.** Women who work outside the home are less likely to become problem drinkers or alcoholics than those without paying jobs. The one exception: women in occupations still dominated by men, such as engineering, science, law enforcement, and top corporate management. "Often women in these fields drink as a way of fitting in," observes Wilsnack. "Drinking takes on symbolic value. It's a way of signaling power, equality, status."

✓ **A lack or loss of roles.** Women of all ages, regardless of marital or employment status, tend to drink more and lean on alcohol when they lose a valued role, for example, when they're laid off from a job or their marriage ends in divorce.

✓ **Self-medication.** Some women feel it's permissible to use alcohol as if it were a medicine. As long as they're taking it for a reason, it seems acceptable to them, even if they're drifting into a drinking problem.

## Alcohol's Effects on Women

Problems directly related to a woman's alcohol use range from the consequences of risky sexual behavior after alcohol consumption (such as unwanted pregnancy or STDs) to severe physiological problems related to fertility and pregnancy. Because they have a far smaller quantity of a protective enzyme in the stomach to break down alcohol before it's absorbed into the bloodstream, women absorb about 30 percent more alcohol into their bloodstream than men. The alcohol travels through the blood to the brain, so women become intoxicated much more quickly. And because there's more alcohol in the bloodstream to break down, the liver may also be adversely affected. In alcoholic women, the stomach seems to completely stop digesting alcohol, which may explain why women alcoholics are more likely to suffer liver damage than men.

Alcohol brings many other health dangers to women:

✓ **Gynecologic problems.** Moderate to heavy drinking may contribute to infertility, menstrual problems, sexual dysfunction, and premenstrual syndrome.

✔ **Pregnancy and fetal alcohol syndrome.** When a woman drinks during pregnancy, her unborn child drinks, too. According to CDC estimates, more than 8,000 alcohol-damaged babies are born every year. Women of all ages may be using alcohol and tobacco when they get pregnant; younger women are less likely to quit.[45]

One of every 750 newborns has a cluster of physical and mental defects called **fetal alcohol syndrome (FAS)**: small head, abnormal facial features, jitters, poor muscle tone, sleep disorders, sluggish motor development, failure to thrive, short stature, delayed speech, mental retardation, and hyperactivity. As a result of their mother's alcohol consumption, many more babies suffer **fetal alcohol effects (FAE)**: low birthweight, irritability as newborns, and permanent mental impairment.

Labels on alcoholic beverages have had a proven but modest effect on reducing drinking during pregnancy, while community-based education efforts have been much more effective. Drug and alcohol abuse also can affect the quality of a woman's mothering.

✔ **Breast cancer.** Numerous studies have suggested an increased risk of breast cancer among women who drink, and many physicians feel that those at high risk for breast cancer should stop, or at least reduce, their consumption of alcohol.

✔ **Osteoporosis.** As women age, their risk of osteoporosis, a condition characterized by calcium loss and bone thinning, increases. Alcohol can block the absorption

of many nutrients, including calcium, and heavy drinking may worsen the deterioration of bone tissue.

✔ **Heart disease.** Women who are very heavy drinkers are more at risk of developing irreversible heart disease than men who drink even more.

## Alcohol Treatment for Women

Women who abuse alcohol also face a special burden: intense social disapproval. Many become cross-addicted to prescription medicines, or they develop eating disorders or sexual dysfunctions. Women often don't get the same care men do, frequently because of financial limitations and child-care responsibilities. Also, women are more likely to blame their symptoms on depression or anxiety, whereas men attribute them directly to alcohol. As a result, women often obtain treatment later in the course of their illness, at a point when their problems are more severe. Increasingly, prevention programs are targeting high-risk women to recognize alcohol problems early and to tackle underlying problems, such as depression and low self-esteem.

One of the most effective programs for women is Women for Sobriety, founded in 1975 by sociologist Jean Kirkpatrick, Ph.D. Its meetings focus on building self-esteem, self-confidence, and responsibility. "AA was started by men, and its message is very disempowering for women," says Kirkpatrick. "We view members as competent women who are struggling with issues that all women must face. Women don't need to recall the painful process of becoming alcoholics. They need to put the past behind them and move on, upward and onward."[46]

## Drinking and Driving

Drunk driving is the most frequently committed crime in the United States. In the last two decades, families of the victims of drunk drivers have organized to change the way the nation treats its drunk drivers. Because of the efforts of MADD (Mothers Against Drunk Driving), SADD (Students Against Destructive Decisions), and other lobbying groups, cities, counties, and states are cracking down on drivers who drink. Since courts have held establishments that serve alcohol liable for the consequences of allowing drunk customers to drive, many bars and restaurants have joined the campaign against drunk driving. Many communities also provide free rides home on holidays and weekends for people who've had too much to drink.

To keep drunk drivers off the road, many cities have set up checkpoints to stop automobiles and inspect drivers for intoxication. The U.S. Supreme Court has ruled that a driver's refusal to submit to a blood-alcohol concentration test at checkpoints or at any other time can be used as evi-

▲ A child with fetal alcohol syndrome (FAS) has distinctive facial characteristics that vary with the severity of the disease, including droopy eyelids, a thin upper lip, and a wide space between the nose and upper lip.

© K. L. Jones/LLResearch

## STRATEGIES FOR PREVENTION

### How to Prevent Drunk Driving

▲ When going out in a group, always designate one person who won't drink at all to serve as the driver.

▲ Never get behind the wheel if you've had more than two drinks within two hours, especially if you haven't eaten.

▲ Never let intoxicated friends drive home. Call a taxi, drive them yourself, or arrange for them to spend the night in a safe place.

dence to prosecute him or her for drunk driving. An increasing number of states have toughened their enforcement of drunk-driving penalties. Some suspend a driver's license for several months for a first offense; repeat offenders can lose their license for a year or more.

The National Highway Traffic Safety Administration estimates that setting the legal age limit for drinking at 21 has saved 16,500 lives in traffic crashes alone since 1975. The majority of states have made it illegal for people younger than 21 to drive with a measurable amount of alcohol in their blood. Research comparing states that adopted such zero tolerance laws to those that did not have such laws found that zero tolerance states experienced 20 percent declines in the proportions of fatal single-vehicle, night crashes (the type most often alcohol-related) involving young drivers. Nationwide, alcohol-related traffic deaths among 15- to 20-year-olds have declined 57 percent. Raising the drinking age also has lowered the rate of pedestrian injuries.[47]

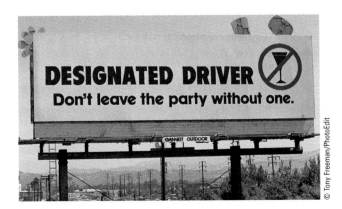

© Tony Freeman/PhotoEdit

▲ Public awareness campaigns like this one for designated drivers can help prevent the high incidence of fatalities caused by drunk drivers.

## Alcohol-Related Problems

About 20 percent of Americans are at-risk drinkers whose alcohol consumption exceeds the limits recommended by government studies (two drinks a day for men, one for women). These individuals are at increased risk of high blood pressure, stroke, violence, motor vehicle accidents, injury, and certain types of cancer.

By the simplest definition, problem drinking is the use of alcohol in any way that creates difficulties, potential difficulties, or health risks for an individual. Like alcoholics, problem drinkers are individuals whose lives are in some way impaired by their drinking. The only difference is one of degree. Alcohol becomes a problem, and a person becomes an alcoholic, when the drinker can't "take it or leave it." He or she spends more and more time anticipating the next drink, planning when and where to get it, buying and hiding alcohol, and covering up secret drinking. (See Table 12-2.)

**Alcohol abuse** involves continued use of alcohol despite awareness of social, occupational, psychological, or physical problems related to drinking, or drinking in dangerous ways or situations (before driving, for instance). A diagnosis of alcohol abuse is based on one or more of the following occurring at any time during a 12-month period:

✔ A failure to fulfill major role obligations at work, school, or home (such as missing work or school).
✔ The use of alcohol in situations in which it is physically hazardous (such as before driving).
✔ Alcohol-related legal problems (such as drunk-driving arrests).
✔ Continued alcohol use despite persistent or recurring social or interpersonal problems caused or exacerbated by alcohol (such as fighting while drunk).

**Alcohol dependence** is a separate disorder in which individuals develop a strong craving for alcohol because it produces pleasurable feelings or relieves stress or anxiety. Over time they experience physiological changes that lead to *tolerance* of its effects; this means that they must consume larger and larger amounts to achieve intoxication. If they abruptly stop drinking, they suffer *withdrawal*, a state of acute physical and psychological discomfort. A diagnosis of alcohol dependence is based on three or more of the following symptoms occurring during any 12-month period:

✔ Tolerance, as defined by either a need for markedly increased amounts of alcohol to achieve intoxication or desired effect, or a markedly diminished effect with continued drinking of the same amount of alcohol as in the past.
✔ Withdrawal, including at least two of the following symptoms: sweating, rapid pulse, or other signs of

▼ **Table 12-2 Recognizing the Warning Signs of Alcoholism**

| | | |
|---|---|---|
| • Experiencing the following symptoms after drinking: frequent headaches, nausea, stomach pain, heartburn, gas, fatigue, weakness, muscle cramps, irregular or rapid heartbeats.<br><br>• Needing a drink in the morning to start the day. | • Denying any problem with alcohol.<br><br>• Doing things while drinking that are regretted afterward.<br><br>• Dramatic mood swings, from anger to laughter to anxiety.<br><br>• Sleep problems. | • Depression and paranoia.<br><br>• Forgetting what happened during a drinking episode.<br><br>• Changing brands or going on the wagon to control drinking.<br><br>• Having five or more drinks a day. |

autonomic hyperactivity; increased hand tremor; insomnia; nausea or vomiting; temporary hallucinations or illusions; physical agitation or restlessness; anxiety; or grand mal seizures.

✔ Drinking to avoid or relieve the symptoms of withdrawal.

✔ Consuming larger amounts of alcohol, or drinking over a longer period than was intended.

✔ Persistent desire or unsuccessful efforts to cut down or control drinking.

✔ A great deal of time spent in activities necessary to obtain alcohol, drink it, or recover from its effects.

✔ Important social, occupational, or recreational activities given up or reduced because of alcohol use.

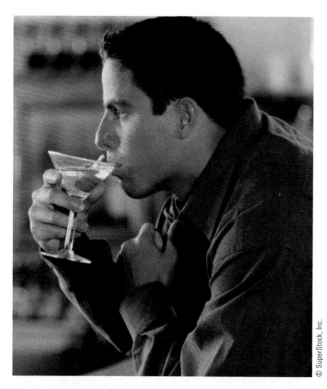

© SuperStock, Inc.

▲ Alcohol dependence may spring from the perception that alcohol relieves stress and anxiety, or creates a pleasant feeling. Chronic drinking—especially daytime drinking and drinking alone—can be a sign of serious problems, even though the drinker may otherwise appear to be in control.

✔ Continued alcohol use despite knowledge that alcohol is likely to cause or exacerbate a persistent or recurring physical or psychological problem.

**Alcoholism,** as defined by the National Council on Alcoholism and Drug Dependence and the American Society of Addiction, is a primary, chronic disease in which genetic, psychosocial, and environmental factors influence its development and manifestations. The disease is often progressive and fatal. Its characteristics include an inability to control drinking, a preoccupation with alcohol, continued use of alcohol despite adverse consequences, and distorted thinking, most notably denial. Like other diseases, alcoholism is not simply a matter of insufficient willpower, but a complex problem that causes many symptoms, can have serious consequences, yet can improve with treatment.

A lack of obvious signs of alcoholism can be deceiving. A person who doesn't drink in the morning but feels that he or she must always have a drink at a certain time of the day may have lost control over his or her drinking. A person who never drinks alone but always drinks socially with others may be camouflaging loss of control. A person who is holding a job or taking care of the family may still spend every waking hour thinking about that first drink at the end of the day (preoccupation).

 According to a recent survey of more than 14,000 undergraduates at four-year colleges, 6 percent of college students met criteria for a diagnosis of alcohol dependence or alcoholism, 31 percent for alcohol abuse. More than two of every five students reported at least one symptom of these conditions and were at increased risk of developing a true alcohol disorder. Few reported seeking treatment since coming to college.[48]

 **What Causes Alcohol Dependence and Abuse?**

Although the exact causes of alcohol dependence and alcohol abuse are not known, certain factors—including biochemical imbalances in the brain, heredity, cultural acceptability, and stress—all seem to play a role. They include the following:

✔ **Genetics.** Scientists who are working toward mapping the genes responsible for addictive disorders have not yet been able to identify conclusively a specific gene that puts people at risk for alcoholism. However, epidemiological studies have shown evidence of heredity's role. Studies of twins suggest that heredity accounts for two-thirds of the risk of becoming alcoholic in both men and women. An identical twin of an alcoholic is twice as likely as a fraternal twin to have an alcohol-related disorder. The incidence of alcoholism is four times higher among the sons of Caucasian alcoholic fathers, regardless of whether they grow up with their biological or adoptive parents.

✔ **Stress and traumatic experiences.** Many people start drinking heavily as a way of coping with psychological problems. About half of all individuals who abuse or are dependent on alcohol also have another mental disorder. Alcohol often is linked with depressive and anxiety disorders. Men and women with these problems may start drinking in an attempt to alleviate their anxiety or depression.

✔ **Parental alcoholism.** According to researchers, alcoholism is four to five times more common among the children of alcoholics, who may be influenced by the behavior they see in their parents. The sons and daughters of alcoholics share certain characteristics, including early onset of problem drinking with severe social consequences, an unstable family, poor academic and social performance in school, and antisocial behavior.

✔ **Drug abuse.** Alcoholism is associated with the abuse of other psychoactive drugs, including marijuana, cocaine, heroin, amphetamines, and various antianxiety medications. Adults under age 30 and adolescents are most likely to use alcohol plus several drugs of abuse, such as marijuana and cocaine. Middle-aged men and women are more likely to combine alcohol with benzodiazepines, such as antianxiety medications or sleeping pills, which may be prescribed for them by a physician.

Whatever the reason they start, some people keep drinking out of habit. Once they develop physical tolerance and dependence, they may not be able to stop drinking on their own.

## Medical Complications of Alcohol Abuse and Dependence

Excessive alcohol use adversely affects virtually every organ system in the body, including the brain, the digestive tract, the heart, muscles, blood, and hormones. In addition, because alcohol interacts with many drugs, it can increase the risk of potentially lethal overdoses and harmful interactions. Among the major risks and complications are:

✔ **Liver disease.** Because the liver is the organ that breaks down and metabolizes alcohol, it is especially vulnerable to its effects. Chronic heavy drinking can lead to alcoholic hepatitis (inflammation and destruction of liver cells) and, in the 15 percent of people who continue drinking beyond this stage, cirrhosis (irreversible scarring and destruction of liver cells). The liver eventually may fail completely, resulting in coma and death.

✔ **Cardiovascular disease.** Heavy drinking can weaken the heart muscle (causing cardiac myopathy), elevate blood pressure, and increase the risk of stroke. The combined use of alcohol and tobacco greatly increases the likelihood of damage to the heart.

✔ **Cancer.** Heavy alcohol use may contribute to cancer of the liver, stomach, and colon, as well as malignant melanoma, a deadly form of skin cancer. Alcohol, in combination with tobacco use, also increases the risk of cancer of the mouth, tongue, larynx, and esophagus. Several major studies have implicated alcohol as a possible risk factor in breast cancer, particularly in young women, although the degree of danger remains unclear.

✔ **Brain damage.** Chronic brain damage resulting from alcohol consumption is second only to Alzheimer's disease as a cause of cognitive deterioration in adults. Long-term heavy drinkers may suffer memory loss, and be unable to think abstractly, recall names of common objects, and follow simple instructions.

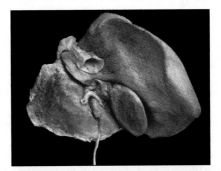
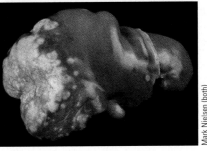

Mark Nielsen (both)

▲ A normal liver (top) compared to one with cirrhosis.

✔ **Vitamin deficiencies.** Alcoholics often tend to have very poor nutrition. Alcoholism is associated with vitamin deficiencies, especially of thiamin ($B_1$), which may be responsible for certain diseases of the neurological, digestive, muscular, and cardiovascular systems. Lack of thiamin may result in Wernicke-Korsakoff syndrome, which is characterized by disorientation, memory failure, hallucinations, and jerky eye movements, and can be disabling enough to require life-long custodial care.

✔ **Digestive problems.** Alcohol triggers the secretion of acids in the stomach that irritate the mucous lining and cause gastritis. Chronic drinking may result in peptic ulcers (breaks in the stomach lining) and bleeding from the stomach lining.

✔ **Reproductive and sexual dysfunction.** Alcohol interferes with male sexual function and fertility through direct effects on testosterone and the testicles. In half of alcoholic men, increased levels of female hormones lead to breast enlargement and a feminine pubic hair pattern. Damage to the nerves in the penis by heavy drinking can lead to impotence. In women who drink heavily, a drop in female hormone production may cause menstrual irregularity and infertility.

✔ **Fetal alcohol syndrome.** The risk of this condition, discussed earlier in the chapter, is greatest if a mother-to-be drinks 3 ounces or more of pure alcohol (the equivalent of six or seven cocktails) a day. Consumption of lower quantities of alcohol can lead to fetal alcohol effects, including low birthweight, irritability in a newborn, and permanent mental impairment. Because no one knows how much alcohol—if any—is safe during pregnancy, the National Institute of Alcohol Abuse and Alcoholism recommends that pregnant women not drink at all.

✔ **Accidents and injuries.** Alcohol may contribute to almost half of the deaths caused by car accidents, burns, falls, and choking. Nearly half of those convicted and jailed for criminal acts committed these crimes while under the influence of alcohol.

✔ **Higher mortality.** As discussed earlier, the mortality rate for alcoholics is two to three times higher than that for nonalcoholics of the same age. Injury is the leading alcohol-related cause of death, chiefly in auto accidents involving a drunk driver. Digestive disease, most notably cirrhosis of the liver, is second. Alcohol is a factor in about 30 percent of all suicides. Alcoholics who attempt suicide may have other risk factors, including major depression, poor social support, serious medical illness, and unemployment.

✔ **Withdrawal dangers.** Withdrawal can be life-threatening when accompanied by medical problems, such as grand mal seizures, pneumonia, liver failure, or gastrointestinal bleeding.

## Alcoholism Treatments

Almost 600,000 Americans undergo treatment for alcohol-related problems every year. Until recent years, the only options for professional alcohol treatment were, as one expert puts it, "intensive, extensive, and expensive," such as residential programs at hospitals or specialized treatment centers. Today individuals whose drinking could be hazardous to their health may choose from a variety of approaches. Treatment that works well for one person may not work for another. As research into the outcomes of alcohol treatments has grown, more attempts have been made to match individuals to approaches tailored to their needs and more likely to help them overcome their alcohol problems.

In a study of 222 men and women who had seriously abused alcohol, those who remained sober for more than a decade credited a variety of approaches, including Alcoholics Anonymous, individual psychotherapy, and other groups such as Women for Sobriety. There is no one sure path to sobriety—a wide variety of treatments may offer help and hope to those with alcohol-related problems.[49] In one of the few studies to follow adolescents for four years after alcohol treatment, about half either completely stopped drug and alcohol involvement or substantially reduced their use. Very few abstained entirely from any substances; over a third of youth treated showed fluctuations in their usage patterns over four years.[50]

## Tobacco and Its Effects

Tobacco, an herb that can be smoked or chewed, directly affects the brain. While its primary active ingredient is nicotine, tobacco smoke contains almost 400 other compounds and chemicals, including gases, liquids, particles, tar, carbon monoxide, cadmium, pyridine, nitrogen dioxide, ammonia, benzene, phenol, acrolein, hydrogen cyanide, formaldehyde, and hydrogen sulfide.

### How Nicotine Works

A colorless, oily compound, **nicotine** is poisonous in concentrated amounts. If you inhale while smoking, 90 percent of the nicotine in the smoke is absorbed into your body. Even if you draw smoke only into your mouth and not into your lungs, you still absorb 25 to 30 percent of the nicotine. The FDA has concluded that nicotine is a dangerous, addictive drug that should be regulated. (See Figure 12-5.)

Nicotine stimulates the cerebral cortex, the outer layer of the brain that controls complex behavior and mental

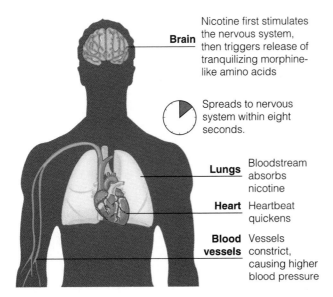

**Brain** Nicotine first stimulates the nervous system, then triggers release of tranquilizing morphine-like amino acids

Spreads to nervous system within eight seconds.

**Lungs** Bloodstream absorbs nicotine

**Heart** Heartbeat quickens

**Blood vessels** Vessels constrict, causing higher blood pressure

▲ **Figure 12-5** The Immediate Effects of Nicotine on the Body The primary active ingredient in tobacco is nicotine, a fast-acting and potent drug.

Sources: American Cancer Society, National Cancer Institute.

activity, and enhances mood and alertness. Investigators have shown that nicotine may enhance smokers' performance on some tasks but leaves other mental skills unchanged. Nicotine also acts as a sedative. How often you smoke and how you smoke determine nicotine's effect on you. If you're a regular smoker, nicotine will generally stimulate you at first, then tranquilize you. Shallow puffs tend to increase alertness because low doses of nicotine facilitate the release of the neurotransmitter *acetylcholine,* which makes the smoker feel alert. Deep drags, on the other hand, relax the smoker because high doses of nicotine block the flow of acetylcholine.

Nicotine stimulates the adrenal glands to produce adrenaline, a hormone that increases blood pressure, speeds up the heart rate by 15 to 20 beats a minute, and constricts blood vessels (especially in the skin). Nicotine also inhibits the formation of urine, dampens hunger, irritates the membranes in the mouth and throat, and dulls the taste buds so foods don't taste as good as they would otherwise. Nicotine is a major contributor to heart and respiratory diseases.

## Tar and Carbon Monoxide

As it burns, tobacco produces **tar,** a thick, sticky dark fluid made up of several hundred different chemicals—many of them poisonous, some of them *carcinogenic* (enhancing the growth of cancerous cells). As you inhale tobacco smoke, tar and other particles settle in the forks of the branchlike

bronchial tubes in your lungs, where precancerous changes are apt to occur. In addition, tar and smoke damage the mucus and the cilia in the bronchial tubes, which normally remove irritating foreign materials from your lungs.

Smoke from cigarettes, cigars, and pipes also contains **carbon monoxide,** the deadly gas that comes out of the exhaust pipes of cars, in levels 400 times those considered safe in industry. Carbon monoxide interferes with the ability of the hemoglobin in the blood to carry oxygen, impairs normal functioning of the nervous system, and is at least partly responsible for the increased risk of heart attacks and strokes in smokers.

# Health Effects of Cigarette Smoking

Figure 12-6 shows a summary of the physiological effects of tobacco and the other chemicals in tobacco smoke. If you're a smoker who inhales deeply and started smoking before the age of 15, you're trading a minute of future life for every minute you now spend smoking. On average smokers die nearly seven years earlier than nonsmokers.[51] Smoking not only eventually kills, it also ages you: Smokers get more wrinkles than nonsmokers.

But the effects of smoking are far more than skin-deep. A cigarette smoker is 10 times more likely to develop lung cancer than a nonsmoker, and 20 times more likely to have a heart attack. Those who smoke two or more packs a day are 15 to 25 times more likely to die of lung cancer than nonsmokers. Moreover, the danger of lung cancer skyrockets when smokers are also exposed to other carcinogens, such as asbestos. This double threat increases the risk of lung cancer to as much as 92 times that for nonsmokers not exposed to asbestos.

## Heart Disease and Stroke

Although a great deal of publicity has been given to the link between cigarettes and lung cancer, heart attack is actually the leading cause of deaths for smokers. Smoking doubles the risk of heart disease, and smokers who suffer heart attacks have only a 50 percent chance of recovering. Smokers have a 70 percent higher death rate from heart disease than nonsmokers, and those who smoke heavily have a 200 percent higher death rate.

The federal Office of the Surgeon General blames cigarettes for one of every ten deaths attributable to heart disease. Smoking is more dangerous than the two most notorious risk factors for heart disease: high blood pressure and high cholesterol. If smoking is combined with one of these, the chances of heart attack are four times greater. Women who smoke and use oral contraceptives have a ten times higher risk of suffering heart attacks than women who do neither.

Smoking also causes a condition called *cardiomyopathy,* which weakens the heart's ability to pump blood and results in the death of about 10,000 people a year. Although researchers don't know precisely how smoking poisons the heart muscle, they speculate that either nicotine or carbon monoxide has a direct toxic effect. Other coronary diseases may be associated with smoking. *Aortic aneurysm* is a bulge in the aorta (the large artery attached to the heart) caused by a weakening of its walls. *Pulmonary heart disease* is a heart disorder caused by changes in blood vessels in the lungs.

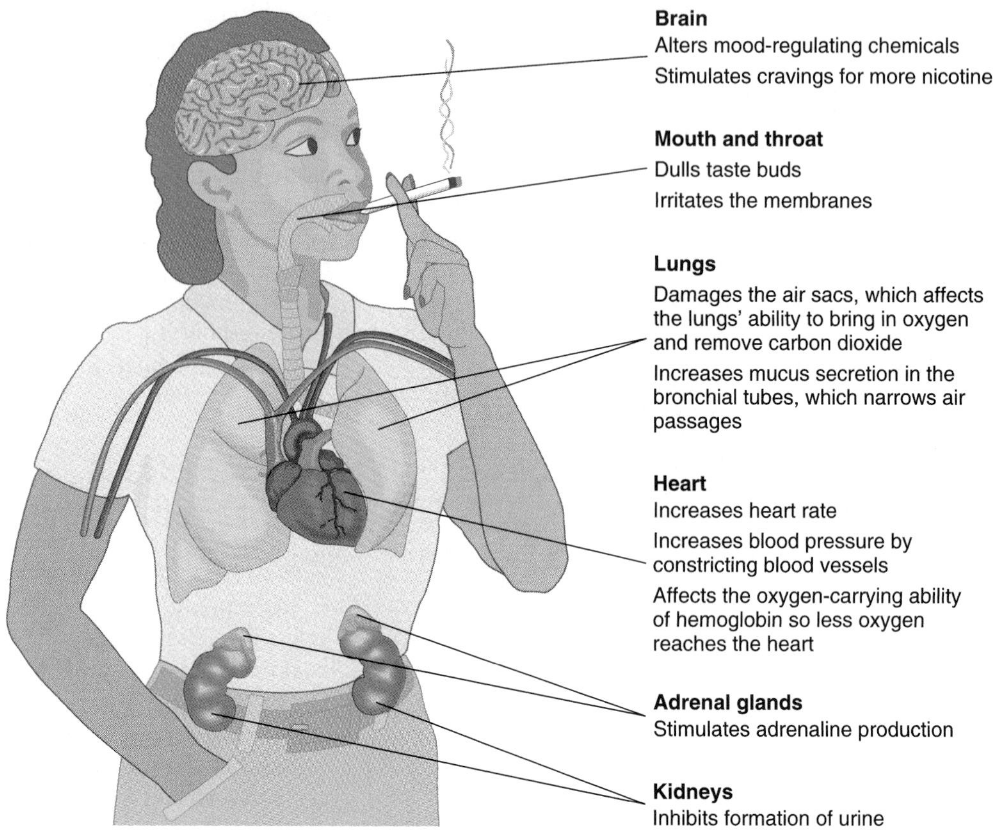

**Brain**
Alters mood-regulating chemicals
Stimulates cravings for more nicotine

**Mouth and throat**
Dulls taste buds
Irritates the membranes

**Lungs**
Damages the air sacs, which affects the lungs' ability to bring in oxygen and remove carbon dioxide
Increases mucus secretion in the bronchial tubes, which narrows air passages

**Heart**
Increases heart rate
Increases blood pressure by constricting blood vessels
Affects the oxygen-carrying ability of hemoglobin so less oxygen reaches the heart

**Adrenal glands**
Stimulates adrenaline production

**Kidneys**
Inhibits formation of urine

▲ **Figure 12-6** Some Effects of Smoking on the Body

Even people who have smoked for decades can reduce their risk of heart attack if they quit smoking. However, recent studies indicate some irreversible damage to blood vessels. Progression of atherosclerosis (hardening of the arteries) among former smokers continues at a faster pace than among those who never smoked.

In addition to contributing to heart attacks, cigarette smoking increases the risk of stroke two to three times in men and women, even after other risk factors are taken into account. According to one study of middle-aged men, giving up smoking leads to a considerable decrease in the risk of stroke within five years of quitting, particularly in smokers of fewer than 20 cigarettes a day. Those with hypertension show the greatest benefit. The risk for heavy smokers declines but never reverts back to that of men who never smoked.

## Cancer

The American Cancer Society estimates that tobacco smoking is the cause of 28 percent of all deaths from cancer and the cause of more than 85 to 90 percent of all cases of lung cancer. The more people smoke, the longer they smoke, and the earlier they start smoking, the more likely they are to develop lung cancer.

Smokers of two or more packs a day have lung cancer mortality rates 15 to 25 times greater than nonsmokers. If smokers stop smoking before cancer has started, their lung tissue tends to repair itself, even if there were already precancerous changes. Former smokers who haven't smoked for 15 or more years have lung cancer mortality rates only somewhat above those for nonsmokers.

Chemicals in cigarette smoke and other environmental pollutants switch on a particular gene in the lung cells of some individuals. This gene produces an enzyme that helps manufacture powerful carcinogens, which set the stage for cancer. The gene seems more likely to be activated in some people than others, and people with this gene are at much higher risk of developing lung cancer. However, smokers without the gene still remain at risk, because other chemicals and genes also may be involved in the development of lung cancer.

Smokers who are depressed are more likely to get cancer than nondepressed smokers. Although researchers don't know exactly how smoking and depression may work together to increase the risk of cancer, one possibility is that stress and depression cause biological changes that lower immunity, such as a decline in natural killer cells that fight off tumors.

Despite some advances in treating lung cancer, the prognosis for sufferers is not good. Even with vigorous therapy, fewer than 10 percent survive for five years after diagnosis. This is one of the lowest survival rates of any type of cancer. And if the cancer has spread from the lungs to other parts of the body, only 1 percent survive for five years after diagnosis.

## Respiratory Diseases

Smoking quickly impairs the respiratory system. Even some teenage smokers show signs of respiratory difficulty—breathlessness, chronic cough, excess phlegm production—when compared with nonsmokers of the same age. Cigarette smokers are up to 18 times more likely than nonsmokers to die of noncancerous diseases of the lungs.

Cigarette smoking is the major cause of chronic obstructive lung disease (COLD), which includes emphysema and chronic bronchitis. COLD is characterized by progressive limitation of the flow of air into and out of the lungs. In emphysema, the limitation of air flow is the result of disease changes in the lung tissue, affecting the bronchioles (the smallest air passages) and the walls of the alveoli (the tiny air sacs of the lung), as shown in Figure 12-7.

Eventually, many of the air sacs are destroyed, and the lungs become much less able to bring in oxygen and remove carbon dioxide. As a result, the heart has to work harder to deliver oxygen to all organs of the body.

In chronic bronchitis, the bronchial tubes in the lungs become inflamed, thickening the walls of the bronchi, and the production of mucus increases. The result is a narrowing of the air passages. Smoking is more dangerous than any form of air pollution, at least for most Americans, but exposure to both air pollution and cigarettes is particularly harmful. Although each may cause bronchitis, together they have a synergistic effect—that is, their combined impact exceeds the sum of their separate effects.

## Other Smoking-Related Problems

Smokers are more likely than nonsmokers to develop gum disease, and they lose significantly more teeth. Even those who quit have worse gum problems than people who never smoked at all. Smoking may also contribute to the loss of teeth and teeth supporting bone, even in individuals with good oral hygiene.

Cigarette smoking is associated with stomach and duodenal ulcers; mouth, throat, and other types of cancer; and cirrhosis of the liver. Smoking may worsen the symptoms or complications of allergies, diabetes, hypertension, peptic ulcers, and disorders of the lungs or blood vessels. Some men who smoke ten cigarettes or more a day may experience sexual impotence. Cigarette smokers also tend to miss work one-third more often than nonsmokers, primarily because of respiratory illnesses. In addition, each year cigarette-ignited fires claim thousands of lives.

Cigarette smoking may increase the likelihood of anxiety, panic attacks, and social phobias, according to a study that followed 688 teenagers into adulthood. Those who smoked a pack a day

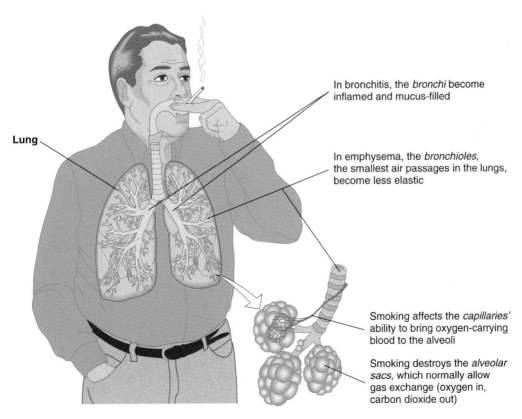

**Lung**

In bronchitis, the *bronchi* become inflamed and mucus-filled

In emphysema, the *bronchioles*, the smallest air passages in the lungs, become less elastic

Smoking affects the *capillaries'* ability to bring oxygen-carrying blood to the alveoli

Smoking destroys the *alveolar sacs*, which normally allow gas exchange (oxygen in, carbon dioxide out)

▲ **Figure 12-7** How Smoking Affects the Lungs

or more were at 6.8 times greater risk of agoraphobia, 5.5 times greater risk of general anxiety disorder, and 15.6 times greater risk of panic disorder. The exact mechanism is unknown, but one theory is that nicotine may have anxiety-generating effects that act on the nervous system.[52]

# Financial Cost of Smoking

The total cost of cigarette smoking to American society includes greater work absenteeism, higher insurance premiums, increased disability payments, and the training costs to replace employees who die prematurely from smoking. In the course of a lifetime, the average smoker can expect to spend tens of thousands of dollars on cigarettes—but that's only the beginning. The potential costs for medical services for a man between the ages of 35 and 39 who smokes heavily may run $60,000 or higher. But the greatest toll—the pain and suffering of cancer victims and their loved ones—obviously cannot be measured in dollars and cents.

# ???? Why Do People Start Smoking?

Most people are aware that an enormous health risk is associated with smoking, but many don't know exactly what that risk is or how it might affect them.

The two main factors linked with the onset of a smoking habit are age and education. The vast majority of white men (93 percent) with less than a high school education are current or former daily cigarette smokers. White women with a similar educational background are also very likely to smoke or to have smoked every day. Hispanic men and women without a high school education are less likely to be or become daily smokers. Other factors associated with the reasons for smoking are discussed in the following sections.

## Genetics

Researchers speculate that genes may account for about 50 percent of smoking behavior, with environment playing an equally important role. Studies have shown that identical twins, who have the same genes, are more likely to have matching smoking profiles than fraternal twins. If one identical twin is a heavy smoker, the other is also likely to be; if one smokes only occasionally, so does the other.

According to Swedish research that has followed 25,000 pairs of same-sex twins since 1886, smoking patterns in men suggested both genetic and environmental influences. The smoking patterns in female twins, however, were quite different. Among those born before 1925, when smoking

was socially unacceptable for women, the overall rate of smoking was low and the genetic influence was absent. However, among those born after 1940, when smoking had become much more acceptable for women, rates of tobacco use increased and the role of genetic influences rose as well—essentially to the same level as that among men. This suggests that some individuals do have a strong genetic predisposition toward tobacco use. However, when smoking is strongly discouraged, they do not express that genetic tendency. On the other hand, if smoking is socially acceptable, the genetic tendency to smoke emerges.

## Parental Role Models

Children who start smoking are 50 percent more likely than youngsters who don't smoke to have at least one smoker in their family. A mother who smokes seems a particularly strong influence on making smoking seem acceptable. The majority of youngsters who smoke say that their parents also smoke and are aware of their own tobacco use.

## Adolescent Experimentation and Rebellion

Young people who are trying out various behaviors may take up smoking because they're curious or because they want to defy adults. Others simply want to appear grown-

---

### STRATEGIES FOR PREVENTION

#### Why Not to Light Up

Before you start smoking—before you ever face the challenge of quitting—think of what you have to gain by *not* smoking:

▲ A significantly reduced risk of cancer of the lungs, larynx, mouth, esophagus, pancreas, and bladder.

▲ Half the risk of heart disease that smokers face.

▲ A lower risk of stroke, chronic obstructive lung disease (COLD), influenza, ulcers, and pneumonia.

▲ A lower risk of having a low-birthweight baby.

▲ A longer lifespan.

▲ Potential savings of tens of thousands of dollars that you would otherwise spend on tobacco products and medical care.

up or cool. Teens often misjudge the addictive power of cigarettes. Many, sure that they'll be able to quit any time they want, figure that smoking for a year or two won't hurt them. But when they try to quit, they can't. Like older smokers, most young people who smoke have tried to quit at least once. The American Cancer Society has found that young smokers tend to become heavy smokers and that the longer anyone is exposed to smoke, the greater the health dangers.

A comprehensive, youth-led prevention program in Florida that emphasizes the truth about tobacco has significantly reduced smoking among middle and high school students.[53] In studies conducted by the CDC, about seven out of ten high school students said they wanted to stop smoking, but only a small percentage were successful.

## Limited Education

People who have graduated from college are much less likely to smoke than high school graduates; those with fewer than 12 years of education are most likely to smoke. An individual with 8 years or less of education is 11 times more likely to smoke than someone with postgraduate training.

## Weight Control

Smokers burn up an extra 100 calories a day—the equivalent of walking a mile—probably because nicotine increases metabolic rate. Once they start smoking, many individuals say they cannot quit because they fear they'll gain weight. The CDC estimates that women who stop smoking gain an average of 8 pounds, while men put on an average of 6 pounds. One in eight women and one in ten men who stop smoking put on 29 pounds or more. The reasons for this weight gain include nicotine's effects on metabolism as well as emotional and behavioral factors, such as the habit of frequently putting something into one's mouth. Yet as a health risk, smoking a pack and a half to two packs a day is a greater danger than carrying 60 pounds of extra weight.

Weight gain for smokers who quit is not inevitable. Aerobic exercise helps increase metabolic rate, and limiting alcohol and foods high in sugar and fat can help smokers control their weight as they give up cigarettes.

## Aggressive Marketing

Cigarette companies spend billions of dollars each year on advertisements and promotional campaigns, with manufacturers targeting ads especially at women, teens, minorities, and the poor. Most controversial are cigarette advertisements in magazines and media aimed at teenagers and even younger children. As part of a nationwide antismoking campaign, health and government officials have called for restrictions on cigarette ads, and manufacturers have agreed not to aim their sales efforts at children and teens.

## Stress

In studies that have analyzed the impact of life stressors, depression, emotional support, marital status, and income, researchers have concluded that an individual with a high stress level is approximately 15 times more likely to be a smoker than a person with low stress. About half of smokers identify workplace stress as a key factor in their smoking behavior.

## Addiction

According to recent research, the first symptoms of nicotine addiction can begin within a few days of starting to smoke and after just a few cigarettes, particularly in teenagers.[54] The findings, based on a study of almost 700 adolescents, challenges the conventional belief that nicotine dependence is a gradual process that takes hold after prolonged daily smoking.

## Smoking in America

Tobacco use remains the most serious and widespread addictive behavior in the world and the major cause of preventable deaths in our society. About one in three Americans (29.3 percent) currently use tobacco products. In a recent national survey of more than 32,000 adults, 23.3 percent were current smokers—down slightly from 25 percent a decade ago.[55] The federal goal is to reduce adult smoking to 12 percent by the year 2010.

## Tobacco Use on Campus

College-age individuals make up the youngest age group that tobacco manufacturers can legally target with their marketing efforts. Smoking by college students rose dramatically during the 1990s and has remained high. The actual percentage of students who smoke varies in different surveys, ranging from 29 percent to as high as 50 percent.[56] Today's students also use a broader range of tobacco products: cigarettes, cigars, pipes, and smokeless tobacco. In a recent survey of students at four-year colleges and universities in Massachusetts, one-third had used a tobacco product, mostly cigarettes, in the past month; 46.4 percent had used tobacco in the past year. Total tobacco use was higher among males than females, but cigarette smoking did not differ by sex. Tobacco use was lower among althletes and higher among students who used alcohol or marijuana.[57]

 Among African-American students, almost half (49 percent) have tried smoking (that is, smoked at least one cigarette but less than 100 during their lifetime); 9.3 percent were "lifetime smokers" (smoked more than 100 cigarettes during their lifetime). More black women than men have tried smoking.[58]

College men and women have nearly identical rates for cigarette smoking, but more men used cigars and smokeless tobacco. White students used more cigarettes and smokeless tobacco than Hispanics, African Americans, or Asians. Among tobacco users, 51.3 percent used more than one tobacco product in the past year; the most frequent combination was cigars and cigarettes. The median age of first cigarette use for students of both genders was 14 years; for first cigar use, it was 17 years for men and 18 years for women.

Students who use tobacco are more likely to smoke marijuana, binge drink, have more sexual partners, have lower grades, rate parties as important, and spend more time socializing with friends. They are less likely than nonusers to rate athletics or religion as important. Tobacco use is lower in western colleges. Unlike cigarette smokers, cigar users rate fraternities, sororities, and sporting events as important. College students who use smokeless tobacco tend to be white men attending schools in rural areas.

 In a survey of 393 colleges and universities, 85 percent of student health center directors considered student smoking a problem or a major problem. Those at public institutions were more likely to perceive smoking as a major problem, while those at religiously affiliated schools were less likely to do so. Most schools—97 percent—restricted smoking in

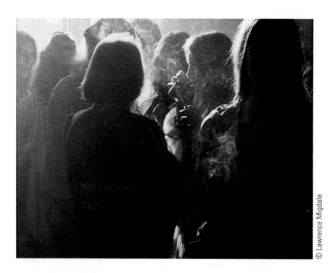

▲ Smoking often goes hand in hand with drinking.

some way, usually in public areas but not in offices or student residences. Schools in the northeast and north-central regions of the country were significantly less likely to prohibit smoking than those in the west.

An estimated 44 percent of students live in smoke-free dorms, while another 29 percent who don't would like to move into one. Freshmen who did not smoke regularly in high school and who live in smoke-free dorms are 40 percent less likely to take up smoking than those in unrestricted housing, according to a study of the smoking behavior of 4,495 students at 101 schools.[59]

Despite concern about student smoking, more than 40 percent of schools do not offer smoking cessation programs to students who want to quit. Those that do primarily refer students to campus support groups or community-based programs like Nicotine Anonymous; they report little student demand for these options. Colleges are much less likely to offer individualized support, medical screening and assistance, or FDA-approved cessation products. Few provide smoking awareness programs, peer education, or quitting incentive programs.[60]

Researchers warn that experimentation with tobacco products in college could evolve into nicotine dependence and daily cigarette smoking. The American College Health Association has adopted a no-smoking policy that encourages all schools to work toward a campuswide tobacco/smoke-free environment. Among its recommendations to the nation's institutions of higher learning are the following:

- ✔ Prohibition of campus-controlled advertising, sales, or free sampling of tobacco products, and of sponsorship of campus events by tobacco-promoting organizations.
- ✔ Prohibition of smoking in all public areas, including classrooms, auditoriums, laboratories, libraries, gymnasiums, meeting rooms, stadiums, buses, vans, meeting rooms, private offices, and dining facilities.
- ✔ Prohibition of smoking in all residence halls, dormitories, and campus housing, including lounges, stairwells, hallways, restrooms, and bedrooms.
- ✔ Prevention and education initiatives directed against tobacco use.
- ✔ Programs that include practical steps to quit tobacco use.[61]

 ## Smoking and Race

Cigarette smoking is a major cause of disease and death in all population groups. However, tobacco use varies within and among racial and ethnic minority groups. Among adults, Native Americans and Alaska Natives have the highest rates of tobacco use—37.9 percent of the men smoke cigarettes, compared with about 25 percent of adults in the overall U.S. population. African-

American men (32.1 percent)and Southeast Asian men also have a high smoking rate. Asian-American and Hispanic women have the lowest rates of smoking. Tobacco use is significantly higher among white college students than among Hispanic, African-America, and Asian students.[62]

Tobacco has taken the greatest toll on the health of African Americans. Middle-aged and older African Americans are far more likely than their counterparts in other major racial and ethnic minority groups to die from coronary heart disease, stroke, or lung cancer. In the 1970s and 1980s, death rates from respiratory cancers (mainly lung cancer) increased among both African-American men and women. In the last decade, these rates declined substantially among African-American men and leveled off in African-American women.

As several studies have shown, many African-American adolescents experiment with smoking but then stop. Among black college students, the risk factors for smoking include friends who smoke, parents who smoked, and a view of religion as unimportant. For lifetime smoking, being single, having had no or few childhood friends who smoked, and having no current friends who smoke decrease the likelihood that an African American would continue to smoke.[63]

African-American teens who smoke are at greater risk of developing long-term consequences than other youths, even when they smoke less. The reason for their increased susceptibility to asthma, allergies, and depression may be potential differences in the way ethnic groups metabolize nicotine.[64]

Tobacco is the substance most abused by Hispanic youth, whose smoking rates have soared in the last ten years.[65] In general, smoking rates among Hispanic adults increase as they adopt the values, beliefs, and norms of American culture. Recent declines in the prevalence of smoking have been greater among Hispanic men with at least a high school education than among those with less education.

According to the U.S. Surgeon General, "adverse infant health outcomes," such as low-birthweight babies, sudden infant death syndrome (SIDS), and infant mortality, are especially high for African Americans, Native Americans, and Alaska Natives who smoke. Cigarette smoking also increases these risks, especially for SIDS, among Asian Americans, Pacific Islanders, and Hispanics.

## Smoking and Women

Approximately one in five women (22 percent) smoke. Smoking rates are even higher among teenage girls; 30 percent of female high school seniors report having smoked within the past 30 days. Globally, smoking prevalence among women varies from as low as 7 percent in developing countries to 24 percent in developed countries.[66]

Women with less than a high school education are three times more likely to smoke than those with a college degree.[67] As discussed in The X & Y Files: "Alcohol, Tobacco, and Gender" (p. 311), women smoke for different reasons and in different ways than men. They also suffer unique consequences.

According to the U.S. Surgeon General, women account for 39 percent of smoking-related deaths each year, a proportion that has doubled since 1965. Since 1980 approximately 3 million women in the United States have died from smoking-related diseases. Each year, American women lose an estimated 2.1 million years of life due to premature deaths attributable to smoking.

If she smokes, a woman's annual risk of dying more than doubles after age 45 compared with a woman who has never smoked. Lung cancer now claims more women's lives than breast cancer. Smoking also is a major cause of cancer of the pharynx and bladder, and may increase the risk of liver, colon, cervical, kidney, and pancreatic cancer.

Women who smoke face an increased risk of depression, stroke, bleeding in the brain, diseases of the blood vessels, and respiratory diseases such as chronic obstructive pulmonary disease. The risk of heart attack in women who smoke 25 or more cigarettes a day is more than 500 percent greater than the risk in women who don't smoke. Even smoking just one to four cigarettes a day doubles the risk. Women who smoke low-nicotine cigarettes are four times more likely to have a first heart attack than women who don't smoke—the same risk as for those who smoke high-nicotine cigarettes.

Women who smoke also are more likely to develop osteoporosis, a bone-weakening disease. They tend to be thin, which is a risk factor for osteoporosis, and they enter menopause earlier, thus extending the period of jeopardy from estrogen loss.

Smoking directly affects women's reproductive organs and processes. Women who smoke are less fertile and experience menopause one or two years earlier than women who don't smoke. Smoking also greatly increases the possible risks associated with taking oral contraceptives. Older women who smoke are weaker, have poorer balance, and are at greater risk of physical disability than nonsmokers.

Women who smoke during pregnancy increase their risk of miscarriage and pregnancy complications, including bleeding, premature delivery, and birth defects such as cleft lip or palate. Women who smoke are twice as likely to have an ectopic pregnancy (in which a fertilized egg develops in the fallopian tube rather than in the uterus) and to have babies of low birthweight as those who have never smoked. However, women who stop smoking before pregnancy reduce their risk of having a low-birthweight baby to that of women who don't smoke. Even those who quit three or four months into the pregnancy have babies with higher birthweights than those who continue smoking throughout pregnancy.

# Other Forms of Tobacco

Some 10.7 million Americans smoke cigars; 7.6 million use smokeless tobacco, and 2.1 million smoke pipes.[68] Ingesting tobacco may be less deadly than smoking cigarettes, but it is dangerous. Smoking cigars, clove cigarettes, and pipes, and chewing or sucking on smokeless tobacco all put the user at risk of cancer of the lip, tongue, mouth, and throat, as well as other diseases and ailments.

## Cigars

Cigar use has declined in the last few years. However, after cigarettes, cigars are the tobacco product most widely used by college students. According to the first national survey to report on undergraduate cigar use, more than a third reported ever smoking a cigar (more than half of men and a quarter of women); 23 percent had smoked a cigar within the past year and 8.5 percent had smoked one within the previous 30 days. About one in five students smoked both cigars and cigarettes. Most cigar use was occasional; fewer than 1 percent of current cigar users on campus smoked daily. Cigar use was similar in white and black students but lower in Hispanics and Asians. In contrast to the ratio for men, more African-American than white women reported smoking cigars (6.8 versus 4 percent).[69]

Cigar smoking is as dangerous even though smokers do not inhale. Cigars are known to cause cancer of the lung and the digestive tract. The risk of death related to cigars approaches that of cigarettes, as the number of cigars smoked and the amount of cigar smoke inhaled increases. (See Figure 12-8.) Cigar smoking can lead to nicotine addiction, even if the smoke is not inhaled. The nicotine in the smoke from a single cigar can vary from an amount roughly equivalent to that in a single cigarette to that in a pack or more of cigarettes.

## Clove Cigarettes

Sweeteners have long been mixed with tobacco, and clove, a spice, is the latest ingredient to be added to the recipe for cigarettes. Clove cigarettes typically contain two-thirds tobacco and one-third clove. Consumers of these cigarettes are primarily teenagers and young adults.

Many users believe that clove cigarettes are safer because they contain less tobacco, but this isn't necessarily the case. The CDC reports that people who smoke clove cigarettes may be at risk of serious lung injury. Smoking clove cigarettes during a mild upper respiratory tract illness can lead to severe breathing difficulty. And clove ciga-

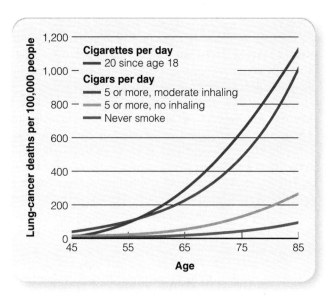

▲ **Figure 12-8** The Dangers of Cigarettes Versus Cigars

Sources: American Cancer Society, National Cancer Institute.

rette smokers, like other cigarette smokers, can become addicted to the tobacco.

Clove cigarettes may be more harmful than conventional cigarettes. They deliver twice as much nicotine, tar, and carbon monoxide as moderate-tar American brands. Eugenol, the active ingredient in cloves (which dentists have used as an anesthetic for years), deadens sensation in the throat, allowing smokers to inhale more deeply and hold smoke in their lungs for a longer time. Chemical relatives of eugenol can produce the kind of damage to cells that may lead to cancer.

## ???? What Are Bidis?

Skinny, sweet-flavored cigarettes called **bidis** (pronounced "beedees") have become a smoking fad among teens and young adults. For centuries, bidis were popular in India, where they are known as the poor man's cigarette and sell for less than five cents a pack. They look strikingly like clove cigarettes or marijuana joints, and are available in flavors like grape, strawberry, and mandarin orange. Bidis are legal for adults and even minors in some states, and are sold on the Internet as well as in stores.

Although bidis contain less tobacco than regular cigarettes, their unprocessed tobacco is more potent. Smoke from bidis has about three times as much nicotine and carbon monoxide and five times as much tar as smoke from regular filtered cigarettes.[70] Because bidis are wrapped in nonporous brownish leaves, they don't burn as easily as cigarettes, and smokers have to inhale harder and more often to keep them lit. In one study, smoking a single bidi required 28 puffs, compared to 9 puffs for cigarettes.

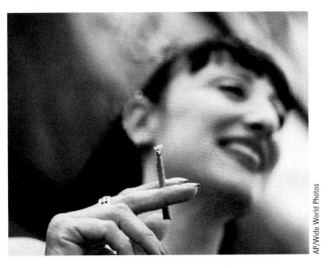

▲ The smoke produced by bidis—skinny, flavored cigarettes—can contain higher concentrations of toxic chemicals than the smoke from regular cigarettes.

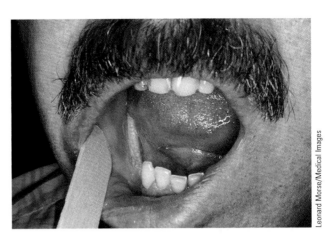

▲ Chewing smokeless tobacco can damage the tissues of the mouth and lead to cancer of the larynx, esophagus, kidney, pancreas, and bladder.

Health authorities view bidis as "cigarettes with training wheels," products that can lead to a lifetime of nicotine addiction because they are easy to buy and lack the health-warning labels required of cigarettes. Unlike regular cigarettes, which are smoked mostly by white youths, bidis also are popular among young Hispanics and blacks.

## Pipes

Many cigarette smokers switch to pipes to reduce their risk of health problems. But former cigarette smokers may continue to inhale, even though pipe smoke is more irritating to the respiratory system than cigarette smoke. People who have only smoked pipes and who do not inhale are much less likely to develop lung and heart disease than cigarette smokers. However, they are as likely as cigarette smokers to develop—and die of—cancer of the mouth, larynx, throat, and esophagus.

## Smokeless Tobacco

The consumption of smokeless tobacco products is rising, particularly among young males. These substances include snuff, finely ground tobacco that can be sniffed or placed inside the cheek and sucked, and chewing tobacco, tobacco leaves mixed with flavoring agents such as molasses. With both, nicotine is absorbed through the mucous membranes of the nose or mouth.

Every day approximately 2,200 U.S. youths, ages 11 to 19, try smokeless tobacco for the first time. About 830 become regular users. Many are emulating professional baseball players who keep wads of tobacco jammed in their cheeks. These young users often lack awareness of its dangers.[71] Smokeless tobacco can cause cancer and noncancerous oral conditions and lead to nicotine addiction and dependence. Smokeless tobacco users are more likely than nonusers to become cigarette smokers. Powerful carcinogens in smokeless tobacco include nitrosamines, polycyclic aromatic hydrocarbons, and radiation-emitting polonium. Its use can lead to the development of white patches on the mucous membranes of the mouth, particularly on the site where the tobacco is placed. Most lesions of the mouth lining that result from the use of smokeless tobacco dissipate six weeks after the use of the tobacco products is stopped, according to a U.S. Air Force study. However, when first found, about 5 percent of these lesions are cancerous or exhibit changes that progress to cancer within ten years if not properly treated. Cancers of the lip, pharynx, larynx, and esophagus have all been linked to smokeless tobacco.

More than 7 million people, many of them young, use snuff and chewing tobacco. In a national survey of 5,894 men and women from 72 colleges and universities, 22 percent of college men and 2 percent of college women used smokeless tobacco. The lowest percentage was in the northeast, the highest in the south-central region. In different regions, 8 to 36 percent of male high school students were regular users. Even when they spot lesions in their mouths, most do not seek medical help but continue to use smokeless tobacco.

In recent years, there has been a decline in chewing tobacco, but an increase in the use of moist snuff, a product that is higher in nicotine and potential cancer-causing chemicals. The use of snuff increases the likelihood of oral cancer by more than four times. Other effects include bad breath, discolored or missing teeth, cavities, gum disease, and nicotine addiction. In a study by the Oregon Research Institute, dental patients were three times more likely to quit snuff and chewing tobacco after hygienists taught them that smokeless tobacco was responsible for their mouth sores, bleeding gums, and receding gums.

## Environmental Tobacco Smoke

Maybe you don't smoke—never have, never will. That doesn't mean you don't have to worry about the dangers of smoking, especially if you live or work with people who smoke. **Environmental tobacco smoke,** or secondhand cigarette smoke, the most hazardous form of indoor air pollution, ranks behind cigarette smoking and alcohol as the third-leading preventable cause of death.

On average, a smoker inhales what is known as **mainstream smoke** eight or nine times with each cigarette, for a total of about 24 seconds. However, the cigarette burns for about 12 minutes, and everyone in the room (including the smoker) breathes in what is known as **sidestream smoke.**

According to the American Lung Association, incomplete combustion from the lower temperatures of a smoldering cigarette makes sidestream smoke dirtier and chemically different from mainstream smoke. It has twice as much tar and nicotine, five times as much carbon monoxide, and 50 times as much ammonia. And because the particles in sidestream smoke are small, this mixture of irritating gases and carcinogenic tar reaches deeper into the lungs. If you're a nonsmoker sitting next to someone smoking seven cigarettes an hour, even in a ventilated room, you'll take in almost twice the maximum amount of carbon monoxide set for air pollution in industry—and it will take hours for the carbon monoxide to leave your body.

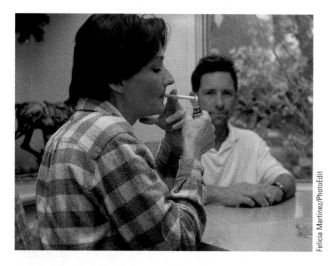

Felicia Martinez/PhotoEdit

▲ Secondhand smoke is the most hazardous form of indoor air pollution.

## What Are the Risks of Secondhand Smoke?

Even a little secondhand smoke is dangerous.[72] According to the Centers for Disease Control and Prevention, every year environmental tobacco smoke causes 3,000 deaths from lung cancer. In a ten-year Harvard University study that tracked 10,000 healthy women who never smoked, regular exposure to other people's smoke at home or work almost doubled the risk of heart disease. On the basis of their findings, the researchers estimated that up to 50,000 Americans may die every year of heart attacks from environmental tobacco smoke, and another 3,000 to 4,000 die of other forms of heart disease caused by secondhand smoke. As a cancer-causing agent, secondhand smoke may be twice as dangerous as radon gas and more than a hundred times more hazardous than outdoor pollutants regulated by federal law. Secondhand smoke also increases the sick leave rates among employees.[73]

## Politics of Tobacco

More than three decades after government health authorities began to warn of the dangers of cigarette smoking, tobacco remains a politically hot topic. After many years of difficult negotiations, the tobacco industry and attorneys general from nearly 40 states reached a historic settlement. Major tobacco companies have agreed to pay more than $200 billion to settle smoking-related lawsuits filed by 46 states, to finance antismoking campaigns, to restrict marketing, to permit federal regulation of tobacco, and to pay fines if tobacco use by minors does not decline.

The federal government has launched a seven-year grassroots antismoking coalition called Americans Stop Smoking Intervention Study (ASSIST) to combat cigarette smoking. Community leaders in some neighborhoods have whitewashed billboard ads for cigarettes. Some civic and consumer associations have proposed boycotting athletic events sponsored by tobacco companies. In some states, school-based tobacco prevention campaigns and tough antismoking campaigns, financed by taxes on cigarettes, have led to impressive declines in cigarette sales.[74]

Nonsmokers, realizing that their health is being jeopardized by environmental tobacco smoke, have increasingly turned to legislative and administrative measures to clear the air and protect their rights. (See Figure 12-9 on p. 332.) Thousands of cities, towns, and counties now restrict smoking in public places and/or regulate the sale of tobacco to minors. Nationally, the airlines have banned smoking on domestic flights. Many institutions, including medical centers and some universities, no longer allow smoking on their premises. Some cities restrict smoking in bars, restaurants, and other public places.

Supporters of smoking restrictions argue that no one should be subjected involuntarily to the dangers of environmental tobacco smoke. Besides the health hazards, smokers jeopardize nonsmokers by increasing the danger of fire. Opponents of smoking restrictions contend that banning smoking on the job might impair rather than enhance productivity, because employees would take more frequent breaks to go to lounges where smoking is permitted—or else would suffer the negative effects of nicotine withdrawal.

# Quitting

Seven in ten adult smokers in the United States say they want to quit, but their success varies widely by race and education. About half of whites who have smoked were able to kick the habit, compared with 45 percent of Asian Americans, 43 percent of Hispanics, and 37 percent of African Americans. Men and women with college and graduate degrees were much more likely to quit successfully than high-school dropouts.[75]

Most people who eventually quit on their own have already tried other methods. Nicotine withdrawal symptoms can behave like characters in a bad horror flick: Just when you think you've killed them, they're back with a vengeance. In recent studies, some people who tried to quit smoking reported a small improvement in withdrawal symptoms over two weeks, but then their symptoms leveled off and persisted. Others found that their symptoms intensified rather than lessened over time. For reasons scientists cannot yet explain, former smokers who start smoking again put their lungs at even greater jeopardy than smokers who never quit.[76]

According to therapists, quitting usually isn't a one-time event but a dynamic process that may take several years and four to ten attempts. The good news is that half of all living Americans who ever smoked have managed to quit. And thanks to new products and programs, it may be easier now than ever before to become an ex-smoker.

## Quitting on Your Own

More than 90 percent of former smokers quit on their own—by throwing away all their cigarettes, by gradually cutting down, or by first switching to a less potent brand. One characteristic of successful quitters is that they see themselves as active participants in health maintenance and take personal responsibility for their own health. Often they experiment with a variety of strategies, such as learning relaxation techniques. In women, exercise has proven especially effective for quitting and avoiding weight gain. Making a home a smoke-free zone also increases a smoker's likelihood of successfully quitting.

## Stop-Smoking Groups

Joining a support group doubles your chances of quitting for good. The American Cancer Society's FreshStart program runs about 1,500 stop-smoking clinics, each with about 8 to 18 members meeting for eight two-hour sessions over four weeks. Instructors explain the risks of smoking, encourage individuals to think about why they smoke, and suggest ways of unlearning their smoking habit. A quitting day is set for the third or fourth session.

The American Lung Association's Freedom from Smoking program consists of eight one- to two-hour sessions over seven weeks. The approach is similar to the American Cancer Society's, but smokers keep diaries and team up with buddies. Ex-smokers serve as advisers on quitting day. Both groups estimate that 27 or 28 percent of their participants successfully stop smoking.

Stop-smoking classes are also available through health-science departments and student-health services on many college campuses, as well as through community public health departments. The Seventh-Day

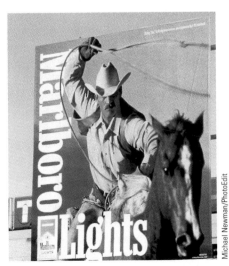
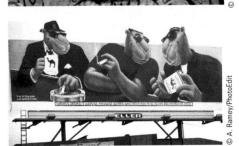

▲ Tobacco advertising is aggressive, but tough antismoking campaigns have led to declines in cigarette sales.

Adventists sponsor a four-week Breathe Free Plan, in which smokers commit themselves to clean living (no smoking, alcohol, tea, or coffee, along with a balanced diet and regular exercise). Many businesses sponsor smoking-cessation programs for employees, which generally follow the approaches of professional groups. Motivation may be even higher in these programs than in programs outside the workplace because some companies offer attractive incentives to participants, such as lower rates on their health insurance.

Some smoking-cessation programs rely primarily on **aversion therapy,** which provides a negative experience every time a smoker has a cigarette. This may involve taking drugs that make tobacco smoke taste unpleasant, undergoing electric shocks, having smoke blown at you, or rapid smoking (the inhaling of smoke every six seconds until you're dizzy or nauseated).

## Nicotine Replacement Therapy

This approach uses a variety of products that supply low doses of nicotine in a way that allows smokers to taper off gradually over a period of months. Nicotine replacement therapies include prescription products (nicotine nasal spray and nicotine inhaler) and nonprescription products (nicotine gum and nicotine patches). The nasal spray, dispensed from a pump bottle, delivers nicotine to the nasal membranes and reaches the bloodstream faster than any other nicotine replacement therapy product. The inhaler delivers nicotine into the mouth and enters the bloodstream much more slowly than the nicotine in cigarettes.

Nonprescription nicotine replacement products, such as patches and gum, are not effective as long-term approaches, according to a recent study from the University of California, San Diego.[77] However, these products may help smokers quit, especially when combined with a support group or counseling.

Because nicotine is a powerful, addictive substance, using nicotine replacements for a prolonged period is not advised. Pregnant women and individuals with heart disease shouldn't use them.

Nicotine replacement therapies don't affect the psychological dependence that makes quitting smoking so

---

> ### *Nonsmoker's Bill of Rights*
>
> Nonsmokers Help Protect the Health, Comfort, and Safety of Everyone by Insisting on the Following Rights:
>
> #### The Right to Breathe Clean Air
> *Nonsmokers have the right to breathe clean air, free from harmful and irritating tobacco smoke. This right supersedes the right to smoke when the two conflict.*
>
> #### The Right to Speak Out
> *Nonsmokers have the right to express — firmly but politely — their discomfort and adverse reactions to tobacco smoke. They have the right to voice their objections when smokers light up without asking permission.*
>
> #### The Right to Act
> *Nonsmokers have the right to take action through legislative means — as individuals or in groups — to prevent or discourage smokers from polluting the atmosphere and to seek the restriction of smoking in public places.*

▲ **Figure 12-9** Nonsmoker's Bill of Rights

hard. That's why the key to long-term success in quitting smoking is getting support.

## Nicotine Gum

Nicotine gum, sold as Nicorette, contains a nicotine resin that's gradually released as the gum is chewed. Absorbed through the mucous membrane of the mouth, the nicotine doesn't produce the same rush as a deeply inhaled drag on a cigarette. However, the gum maintains enough nicotine in the blood to diminish withdrawal symptoms. A month's supply of Nicorette costs roughly $45.

Although this gum is lightly spiced to mask nicotine's bitterness, many users say that it takes several days to become accustomed to its unusual taste. Its side effects include mild indigestion, sore jaws, nausea, heartburn, and stomachache. Also, because Nicorette is heavier than regular chewing gum, it may loosen fillings or cause problems with dentures. Drinking coffee or other beverages may block absorption of the nicotine in the gum; individuals trying to quit smoking shouldn't ingest any substance immediately before or while chewing nicotine gum.

Most people use nicotine gum as a temporary crutch and gradually taper off until they can stop chewing it relatively painlessly. However, 5 to 10 percent of users transfer their dependence from cigarettes to the gum. When they stop using Nicorette, they experience withdrawal symptoms, although the symptoms tend to be milder than those prompted by quitting cigarettes. Intensive counseling to

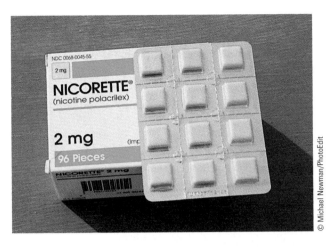

▲ Nicorette gum, when chewed, gradually releases a nicotine resin and helps some smokers break their habit. Nicorette is now available without a prescription.

teach smokers coping methods can greatly increase the success rates.

## Nicotine Patches

Nicotine transdermal delivery system products, or patches, provide nicotine, their only active ingredient, via a patch attached to the skin by an adhesive. Like nicotine gum, the nicotine patch minimizes withdrawal symptoms, such as intense craving for cigarettes. Some insurance programs pay for patch therapy. Nicotine patches, which cost between $3.25 and $4 each, are replaced daily during therapy programs that run between 6 and 16 weeks. There is no evidence that continuing their use for more than 8 weeks provides added benefit.

Some patches deliver nicotine around the clock and others for just 16 hours (during waking hours). Those most likely to benefit from nicotine patch therapy are people who smoke more than a pack a day, are highly motivated to quit, and participate in counseling programs. While using the patch, 37 to 77 percent of people are able to abstain from smoking. When combined with counseling, the patch can be about twice as effective as a placebo, enabling 26 percent of smokers to abstain for six months.

Patch wearers who smoke or use more than one patch at a time can experience a nicotine overdose; some users have even suffered heart attacks. Occasional side effects include redness, itching, or swelling at the site of the patch application; insomnia; dry mouth; and nervousness.

 Why are teen smokers at a greater risk for cancer and other diseases?

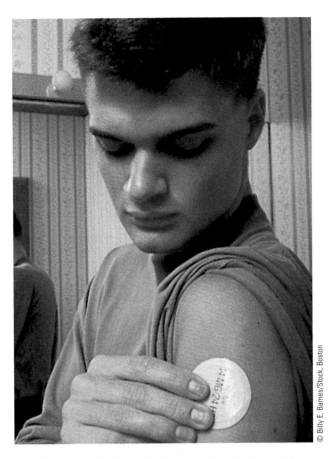

▲ A nicotine patch releases nicotine transdermally (through the skin) in measured amounts, which are gradually decreased over time.

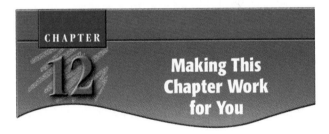

CHAPTER

**12**

**Making This Chapter Work for You**

1. Which of the following statements about the effects of alcohol on the body systems is true?
   a. In most individuals, alcohol sharpens the responses of the brain and nervous system, enhancing sensation and perception.
   b. Moderate drinking may have a positive effect on the cardiovascular system.
   c. French researchers have found that drinking red wine with meals may have a positive effect on the digestive system.
   d. The leading alcohol-related cause of death is liver damage.

2. Which of the following statements about drinking on college campuses is true?

a. The percentage of students who frequently binge drink has increased.

b. The number of women who binge drink has decreased.

c. Because of peer pressure, students in fraternities and sororities tend to drink less than students in dormitories.

d. Students who live in substance-free dormitories tend to binge drink when alcohol is available.

3. Racial and ethnic patterns related to alcohol use include which of the following?

a. Asian-American women tend to have higher rates of alcoholism than Asian-American men.

b. Socioeconomic conditions increase the likelihood of alcohol problems in African Americans and Native Americans.

c. White Americans tend to have higher rates of cirrhosis of the liver than African Americans or Native Americans.

d. The Hispanic culture discourages men from drinking because heavy drinking indicates a lack of machismo.

4. Women who have drinking problems

a. often have suffered from fetal alcohol syndrome as a result of their mother's alcohol consumption.

b. are less likely to have an alcoholic parent than men with drinking problems.

c. are at higher risk for osteoporosis than women who are not heavy drinkers.

d. are less likely to suffer liver damage than men.

5. Which of the following statements about alcohol abuse and dependence is false?

a. Alcohol dependence involves a persistent craving for and an increased tolerance to alcohol.

b. An individual may have a genetic predisposition for developing alcoholism.

c. Alcoholics often abuse other psychoactive drugs.

d. Alcohol abuse and alcohol dependence are different names for the same problem.

6. Which of the following statements about tobacco and its components is true?

a. Nicotine settles in the lungs, eventually causing precancerous changes.

b. Tobacco stimulates the kidneys to form urine.

c. Carbon monoxide contained in tobacco smoke impairs oxygen transport in the body.

d. Tar is the addictive substance in tobacco.

7. Cigarette smokers

a. are more likely to die of lung cancer than heart disease.

b. usually develop lung problems after years of tobacco use.

c. have two to three times the risk of suffering a stroke than nonsmokers.

d. may completely reverse the damage to their blood vessels if they quit smoking.

8. Tobacco use on college campuses

a. is most often in the form of smokeless tobacco products used by students to avoid detection.

b. is more prevalent among those students who also use marijuana, binge drink, and spend more time socializing with friends.

c. has decreased in the past 10 years because almost all schools have adopted a no-smoking policy on their premises.

d. is considered a minor problem by most student health center directors, since less than a third of students smoke.

9. Secondhand tobacco smoke is

a. the smoke inhaled by a smoker.

b. more hazardous than outdoor pollution as a cancer-causing agent.

c. less hazardous than mainstream smoke.

d. less likely to cause serious health problems in children than in adults.

10. Quitting smoking

a. usually results in minor withdrawal symptoms.

b. will do little to reverse the damage to the lungs and other parts of the body.

c. can be aided by joining a support group.

d. is best done by cutting down on the number of cigarettes you smoke over a period of months.

Answers to these questions can be found on page 415.

## Critical Thinking

1. Driving home from his high school graduation party, 18-year-old Rick has had too much to drink. As he crosses the dividing line on the two-lane road, the driver of an oncoming car—a young mother with two young children in the backseat—swerves to avoid an accident. She hits a concrete wall and dies instantly, but her children survive. Rick has no record of drunk driving. Should he go to prison? Is he guilty of manslaughter? How would you feel if you were the victim's husband? If you were Rick's friend?

2. Have you ever been around people who have been intoxicated when you have been sober? What did you think of their behavior? Were they fun to be around? Was the experience not particularly enjoyable, boring, or difficult in some way? Have you ever been intoxicated? How do you behave when you are drunk? Do you find the experience enjoyable? What do the people around you think of your actions when you are drunk?

3. Has smoking become unpopular among your friends or family? What social activities continue to be associated with smoking? Can you think of any situation in which smoking might be frowned upon?

4. How would you motivate someone you care about to stop smoking? What reasons would you give for them to stop? Describe your strategy.

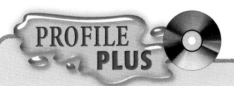

## PROFILE PLUS

Excessive drinking and smoking can cause long-term health problems. How are they affecting you? Find out with these activities on your Profile Plus CD-ROM:

Do You Have a Drinking Problem?

Addictive Behavior Questionnaires

Smoking Cessation Questionnaire

## SITES & BYTES

### Facts on Tap: Alcohol and Your College Experience
www.factsontap.org

This colorful and interactive web site features a variety of activities and straightforward information specifically written for college students. Some of the topics include alcohol and the college experience, the effects of alcohol on the nondrinker, alcohol and the family, and a true-false quiz to test your knowledge of alcohol and its effects.

### Truth—Smoking Awareness and Prevention
www.wholetruth.com

This interactive site provides answers to common myths and questions pertaining to cigarette smoking in an entertaining way, targeted at teens and young adults.

### Bacchus and Gamma Peer Education Network
www.bacchusgamma.org

Designed for college students and college health professionals, this site features information about alcohol use and abuse, smoking prevention and cessation, sexual health, and campus peer-educator groups. An online interactive alcohol responsibility course is offered for campus policy offenders.

### InfoTrac College Edition Activity   John R. Knight, et al. "Alcohol Abuse and Dependence Among U.S. College Students." *Journal of Studies on Alcohol,* Vol. 63, No. 3, May 2002, p. 263.

1. According to the study design, what is the gender difference in the definition of "heavy episodic drinker"?

2. Which risky behaviors are associated with a diagnosis of alcohol abuse or dependence?

3. What were some of the limitations of the study?

You can find additional readings relating to alcohol and tobacco use with InfoTrac College Edition, an online library of more than 900 journals and publications. Follow the instructions for accessing InfoTrac that were packaged with your textbook; then search for articles using a keyword search.

For additional links, resources, and suggested readings on InfoTrac, visit our Health & Wellness Resource Center at http://health.wadsworth.com.

## Key Terms

The terms listed here are used within the chapter on the page indicated. Definitions of terms are in the Glossary at the end of the book.

alcohol abuse  317
alcohol dependence  317
alcoholism  318
aversion therapy  332
bidis  328
binge drinking  310

blood-alcohol concentration
  (BAC)  304
carbon monoxide  321
environmental tobacco
  smoke  330
ethyl alcohol  304

fetal alcohol effects
  (FAE)  316
fetal alcohol syndrome
  (FAS)  316
intoxication  305

mainstream smoke  330
nicotine  320
proof  304
sidestream smoke  330
tar  321

## References

1. Wechsler, Henry, and Bernice Wuethrich. *Dying to Drink: Confronting Binge Drinking on College Campuses.* Emmaus, PA: Rodale Press, 2002.

2. Rigotti, Nancy, et al. "U.S. College Students' Use of Tobacco Products: Results of a National Survey." *Journal of the American Medical Association,* Vol. 284, No. 6, August 9, 2000.

3. National Institute on Alcohol Abuse and Alcoholism, www.niaaa.nih.gov.

4. Mukamal, Kenneth, et al. "Prior Alcohol Consumption and Mortality Following Acute Myocardial Infarction." *Journal of the American Medical Association,* Vol. 285, No. 15, April 18, 2001, p. 1965.

5. "New Study Shows Alcohol May Affect Cognition in Young People." *Dana Brain Daybook,* Vol. 4, No. 2, March–April 2000.

6. Mukamal et al., "Prior Alcohol Consumption and Mortality Following Acute Myocardial Infarction."

7. "Targeting the At-Risk Drinker with Screening and Advice." *Facts of Life: Issue Briefing for Health Reporters,* Vol. 6, No. 1, January 2001.

8. Schulenberg, John, and Jennifer Maggs. "A Developmental Perspective on Alcohol Use and Heavy Drinking During Adolescence and the Transition to Young Adulthood." *Journal of Studies on Alcohol,* Vol. 63, No. 2, March 2002, p. 54.

9. Wechsler, Henry, et al. "Trend in College Binge Drinking During a Period of Increased Prevention Efforts." *Journal of American College Health,* Vol. 50, No. 5, March 2002, p. 203.

10. Wechsler, Henry, et al. "Underage College Students' Drinking Behavior, Access to Alcohol, and the Influence of Deterrence Policies." *Journal of American College Health,* Vol. 50, No. 5, March 2002, p. 223.

11. Gose, Ben. "Harvard Researchers Note a Rise in College Students Who Drink Heavily and Often." *Chronicle of Higher Education,* Vol. 46, No. 20, March 24, 2000, p. A55.

12. Anding, Jenna, et al. "Dietary Intake, Body Mass Index, Exercise, and Alcohol." *Journal of American College Health,* Vol. 49, January 2001, p. 167.

13. Carter, Colleen, and William Kahnweiler. "The Efficacy of the Social Norms Approach to Substance Abuse Prevention Applied to Fraternity Men." *Journal of American College Health,* Vol. 49, No. 20, September 2000, p. 66.

14. Minto, Scott, et al. "A New Approach to Student Alcohol Abuse at Georgetown University." *Journal of American College Health,* Vol. 51, No. 2, September 2002, p. 81.

15. Wood, Mark, et al. "Social Influence Processes and College Student Drinking: The Mediational Role of Alcohol Outcome Expectancies." *Journal of Studies on Alcohol,* Vol. 62, No. 1, January 2001, p. 32.

16. Hildebran, Kathryn, and Dewaynef Johnson. "Comparison of Patterns of Alcohol Use Between High School and College Athletes and Nonathletes." *Research Quarterly for Exercise and Sport,* Vol. 72, No. 1, March 2001, p. A-30.

17. O'Malley, Patrick, et al. "Epidemiology of Alcohol and Other Drug Use Among American College Students." *Journal of Studies on Alcohol,* Vol. 63, No. 2, March 2002, p. 23.

18. McCabe, Sean. "Gender Differences in Collegiate Risk Factors for Heavy Episodic Smoking." *Journal of Studies on Alcohol,* Vol. 63, No. 1, p. 49.

19. Wechsler et al. "Trend in College Binge Drinking During a Period of Increased Prevention Efforts."

20. Harford, T. C., et al. "The Impact of Current Residence and High School Drinking on Alcohol Problems Among College Students." *Journal of Studies on Alcohol,* Vol. 63, No. 3, May 2002, p. 271.

21. "NIAAA Study Finds Extensive Damage from College Drinking." *Alcoholism & Drug Abuse Weekly,* Vol. 14, No. 15, April 15, 2002, p. 6.

22. "Binge Drinkers More Likely to Abuse Additional Substances." *Brown University Digest of Addiction Theory and Application,* Vol. 21, No. 3, March 2002, p. 2.

23. Wechsler, Henry, et al. "Binge Drinking on America's College Campuses." Harvard School of Public Health, 2001. Available at www.hsph.harvard.edu/cas.

24. Wechsler et al. "Trend in College Binge Drinking During a Period of Increased Prevention Efforts."

25. Cariati, Sophia. "More Young Women Drinking, Suffering Disporportionate Consequences." News Release, Society for Women's Health Research, April 12, 2002.

26. Keeling, Richard. "Binge Drinking and the College Environment." *Journal of American College Health,* Vol. 50, No. 5, March 2002, p. 197.

27. Brower, Aaron. "Are College Students Alcoholics?" *Journal of American College Health,* Vol. 50, No. 5, March 2002, p. 253.

28. "Report Gives Colleges Failing Grades for Reducing College Binge Drinking." *Alcoholism & Drug Abuse Weekly,* Vol. 14, No. 13, April 1, 2002, p. 1.

29. "Colleges Report More Alcohol, Drug Violations." *Alcoholism & Drug Abuse Weekly,* Vol. 14, No. 14, April 8, 2002, p. 7.

30. Harris, Rebecca. "Party Patrol: Squad Fights for Alcohol-Free Fun." *Careers & Colleges,* Vol. 22, No. 4, March 2002, p. 5.

31. Wilenz, Pam. "Greek Membership Does Not Predict Post-College Drinking Levels." *American Psychological Association,* March 1, 2001.

32. Jones, Sherry, et al. "Binge Drinking Among Undergraduate College Students in the United States: Implications for Other Substance Use." *Journal of American College Health,* Vol. 50, No. 1, July 2001, p. 33.

33. Wechsler, Henry, et al. "Drinking Levels, Alcohol Problems, and Secondhand Effects in Substance-Free College Residences: Results of a National Study." *Journal of Studies on Alcohol,* Vol. 62, No. 1, January 2001, p. 23.

34. "Many Students Suffer Alcohol-Related Injuries." *Brown University Digest of Addiction Theory and Application,* Vol. 21, No. 1, January 2002, p. S1.

35. Hingson, R., et al. "Magnitude of Alcohol-Related Mortality and Morbidity Among U.S. College Students Ages 18–24." *Journal of Studies on Alcohol,* Vol. 63, No. 2, April 2002, p. 136.

36. Juhnke, Gerald, et al. "Establishing an Alcohol and Other Drug Assessment and Intervention Program Within an On-Site Counselor Education Research and Training Clinic." *Journal of Addictions & Offender Counseling,* Vol. 22, No. 2, April 2002, p. 83.

37. Jones et al., "Binge Drinking Among Undergraduate College Students in the United States."

38. *Substance Use and Risky Sexual Behavior.* Menlo Park, CA: Henry J. Kaiser Family Foundation, 2002.

39. Wechsler, Henry, et al. "Secondhand Effects of Student Alcohol Use Reported by Neighbors of Colleges." *Social Science & Medicine,* Vol. 55, No. 3, July 2002, p. 425.

40. Ziemelis, Andris, et al. "Prevention Efforts Underlying Decreases in Binge Drinking at Institutions of Higher Education." *Journal of American College Health,* Vol. 50, No. 5, March 2002, p. 238.

41. O'Malley et al. "Epidemiology of Alcohol and Other Drug Use Among American College Students."

42. National Institute on Alcohol Abuse and Alcoholism, www.niaaa.nih.gov.

43. Hales, Dianne. *Just Like a Woman.* New York: Bantam Books, 2000.

44. Wilsnack, Sharon. Personal interview.

45. "Younger Women Less Likely to Stop Using Alcohol and Tobacco During Pregnancy." *Medical Letter on the CDC & FDA,* November 26, 2000.

46. Kirkpatrick, Jean. Personal interview.

47. "10th Special Report to Congress on Alcohol and Health." National Institute on Alcohol and Alcohol Abuse, December 2000.

48. Knight, J. R., et al. "Alcohol Abuse and Dependence Among U.S. College Students." *Journal of Studies on Alcohol,* Vol. 63, No. 3, May 2002, p. 263.

49. Fletcher, Anne. *Sober for Good.* New York: Houghton Mifflin, 2001.

50. Brown, Sandra, et al. "Four-Year Outcomes from Adolescent Alcohol and Drug Treatment." *Journal of Studies on Alcohol,* Vol. 62, No. 3, May 2001, p. 381.

51. "Reducing Tobacco Use: The Quest to Quit." *Facts of Life: Issue Briefing for Health Reporters,* Vol. 6, No. 3, March–April 2001.

52. Johnson, Jeffrey, et al. "Association Between Cigarette Smoking and Anxiety Disorders During Adolescence and Early Adulthood." *Journal of the American Medical Association,* Vol. 284, No. 18, November 8, 2000, p. 2348.

53. Bauer, Ursula, et al. "Changes in Youth Cigarette Use and Intentions Following Implementation of a Tobacco Control Program." *Journal of the American Medical Association,* Vol. 284, No. 6, August 9, 2000, p. 723.

54. DiFranza, Joseph. "Initial Symptoms of Nicotine Dependence in Adolescents." *Tobacco Control,* Vol. 9, 2000.

55. Centers for Disease Control and Prevention, www.cdc.gov.

56. Wechsler, Henry, et al. "College Smoking Policies and Smoking Cessation Programs: Results of a Survey of College Health Center Directors." *Journal of American College Health,* Vol. 49, No. 5, March 2001, p. 205.

57. Rigotti, N. A., et al. "Tobacco Use by Massachusetts Public College Students: Long-Term Effect of the Massachusetts Tobacco Control Program." *Tobacco Control,* Vol. 11, No. 2, June 2002, p. ii20.

58. Hestick, Henrietta, et al. "Trial and Lifetime Smoking Risks Among African-American College Students." *Journal of American College Health,* Vol. 49, No. 5, March 2001, p. 205.

59. Wechsler et al., "College Smoking Policies and Smoking Cessation Programs."

60. Mooney, Debra. "Facilitating Student Use of Campus Smoking Cessation Services." *Journal of American College Health,* Vol. 50, No. 3, November 2001, p. 137.

61. "Position Statement on Tobacco on College and University Campuses." American College Health Association, www.acha.org.

62. Rigotti, et al. "U.S. College Students' Use of Tobacco Products."

63. Hestick et al., "Trial and Lifetime Smoking Risks Among African-American College Students."

64. "African-American Teens at High Risk from Smoking." *Alcoholism & Drug Abuse Weekly,* Vol. 13, No. 10, March 5, 2001, p. 8.

65. Guinn, Bobby, et al. "Association of Tobacco Use with Acculturative Status, Knowledge, and Attitudes Among Early Adolescent Mexican Americans." *Research Quarterly for Exercise and Sport,* Vol. 72, No. 1, March 2001, p. A-29.

66. "Report: Tobacco-Related Deaths Increase Among Women." *Alcoholism & Drug Abuse Weekly,* Vol. 13, No. 14, April 2, 2001, p. 5.

67. *Women and Smoking: A Report of the Surgeon General—2001.* Washington, DC: U.S. Department of Health and Human Services, 2001.

68. "HHS Report Shows Drug Use Rates Stable, Youth Tobacco Use Declines." *Medical Letter on the CDC & FDA,* October 21, 2001, p. 2.

69. Rigotti et al., "U.S. College Students' Use of Tobacco Products."

70. Malson, Jennifer, et al. "Comparison of the Nicotine Content of Tobacco Used in Bidis and Conventional Cigarettes." *Tobacco Control,* Vol. 10, No. 2, June 2001, p. 181.

71. Goebal, Lynne, et al. "Young Users of Smokeless Tobacco Lack Awareness of Its Dangers." *Nicotine & Tobacco Research,* December 2000.

72. Glantz, Stanton, and William Parmley. "Even a Little Secondhand Smoke Is Dangerous." *Journal of the American Medical Association,* Vol. 286, No. 4, July 25, 2001, p. 436.

73. Heloma, Antero, et al. "The Short-Term Impact of National Smoke-Free Workplace Legislation on Passive Smoking and Tobacco Use." *American Journal of Public Health,* Vol. 91, No. 9, September 2001, p. 1416.

74. Wang, Li Yan, et al. "Cost-Effectiveness of a School-Based Tobacco-Use Prevention Program." *Archives of Pediatrics & Adolescent Medicine,* Vol. 155, No. 9, September 2001, p. 1043.

75. Centers for Disease Control and Prevention, www.cdc.gov.

76. "Study Shows Dangers of Resuming Smoking." *Alcoholism & Drug Abuse Weekly,* Vol. 13, No. 40, October 22, 2001, p. 8.

77. Pierce, John, and Elizabeth Gilpin. "Impact of Over-the-Counter Sales on Effectiveness of Pharmaceutical Aids for Smoking Cessation." *Journal of the American Medical Association,* Vol. 288, No. 10, September 11, 2002, p. 1260.

# Consumerism, Complementary and Alternative Medicine, and the Health-Care System

After studying the material in this chapter, you should be able to:

- **Discuss** strategies for self-care.
- **List** ways of evaluating health news and online medical advice.
- **List** your rights as a medical consumer.
- **Describe** the different types of complementary and alternative therapies and **explain** what research has shown about their effectiveness.
- **Explain** what managed care is.

You have more health-care options than previous generations could have imagined. Americans use more health-care services, see more health practitioners, undergo more surgery, take more prescription drugs, and spend more time in hospitals than the citizens of any other nation. Not surprisingly, our medical costs also are higher than in any other country: National health expenditures are expected to reach $2.2 trillion in 2008, 16.2 percent of the gross domestic product.[1]

Millions of Americans are turning to *complementary and alternative medicine (CAM)*, a term that includes a broad range of healing philosophies, approaches, and therapies not traditionally taught in medical schools or provided in hospitals. But consumers are learning that they have to be just as savvy—and as skeptical—about these therapies and practitioners as they are with any other form of health care.

*College health* has been defined as "the caring intersection between health and education."[2] As a college student, you are concerned with and responsible for both. This chapter will help prepare you for a lifetime of making health-care choices. Whether you are monitoring your blood pressure, considering elective surgery, or deciding whether to try an alternative therapy, you need to take charge of your health. The reason: No one cares more about your health than you do.

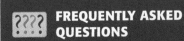

**FREQUENTLY ASKED QUESTIONS**

**FAQ:** How can I evaluate online health advice? p. 340

**FAQ:** Is alternative medicine effective? p. 346

**FAQ:** What is managed care? p. 351

## Becoming a Savvy Health-Care Consumer

It's up to you. Knowing how to spot health problems, how to evaluate health news, what to expect from health-care professionals, and where to turn for appropriate treatment can ensure you receive the best possible care, while keeping your own costs down. (See Student Snapshot: "How Well Informed Are College Students?")

### Self-Care

Most people do treat themselves. You probably prescribe aspirin for a headache, chicken soup or orange juice for a cold, or a weekend trip to unwind from stress. At the very least, you should know what your **vital signs** are and how they compare against normal readings. (See Table 13-1.)

Once a thermometer was the only self-testing equipment found in most American homes. Now an estimated 300 home tests are available to help consumers monitor everything from fertility to blood pressure to cholesterol

levels. (See Table 13-2.) More convenient and less expensive than a visit to a clinic or doctor's office, the new tests are generally as accurate as those administered by a professional. Always follow directions precisely, and if your concerns persist, see your doctor.

### ???? How Can I Evaluate Online Health Advice?

The Internet has become a major source of health information—and misinformation—with more than 10,000 health-related sites. An estimated 41 million Americans go online for medical information every year. Many people want to learn more about medications and treatments; others share experiences with people with similar problems via chat rooms and bulletin boards.

The Internet permits ease of access to cutting-edge medical knowledge and bridges the communication gap created by high-tech medicine. However, it also has serious drawbacks. According to a recent analysis, simple queries for terms such as *obesity* or *depression* often lead to irrelevant sites, relevant sites with incomplete information, or

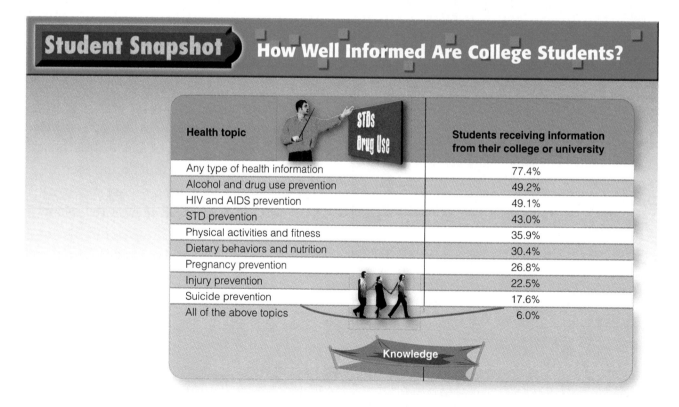

### Student Snapshot — How Well Informed Are College Students?

| Health topic | Students receiving information from their college or university |
|---|---|
| Any type of health information | 77.4% |
| Alcohol and drug use prevention | 49.2% |
| HIV and AIDS prevention | 49.1% |
| STD prevention | 43.0% |
| Physical activities and fitness | 35.9% |
| Dietary behaviors and nutrition | 30.4% |
| Pregnancy prevention | 26.8% |
| Injury prevention | 22.5% |
| Suicide prevention | 17.6% |
| All of the above topics | 6.0% |

Source: Data based on a survey conducted by the Centers for Disease Control and Prevention of 4,609 undergraduates at 136 colleges and universities. Brener, Nancy, and Vani Gowda. "U.S. College Students' Reports of Receiving Health Information on College Campuses." *Journal of American College Health,* Vol. 49, No. 5, March 2001, p. 223.

## ▼ Table 13-1 Take Your Own Vital Signs

| Vital Sign | Normal Values |
| --- | --- |
| **Temperature** | 98.9°F in the morning or 99.9°F later in the day is upper limit of the normal oral tempeature for people 40 years old or younger.<br><br>• Women's temperatures are slightly higher than men's.<br>• African Americans' temperatues are slightly higher than white Americans.<br><br>Measure your temperature with a mercury or digital thermometer. |
| **Blood pressure** | 120/70 to 140/90, depending on age and gender.<br>You can measure your own blood pressure if you want to invest in blood pressure equipment. Check your local drugstore to purchase a blood pressure cuff or digital blood pressure monitor. |
| **Pulse** | 72 beats per minute. Take your pulse rate at your wrist or at the carotid artery in your neck. |
| **Respiration rate** | 15–20 breaths per minute. |

sites that are difficult for most consumers to understand.[3] Many sites are used to promote products or people. Some chat rooms can lead to encounters with unpleasant people. Even when information is technically precise, laypeople may not know how to interpret it properly. Although peer-reviewed websites do offer high-quality information, fewer patients than clinicians reported that they looked for health information on these sites.[4]

Some doctors have set up websites for the sole purpose of selling drugs such as Viagra—a practice state and federal regulators have deemed unethical, though not illegal. The American Medical Association has called for disciplinary action for doctors who prescribe drugs to people they have never met or examined. Other "cyberdocs" offer "virtual house calls" with board-certified physicians who engage in private chat sessions on minor illnesses and prescribe medicine (except controlled drugs like narcotics). In the future, videoconferencing may allow doctors to examine patients in cyberspace. However, there are no professional standards for doctors on the Internet, and experts advise cau-

## ▼ Table 13-2 Home Health Tests: A Consumer's Guide

| Type of Test | What It Does |
| --- | --- |
| **Pregnancy** | Determines if a woman is pregnant by detecting the presence of human chorionic gonadotropin in urine. Considered 99 percent accurate. |
| **Fertility** | Measures levels of luteinizing hormone (LH), which rise 24 to 36 hours before a woman conceives. Can help women increase their odds of conceiving. |
| **Blood pressure** | Measures blood pressure by means of an automatically inflating armband or a cuff for the finger or wrist; helps people taking hypertension medication or suffering from high blood pressure monitor their condition. |
| **Cholesterol** | Checks cholesterol in blood from a finger prick; good for anyone concerned about cholesterol. |
| **Colon cancer** | Screening test to detect hidden blood in stool; recommended for anyone over 40 or concerned about colorectal disease. |
| **Urinary tract infection** | Diagnoses infection by screening for certain white blood cells in urine; advised for women who get frequent UTIs and whose doctors will prescribe antibiotics without a visit. |
| **HIV infection** | Detects antibodies to HIV in a blood sample sent anonymously to a lab. Controversial because no face-to-face counseling is available for those who test positive. |

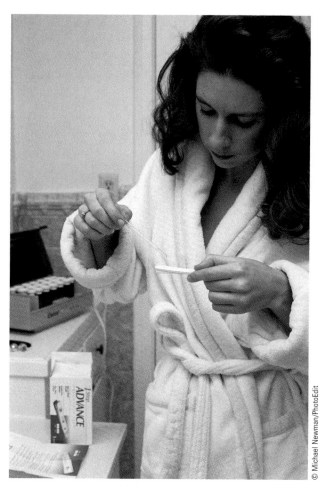

▲ Home health tests can be more convenient and less expensive than a trip to a clinic or doctor's office.

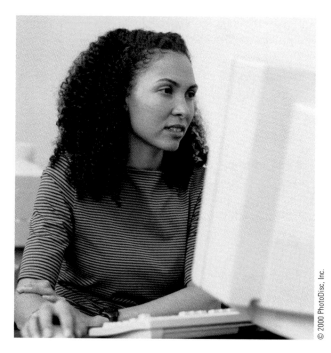

▲ Millions of Americans go online to learn about medical problems and treatments and to chat with others who have similar questions or problems.

✔ Check the references. As with other health-education materials, web documents should provide the reader with references. Unreferenced suggestions may be unwarranted, scientifically unsound, and possibly unsafe.

✔ Consider the author. Is he or she recognized in the field of health education or otherwise qualified to publish a health-information web document? Does the author list his or her occupation, experience, and education?

## Evaluating Health News

Cure! Breakthrough! Medical miracle! These words make catchy headlines. Remember that although medical breakthroughs and cures do occur, most scientific progress is made one small step at a time. Even though medicine is considered a science, some experts estimate that no more than 15 percent of medical interventions can be supported by reliable scientific evidence.

Medical opinions invariably change over time, sometimes going from one extreme to another. For instance, several decades ago the treatment of choice for breast cancer was radical mastectomy—removal of the woman's breast, lymph nodes, and chest wall. Since then much less extensive surgery (lumpectomy), coupled with chemotherapy or radiation, or both, has proven equally effective. Once individuals who'd suffered heart attacks were advised

tion. The doctor who treats your allergies may be a urologist or pathologist who is not up-to-date on new therapies or is unaware of potential side effects.

Here are some specific guidelines for evaluating online health sites:

✔ Check the creator. Websites are produced by health agencies, health support groups, school health programs, health-product advertisers, health educators, and health-education organizations. Read site headers and footers carefully to distinguish biased commercial advertisements from unbiased sites created by scientists and health agencies.

✔ Look for possible bias. Websites may be attempting to provide healthful information to consumers, but they also may be attempting to sell a product. Many sites are merely disguised advertisements.

✔ If you are looking for the most recent research, check the date the page was created and last updated as well as the links. Several nonworking links signal that the site isn't carefully maintained or updated.

to limit all physical activity. Today a progressive exercise program is a standard component of rehabilitation.

Health researchers are struggling to find better ways of assessing what they know and need to know in order to offer more complete and balanced information to consumers. However, sometimes the only certainty is uncertainty. Rather than putting your faith in the most recent report or the hottest trend, try to gather as much background information and as many opinions as you can. Weigh them carefully—ideally with a trusted physician—and make the decision that seems best for you.

When reading a newspaper or magazine article or listening to a radio or television report about a medical advance, look for answers to the following questions:

✔ Who are the scientists involved? Are they recognized, legitimate health professionals? What are their credentials? Are they affiliated with respected medical or scientific institutions? Be wary of individuals whose degrees or affiliations are from institutions you've never heard of, and be sure that the person's educational background is in a discipline related to the area of research reported.

✔ Where did the scientists report their findings? The best research is published in peer-reviewed professional journals, such as the *New England Journal of Medicine*. Research developments also may be reported at meetings of professional societies.

✔ Is the information based on personal observations? Does the report include testimonials from cured patients or satisfied customers? If the answer to either question is yes, be wary.

✔ Does the article, report, or advertisement include words like *amazing, secret,* or *quick?* Does it claim to be something the public has never seen or been offered before? Such sensationalized language is often a tip-off to a dubious treatment.

✔ Is someone trying to sell you something? Manufacturers who cite studies to sell a product have been known to embellish the truth.

✔ Does the information defy all common sense? Be skeptical. If something sounds too good to be true, it probably is.

## Your Medical Rights

As a consumer, you have basic rights to help ensure that you know about any potential dangers, receive competent diagnosis and treatment, and retain control and dignity in your interactions with health-care professionals. Many hospitals publish a patient's bill of rights, including your rights to know whether a procedure is experimental; to refuse to undergo a specific treatment; to designate some-

one else to make decisions about your care if and when you cannot; and to leave the hospital, even against your physician's advice.

You have the right to be treated with respect and dignity, including being called "Mr." or "Ms." or whatever you wish, rather than by your first name. Make clear your preferences. If you feel that health-care professionals are being condescending or inconsiderate, say so—in the same tone and manner that you would like others to use with you. If you're hospitalized, find out if there's a patient advocate or representative at your hospital. These individuals can help you communicate with physicians, make any special arrangements, and get answers to questions or complaints.

You have the right to good, safe care. More than one in five Americans or a family member have experienced a medical or prescription drug error, according to a report by the Commonwealth Fund. One in ten got sicker as a result of the mistake.[5]

You have the right to give consent to donate an organ while alive, or have your organs removed in the event of an accident, injury, or illness that leaves you brain-dead. However, you cannot agree to donate a body part for money or other compensation. Congress has prohibited the marketing of organs; any attempt to do so is a felony punishable by up to five years in jail and a $50,000 fine.

## Your Right to Information

By law, a patient must give consent for hospitalization, surgery, and other major treatments. **Informed consent** is a right, not a privilege. Use this right to its fullest. Ask questions. Seek other opinions. Make sure that your expectations are realistic and that you understand the potential risks, as well as the possible benefits, of a prospective treatment. Informed consent is required for research studies, but patients often don't realize that they have the right not to participate and to get complete information on the purpose and nature of the study.

## Your Medical Records

You have a right to know what is in your medical records. Some states have laws assuring patient access to records. Consumer advocates advise that you routinely request records from physicians, hospitals, and laboratories—first verbally, then in writing. Privacy has become an increasing concern as patients' records have been computerized in large databases. The Medical Information Bureau (MIB) obtains information on individuals' medical claims and conditions from about 750 life insurance companies and combines it into the equivalent of a credit report. Anytime you fill out an application for insurance or file a claim for disability or reimbursement, your insurance company or health-care plan can contact MIB to review every medical claim you've made in the previous seven years.

To protect your privacy, don't routinely fill out medical questionnaires or histories. Always ask the purpose and find out who will have access to the information you provide. Specifically ask if your history may be entered into a database. Tell your physician or health-care group that you do not want your records to leave their offices without your approval. Put it in writing. When you do have to authorize the release of your records, limit the information to a specific condition, physician, and hospital rather than authorizing release of all your records. Contact the MIB (www.mib.com) to find out if there is a file on you and ask to review it. Be sure to correct any inaccuracies.

## Quackery

Every year millions of Americans search for medical miracles that never happen. In all, they spend more than $10 billion on medical **quackery,** unproven health products

and services. Those who lose only money are the lucky ones. Many also waste precious time, during which their conditions worsen. Some suffer needless pain, along with crushed expectations. Far too many risk their lives on a false hope—and lose.

The peddlers of such false hopes are quacks, who, by definition, promote for profit worthless or unproven treatments. The Internet has become a popular medium for quacks to promote themselves and their wares. Nations have joined together in Operation Cure All, a law enforcement and public education campaign to stop Internet health fraud. This group has targeted various devices, herbal products, and dietary supplements purported to treat or cure cancer, AIDS, arthritis, hepatitis, Alzheimer's disease, diabetes, and other chronic conditions.

## STRATEGIES FOR PREVENTION

### Protecting Yourself Against Quackery

▲ Arm yourself with up-to-date information about your condition or disease from appropriate organizations, such as the American Cancer Society or the Arthritis Foundation, which keep track of unproven and ineffective methods of treatment.

▲ Ask for a written explanation of what a treatment does and why it works, evidence supporting all claims (not just testimonials), and published reports of the studies that have been done, including specifics on numbers treated, doses, and side effects.

▲ Be skeptical of self-styled "holistic practitioners," treatments supported by crusading groups, and endorsements from self-proclaimed experts or authorities.

▲ Don't quickly part with your money. Be especially careful because insurance companies won't reimburse for unproven therapies.

▲ Don't discontinue your current treatment without your physician's approval. Many physicians encourage supportive therapies—such as relaxation exercises, meditation, or visualization—as a supplement to standard treatments.

## Complementary and Alternative Medicine

The last decade has seen an enormous increase in the use of a broad range of therapies sometimes called complementary, alternative, unconventional, or holistic. Complementary therapies are adjuncts to conventional therapy, usually intended to improve quality of life rather than stop the progression of disease. Alternative treatments are typically given outside the mainstream medical system, have usually not been corroborated by clinical trials, and are often hoped to be curative.[6]

The medical research community uses the term **complementary and alternative medicine (CAM)** to apply to all health-care approaches, practices, and treatments not widely taught in medical schools and not generally used in hospitals.[7] CAM is not usually reimbursed by medical insurance companies.[8] More than two-thirds of health maintenance organizations cover at least one form of CAM, but the majority of patients pay with their own funds.[9]

CAM includes many healing philosophies, approaches, and therapies, including preventive techniques designed to delay or prevent serious health problems before they start and **holistic** methods that focus on the whole person and the physical, mental, emotional, and spiritual aspects of well-being. Some approaches are based on the same physiological principles as traditional Western methods; others, such as acupuncture, are based on different healing systems.

According to national surveys, 40 to 45 percent of Americans say they have tried at least one nontraditional treatment.[10] Americans make more visits (an estimated 629 million) to alternative practitioners than they do to primary care physicians and spend about as much in annual out-of-pocket expenditures, including money for practitioners, herbal remedies, megavitamins, diet products, books, classes, and equipment. Most people use CAM along with their traditional medical care.[11] (See The X & Y Files: "Men and Women As Health-Care Consumers.")

## Why People Use Complementary and Alternative Therapies

According to several surveys, people don't turn to CAM because they are dissatisfied with conventional care, but because they want more than conventional medicine has to offer. Those who've used CAM believed that most physicians rely too heavily on prescription drugs, don't provide enough information on nutrition and exercise, and ignore the social and spiritual aspects of care.[12] People who use CAM tend to have more education, an interest in personal and spiritual growth, and a belief that body, mind, and spirit are all involved in health.[13] Compared to those who don't use CAM, users often report poorer health and see alternative health care as more in tune with their own values, beliefs, and philosophies about life. The main benefit they report is relief from symptoms of an illness.[14]

An estimated 10 to 50 percent of cancer patients try alternative treatments, many without their physician's knowledge.[15] The American Cancer Society and the National Cancer Institute are supporting research into various alternative approaches in cancer care, such as the use of vitamin A derivatives, green tea, melatonin, shark cartilage, and detoxification with coffee enemas.[16]

Cancer patients seek out alternatives as a way of taking an active role in their treatment and to be sure that "everything possible is being done," according to one survey. In one study of prostate cancer patients, 37 percent of those undergoing treatment with conventional therapies also turned to one or more complementary practices.[17] Other research suggests that cancer patients in the greatest emotional distress may seek out alternative treatments. For example, women who tried alternative as well as conventional treatments for early-stage breast cancer tended to have more depression, greater fear of recurrence, and less robust mental health.[18]

## Doctors and CAM

**Integrative medicine,** which combines selected elements of both conventional and alternative medicine in a comprehensive approach to diagnosis and treatment, is gaining

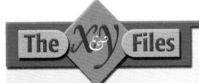

## The X & Y Files  Men and Women As Health-Care Consumers

The genders differ significantly in the way they use health-care services in the United States. Women see more doctors than men, take more prescription drugs, are hospitalized more, and control the spending of three of every four health-care dollars. In a national telephone poll, 76 percent of American women—but only 60 percent of men—said they had had a health exam in the last 12 months.

Many experts believe that the need for birth control and reproductive health services gets women into the habit of making regular visits to health-care professionals, primarily gynecologists. There are no comparable specialists for men, who tend to visit urologists, specialists in male reproductive organs, only when they develop problems. Men also are conditioned to take a stoic, tough-it-out attitude to early symptoms of a disease.

Men feel they are not allowed to manifest illness unless it's overt, says family practitioner Martin Miner, M.D., who has conducted research on men and health care. One reason men die earlier than women is because of the length of time they wait to go for treatment.

The genders also differ in the symptoms and syndromes they develop. For instance, men are more prone to back problems, muscle sprains and strains, allergies, insomnia, and digestive problems. Men develop heart disease about a decade earlier in life than women. More men develop ulcers and hernias; women are more likely to get gallbladder disease and irritable bowel syndrome. An estimated 3 to 6 percent of men suffer from migraines, compared with 15 to 17 percent of women. Yet women and men spend similar proportions of their lifetimes—about 81 percent—free of disability. For men, whose lifespans are shorter, this translates into an average of 58.8 years; for women, 63.9 years.

The genders also differ in access to health services. Women are more likely than men to lack health insurance, and the lower a woman's income and education, the less her likelihood of getting important preventive services, such as an annual Pap smear or prenatal care. Women and men are about equally likely to use complementary and alternative medicine—but different types. Men outnumber women in use of chiropractic services and acupuncture, while women are more likely to try herbal medicine, mind-body remedies, folk remedies, movement and exercise techniques, and prayer or spiritual practices. Both sexes turn to alternative treatments for the same reason: a desire for greater control over their health.

greater acceptance within the medical community.[19] Approximately 1,500 articles on CAM are published annually in medical literature; recent international surveys found that the prevalence of CAM use ranges from 9 percent to 65 percent.[20] More medical schools are teaching courses in CAM, and more than 60 percent of physicians say they've recommended alternative therapies to their patients at least once in the preceding year.[21]

Many doctors are calling upon their colleagues not to dismiss or embrace CAM but to consider each approach thoroughly and evaluate its potential to benefit patients. In a survey of physicians, most—60 percent, more women than men—wanted to learn more about CAM. The most common reasons were "to dissuade patient if alternative method is unsafe and/or ineffective" and "to recommend method to patient if safe and effective." The physicians who felt "very positive" or "somewhat positive" about CAM therapies were more interested in education but no more comfortable in discussing CAM with patients.[22]

The World Health Organization has released a global plan to address the safety of traditional and complementary medicines. The strategy aims to help countries regulate such medicines and to make them safer and more accessible to their populations.[23]

## ???? Is Alternative Medicine Effective?

Many have criticized health-care providers for giving alternative therapies "a free ride" by not demanding the same proof and regulation required to traditional treatments.[24] Under current FDA regulations, testing required for natural health products is the same as required for food, not drugs, which allows them to be marketed without proof of purity, standardization of ingredients, or proof of medicinal efficacy.

However, the National Center for Complementary and Alternative Medicine (NCCAM), part of the National Institutes of Health, conducts and supports studies using the same rigorous standards applied to conventional medicine and disseminates information to patients and health-care consumers. Its three goals are evaluating the safety and efficacy of natural products, supporting their scientific study, and evaluating the practices that implement them. Its budget has grown dramatically, jumping from $2 million in 1993 to $68.7 million in 2000.[25] Current studies are investigating shark cartilage as a cancer treatment, St. John's wort for depression, and a complex nutritional approach to pancreatic cancer.

As studies are conducted, some alternative therapies are gaining acceptance, while others have shown little or no demonstrable benefits.[26] (See Savvy Consumer: "Evaluating Complementary and Alternative Medicine.")

Among the forms of CAM that have proven effective are the following:[27]

- ✔ Moxibustion (burning of Chinese herbs) directly over a specific acupuncture point to help a breech fetus turn around in the womb.
- ✔ Chinese herbs for irritable bowel syndrome. Chinese herbs (including dang shen, huo xiang, and wu wei zi) proved more effective than a placebo in relieving diarrhea, abdominal pain, and other symptoms.
- ✔ Saw palmetto for enlarged prostate gland. In 18 studies with a total sample size of nearly 3,000 patients, men with benign prostatic hyperplasia who took this herbal remedy were twice as likely to report improvement as those taking a placebo.

NCCAM has classified CAM practices into five categories (see Table 13-3). The three most widely used approaches are chiropractic, herbal medicine, and acupuncture.

## Chiropractic

**Chiropractic** is a treatment method based on the theory that many human diseases are caused by misalignment of the bones (subluxation). Chiropractors are licensed in all 50 states, but chiropractic is considered a mainstream therapy by some and a form of CAM by others. Significant research in the last ten years has demonstrated its efficacy for acute lower-back pain. NIH is funding research on other potential benefits, including headaches, asthma, middle ear inflammation, menstrual cramps, and arthritis.

Chiropractors, who emphasize wellness and healing without drugs or surgery, may use X rays and magnetic resonance imaging (MRI), as well as orthopedic, neurological,

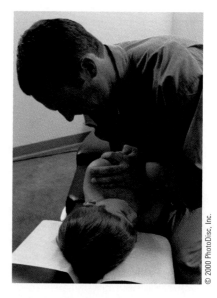

▲ A chiropractor can help relieve shoulder and back pain.

## *Savvy* Consumer

### Evaluating Complementary and Alternative Medicine

You should never decide on any treatment—traditional or complementary/alternative medicine (CAM)—without fully evaluating it. Here are some key questions to ask:

- **Is it safe?** The fact that a substance is "natural" or that a treatment does not require hospitalization or surgery doesn't mean it is safe. Talk to your medical doctor so you understand any particular risks to your overall health or any unknown long-term effects. Be particularly wary of unregulated products.

- **Is it effective?** We know far less about the efficacy of many alternative treatments than we do about traditional therapies. You can obtain information on what is known about the effectiveness of specific treatments from the National Center for Complementary and Alternative Medicine through its website and information clearinghouse (http://nccam.nih.gov).

- **Will it interact with other medicines or conventional treatments?** This is an important question to discuss with your doctor and to investigate by doing research online or in the library. Some combinations—such as the use of a prescription sleeping pill and sleep-inducing melatonin—can be dangerous, and some herbal remedies can interfere with hypertension drugs and increase the risks of anesthesia. Many widely used alternative remedies can interact with prescription medications in dangerous ways.

- **Is the practitioner qualified?** Many states license practitioners who provide acupuncture, chiropractic services, naturopathy, herbal medicine, homeopathy, and other treatments. Find out if yours does, and always choose a licensed professional. You also can contact medical regulatory agencies and consumer affairs departments, which provide information about a specific practitioner's license, education, and accreditation, and will let you know if any complaints have been filed against him or her. Many organizations of specific types of practitioners have websites. However, remember that they are presenting information from an advocate's point of view.

- **What has been the experience of others?** Talk to people who have used CAM for a similar problem, both recently and in the past. Keep in mind that their perspectives—positive or negative—are subjective and should not be your only criterion for selecting a therapy. Also try to find people who have been cared for by the practitioner you are considering.

- **Can you talk openly and easily with the practitioner?** Your relationship with your CAM practitioner is as important as your relationship with your medical doctor. You should feel comfortable asking questions and confident in the answers you receive. What is his or her educational background, principles, and beliefs?

- **Are you comfortable with the CAM care setting?** Visit the practitioner's office, clinic, or hospital. Does it put you at ease, or make you feel out-of-place or anxious? How do conditions such as cleanliness and staff professionalism compare with the health-care settings with which you are more familiar? Find out how many clients a practitioner sees every week and how much time is spent with each one.

- **What are the costs?** Many CAM services are not covered by HMOs or health insurers. Find out if your plan will cover any treatments. Also check what other practitioners charge for the same service so you can decide if a fee is appropriate. Regulatory agencies and professional associations often provide cost information.

and manual examinations in making diagnoses. However, chiropractic treatment consists solely of the manipulation of misaligned bones that may be putting pressure on nerve tissue and affecting other parts of the body. Many HMOs offer chiropractic services, which are the most widely used alternative treatment among managed-care patients.

## Herbal or Botanical Medicine

About one in three Americans has tried an herbal remedy at least once.[28] In the last decade the market for **herbal** or botanical **medicines** has grown to an estimated $12 billion.[29]

Herbal medicines can pose serious risks, particularly when taken along with prescription medications. St. John's wort affects the action of drugs like the anticlotting agent warfarin (Coumadin). When taken with dextromethrophan, an ingredient in cough syrup, St. John's wort can cause serotonin syndrome, a potentially fatal condition characterized by rapid pulse, high fever, and convulsions. Ginkgo biloba and ginseng also interact with warfarin. Kava interacts with sedatives and other agents. Because of the potential of dangerous interactions, you

▼ **Table 13-3 Complementary and Alternative Medicine Practices**

The National Center for Complementary and Alternative Medicine (NCCAM) developed the following classifications:

**Alternative Medical Systems**

These include acupuncture, Oriental medicine, tai chi, external and internal Qi, Ayurvedic medicine, naturopathy, and unconventional Western systems, such as homeopathy and orthomolecular medicine.

**Mind-Body Interventions**

These approaches include many behavioral medicine techniques, such as journaling, as well as hypnosis, yoga, meditation, biofeedback, imagery, music, art and dance therapy, spiritual healing, and community-based approaches (for example, Alcoholics Anonymous and Native American sweat rituals).

**Biologically Based Therapies**

These include botanical medicine or phytotherapy, the use of individual herbs or combinations; special diet therapies, such as macrobiotics, Ornish, McDougall, and high fiber; Mediterranean orthomolecular medicine (use of nutritional and food supplements for preventive or therapeutic purposes); and use of other products (such as shark cartilage) and procedures applied in an unconventional manner not covered in other categories.

**Manipulative and Body-Based Methods**

These are systems based on manipulation and/or movement of the body, divided into three subcategories: chiropractic medicine; massage and body work (including osteopathic manipulation, Swedish massage, Alexander technique, reflexology, Pilates, acupressure, and rolfing); and unconventional physical therapies (including colonics, hydrotherapy, and light and color therapies).

**Energy Therapies**

These therapies focus either on energy fields originating within the body (biofields) or those from other sources (electromagnetic fields). Biofields include therapeutic touch, SHEN, and biorelax methods.

Source: NCCAM. For more information on complementary and alternative treatments, visit http://nccam.nih.gov.

should always tell your doctor if you're taking an alternative medicine.

Even when used alone, herbs and natural substances, just like synthetic drugs, can have side effects and risks. (See Table 13-4.) Some users experience allergic reactions. Studies have connected some herbs, including St. John's wort, echinacea, and ginkgo, with blocking contraception and, in other cases, with infertility. St. John's wort has also been linked to high blood pressure. Echinacea, used for

© Kevin R. Morris/CORBIS

▲ Herbal medicines are a popular form of alternative medicine.

fighting off cold and flu symptoms, may exacerbate autoimmune disorders, such as lupus, rheumatoid arthritis, and multiple sclerosis. There also are suggestions of genetic damage to sperm with several popular herbs.

Unlike over-the-counter and prescription drugs, "natural" remedies have not been subject to rigorous testing. The FDA categorizes herbs as dietary supplements, which are not subject to the same efficacy and safety trials that all new drugs must undergo. Under the provisions of the 1994 Dietary Supplement Health and Education Act, herbal medicine manufacturers can advertise the supposed benefits of their wares as long as they don't claim that the products affect a specific illness.

Some botanicals used for weight loss are particularly dangerous. When a Belgian weight loss clinic using a combination of appetite suppressants and Chinese herbs switched to an herb containing aristolochic acid, dozens of patients suffered kidney failure. Belgian researchers have since found that the clinic's patients have high rates of cancer of the lining of the bladder and ureter.[30] The amphetamine-like herb called *ephedra,* or Ma huang, sold as an energy booster and weight loss aid, can cause dangerous rises in blood pressure and speed up the heart rate. More than 800 injuries and 17 deaths have been linked to this herb.[31] The FDA has proposed a limit on the amount of ephedra that can be added to supplements and has issued warnings on other potentially dangerous herbs, including chaparral, comfrey, yohimbe, lobelia, germander, willow bark, jin bu huan, and products containing magnolia or stephania.

Another problem with wisely using herbal preparations is that potency varies greatly, depending on the form

## ▼ Table 13-4 Some Popular Herbal Remedies

| Herb | Used For | Does It Work? | Warning |
|------|----------|---------------|---------|
| **Acidophilus** | Diarrhea, digestive problems, upset stomach, or yeast infections caused by use of antibiotics | Acidophilus, either in live lactobacillus acidophilus cultures in yogurt or in capsules, can restore the body's normal bacterial balance. | Refrigerate to preserve potency. |
| **Aloe vera** | Sunburn, cuts, burns, eczema, psoriasis | In studies on both humans and animals, aloe vera applied directly to the skin has been shown to speed healing and have antibacterial, anti-inflammatory, and mild anesthetic effects. | Refrigerate gel to extend its shelf life. |
| **Chamomile** | Relaxation, better sleep, stomach aches, menstrual cramps | Laboratory and animal studies indicate that chamomile's active compounds have properties that combat inflammation, bacterial infection, and spasms. | People allergic to plants in the daisy family, such as ragweed, may have an allergic reaction. |
| **Echinacea** | Colds and flu | Inconsistent findings, although one study found that flu sufferers who used echinacea extract recovered more quickly than others. | Use for more than eight weeks at a time may lessen its effectiveness and suppress immunity. Should not be taken by pregnant women and those with diabetes, tuberculosis, or autoimmune disorders. |
| **Garlic** | Fighting infection, preventing heart disease and cancer, stimulating the immune system | Extensive laboratory and animal studies and a review of clinical trials have shown that the active ingredient in garlic has anti-infective and anti-tumor properties and lowers cholesterol. | Check with your doctor if you take blood-thinning medication, including aspirin or ibuprofen, because garlic also is an anticoagulant. |
| **Ginkgo biloba** | Improving memory, cognition, and circulation | There is some evidence that ginkgo biloba can help stabilize mental deterioration in patients with early Alzheimer's disease or stroke-related dementia. One study found that healthy seniors who took ginkgo performed mental tasks better. | Do not take with aspirin because of risk of excessive bleeding. Should not be used during pregnancy. Side effects include upset stomach, headache, and an allergic skin reaction. |
| **Ginseng** | Improving mental and physical energy and stamina | Small studies have shown that ginseng can help improve mental performance and respiratory function during exercise. | If used for more than two weeks, ginseng can cause nervousness and heart palpitations, especially in those with high blood pressure. |
| **Goldenseal** | Colds, allergies, upper respiratory tract infections | Little research has been done, but some laboratory and animal studies suggest that one of goldenseal's components may have some antibiotic and antihistamine effects. | Goldenseal should not be used instead of traditional antibiotics and should never be used for more than ten days at a time. Long-term use may interfere with the normal bacterial balance in the digestive system. |
| **St. John's wort** | Anxiety and depression | Older studies showing benefits had serious flaws. Recent, more rigorous research has shown that St. John's wort is not effective against major depression. | Side effects include stomach pain, bloating, constipation, nausea, fatigue, dry mouth. St. John's wort should never be taken in combination with prescription antidepressants. |

in which they're used. The U.S. Pharmacopeia, a nonprofit organization that sets strength and purity standards for prescription and over-the-counter drugs, has published standards for some popular botanicals. Those that meet these standards have "NF" (National Formulary) on the package. The FDA also now requires a supplements facts panel on the label, similar to the nutritional facts panel on most foods. It contains information on which part of the plant was used to make the product and how much is an appropriate amount to use.

## Acupuncture

An ancient Chinese form of medicine, **acupuncture** is based on the philosophy that a cycle of energy circulating through the body controls health. Pain and disease are the result of a disturbance in the energy flow, which can be corrected by inserting long, thin needles at specific points along longitudinal lines, or *meridians,* throughout the body. Each point controls a different corresponding part of the body. Once inserted, the needles are rotated gently back and forth or charged with a small electric current for a short time. Western scientists aren't sure exactly how acupuncture works, but some believe that the needles alter the functioning of the nervous system.

In *acupressure,* the therapist uses his or her finger and thumb to stimulate certain points, relieve pain, and relax muscles. **Reflexology** is based on the theory that massaging certain points on the foot or hand relieves stress or pain in corresponding parts of the body. These methods seem most effective in easing chronic pain, arthritis, and withdrawal from nicotine, alcohol, or drugs.

An NIH consensus development panel that evaluated current research into acupuncture concluded that there is "clear evidence" that acupuncture can control nausea and vomiting in patients after surgery or while undergoing chemotherapy and relieve postoperative dental pain. The panel said that acupuncture is "probably" also effective in the control of nausea in early pregnancy and that there were "reasonable" studies, some using "sham" needles that make it more difficult for patients to know if they are or are not undergoing acupuncture,[32] showing that the use of acupuncture, by itself or as an adjunct to other therapies,

resulted in satisfactory treatment of a number of other conditions, even though there was not "firm evidence of efficacy at this time." These conditions include addiction to illicit drugs and alcohol (but not to tobacco), stroke rehabilitation, headache, menstrual cramps, tennis elbow, general muscle pain, low-back pain, carpal tunnel syndrome, and asthma. Ongoing studies are evaluating the efficacy of acupuncture for chronic headaches and migraines.

## Other Alternative Treatments

Considered alternative here, **ayurveda** is a traditional form of medical treatment in India, where it has evolved over thousands of years. Its basic premise is that illness stems from incorrect mental attitudes, diet, and posture. Practitioners use a discipline of exercise, meditation, herbal medication, and proper nutrition to cope with such stress-induced conditions as hypertension, the desire to smoke, and obesity. The best known advocate of ayurvedic medicine is Deepak Chopra, M.D., an endocrinologist (specialist in hormone-related disorders) who has written several books on ayurveda and the intimate relationship between consciousness and health.

**Biofeedback** uses machines that measure temperature or skin responses and then relays this information to the subject. In this way, people can learn to control usually involuntary functions, such as circulation to the hands and feet, tension in the jaws, and heartbeat rates. Biofeedback has been used to treat dozens of ailments, including asthma, epilepsy, pain, and Reynaud's disease (a condition in which the fingers become painful and white when exposed to cold). Many health insurers now cover biofeedback treatments.

**Homeopathy** is based on three fundamental principles: "like cures like"; treatment must always be individualized; and less is more—the idea that increasing dilution (and lowering the dosage) can increase efficacy. By administering doses of animal, vegetable, or mineral substances to a large number of healthy people to see if they all develop the same symptoms, homeopaths determine which substances may be given, in small quantities, to alleviate the symptoms. Some of these substances are the same as those used in conventional medicine: nitroglycerin for certain heart conditions, for example, although the dose is minuscule.

**Naturopathy** emphasizes natural remedies, such as sun, water, heat, and air, as the best treatments for disease. Therapies might include dietary changes (such as more vegetables and no salt or stimulants), steam baths, and exercise. Some naturopathic physicians (who are not M.D.s) work closely with medical doctors in helping patients.

Carl Simonton, M.D., a cancer specialist, developed the technique of creative **visualization,** or imaging, to help heal cancer patients, including some diagnosed as terminally ill. On the premise that positive and negative beliefs and attitudes have a great deal to do with whether people

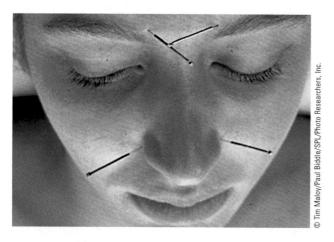

▲ The ancient Chinese practice of acupuncture produces healing through the insertion and manipulation of needles at specific points throughout the body. The procedure is not painful.

© Tim Maloy/Paul Biddle/SPL/Photo Researchers, Inc.

get well or die of disease, patients imagine themselves getting well. They "see," for instance, their immune-system cells marching to conquer the cancer cells. Or they use visualization to create a clear idea of what they want to achieve, whether the goal is weight loss or relaxation.

**Massage therapy** involves the use of the hands to rub, stroke, or knead the body to "positively affect the health and well-being of the individual." Some states have created licensing statutes for massage therapy; others allow local jurisdictions to regulate massage professionals.[33]

# The Health-Care System

In the past, getting health care was fairly simple. When people were sick, they went to their family physician and paid in cash. If they didn't have enough money, the physician would still provide care. Today health care involves many more people, places, and processes. As a college student, you can turn to the student health service if you get sick. There, a nurse, nurse practitioner, physician's assistant, or medical doctor may evaluate your symptoms and provide basic care. However, you may rely on a primary care physician in your hometown to perform regular checkups or manage a chronic condition like asthma. If you're injured in an accident, you probably will be treated at the nearest emergency room. If you become seriously ill and require highly specialized care, you may have to go to a university-affiliated medical center to receive a state-of-the-art treatment.

## What Is Managed Care?

**Managed care** has become the predominant form of health care in the United States. More than 180 million Americans are enrolled in managed care.[34] Managed-care organizations, which take various forms, deliver care through a network of physicians, hospitals, and other health-care professionals who agree to provide their services at fixed or discounted rates.

Consumers in a managed-care group must follow certain procedures in advance of seeking care (for example, getting prior approval for a test or treatment) and must abide by a limit on reimbursement for certain services. Some procedures may be deemed unnecessary and not be covered at all. Patients who choose to see a physician who is not a participating member of the medical-insurance coverage group may have to pay the entire fee themselves.

Managed-care plans have been criticized for pressuring providers to undertreat patients—for example, sending them home from the hospital too soon or denying them costly tests or treatments. Members have complained of long waits, the need to switch primary physicians if their doctor leaves the plan, difficulty getting approval for needed services, and a sense that providers pay more attention to the bottom line than to the health needs of their patients.

As dissatisfaction with managed care has grown, consumers have demanded more choice of physicians, direct access to specialists, and the ability to go "out of network." In response to patients' complaints, many states have approved patient protection acts or comprehensive consumer bills of rights. Federal legislators also have debated a national patient's bill of rights for years, but have disagreed over controversial provisions, such as allowing patients to sue their insurers or employers in either state or federal courts if they feel their rights have been violated.[35]

According to the National Committee for Quality Assurance, managed-care plans have shown improvement in the delivery of care, but health-care costs continue to rise.[36] As a result, employers are cutting back coverage and asking employees to shoulder more of the burden of their health care in the belief that consumers will seek more efficient care when they are required to pay more out of pocket.[37]

## Health Maintenance Organizations

**Health maintenance organizations (HMOs)** are managed-care plans that emphasize routine care and prevention by providing complete medical services in exchange for a predetermined monthly payment. In a *group-model HMO*, physicians provide care in offices at a clinic run by the HMO. In an *individual practice association (IPA)*, or network HMO, independent physicians provide services in their own offices. HMOs generally pay a fixed amount per patient to a physician or hospital, regardless of the type and number of services actually provided. This is called *capitation*.[38]

Members of HMOs pay a regular, preset fee that usually includes diagnostic tests, routine physical exams, vaccinations, and treatment of illnesses. HMOs usually do not require a deductible, and copayments for medications or services are small. The primary drawback of standard HMOs is that the consumer is limited to a particular health-care facility and staff. Open-ended or point-of-service HMOs charge more but let members seek treatment elsewhere if they prefer. These hybrid plans have proven the most popular. Although some large HMOs have earned profits, the HMO industry as a whole consistently lost money in the last decade. Enrollment in HMOs rose steadily in the early 1990s but has declined in more recent years. The total number of HMOs also has dropped.[39]

Although HMOs have been accused of undermining the quality of patient care, recent studies of the outcomes of cancer patients in HMOs and in traditional fee-for-service practices have found little difference. HMOs are, on average, more likely to detect breast cancer early and just as likely to offer a breast-saving lumpectomy rather than a mastectomy. Prostate cancer patients treated in HMOs also had similar ten-year survival rates as those receiving fee-for-service care.

## Preferred Provider Organizations

In a **preferred provider organization (PPO),** a third party—a union, an insurance company, or a self-insured business—contracts with a group of physicians and hospitals to treat members at a discount. PPO members may choose any physician within the network, and usually pay a 10 percent copayment for care within the system and a higher percentage (20 to 30 percent) for care elsewhere. PPOs generally require prior approval for expensive tests or major procedures.

A *point-of-service (POS)* plan is a PPO that permits patients to use physicians outside the network. Consumers pay the difference between the preferred provider's discounted fee and the outside physician's fee. A *gatekeeper plan* requires members to choose a primary physician, as in an HMO, who must approve all referrals to specialists.

## Government-Financed Insurance Plans

The government provides two major forms of health financing: Medicare and Medicaid. Under Medicare, the federal government pays 80 percent of most medical bills, after a deductible fee, for people over age 65. Medicare doesn't cover drugs, eyeglasses, or dental work.

Medicaid, a federal and state insurance plan that protects people with very low or no incomes, is the chief source of coverage for the unemployed. However, many unemployed Americans don't qualify because their family incomes are above the poverty line. Publicly insured patients are more likely than those with private insurance to receive inadequate care and to experience adverse health outcomes.

## The Uninsured

As many as 33 million Americans lack health insurance. Many others are underinsured, meaning that they don't have adequate coverage and are less likely to receive preventive care or routine checkups. According to the Commonwealth Fund, women, who are more likely to be caring for children or aging parents, are themselves less likely than men to have good access to health care. The number of uninsured women has grown three times faster than the number of uninsured men and, if this trend continues, will exceed that of uninsured men by the year 2005.[40] (See Figure 13-1).

Eleven million children under age 19 do not have insurance coverage. Nearly one in three young adults between ages 18 and 24 has no health insurance—the highest proportion of any age group.[41] Some universities, such as those in the University of California system, are requiring all students to purchase insurance that can be used to cover services beyond those provided in university clinics.[42]

Uninsured patients have shorter hospital stays, cannot undergo costly therapies, and have a greater risk of dying in

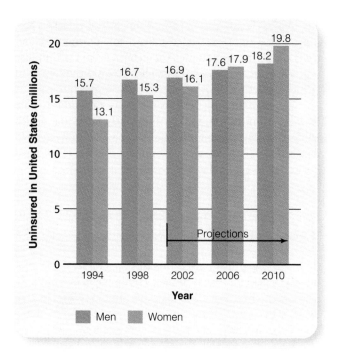

▲ **Figure 13-1** The Number of Uninsured (in Millions) in the United States

Source: Jeanne M. Lambrew. "Diagnosing Disparities in Health Insurance for Women: A Prescription for Change." New York: Commonwealth Fund, August 2001.

the hospital than insured patients. About 85 percent of uninsured Americans are from families in which the head of the family works but can't get insurance through his or her employer.[43] Some of these people work part-time and do not qualify for insurance. Others work for businesses too small to qualify for group insurance. The availability of insurance affects both access to care and the way care is delivered.

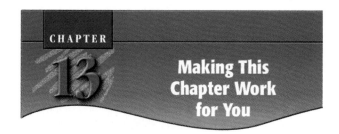

1. Which of the following statements is false?
   a. Home health tests are available for pregnancy, colon cancer, and HIV infection.
   b. Vital signs include temperature, blood pressure, pulse, and cholesterol level.
   c. Health expenditures in the United States are expected to continue to rise in the next five years.

d. Most college students have received some type of health information from their college or university.

2. Which of the following statements about health information on the Internet is true?
   a. Chat rooms are the most reliable source of accurate medical information.
   b. Physicians who have websites must adhere to a strict set of standards set by the American Medical Association.
   c. Government-sponsored sites such as that of the Centers for Disease Control and Prevention are excellent sources of accurate health-care information.
   d. The Internet is a safe and cost-effective source of prescription drugs.

3. Patients have all the rights below except which of the following?
   a. access to their medical records
   b. medical care that meets accepted standards of quality
   c. to donate a body part for compensation
   d. to leave the hospital against their physician's advice

4. Informed consent means
   a. the patient has informed the doctor of his or her symptoms and has consented to treatment.
   b. the physician has informed the patient about the treatment to be given and has consented to administer the treatment.
   c. the patient has informed the doctor of his or her symptoms, and the doctor has consented to administer treatment.
   d. the physician has informed the patient about the treatment to be given, and the patient has consented to the treatment.

5. People use complementary and alternative therapies
   a. to spend less money on health care.
   b. to take an active role in their own treatment.
   c. to show their disdain for the medical establishment.

d. to take more prescription drugs.

6. Examples of complementary and alternative therapies include all of the following *except*
   a. psychiatry
   b. acupuncture
   c. chiropractic
   d. homeopathy

7. Herbal remedies that appear to have positive health effects include
   a. ayurveda for controlling asthma.
   b. acidophilus for improving memory.
   c. aloe vera for diabetes.
   d. garlic for preventing infection and tumor growth.

8. Which statement is false?
   a. Acupuncture has been shown to control nausea in patients after surgery.
   b. Reflexologists massage points on the foot or hand to relieve stress or pain in corresponding parts of the body.
   c. People can learn to control involuntary functions through biofeedback.
   d. Naturopathy is based on the premise that "like cures like."

9. Americans receive their health care in many forms. Which is true?
   a. Medicaid covers people over 65 years of age.
   b. Managed-care plans cover the cost of all physician visits.
   c. About 40 million Americans lack health insurance.
   d. Unemployed Americans receive Medicare.

10. Managed care features all of the following except
    a. health maintenance organizations.
    b. a fee-for-service system of insurance.
    c. preferred provider organizations.
    d. limitations on reimbursement for certain health services.

Answers to these questions can be found on page 415.

## Critical Thinking

1. Have you used any complementary or alternative approaches to health care? If so, were you satisfied with the results? How did your experience with the CAM therapist compare with your most recent experience with a traditional medical practitioner? Do you feel confident that you know the difference between alternative care and quackery?

2. If you're young and healthy, you'll have little problem getting health insurance. However, if you develop a chronic illness, sustain serious injuries in an accident, or simply get older, you may find insurance harder to get and more expensive to keep. What is your insurance coverage? Do you believe insurance companies have the right to turn down applicants with preexisting conditions, such as high blood pressure? Do they have the right to require screening for potentially serious health problems, such as HIV infection, or to cancel the policies of individuals who have run up high medical bills in the past?

3. Jocelyn has been experiencing a great deal of fatigue and frequent headaches for the past couple of months. She doesn't have health insurance and doesn't want to spend money on a doctor visit. So she did some research on the Internet about ways to relieve her symptoms and was considering taking a couple of herbal supplements that were touted as potential treatments. If she asked you for your advice, what would you tell her? Do you think self-care is appropriate in this situation?

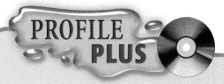

How do you make intelligent choices about health care? Be an informed consumer with help from the guide on Profile Plus CD-ROM.

Guide to Choosing Medical Treatment

## SITES & BYTES

### National Health Information Center
**www.health.gov/nhic**

This excellent site, sponsored by the National Health Information Center (NHIC) of the U.S. Office of Disease Prevention and Health Promotion, is a health information referral service providing health professionals and consumers with a database of various health organizations. The site provides a searchable database, publications, and a list of toll-free numbers for health information.

### National Center for Complementary and Alternative Medicine
**http://nccam.nih.gov/**

This National Institutes of Health site features a variety of fact sheets on alternative therapies and dietary supplements, research, current news, and databases for the public as well as for practitioners.

### Federal Citizen Information Center
**www.pueblo.gsa.gov**

This site is an excellent resource for all types of consumer information, including a variety of health topics: general health, mental health, health-care consumerism, current health news, medications, vaccines, alternative therapies, men's and women's health, children's health, and more. All the information here is free; you can read online or print out any publication in the Consumer Information Catalog.

Please note that links are subject to change. If you find a broken link, use a search engine such as www.yahoo.com and search for the website by typing in keywords.

**InfoTrac College Edition Activity** Carrie Bodane and Kenneth Brownson. "The Growing Acceptance of Complementary and Alternative Medicine." *Health Care Manager,* Vol. 20, No. 3, p. 11.

1. Why is there a growing patient demand for greater use and acceptance of alternative therapies by the professional medical community?

2. What is the significance of the 1994 Dietary Supplement Act? How does the FDA protect consumers with regard to dietary supplements versus medications?

3. What is the major therapeutic emphasis of conventional medicine? How does this contrast with the health claims of alternative (complementary) therapies? Provide a specific example.

For additional links, resources, and suggested readings on InfoTrac College Edition, visit our Health & Wellness Resource Center at http://health.wadsworth.com.

## Key Terms

The terms listed here are used within the chapter on the page indicated. Definitions of the terms are in the Glossary at the end of this book.

**acupuncture** 350        **ayurveda** 350        **biofeedback** 350        **chiropractic** 346

## References

1. "Sharp Rise in Healthcare Costs Projected." *Healthcare Financial Management,* Vol. 54, No. 11, November 2000.

2. Swinford, Paula. "Advancing the Health of Students: A Rationale for College Health Programs." *Journal of American College Health,* Vol. 50, No. 6, May 2002, p. 261.

3. "Good Health Is Hard to Find on the Internet." *Medicine & Health,* Vol. 55, No. 21, May 28, 2001, p. 5.

4. Sigouin, Christopher, and Alejandro R. Jadad. "Awareness of Sources of Peer-Reviewed Research Evidence on the Internet." *Journal of the American Medical Association,* Vol. 287, No. 21, June 5, 2002, p. 2867.

5. Davis, Karen, et al. "Room for Improvement: Patients' Report on the Quality of Their Health Care." New York: Commonwealth Fund, April 2002.

6. Cassileth, Barrie, et al. "Integrative Cancer Therapy: Best of 2 Worlds." *Patient Care,* Vol. 36, No. 10, August, 2002, p. 47.

7. National Center for Complementary and Alternative Medicine, website: http://nccam.nih.gov.

8. Tillman, Robert. "Paying for Alternative Medicine: The Role of Health Insurers." *Annals of the American Academy of Political and Social Science,* September 2002, p. 64.

9. Ernst, E. "The Role of Complementary and Alternative Medicine." *British Medical Journal,* Vol. 321, No. 7269, November 4, 2000.

10. Silverstein, Daniel, and Allen Spiegel. "Are Physicians Aware of the Risks of Alternative Medicine?" *Journal of Community Health,* Vol. 26, No. 3, June 2001, p. 159.

11. Goldstein, Michael. "The Emerging Socioeconomic and Political Support for Alternative Medicine in the United States." *Annals of the American Academy of Political and Social Science.* September 2002, p. 44.

12. Vernarec, Emil. "Why Do Patients Turn to CAM?" *RN,* Vol. 65, No. 5, May 2002, p. 25.

13. Barrett, Bruce, et al. "Bridging the Gap Between Conventional and Alternative Medicine." *Journal of Family Practice,* Vol. 49, No. 3, March 2000, p. 234.

14. Lamarine, Roland. "Alternative Medicine: More Than a Harmless Option." *Current Health 2,* Vol. 27, No. 6, February 2001, p. 19.

15. "When Cancer Patients Keep Alternative Medicine Secrets." *Tufts University Health & Nutrition Letter,* Vol. 18, No. 2, April 2000.

16. Josefson, Deborah. "U.S. Cancer Institute Funds Trials of Complementary Therapy." *British Medical Journal,* Vol. 320, No. 7251, June 24, 2000.

17. "Complementary Health Practices Much More Widespread Than Is Suspected by Doctors." *Cancer Weekly,* February 15, 2000.

18. Lamarine. "Alternative Medicine: More Than a Harmless Option."

19. Rees, Lesley, and Andrew Weil. "Integrated Medicine Imbues Orthodox Medicine with the Values of Complementary Medicine." *British Medical Journal,* Vol. 322, No. 7279, January 20, 2001, p. 119.

20. Ernst, E. "Prevalence of Use of Complementary/Alternative Medicine: A Systematic Review." *Bulletin of the World Health Organization,* Vol. 78, No. 2, February 2000.

21. Berman, Brian. "Complementary Medicine and Medical Education: Teaching Complementary Medicine Offers a Way of Making Teaching More Holistic." *British Medical Journal,* Vol. 33, No. 7279, January 20, 2001, p. 121.

22. Winslow, Lisa Corbin, and Howard Shapiro. "Physicians Want Education About Complementary and Alternative Medicine to Enhance Communication with Their Patients." *Archives of Internal Medicine,* Vol. 162, No. 10, May 27, 2002, p. 1176.

23. "WHO Considers Traditional and Complementary Medicine." *British Medical Journal,* Vol. 324, No. 7348, May 25, 2002, p. 1234.

24. Nahin, Richard, and Stephen Straus. "Research into Complementary and Alternative Medicine: Problems and Potential." *British Medical Journal,* Vol. 33, No. 7279, January 20, 2001, p. 161.

25. Dworkin, Norine. "Doing What Comes Naturally." *Psychology Today,* Vol. 34, No. 2, March 2001, p. 39.

26. Jonas, Wayne. "Policy, the Public, and Priorities in Alternative Medicine Research." *Annals of the American Academy of Political and Social Science.* September 2002, p. 29.

27. Vickers, Andrew. "Complementary Medicine." *British Medical Journal,* Vol. 321, No. 7262, September 16, 2000.

28. Vickers, Andrew, et al. "Herbal Medicine." *Western Journal of Medicine,* Vol. 175, No. 2, August 2001, p. 125.

29. Grant, Michael, et al. "Alternative Pharmacotherapy." *Journal of Family Practice,* Vol. 49, No. 10, October 2000, p. 927.

30. Kessler, David. "Cancer and Herbs." *New England Journal of Medicine,* Vol. 342, No. 23, June 8, 2000, p. 1742.

31. Haller, Christine, and Neal Benowitz. "Adverse Cardiovascular and Central Nervous System Events Associated with Dietary Supplements Containing Ephedra Alkaloids." *New England Journal of Medicine,* Vol. 343, No. 25, December 21, 2000, p. 1833.

32. Cummings. Mike. "Commentary: Controls for Acupuncture—Can We Finally See the Light?" *British Medical Journal,* Vol. 322, No. 7302, June 30, 2001, p. 1578.

33. Josefek, Kristen. "Alternative Medicine's Roadmap to the Mainstream." *American Journal of Law & Medicine,* Summer–Fall, 2000, p. 295.

34. Cauchi, Richard. "Making the Best of Managed Care." *State Legislatures,* Vol. 27, No. 6, June 2001, p. 22.

35. Loiacono, Kristin. "Patients' Rights Legislations: What the Senators Said." *Trial,* Vol. 37, No. 8, August 2001, p. 11.

36. "Managed Care Quality Makes Gains." *Business Insurance,* Vol. 36, No. 38, September 23, 2002, p. 8.

37. Iglehart, John K. "Changing Health Insurance Trends." *New England Journal of Medicine,* Vol. 347, No. 12, September 19, 2002, p. 956.

38. Roberts, Shauna. "Health Maintenance Organizations Part 1: Kinds of HMOs." *Diabetes Forecast,* Vol. 53, No. 11, November 2000.

39. "HMO Enrollment Grows Slowly, Steadily." *Healthcare Financial Management,* Vol. 54, No. 7, July 2000.

40. Lambrew, Jeanne. "Expanding Health Insurance for Working Americans." New York: Commonwealth Fund, August 2001.

41. Siskos, Catherine. "Don't Get Sick." *Kiplinger's Personal Finance Magazine,* Vol. 54, No. 4, July 2000.

42. "UC Set to Require Student Insurance." *Policy & Practice of Public Human Services,* Vol. 58, No. 4, December 2000.

43. Wyn, Roberta, et al. "Falling Through the Cracks." Menlo Park, CA: Henry J. Kaiser Family Foundation, February 2001.

# Staying Safe: Preventing Injury, Violence, and Victimization

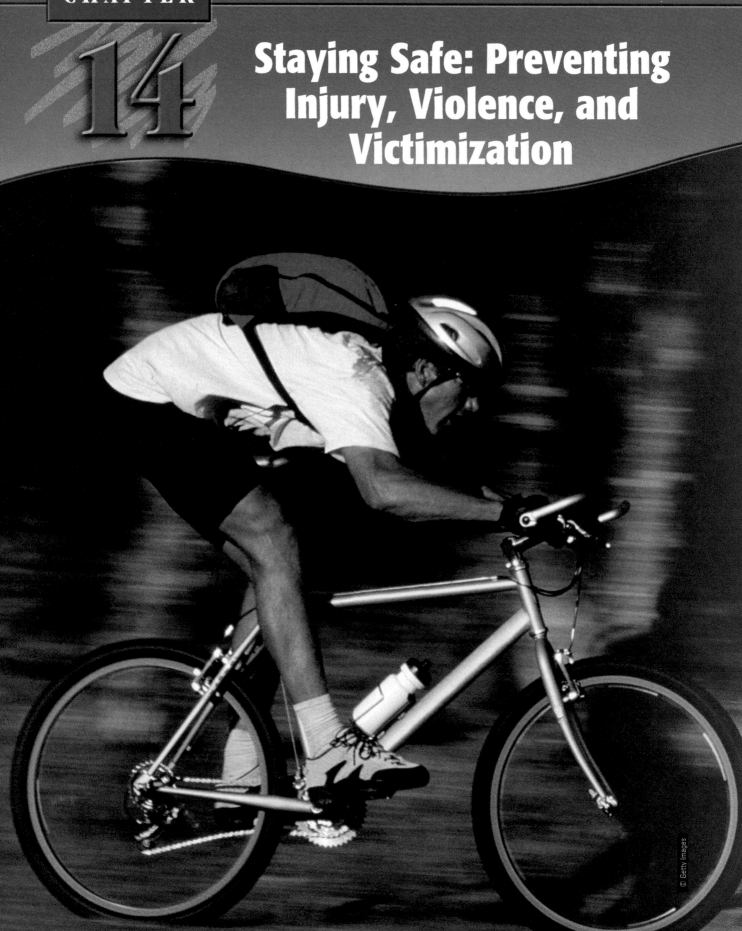

After studying the material in this chapter, you should be able to:

- **List** and **explain** factors that increase the likelihood of an accident.
- **Describe** safety procedures for road, residential, and outdoor safety.
- **Define** sexual victimization, sexual harassment, and sexual coercion.
- **Describe** recommended actions for preventing rape.

Accidents, injuries, assaults, and crimes may seem like things that happen only to other people, only in other places. But no one, regardless of how young, healthy, or strong, is immune from danger. The risks to college students include alcohol-associated injuries and illnesses, traffic accidents, and physical and sexual assaults.[1]

Recognizing the threat of intentional and unintentional injury is the first step to ensuring your personal safety. You may think that the risk of something bad happening is simply a matter of chance, of being in the wrong place at the wrong time. That's not the case. Certain behaviors, such as using alcohol or drugs and not buckling your seat belt, greatly increase the risk of harm. Ultimately, you have more control over your safety than anyone or anything else in your life.

This chapter is a primer in self-protection that could help safeguard—perhaps even save—your life. Included are recommendations for common sense safety on the road, at home, and outdoors. This chapter also explores other serious threats to personal safety in our society: violence and sexual victimization.

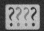 **FREQUENTLY ASKED QUESTIONS**

**FAQ: What is sexual harassment? p. 366**

**FAQ: How can I prevent date rape? p. 369**

# Unintentional Injury: Why Accidents Happen

The major threat to the lives of college students isn't illness but injury. Almost 75 percent of deaths among Americans 15 to 24 years old are caused by "unintentional injuries" (a term public health officials prefer), suicides, and homicides.[2] The odds of dying from an injury in any given year are about one in 765; over a lifetime they rise to one in 23.[3] In all, injuries—intentional and unintentional—claim  almost 150,000 lives a year. Accidents, especially motor vehicle crashes, kill more college-age men and women than all other causes combined; the greatest number of lives lost to accidents is among those 25 years of age.

Many factors influence an individual's risk of accident or injury, including age, alcohol and drug use, stress, inherently dangerous situations, and thrill seeking.

## Age

Injury is the leading cause of death in the United States during the first four decades of life. Each year violence and unintentional injuries cause more than 146,000 deaths and cost more than $260 billion.[4] Most victims of fatal accidents are males, often in their teens and twenties. Feeling full of life and energy, they may take dangerous risks because they think they're invulnerable.

## Alcohol and Drugs

An estimated 40 percent of Americans are involved in an alcohol-related accident sometime during their lives. In nearly half of motor-vehicle deaths, either the driver or a pedestrian was intoxicated at the time of the crash.

## Stress

In times of tension and anxiety, we all pay less attention to what we're doing. One common result is an increase in accidents. If you find yourself having a series of small mishaps or near-misses, do something to lower your stress level, rather than wait for something more harmful to happen. (See Chapter 2 on stress.)

## Situational Factors

Some situations—such as driving on a curvy, wet road in a car with worn tires—are so inherently dangerous that they greatly increase the odds of an accident. But even when there's greater risk, you can lower the danger: For instance, you can make sure your tires and brakes are in good condition.

## Thrill Seeking

To some people, activities that others might find terrifying—such as skydiving or parachute jumping—are stimulating. These thrill seekers may have lower-than-normal levels of the brain chemicals that regulate excitement. Because the stress of potentially hazardous sports may increase the levels of these chemicals, they feel pleasantly aroused rather than scared.

# Safety on the Road

After a five-year decline, the number of people killed on American highways appears to be rising, particularly for motorcycle riders and teenagers between the ages of 16 and 20.[5] Every 14 seconds someone in America is injured in a traffic crash; every 12 minutes someone is killed. Motor vehicle accidents in the United States annually claim about 42,000 lives, more than any other form of unintentional injury. They are the leading cause of all deaths for people ages 1 to 24; only cancer and heart attacks claim more American lives.[6] Far more people—more than 3.5 million annually—are injured in motor vehicle accidents.

According to the National Highway Traffic Safety Administration (NHTSA), motor vehicle crashes on America's roadways cost $230.6 billion per year—an average of $820 for every person in the United States. This is based on an estimated cost of $977,000 for a fatality and $1.1 million for a critically injured crash survivor.[7]

In various studies, posttraumatic stress disorder (PTSD), discussed in Chapter 3, has developed in 8 to 39 percent of individuals injured in motor vehicle crashes or other accidents. It is more likely to develop after a motor vehicle accident when other distressing events occur at the same time, when the victim feared death, when the accident was extremely serious, or when the victim was socially isolated afterward. Children injured in traffic accidents and their parents are at high risk of stress-related symptoms, particularly immediately after a crash.[8]

## Safe Driving

Basic precautions can greatly increase your odds of reaching a destination alive. (See Table 14-1.) According to a recent NHTSA study, excessive driving speed is associated with 12,350 fatalities a year. Speed also contributes to 690,000 nonfatal injuries.[9]

## STRATEGIES FOR PREVENTION

### How to Drive Safely

▲ Don't drive while under the influence of alcohol or other drugs, including medications that may impair your reflexes, cause drowsiness, or affect your judgment.

▲ Never get into a car if you suspect the driver may be intoxicated or affected by a drug.

▲ Remain calm when dealing with drivers who are reckless or rude. If someone cuts you off, back off to a safe distance. When you can, drive so that you have enough space around you.

▲ Be alert and anticipate possible hazards. Don't let yourself be distracted by conversations, children's questions, arguments, food or drink, or scenic views. If you become exhausted, pull over and rest.

▲ Don't get too comfortable. Alertness matters. Use the rearview mirror often. Don't let passengers or packages obstruct your view. Use the turn signals when changing lanes or making a turn.

▲ Make sure small children are in safety seats. Unless pets are trained to ride quietly in a car, keep them in carrying cases.

▲ Drive more slowly if weather conditions are bad. Avoid driving during heavy rain, snow, or other conditions that affect visibility and road conditions. If you must drive in hazardous conditions, make sure that your car has the proper equipment, such as chains or snow tires, and that you know how to respond in case of a skid.

▲ Properly maintain your car, replacing windshield wipers, tires, and brakes when necessary. Keep flares and a fire extinguisher in your car for use in emergencies.

▲ To avoid a head-on collision, generally veer to the right—onto a shoulder, lawn, or open space. Steer your way to safety; avoid hitting the brakes hard once you leave the pavement. If you have to hit something stationary, look for a soft target— bushes, parked cars, woodframe buildings—as opposed to hard boulders, brick walls, trees, and concrete abutments.

### ▼ Table 14-1 Staying Alive

| Strategy | Reduction in Risk of Death |
|---|---|
| **Motor vehicle passengers** | |
| Properly wear three-point restraints | 47% |
| Always use lap belt if car has automatic seat belts | 58% |
| Choose a car with an air bag | 20% |
| Do not ride with an intoxicated driver | Greater than 90% |
| **Drivers** | |
| Avoid driving at night for first year after getting license | Greater than 50% |
| **Cyclists** | |
| Wear a helmet | 85% (bicycle) 55% (motorcycle) |
| **Boaters** | |
| Do not drink alcohol while boating | Greater than 90% |

Source: Grossman, David. "Adolescent Injury Prevention and Clinicians: Time for Instant Messaging." *Western Journal of Medicine,* Vol. 172, No. 3, March 2000, p. 151.

Vehicles equipped with seat belts, air bags, padded dashboards, safety glass windows, a steel frame, and side-impact beams all help protect against injury or death. The size and weight of a vehicle also matter. According to the National Highway Traffic Safety Administration, sport-utility vehicles (SUVs) are two-and-a-half times as likely as other vehicles to kill the occupants of another vehicle in a collision.

## Seat Belts

Seat belts save an estimated 9,500 lives in the United States each year. When lap-shoulder belts are used properly, they reduce the risk of fatal injury to front-seat passengers by 45 percent and the risk of moderate-to-critical injury by 50 percent. The risk of death or severe injury increases nearly fivefold for front-seat passengers when backseat passengers aren't wearing seat belts. In a collision, unbelted backseat passengers may be thrown forward, pushing the front-seat passengers into the dashboard and the windshield.[10]

A significant percentage of drivers do not regularly use seat belts. Although nonusers come from all segments of society, they are frequently male, younger than 30 years of age, unmarried, have little or no postsecondary education, and often drive pickup trucks or sport-utility vehicles. In

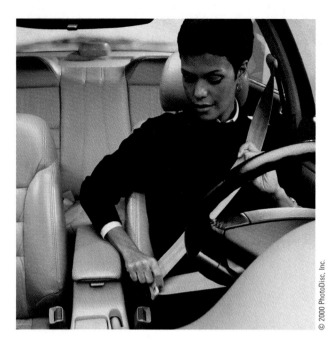

© 2000 PhotoDisc, Inc.

▲ Buckling up is one of the simplest and most effective ways of protecting yourself from injury.

NHTSA surveys, the female seat belt use rate is generally 10 percentage points higher than the male use rate. Overall seat belt use rates are highest in the suburbs, followed by cities, then rural areas.

## Air Bags

An air bag, either with or without a seat belt, has proven the most effective means of preventing adult death, somewhat more so for women than for men.[11] Because there is controversy over the potential hazard they pose to children, the American Academy of Pediatrics recommends that children be placed in the backseat, whether or not the car is equipped with a passenger air bag.

## Safe Cycling

Mile for mile, motorcycling is far more risky than automobile driving. The most common motorcycle injury is head trauma, which can lead to physical disability, including paralysis and general weakness, as well as problems reading and thinking. It can also cause personality changes and psychiatric problems, such as depression, anxiety, uncontrollable mood swings, and anger. Complete recovery from head trauma can take four to six years, and the costs can be staggering. Head injury can also result in permanent disability, coma, and death. To prevent head trauma, motorcycle helmets are required in most states.

Approximately 80.6 million people ride bicycles. Each year, bicycle crashes kill about 900 of these individuals; about 200 of those killed are children under age 15. Men are more likely to suffer cycling injuries. The risk increases with high speed; collisions with motor vehicles are most likely to be fatal.[12]

According to a national survey, 50 percent of all bicycle riders in the United States regularly wear bike helmets—43 percent every time they ride and 7 percent more than half the time. Safety is the primary reason that 98 percent of those surveyed gave for wearing a helmet, followed by the insistence of a parent or spouse. The reasons for not wearing a bike helmet included riding only a short distance, forgetting to put it on, or feeling that the helmet was uncomfortable. (See Savvy Consumer: "Buying a Bicycle Helmet.")

## *Savvy* Consumer

### Buying a Bicycle Helmet

What should you look for when buying a helmet? Here are some basic guidelines:

- A government regulation requires all helmets produced after 1999 to meet the Consumer Product Safety Commission standard; look for a CPSC sticker inside the helmet. The ASTM standard is comparable to CPSC. The Snell Memorial Foundation's B-90 standard is even better.
- Check the fit. The helmet should sit level on your head, touching all around, comfortably snug but not tight. The helmet should not move more than about an inch in any direction, regardless of how hard you tug at it.
- Pick a bright color for visibility. Avoid dark colors, thin straps, or a rigid visor that could snag in a fall.
- Look for a smooth plastic outer shell, not one with alternating strips of plastic and foam.
- Watch out for excessive vents, which put less protective foam in contact with your head in a crash.
- Mirrors should have a breakaway mount; the wire type mounted on eyeglasses can gouge an eye in a fall.

## Safety at Home

Every year home accidents cause nearly 25 million injuries. Poison poses the greatest threat, causing more than 17,000 deaths every year. Half a million children swallow poisonous materials each year; 90 percent are under age 5. Adults may also be poisoned by mistakenly taking someone else's prescription drugs or taking medicines in the dark and swallowing the wrong one. In most cities, you can call a poison control center for advice.

### Falls

Falls of all kinds are the second leading cause of death from unintentional injury in the United States.[13] High heels or worn footgear, poor lighting, slippery or uneven walkways, broken stairs and handrails, loose or worn rugs, and objects left where people walk all increase the likelihood of a slip.

### Fires

You can prevent fires by making sure that the three ingredients of fire—fuel, a heat source, and oxygen—don't get a chance to mix. Almost anything can act as fuel for fire, including paper, wood, and flammable liquids such as oils, gasoline, and some paints. A heat source can be a spark from a lighted match, a pilot light, or an electrical wire. Oxygen is necessary for the chemical reaction between the fuel and heat source that causes combustion.

If a fire starts and it's small, you may be able to put it out with a portable fire extinguisher before it spreads. However, if the fire does get out of control, you might have

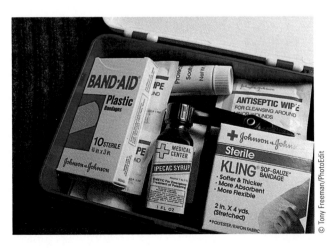

▲ Your home first-aid kit should include (at minimum) bandages, sterile gauze pads, adhesive tape, scissors, cotton, antibiotic ointment, a needle, safety pins, calamine lotion, syrup of ipecac to induce vomiting, and a thermometer.

only two to five minutes to get out of the house or building alive. A fire-escape plan can save time and lives. Sketch a plan of your house, apartment building, dormitory, or fraternity or sorority house. Identify two ways out of each room or apartment. Make sure everyone is familiar with these escape routes. Designate an area outside where all family members or dorm residents should meet after escaping from a fire.

In a national survey, 67 percent of colleges had at least one dorm without a sprinkler system.[14] If a fire breaks out in your dorm room, get out as quickly as possible, but don't run. Before opening a room door, place your hand on it. If it's hot, don't open it. If the door feels cool, open it slightly to check for smoke; if there's none, leave by your planned escape route. If you're on an upper floor and your escape routes are blocked, open a window (top and bottom, if possible) and wait or signal from the window for help. Never try to use an elevator in a fire.

## Recreational Safety

According to a study by the Johns Hopkins School of Public Health, every year 750,000 Americans are injured during recreational activities such as horseback riding, skiing, sledding, skating, and playground activities; 82,000 suffer head injuries requiring emergency room or hospital treatment.

### Handling Heat

Each year as many as 1,000 Americans die from heat-caused illnesses that are almost always preventable. Two common heat-related maladies are **heat cramps** and **heat stress.** Heat cramps are caused by hard work and heavy sweating in the heat. Heat stress may occur simultaneously or afterward, as the blood vessels try to keep body temperature down. **Heat exhaustion,** a third such malady, is the result of prolonged sweating with inadequate fluid replacement. (See Table 14-2.)

The first step in treating these conditions is to stop exercising, move to a cool place, and drink plenty of water. Don't resume work or activity until all the symptoms have disappeared; see a doctor if you're suffering from heat exhaustion. **Heat stroke** is a life-threatening medical emergency caused by the breakdown of the body's mechanism for cooling itself. The treatment is to cool the body down: Move to a cooler environment; sponge down with cool water, and apply ice to the back of the neck, armpits, and groin. Immersion in cold water could cause shock. Get medical help immediately.

| ▼ Table 14-2 Heat Dangers |  |  |
| --- | --- | --- |
| **Illness** | **Symptoms** | **Treatment** |
| **Heat cramps** | Muscle twitching or cramping; muscle spasms in arms, legs, and abdomen | Stop exercising; cool off; drink water. |
| **Heat stress** | Fatigue, pale skin, blurred vision, dizziness, low blood pressure | Stop exercising; cool off; drink water. |
| **Heat exhaustion** | Excessive thirst, fatigue, lack of coordination, increased sweating, elevated body temperature | Stop exercising; cool off; drink water. See a doctor. |
| **Heat stroke** | Lack of perspiration, high body temperature (over 105°F), dry skin, rapid breathing, coma, seizures, high pulse | Cool the body; sponge down with cool water; apply ice to the back of the neck, the armpits, and the groin. Get immediate medical help. |

## Coping with Cold

The tips of the toes, fingers, ears, nose, chin, and cheeks are most vulnerable to exposure to high wind speeds and low temperatures, which can result in **frostnip.** Because frostnip is painless, you may not even be aware of it occurring. Watch for a sudden blanching or lightening of your skin. The best early treatment is warming the area by firm, steady pressure with a warm hand; blowing on it with hot breath; holding it against your body; or immersing it in warm (not hot) water. As the skin thaws, it becomes red and starts to tingle. Be careful to protect it from further damage. Don't rub the skin vigorously or with snow, as you could damage the tissue.

More severe is **frostbite,** which can be either superficial or deep. *Superficial frostbite,* the freezing of the skin and tissues just below the skin, is characterized by a waxy look and firmness of the skin, although the tissue below is soft. Initial treatment should be to slowly rewarm the area. As the area thaws, it will be numb and bluish or purple, and blisters may form. Cover the area with a dry, sterile dressing, and protect the skin from further exposure to cold. See a doctor for further treatment. *Deep frostbite,* the freezing of skin, muscle, and even bone, requires medical treatment. It usually involves the tissues of the hands and feet, which appear pale and feel frozen. Keep the victim dry and as warm as possible on the way to a medical facility. Cover the frostbitten area with a dry, sterile dressing.

The gradual cooling of the center of the body may occur at temperatures above, as well as below, freezing—usually in wet, windy weather. When body temperature falls below 95° Fahrenheit, the body is incapable of rewarming itself because of the breakdown of the internal system that regulates its temperature. This state is known as **hypothermia.** The first sign of hypothermia is severe shivering. Then the victim becomes uncoordinated, drowsy, listless, confused, and is unable to speak properly. Symptoms become more severe as body temperature continues to drop, and coma or death can result.

Hypothermia requires emergency medical treatment. Try to prevent any further heat loss: Move the victim to a warm place, cover him or her with blankets, remove wet clothing, and replace it with dry garments. If the victim is conscious, administer warm liquids, not alcohol.

## Drowning

Over the last few decades, deaths from drowning have declined. Possible reasons include less use of alcohol by swimmers and boaters, and an increase in body fat, which makes floating easier. Toddlers under age 4 and teenage boys between 15 and 19 remain at greatest risk. Among young children, 90 percent of drownings occur in residential swimming pools.

Drowning is the second leading cause of unintentional injury death among children ages 1 to 19 years. Young children are most likely to drown in swimming pools; teenagers, in natural bodies of freshwater.[15] The causes of drowning, in order of frequency, are becoming exhausted, being swept into deep water, losing support, becoming trapped or entangled, having a cramp or other attack, and striking an underwater object. Many drowning victims were strong swimmers. Most drownings occur at unorgan-

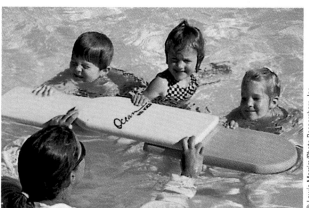

▲ Water safety training can begin in early childhood. Swimming, treading water, and engaging in safe water practices are all important to preventing drownings.

ized facilities, such as ponds or pools with no lifeguard present.

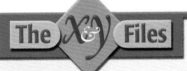

# Intentional Injury: Living in a Dangerous World

Although the United States remains the most violent country in the Western world, the rate of violent crime is going down. The World Health Organization (WHO) defines violence as "the intentional use of physical force or power, threatened or actual, against oneself, another person, or a group or community, that either results in, or has a high likelihood of resulting in, injury, death, psychological harm, maldevelopment, or deprivation."[16] In the first comprehensive review of the global impact of violence, WHO estimated that violence claimed more than 1.6 million lives in 2000.[17] Nearly half of these deaths were suicides, almost a third were homicides, about a fifth were casualties of armed conflict. Men accounted for three-quarters of all victims of homicide, with the highest rates among those between ages 15 and 29.[18]

## Violence in the United States

Gun-related injuries and deaths have declined, but guns remain the second-leading cause of injury-related death in the United States after car accidents. About 260 Americans are injured by firearms every day; one-third die from their wounds.[19] Despite the decline in crime, gun violence annually takes the lives of nearly 30,000 Americans, including 10 children every day. The proportion of youth involved in crime has actually risen. Almost half the victims of violent crime are under 25 years of age.[20]

Although men commit nine times more violent crimes than women, the rates are getting closer. (See The X & Y Files: "Which Gender Is at Greater Risk?") Individuals with mental illness are somewhat more likely to become violent than others. In people with no psychiatric disorder, the prevalence of violence is 2 percent, compared with 8 percent in those with schizophrenia. The risk of violence is highest in people with alcohol or drug misuse or dependence disorders.[21]

 There are ethnic and racial differences in patterns of violence. African Americans are at greater risk of victimization by violent crime than whites or persons of other racial

---

# The X & Y Files    **Which Gender Is at Greater Risk?**

Just like illness, injury doesn't discriminate against either gender. Both men and women can find themselves in harm's way—but for different reasons. Here are some gender differences in vulnerability:

- Men are ten times more likely to die of an occupational injury than women.

- Males are most often the victims and the perpetrators of homicides in the United States. In about 68 percent of cases reported by the Bureau of Justice Statistics, both the offender and the victim were male. In 22 percent, the offender was male and the victim female. In 7.8 percent of all cases, the offender was female and the victim male, while in 2.3 percent both the offender and victim were female.

- Overall, men are 3.6 times more likely than women to be murdered and 9 times more likely to commit murder. Both men and women are more likely to kill or attempt to kill male victims than female victims.

- Boys and men are more likely to be perpetrators of interpersonal violence, including homicide, physical assault, sexual assault, domestic abuse, and hate-related crimes. They are three to five times more likely than women and

girls to carry weapons, thus increasing their risks for homicide and suicide. Men are 1.5 times more likely than women to be assaulted as an adult. Each year 3.2 million men, compared with 1.9 million women, are physically attacked.

- Women are more often the targets of partner violence. Approximately 1.3 million women and 835,000 men are annually assaulted by an intimate partner. At some point in their lifetime, 22.1 percent of women—compared with 7.4 percent of men—report a physical attack by a spouse, partner, boyfriend or girlfriend, or date. About two-thirds (64 percent) of women who report being raped, physically assaulted, or stalked were victimized by a current or former husband, cohabiting partner, boyfriend, or date.

- Physical assaults are more likely to injure women than men. Of female assault victims, 39 percent—compared with 24.8 percent of male assault victims—reported being injured during their most recent attack. Female rape victims also reported more injuries than men who've been raped.

groupings. Hispanics are at greater risk of violent victimization than non-Hispanics. There is little difference between white women and nonwhite women in rape, physical assault, or stalking. Native American and Alaska Native women are significantly more likely than white women or African-American women to report being raped. Mixed-race women also have a significantly higher incidence of rape than white women. Native American and Alaska Native men report significantly more physical assaults than Asian and Pacific Islander men. (See Table 14-3.)

Alcohol availability increases the rates of total crime, violent crime, property crime, and homicides.[22]

## Hate Crimes

Recent years have seen the emergence of violent crimes motivated by hatred of a particular person's (or group of persons') race, religion, sexual orientation, or political values. These hate crimes have included the dragging death of a young African-American man, the beating death of a young gay man, the shooting of children and teachers at a Jewish community center, and the vandalizing of Muslim-owned businesses after the terrorist attacks of September 11, 2001. Politicians and government leaders have called for an expansion of hate-crime laws that would inflict especially severe sentences on those who commit violence on the basis of racism, sexism, homophobia, anti-Semitism, or other forms of prejudice.

### STRATEGIES FOR CHANGE

#### Coping with the Threat of Violence and Terrorism

Uncertainty can be the most difficult aspect of living in a dangerous world. While you cannot eliminate risk, the following strategies can help you deal with it:

▲ Focus on the here-and-now. Make a daily to-do list. Check off each chore as you complete it. Break down large projects into a series of manageable steps.

▲ Act despite fear. Take that first step even if you are anxious, trusting that the second will be easier.

▲ Adjust your attitude. The way you appraise a situation—as a threat that endangers your life or as a challenge that can be overcome—has a tremendous impact on your psychological and physical responses.

▲ Draw on your spiritual beliefs. Faith and values provide a bridge over the unknown.

▲ Dare to hope. This may be the most life-affirming coping strategy of all.

## Crime on Campus

Once considered havens from the meanness of America's streets, colleges and universities have seen a dramatic rise in crime in recent years. However, crime rates in these institutions are lower than in the general community.[23] Property crimes, such as burglary and theft, account for most crimes in campus. However, the

▼ **Table 14-3 Lifetime Victimization (Percentage of People)**

| Type of Victimization | Total | White | African American | Asian and Pacific Islander | Native American and Alaska Native | Mixed Race |
|---|---|---|---|---|---|---|
| **Women** | (n = 7,850) | (n = 6,452) | (n = 780) | (n = 133) | (n = 88) | (n = 397) |
| Rape | 18.2% | 17.7% | 18.8% | 6.8% | 34.1% | 24.4% |
| Physical assault | 51.8% | 51.3% | 52.1% | 49.6% | 61.4% | 57.7% |
| Stalking | 8.2% | 8.2% | 6.5% | 4.5% | 17.0% | 10.6% |
| **Men** | (n = 7,759) | (n = 6,424) | (n = 659) | (n = 165) | (n = 105) | (n = 406) |
| Rape | 3.0% | 2.8% | 3.3% | — | — | 4.4% |
| Physical assault | 66.6% | 66.5% | 66.3% | 58.8% | 75.2% | 70.2% |
| Stalking | 2.3% | 2.1% | 2.4% | — | — | 3.9% |

Source: Tjaden, Patricia, and Nancy Thoennes. *Full Report of the Prevalence, Incidence and Consequences of Violence Against Women.* Washington, DC: National Center for Justice, November 2000.

rates of murder and of hate crimes have risen in recent years.[24] According to the U.S. Department of Education, the criminal homicide rate on campus is 0.07 per 100,000 students—compared with a criminal homicide rate of 5.7 per 100,000 persons overall in the United States and of 14.1 per 100,000 for young people ages 17 to 29.[25]

Colleges must compile annual security reports with statistics on violent crime, as well as drug and alcohol violations.[26] The most recent crime statistics for the nation's 6,269 colleges, universities, and career schools are posted on the Internet at http://ope.ed.gov/security. Under the Federal Student Right to Know and Campus Security Act, all colleges and universities receiving federal funds must publish and make readily available the number of campus killings, assaults, sexual assaults, robberies, burglaries, and other crimes, and their security policies.[27] (See discussions of sexual harassment and assault later in this chapter.)

In a random sample of more than 10,000 undergraduates at four-year schools, 4.3 percent of the students reported that they have a working firearm at college; 1.6 percent had been threatened with a gun. The students most likely to own or to be threatened with a gun are male, live off campus, binge drink, and engage in other risky behavior after drinking. (See Student Snapshot: "Guns on Campus.")[28]

Because of concerns about safety on campus, more schools are taking tougher stands on student behavior. Many have established codes of conduct barring the use of alcohol and drugs, fighting, and sexual harassment. Many also have instituted policies requiring suspension or expulsion for students who violate this code.

As a preventive measure, many campuses have set up public safety programs, which include late-night shuttle buses and escorts, student bicycle patrols, outdoor emergency phones, and increased numbers of police and security guards. Sexual-assault services provide counseling, crisis

## Student Snapshot — Guns on Campus*

| Characteristics | Firearm Owners (Percent) | Victims of Firearm Threat (Percent) |
|---|---|---|
| **Male gender** | 85 | 70 |
| **Race** | | |
| White | 91 | 62 |
| African-American | 3 | 17 |
| Asian | 2 | 10 |
| **Living arrangements** | | |
| Off-campus | 86 | 71 |
| With roommate | 54 | 61 |
| With parent/relative | 19 | 17 |
| With significant other | 16 | 9 |
| Alone | 14 | 15 |
| **Alcohol and driving** | | |
| Binge and drive | 27 | 31 |
| Binge but not drive | 36 | 36 |
| Nonbinge drinker | 23 | 22 |
| Nondrinker | 12 | 10 |
| **Alcohol-related problems** | | |
| Unprotected sex | 17 | 26 |
| Vandalize property | 21 | 23 |
| Trouble with police | 10 | 21 |

*Based on a random sample of 10,000 undergraduates.
Source: Millder, Matthew, et al. "Guns and Gun Threats at College." *Journal of American College Health,* Vol. 51, No. 2, p. 57.

intervention, and educational programs. Students are urged to walk in groups, lock their doors and windows, and limit alcohol consumption. Freshman orientation often includes mandatory sessions on campus safety and sexual assault.

## Family Violence

Violence doesn't stop at the front door of America's homes. According to the Federal Bureau of Investigation, the most common and least-reported violent crime is an attack in which the victim and the perpetrator knew each other at the time of or before the incident. One-third of all murders occur within families. Physical violence may occur in 20 to 30 percent of all American households. As with other forms of violent crime, there has been a decline in assaults and murders by intimates.

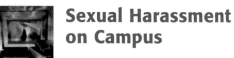

## Sexual Victimization and Violence

Sexual victimization refers to any situation in which a person is deprived of free choice and forced to comply with sexual acts. This is not only a woman's issue; in fact, men are also victimized. In recent years, researchers have come to view acts of sexual victimization along a continuum, ranging from street hassling, stalking, and obscene telephone calls to rape, battering, and incest.

 ## What Is Sexual Harassment?

All forms of sexual harassment or unwanted sexual attention—from the display of pornographic photos to the use of sexual obscenities to a demand for sex by anyone in a position of power or authority—are illegal.

 ## Sexual Harassment on Campus

As many as 30 to almost 50 percent of female undergraduates and 12 to 18 percent of male undergraduates have experienced some form of sexual harassment.[29] Professors or supervisors may pressure students into sexual involvement for the sake of a grade, recommendation, or special opportunity. If a student tries to end a sexual relationship, the professor or supervisor may threaten reprisals. Most harassment comes from male faculty members, but both men and women report having been harassed by either male or female faculty. In a University of Washington study, college men were almost as likely as women to report unwanted sexual contact and coercion.

Sexual harassment can undermine students' well-being and academic performance. Its effects include diminished ambition and self-confidence, reduced ability to concentrate, sleeplessness, depression, physical aches, and numerous other ailments. Some students avoid classes or other contact with certain faculty members because of the risk of sexual advances. However, few victims of sexual harassment file official grievances.

Because college administrations can be held legally responsible for allowing a hostile or offensive sexual environment, many schools have set up committees to handle student complaints and to take action against faculty members. Universities also are discouraging and, in some cases, restricting consensual relationships between teachers and students, especially any dating of students by their academic professors or advisers. Although such relationships may seem consensual, in reality they may not be because of the power faculty members have to determine students' grades and futures. In some cases, students have sued their universities for failing to protect them from professors who pressured them into sexual liaisons.

If you encounter sexual harassment as a student, report it to the department chair or dean. If you don't receive an adequate response to your complaint, talk with the campus representatives who handle matters involving affirmative action or civil rights. Federal guidelines prevent any discrimination against you in terms of grades or the loss of a job or scholarship if you report harassment. Schools that do not take measures to remedy harassment could lose federal funds.

## Sexual Victimization of Students

As the nation has become more aware of issues such as sexual harassment and coercion, there has been growing recognition that college campuses are not ivory towers isolated from these dangers. Recent federal legislation requires colleges and universities to report crimes of all sorts, including sexual victimization.

According to recent estimates, one in eight college women is raped during her years on campus; 84 percent know their assailants.[30] In a national survey, more than a third of attempted rapes (35 percent) took place on a date, as did 22.9 percent of threatened rapes and 12.8 percent of completed rapes. More than half of completed rapes (51.8 percent) took place after midnight, 36.6 percent occurred between 6:00 P.M. and midnight, and 11.8 percent between 6:00 A.M. and 6:00 P.M.[31]

Certain college women are at higher risk of sexual victimization. Among the risk factors are frequently drinking enough to get drunk, being unmarried, and having been a victim of a sexual assault prior to the start of the school year. Fewer than 5 percent of college women reported rapes, either completed or attempted, to law enforcement officials. However, in about two-thirds of rape incidents, the victim did tell another person, most often a friend, about what happened.

The national survey found that the most common forms of sexual victimization on campus involved sexual or sexist remarks, catcalls, and whistles. One in five women reported obscene phone calls or being asked intrusive questions about her sex or romantic life. One in ten had false rumors spread about her sex life. About 6 percent confronted pornographic pictures, while 5 percent encountered a man exposing his sexual organs.

## Sexual Coercion and Rape

At a bar on a weekend night, a group of intoxicated young men grab a woman and squeeze her breasts as she struggles to get free. At a party, a man offers his date drugs and alcohol in the hope of lowering her resistance to sex. Although some people don't realize it, such actions are forms of sexual coercion (forced sexual activity), which is very common on and off college campuses. In fact, about one in five college women report being forced to have sexual intercourse.

**Sexual coercion** can take many forms, including exerting peer pressure, taking advantage of one's desire for popularity, threatening an end to a relationship, getting someone intoxicated, stimulating a partner against his or her wishes, or insinuating an obligation based on the time or money one has expended. Men may feel that they need to live up to the sexual stereotype of taking advantage of every opportunity for sex. Women are far more likely than men to encounter physical force.

**Rape** refers to sexual intercourse with an unconsenting partner under actual or threatened force. Sexual intercourse between a male over the age of 16 and a female under the age of consent (which ranges from 12 to 21 in different states) is called *statutory rape*. In *acquaintance rape*, or *date rape*, discussed in depth later in this chapter, the victim knows the rapist. In *stranger rape*, the rapist is an unknown assailant. Both stranger and acquaintance rapes are serious crimes that can have a devastating impact on their victims.

According to the National Violence Against Women survey, more than half of all women in the United States report an attempted or completed rape and/or physical assault. One in six women, compared with one in 33 men, has experienced an attempted or completed rape in the course of a lifetime.[32] In the previous 12 months, according to the survey, 0.3 percent of the women and 0.1 percent of the men had been raped. These findings indicate that some 302,091 women and 92,748 men are forcibly raped in the United States every year.[33] (See Table 14-3.)

The motives of rapists vary. Those who attack strangers often have problems establishing intimate relationships, have poor self-esteem, feel inadequate, and may have been sexually abused as children. Some rapists report a long his-

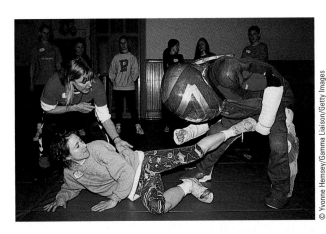

▲ Model mugging courses train women to actively resist assault and rape.

tory of fantasizing about rape and violence, generally while masturbating. Others commit rape out of anger that they can't express toward a wife or girlfriend. The more sexually aggressive men have been, the more likely they are to see such aggression and violence as normal and to believe rape myths, such as that it's impossible to rape a woman who doesn't really want sex. Sexually violent and degrading photographs, films, books, magazines, and videos may contribute to some rapists' assaultive behaviors. Hard-core pornography depicting violent rape has been strongly associated with judging oneself capable of sexual coercion and aggression, and with engaging in such acts.

Alcohol and drugs also play a major role. About 25 percent of both men and women report unwanted sexual experiences as a result of alcohol use. Many rapists drink prior to an assault, and alcohol may interfere with a victim's ability to avoid danger or resist attack.

For many years, the victims of rape were blamed for doing something to bring on the attack. Researchers have since shown that women are raped because they encounter sexually aggressive men, not because they look or act a certain way. Although no woman is immune to attack, many rape victims are children or adolescents. Women who were sexually abused or raped as children are at greater risk than others. Scientists are exploring the reasons for this greater vulnerability.

Women who successfully escape rape attempts do so by resisting verbally and physically, usually by yelling and fleeing. Women who use forceful verbal or physical resistance (screaming, hitting, kicking, biting, and running) are more likely to avoid rape than women who try pleading, crying, or offering no resistance.

## Acquaintance or Date Rape

Most rapes are committed by someone who is known to the victim. Both women and men report having been forced into sexual activity by someone they know. Many college students are in the age group most likely to face this threat: women aged 16 to 25 and men under 25. Women are most vulnerable and men are most likely to commit assaults during their senior year of high school and their first year of college.

Women who describe incidents of sexual coercion that meet the legal definition of rape often don't label it as such. They may have a preconceived notion that true rape consists of a blitzlike attack by a stranger. Or they may blame themselves for getting into a situation in which they couldn't escape. They may feel some genuine concern for others who would be devastated if they knew the truth (for example, if the rapist were the brother of a good friend or the son of a neighbor).

 According to various studies, 25 to 60 percent of college men have engaged in some form of sexual coercion. Most often these men simply ignored a woman when she said no or protested. In addition, many college men reported engaging in sexual activity against their own wishes, most often because of male peer pressure or a desire to be popular.

The same factors that lead to other forms of sexual victimization can set the stage for date rape. Socialization into an aggressive role, acceptance of rape myths, and a view that force is justified in certain situations increase the likelihood of a man's committing date rape. Other factors can also play a role, including the following:

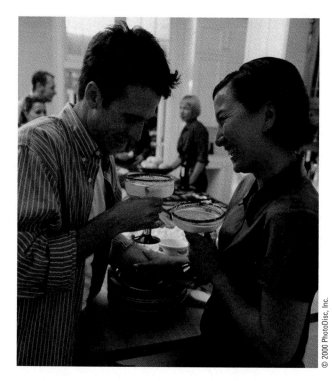

▲ Acquaintance rape and alcohol use are very closely linked. Both men and women may find their judgment impaired or their communications unclear as a result of drinking.

✔ **Personality and early sexual experiences.** Certain factors may predispose individuals to sexual aggression, including first sexual experience at a very young age, earlier and more frequent than usual childhood sexual experiences (both forced and voluntary), hostility toward women, irresponsibility, lack of social consciousness, and a need for dominance over sexual partners.

✔ **Situational variables (what happens during the date).** Men who initiate a date, pay all expenses, and provide transportation are more likely to be sexually aggressive, perhaps because they feel they can call all the shots.

✔ **Acceptance of sexual coercion.** Some social groups, such as fraternities and athletic teams, may encourage the use of alcohol; reinforce stereotypes about masculinity; and emphasize violence, force, and competition. The group's shared values, including an acceptance of sexual coercion, may keep individuals from questioning their behavior.

✔ **Drinking.** Alcohol use is one of the strongest predictors of acquaintance rape. Men who've been drinking may not react to subtle signals, may misinterpret a woman's behavior as a come-on, and may feel more sexually aroused. At the same time, drinking may impair a woman's ability to effectively com-

municate her wishes and to cope with a man's aggressiveness.

✔ **Date rape drugs.** Drugs such as Rohypnol (roofie, La Rocha, rope, Mexican Valium, Rib Roche, R-2), a tranquilizer used overseas, and gamma hydroxybutrate (GHB), a depressant with potential benefits for people with narcolepsy, have been implicated in cases of acquaintance or date rape. Since both are odorless and tasteless, victims have no way of knowing whether their drink has been tampered with. The subsequent loss of memory leaves victims with no explanation for where they've been or what's happened.

Rohypnol—which can cause impaired motor skills and judgment, lack of inhibitions, dizziness, confusion, lethargy, very low blood pressure, coma, and death—has been outlawed in this country. Deaths also have been attributed to GHB overdoses.

✔ **Gender differences in interpreting sexual cues.** In research comparing college men and women, the men typically overestimated the woman's sexual availability and interest, seeing friendliness, revealing clothing, and attractiveness as deliberately seductive. In one study of date rape, the men reported feeling "led on," in part because their female partners seemed to be dressed more suggestively than usual.

## ???? How Can I Prevent Date Rape?

For men:

✔ Remember that it's okay not to "score" on a date.

✔ Don't assume that a sexy dress or casual flirting is an invitation to sex.

✔ Be aware of your partner's actions. If she pulls away or tries to get up, understand that she's sending you a message—one you should acknowledge and respect.

✔ Restrict drinking, drug use, or other behaviors (such as hanging out with a group known to be sexually aggressive in certain situations) that could affect your judgment and ability to act responsibly.

✔ Think of the way you'd want your sister or a close woman friend to be treated by her date. Behave in the same manner.

For women:

✔ If the man pays for all expenses, he may think he's justified in using force to get "what he paid for." If you cover some of the costs, he may be less aggressive.

✔ Back away from a man who pressures you into other activities you don't want to engage in on a date, such as chugging beer or drag racing with his friends.

✔ Avoid misleading messages and avoid behavior that may be interpreted as sexual teasing. Don't tell him to stop touching you, talk for a few minutes, and then resume petting.

✔ Despite your clearly stated intentions, if your date behaves in a sexually coercive manner, use a strategy of escalating forcefulness—direct refusal, vehement verbal refusal, and, if necessary, physical force.

✔ Avoid using alcohol or other drugs when you definitely do not wish to be sexually intimate with your date.

## Male Rape

No one knows how common male rape is because men are less likely to report such assaults than women. In a recent survey in England, nearly 3 percent of men reported non-consensual sexual experiences as adults. Other researchers estimate that the victims in about 10 percent of acquaintance rape cases are men. These hidden victims often keep silent because of embarrassment, shame, or humiliation, as well as their own feelings and fears about homosexuality and conforming to conventional sex roles.

Although many people think men who rape other men are always homosexuals, most male rapists consider themselves to be heterosexual. Young boys aren't the only victims. The average age of male rape victims is 24. Rape is a serious problem in prison, where men may experience brutal assaults by men who usually resume sexual relations with women once they're released.

## Impact of Rape

Rape-related injuries include unexplained vaginal discharge, bleeding, infections, multiple bruises, and fractured ribs. Victims of sexual violence often develop chronic symptoms, such as headaches, backaches, high blood pressure, sleep disorders, pelvic pain, and sexual fertility problems. But sexual violence has both a physical and a psychological impact. The psychological scars of a sexual assault take a long time to heal. Therapists have linked sexual victimization with hopelessness, low self-esteem, high levels of self-criticism, and self-defeating relationships. An estimated 30 to 50 percent of women develop posttraumatic stress disorder following a rape. Many do not seek counseling until a year or more after an attack, when their symptoms ahve become chronic or intensified.[34]

Acquaintance rape may cause fewer physical injuries but greater psychological torment. Often too ashamed to tell anyone what happened, victims may suffer alone, without skilled therapists or sympathetic friends to reassure them. Women raped by acquaintances blame themselves more, see themselves less positively, question their judgment, have greater difficulty trusting others, and have higher levels of psychological distress. Nightmares, anxiety, and flashbacks are common. The women may avoid others, become less capable of protecting themselves, and continue to be haunted by sexual violence for years. A therapist can help these victims begin the slow process of healing.

## What to Do in Case of Rape

If a woman has been raped, she will have to decide whether to report the attack to the police. Even an unsuccessful rape attempt should be reported because the information a woman may provide about the attack—the

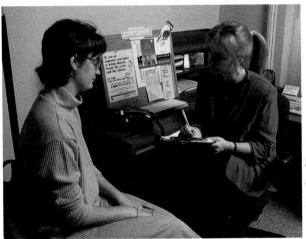

▲ Counseling from a trained professional can help ease the trauma suffered by a rape victim.

assaulter's physical characteristics, voice, clothes, car, even an unusual smell—may prevent another woman from being raped.

Only a small percentage of college women who are raped report their assault to police; many don't even tell a close friend or relative about the assault. Women who are raped should call a friend or a rape crisis center. A rape victim should not bathe or change her clothes before calling the police. Semen, hair, and material under her fingernails or on her apparel all may be useful in identifying the man who raped her.

A rape victim who chooses to go to a doctor or hospital should remember that she may not necessarily have to talk to police. However, a doctor can collect the necessary evidence, which will then be available if she later decides to report the rape to police. All rape victims should talk with a doctor or health-care worker about testing and treatment for sexually transmitted diseases and postintercourse conception.

Many rape victims find it very helpful to contact a rape crisis center, where qualified staff members assist in dealing with the trauma. They can also put victims in touch with other survivors of rape and support groups. Many colleges, universities, and large urban communities in the United States have such programs. Friends and family members should remember that many women mistakenly blame themselves for the rape. However, the victim hasn't committed a crime—the man who raped her has.

police, deans of student affairs, fraternity or sorority representatives, and campus ministers.

While most campuses provide self-defense seminars for potential female victims of rape and general campus safety measures, some have tried innovative approaches, such as Men Against Violence, a peer-education program that confronts male students' conceptions of manhood and appropriate gender roles to reduce their likelihood of sexual or physical violence.[36] Such all-male, peer-guided approaches that challenge myths about rape and rape victims also have proven effective in targeting college fraternity men.

In addition, practical institutional steps—such as providing adequate lighting, escort services, and clear policies against both violence and drug and alcohol abuse—can help. Self-defense classes teach women how to avoid becoming victims either by escaping or protecting themselves. Follow-up studies of college women have found that self-defense training increased their sense of control over their life, confidence, security, independence, and physical prowess.

Campuses are also providing secondary prevention by getting help to victims of sexual violence as soon as possible through rape-crisis teams and emergency mental-health services, and tertiary prevention by working with victims to ameliorate the long-term effects of their experience through psychotherapy, educational services, and medical care.

# Halting Sexual Violence: Prevention Efforts

Sexual violence has its roots in social attitudes and beliefs that demean women and condone aggression. According to international research, much sexual violence takes place within families, marriage, and dating relationships. In many settings, rape is a culturally approved strategy to control and discipline women. In these places, laws and policies to improve women's status are critical to ending sexual coercion.[35]

 As colleges and universities have become more aware of the different forms of sexual danger, many have taken the lead in setting up primary prevention programs (including newspaper articles; seminars in dormitories, fraternities, and sororities; and lectures) to help students examine their attitudes and values, understand cultural influences, and develop skills for avoiding or escaping from dangerous situations. All men and women should recognize misleading rape myths and develop effective ways of communicating to avoid misinterpretation of sexual cues. Students should also know to whom they can turn to learn more about and seek help for sexual victimization: counselors, campus

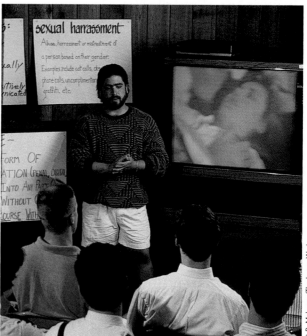

▲ All-male workshops can generate discussions about gender roles and violence, and may also provide positive pressure against rape and other forms of aggression against women.

Are courses in conflict management and peace studies a solution to preventing school violence?

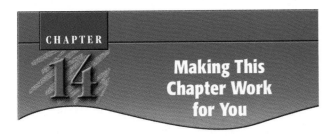

**CHAPTER**

**14**

**Making This Chapter Work for You**

1. You can help keep yourself safe by doing all of the following *except*
   a. using seatbelts when driving or a passenger.
   b. wearing pajamas made of nonflammable materials.
   c. removing or fixing loose carpets.
   d. allowing a spilled liquid to dry on a slippery floor before cleaning it up.

2. Which of the following factors affects an individual's risk of accident or injury?
   a. hunger level
   b. stress level
   c. amount of automobile insurance coverage
   d. knowledge of CPR

3. Safe-driving tips include all of the following *except*
   a. Avoid driving at night for the first year after getting a license.
   b. Make sure your car has snow tires or chains before driving in hazardous snowy conditions.
   c. If riding with an intoxicated driver, keep talking to him so that he doesn't fall asleep at the wheel.
   d. Don't let packages or people obstruct the rear or side windows.

4. Which of the following statements about home safety is true?
   a. Falls pose the greatest threat of injury in the home, followed by poison.
   b. The three ingredients of fire are fuel, a heat source, and oxygen.
   c. The risk of falls is lowest in the elderly.
   d. When using cleaning products, make sure that windows are tightly closed.

5. Which of the following statements about recreational safety hazards is true?
   a. Hypothermia is a life-threatening medical emergency caused by the inability of the body to cool itself.
   b. The most common heat-related conditions are heat stroke and heat exhaustion.

   c. Most drownings occur at organized facilities.
   d. Frostbite usually affects the tissues of the hands and feet.

6. Which of the following statements about violence in the United States is false?
   a. Almost half the victims of violent crime are under 25 years of age.
   b. Risk of violence is highest in people with alcohol or drug misuse or dependence disorders.
   c. Gun-related deaths are the leading cause of death in the United States, followed by car accidents.
   d. Boys and men are most likely to be the perpetrators of homicide, domestic abuse, and hate-related crimes.

7. Which statement about violence on college campuses is false?
   a. Property crimes account for most crimes on campus.
   b. Crime rates at colleges and universities are higher than in the general community.
   c. Students most likely to own a gun are male, live off campus, and binge drink.
   d. Crime statistics for colleges and universities are posted on the Internet.

8. Sexual victimization
   a. includes sexual harassment, sexual coercion, and rape.
   b. is gender-specific, affecting women who are violated emotionally or physically by men.
   c. is rare in academic environments such as college campuses.
   d. most commonly takes the form of physical assault and stalking.

9. Which of the following statements about rape is true?
   a. When a person is sexually attacked by a stranger, it is referred to as *rape*. When a person is sexually attacked by an acquaintance, it is referred to as *sexual coercion.*
   b. Statutory rape is defined as sexual intercourse initiated by a woman under the age of consent.
   c. Men who rape other men usually consider themselves heterosexuals.
   d. Women who flirt and dress provocatively are typically more willing to participate in aggressive sex than women who dress conservatively and do not flirt.

10. Ways to protect or prevent rape include:
    a. Use alcohol and drugs only in familiar surroundings.
    b. Take a self-defense class.

c. To avoid angering a sexually aggressive person, become passive and quiet.

d. Do not discuss your sexual limits on a first or second date because just talking about sex will encourage your date to think you are interested in a sexual relationship.

Answers to these questions can be found on page 415.

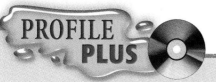

## Critical Thinking

1. Can you name two risk factors in your daily life that might increase the likelihood of accidental injury? What actions have you taken to keep yourself safe? Are there other risk factors you could minimize or eliminate? What might you do about them?

2. A friend of yours, Eric, frequently makes crude or derogatory comments about women. When you finally call him on this, his response is, "I didn't say anything wrong. I like women." What might you say to him?

3. At one college, women raped by acquaintances or dates scrawled the names of their assailants on the walls of women's restrooms on campus. Several young men whose names appeared on the list objected, protesting that they were innocent and were being unfairly accused. How do you feel about this method of fighting back against date rape? Do you think it violates the rights of men? How do you feel about naming women who've been raped in news reports? Are there circumstances in which a woman's identity should be revealed? Would fewer women report a rape if not assured of privacy?

## PROFILE PLUS

Can your world be a safer place? Discover strategies to lessen the risk of injury with the information found on your Profile Plus CD-ROM.

Injury Prevention and Control

## SITES & BYTES

### National Safety Council
**www.nsc.org**

This site provides resources and fact sheets on issues related to public safety, the environment, the community, and the workplace. Topics include auto safety, first aid, air quality, lead poisoning, sun safety, and disaster recovery.

### Occupational Safety and Health (OSHA)
**www.osha.gov**

This U.S. Department of Labor site features a wealth of information on occupational safety and accident prevention, as well as a searchable database. Included is a section on ergonomics.

### The Rape Crisis Center
**www.rapecrisis.com**

This private nonprofit organization provides support to victims of sexual violence and their families, including a 24x7 crisis hotline and several advocacy programs.

**InfoTrac College Edition Activity** Antonia Abbey. "Alcohol-Related Sexual Assault: A Common Problem Among College Students." Journal of Studies on Alcohol, Vol. 63, No. 2, March 2002, p. S118.

1. What percentages of college women report being sexually assaulted or raped? What percentages of college men acknowledge sexually assaulting or raping college women? What percentage of sexual assault cases are reported by college students? What percentage of these involve alcohol? How many are perpetrated by someone the victim knew? About how many occur while on a date?

2. What are the similarities between alcohol-involved sexual assaults and sexual assaults that do not involve alcohol?

3. According to the article, what are some of the explanations for the relationship between alcohol consumption and sexual assault?

You can find additional readings relating to injury and violence with InfoTrac College Edition, an online library of more than 900 journals and publications. Follow the instructions for accessing InfoTrac that were packaged with your textbook; then search for articles using a keyword search.

For additional links, resources, and suggested readings on InfoTrac, visit our Health & Wellness Resource Center at http://health.wadsworth.com.

## Key Terms

The terms listed here are used within the chapter on the page indicated. Definitions of terms are in the Glossary at the end of the book.

## References

1. Keeling, Richard. "Risks to Students' Lives: Setting Priorities." *Journal of American College Health,* Vol. 51, No. 2, September 2002, p. 53.

2. Grossman, David. "Adolescent Injury Prevention and Clinicians: Time for Instant Messaging." *Western Journal of Medicine,* Vol. 172, No. 3, March 2000, p. 151.

3. National Safety Council. www.nsc.org.

4. "CDC to Launch New Injury Research Agenda." *Medical Letter on the CDC & FDA,* July 21, 2002, p. 9.

5. Department of Transportation's National Highway Traffic Safety Administration.

6. Quinlan, Kyran, et al. "Characteristics of Child Passenger Deaths and Injuries Involving Drinking Drivers." *Journal of the American Medical Association,* Vol. 283, No. 17, May 3, 2000, p. 2249.

7. "Study Shows Economic Impact of U.S. Vehicle Crashes Reaches $230.6 Billion." *Public Roads,* Vol. 66, No. 1, July–August 2002, p. 52.

8. Winston, Flaura Koplin, et al. "Acute Stress Disorder Symptoms in Children and Their Parents after Pediatric Traffic Injury." *Pediatrics,* Vol. 109, No. 6, June 2002, p. 1163.

9. Minter, Stephen. "Slow Down, You Move Too Fast." *Occupational Hazards,* Vol. 64, No. 6, June 2002, p. 8.

10. Stephenson, Joan. "Backseat Seat Belts." *Journal of the American Medical Association,* Vol. 287, No. 6, February 13, 2002, p. 706.

11. "Study: Driver Airbags Reduce Risk of Death by 8%." *Automotive News,* Vol. 76, No. 5984, May 20, 2002, p. 20N.

12. Thompson, Matthew, and Fredrick Rivara. "Bicycle-Related Injuries." *American Family Physician,* Vol. 63, No. 10, May 15, 2001, p. 2007.

13. Preboth, Monica. "AAP Statement on Falls in Children." *American Family Physician,* Vol. 64, No. 8, October 15, 2001, p. 1468.

14. Fitzgerald, Nancy. "Safety on Campus." *Careers & Colleges,* Vol. 22, No. 18, March 2002, p. 18.

15. Brenner, Ruth, et al. "Where Children Drown." *Pediatrics,* Vol. 108, No. 1, July 2001, p. 85.

16. Heath, Iona. "Treating Violence As a Public Health Problem: The Approach Has Advantages But Diminishes the Human Rights Perspective." *British Medical Journal,* Vol. 325, No. 7367, October 5, 2002, p. 726.

17. Krug, Etienne, et al. "The World Report on Violence and Health." *Lancet,* Vol. 360, No. 9339, October 5, 2002, p. 1083.

18. Mayor, Susan. "WHO Report Shows Public Health Impact of Violence." *British Medical Journal,* Vol. 325, No. 7367, Ocrober 5, 2002, p. 731.

19. Centers for Disease Control and Prevention (CDC).

20. Puruggganan, Ruth, et al. "Exposure to Violence Among Urban School-Aged Children: Is It Only on Television?" *Pediatrics,* Vol. 106, No. 4, October 2000, p. 949.

21. Walsh, Elizabeth, and Thomas Fahy. "Violence in Society: Contribution of Mental Illness Is Low." *British Medical Journal,* Vol. 325, No. 7363, September 7, 2002, p. 507.

22. Gyimah-Brempong, Kwabena. "Alcohol Availability and Crime: Evidence from Census Tract Data." *Southern Economic Journal,* Vol. 68, No. 1, July 2001, p. 2.

23. Carter, Daniel. "Covering Crime on College Campuses." *Quill,* Vol. 88, No. 8, September 2000, p. 32.

24. Fitzgerald. "Safety on Campus."

25. U.S. Department of Education.

26. Dervarics, Charles. "College Groups Battle Safety Advocates over Reform Plan." *Community College Week,* Vol. 13, No. 26, August 6, 2001, p. 3.

27. "Database Will List Campus Crime Figures." *Black Issues in Higher Education,* Vol. 17, No. 11, July 20, 2000.

28. Millder, Matthew, et al. "Guns and Gun Threats at College." *Journal of American College Health,* Vol. 51, No. 2, p. 57.

29. Murnen, Sarah, and Linda Smolak. "The Experience of Sexual Harassment Among Grade-School Students: Early Socialization of Female Subordination?" *Sex Roles: A Journal of Research,* July 2000.

30. Fitzgerald. "Safety on Campus."

31. Fisher, Bonnie, et al. *The Sexual Victimization of College Women.* Washington, DC: U.S. Department of Justice, December 2000.

32. Hensley, Laura. "Treatment for Survivors of Rape: Issues and Interventions." *Journal of Mental Health Counseling,* Vol. 24, No. 4, October 2002, p. 330.

33. Tjaden, Patricia, and Nancy Thoennes. *Full Report of the Prevalence, Incidence and Consequences of Violence Against Women.* Washington, DC: National Center for Justice, November 2000.

34. Hensley. "Treatment for Survivors of Rape."

35. Jewkes, Rachel. "Preventing Sexual Violence: A Rights-Based Approach." *Lancet,* Vol. 360, No. 9339, October 5, 2002, p. 1092.

36. Hong, Luoluo. "Toward a Transformed Approach to Prevention: Breaking the Link Between Masculinity and Violence." *Journal of American College Health,* Vol. 48, No. 6, May 2000, p. 269.

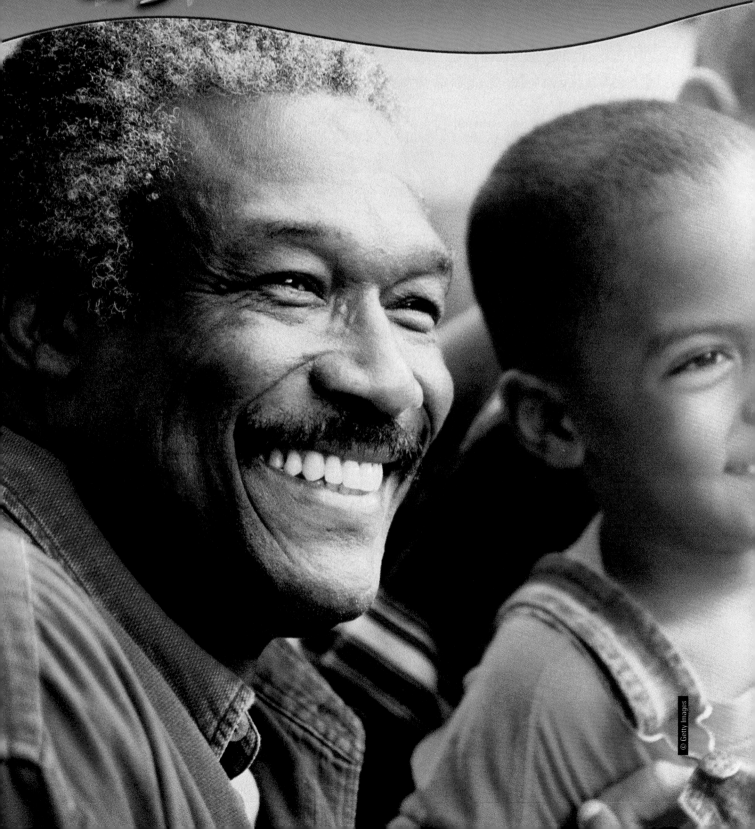

# CHAPTER

## 15

# A Lifetime of Health

**After studying the material in this chapter, you should be able to:**

- **List** the benefits that older Americans can gain from physical activity.
- **Name** three memory skills that diminish with age.
- **Explain** why many elderly people suffer from poor nutrition.
- **Describe** the midlife changes in the female reproductive system.
- **Identify** some of the challenges of aging.
- **Define** death and **explain** the stages of emotional reaction experienced in facing death.
- **Explain** the purposes of advanced directives, a living will, and a holographic will.
- **List** and **explain** factors affecting the length and intensity of grief.

Too young to worry about getting old? Think again. Whether you're in your teens, twenties, thirties, or older, now is the time to start taking the steps that will add healthy, active, productive years to your life.

**Aging**—the characteristic pattern of normal life changes that occurs as humans, plants, and animals grow older—remains inevitable. However, at any age, at any stage of life, at any level of fitness, you can do a great deal to influence the impact that the passage of time has on you. More and more Americans are extending not just their lifespan, but also their *health span*—their years of health and vitality. You can do the same. This chapter provides a preview of the changes age brings, the steps you can take to age healthfully, and the ways you can make the most of all the years of your life.

Invariably, though, no one gets out of this life alive. Death is the natural completion of things, as much a part of the real world as life itself. In time we all lose people we cherish. With each loss, part of us may seem to die, yet each loss also reaffirms how precious life is.

Yet we wonder, as human beings always have, what, if anything, is beyond death. This chapter explores the meaning of death, describes the process of dying, provides practical information on medical and legal arrangements, and offers advice on comforting the dying and helping their survivors.

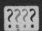 **FREQUENTLY ASKED QUESTIONS**

**FAQ: Does body composition change with age? p. 377**

**FAQ: Do nutritional needs change over time? p. 381**

**FAQ: Is it ever too late to quit smoking? p. 383**

**FAQ: What are advance directives? p. 387**

**FAQ: What is a living will? p. 388**

**FAQ: How can you help survivors of a loss? p. 393**

# Living in an Aging Society

America is turning gray. People age 65 and older make up 13 percent of the U.S. population. By the year 2014, this group will grow to 15 percent.[1] By the midpoint of the twenty-first century, 80 million Americans—one in five—will be seniors (65 or older).[2]

Throughout your life, you will confront a variety of issues related not just to your age, but also to that of the aging American population. These include:

✔ **Retirement costs.** Unless changes are made to decrease the demand on the Social Security system, Social Security taxes on workers may be increased.

✔ **Health costs.** Some experts argue that health costs will soar because people over age 65 use more health services and require more medical care than those who are younger. However, others contend that nations with a large elderly population do not necessarily spend more of their national wealth on health care.

✔ **Gray-power politics.** Senior citizens go to the polls in larger numbers than younger voters. With such voting power, programs for the elderly may make up a larger share of future federal budgets.

✔ **Anti-aging gimmicks.** As the population ages, health hucksters push an every-growing number of unproven anti-aging treatments, such as melatonin or the hormone DHEA. Because some preparations have the potential to harm, consumers must be wary of all claims to turn back or slow down the biological clock. (Chapter 13 offers advice on avoiding health quackery.)

# Successful Aging

The number of Americans living long enough to blow out 100 birthday candles has increased 35 percent from a decade ago. Among senior citizens, the most rapid growth in the last decade has been in the oldest age groups.[3] (See Figure 15-1.)

Americans are not only living longer, but staying healthy and independent longer. More than eight in ten elderly Americans are able to take care of themselves on their own. For the first time, the rate of disability among Americans older than age 85 has dropped below 20 percent. Among the factors contributing to a longer healthspan are improved medical care, diet, exercise, and public health advances.[4]

Genes, as studies of identical twins have revealed, influence only about 30 percent of the rate and ways in which we age. "The rest is up to us," says Michael Roizen, M.D., author of *RealAge,* who notes that it's possible to

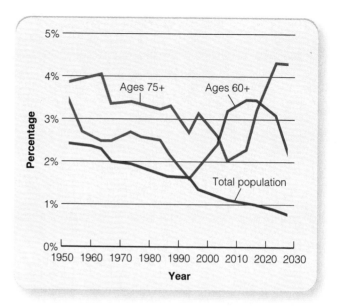

▲ **Figure 15-1** The Graying of America
The percentage of annual growth of the total U.S. population decreases as the senior population increases.

Source: National Institute on Aging.

become healthier, fitter, and biologically younger with time. "With relatively simple changes, someone whose chronological age is 69 can have a physiological age of 45. And the most amazing thing is that it's never too late to live younger—until one foot is 6 feet under."[5]

## Fit for Life

At one time, everyone, even the medical experts, thought that aging meant weakness, frailty, and declining strength. Now we know better: No one is ever too old to get in shape. Rather than telling seniors to take it easy, the American College of Sports Medicine encourages them to engage in the full range of physical activities, including aerobic conditioning. As much as 50 percent of the physiologic declines commonly attributed to aging are due to sedentary living and can be dramatically reversed. With regular conditioning, 60-year-olds can regain the fitness they had at age 40 to 45.

Adults over the age of 72 who exercise more and smoke less than their peers are most likely to enjoy long, healthy, and happy lives, according to a recent study that followed 1,000 seniors for nine years. Proactive health-promoting behaviors, such as exercising and not smoking, contributed to high quality throughout life, even when begun late in life.[6] People who are not physically fit are more likely to die than those who are, even if they are physically healthy, according to another study of 6,213 people.[7] In addition to physical activity, social interactions, such as entertaining friends and getting involved with religious activities, lead to greater life satisfaction as people get older.[8]

Exercise is so effective in preserving well-being that gerontologists describe it as "the closest thing to an anti-aging pill." It slows many changes associated with advancing age, such as loss of lean muscle tissue, increase in body fat, and decreased work capacity. It lowers the risk of heart disease and stroke in the elderly—and greatly improves general health. Male and female runners over age 50 have much lower rates of disability and much lower health-care expenses than less active seniors. Even less intense activities, such as gardening, dancing, and brisk walking, can delay chronic disability.[9] Walking has proven helpful in delaying cognitive decline in older women.[10]

According to the U.S. surgeon general, physical activity offers older Americans additional benefits, including the following:

✔ Greater ability to live independently.
✔ Reduced risk of falling and fracturing bones.
✔ Lower risk of dying from coronary heart disease and of developing high blood pressure, colon cancer, and diabetes.
✔ Reduced blood pressure in some people with hypertension.
✔ Fewer symptoms of anxiety and depression.
✔ Improvements in mood and feelings of well-being.

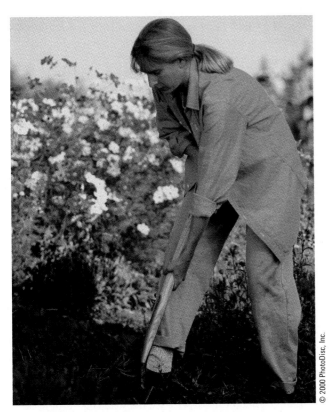

© 2000 PhotoDisc, Inc.

▲ Physical fitness can be enhanced at any age by routine activities such as gardening.

Despite these potential benefits, many seniors are not active. By age 75, about one in three men and one in two women engage in no physical activity. Yet even sedentary individuals in their eighties and nineties can participate in an exercise program—and gain significant benefits.

Federal health officials recommend a moderate amount of physical activity, either in longer sessions of moderately intense activities (such as walking) or in shorter sessions of more vigorous activities (such as race-walking or stair-climbing). Seniors can gain additional health benefits by increasing the duration, intensity, or frequency of their workouts, but should avoid overdoing their training because of the risk of injury. Older adults should always consult with a physician before beginning a new physical activity program.

## ???? Does Body Composition Change with Age?

Both weight and body fat percentage typically increase in adulthood. (See Figure 15-2.) Starting in their twenties, American men and women put on an average of 1 pound of weight a year. By age 65, they have gained about 40 pounds. Because activity levels decline with age, the average individual also loses half a pound of lean body mass a year. The result is a dramatic change in body composition over time: a 20-pound loss of lean tissue and a 40-pound gain in body fat.

Body composition can affect how well older individuals function. In a study of women between the ages of 68 and 75, muscle strength was related to lean mass. The women with the greatest level of disability had higher BMIs and a higher percentage of body fat. Changes in body composition over time are not inevitable. Researchers have documented that physical activity—both aerobic workouts and resistance exercise—can increase and maintain lean body tissue.

## The Aging Brain

Scientists used to think that the aging brain, once worn out, could never be fixed. Now they know that the brain can and does repair itself. When neurons (brain cells) die, the surrounding cells develop "fingers" to fill the gaps and establish new connections, or synapses, between surviving neurons. Although self-repair occurs more quickly in young brains, the process continues in older brains. Even victims of Alzheimer's disease, the most devastating form of senility, have enough healthy cells in the diseased brain to regrow synapses. Scientists hope to develop drugs that someday may help the brain repair itself.

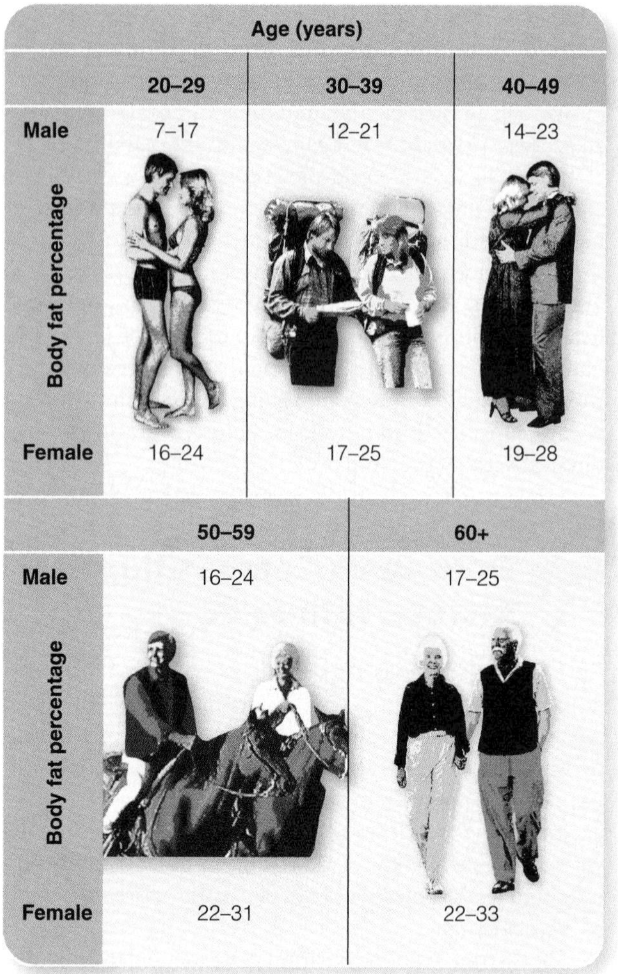

▲ **Figure 15-2** Ideal Body Fat Percentages
As we grow older, body fat percentages tend to increase about 5 to 10 percent every decade. An individual whose body fat percentages are outside the ideal range may have a weight problem.

Source: American College of Sports Medicine.

Mental ability does not decline along with physical vigor. Researchers have been able to reverse the supposedly normal intellectual declines of 60- to 80-year-olds by tutoring them in problem solving. Reaction time, intellectual speed and efficiency, nonverbal intelligence, and maximum work rate for short periods may diminish by age 75. However, understanding, vocabulary, ability to remember key information, and verbal intelligence remain about the same.

## Thinking Young

The healthiest seniors are actively engaged in life, resilient, optimistic, productive, and socially involved, observes John Rowe, M.D., of the MacArthur Foundation Research Network on Successful Aging.[11] While seniors are not immune to life's slings and arrows, successful agers bounce back after a setback and have a can-do attitude about the challenges they face. They also tend to be lifelong learners

who may take up entirely new hobbies late in life—pursuits that stimulate production of more connections between neurons and that may slow aging within the brain.

Just as with muscles, the best advice for keeping your brain healthy as you age is "use it or lose it." Some memory loss among healthy older people is normal, but this is reversible with training in simple methods, such as word associations, that improve recall. The National Institute on Aging has launched a study of Vitamin E and an experimental medication, Aricept (donepezil), as potential treatments for age-related mild cognitive impairment.

## Memory

Some memory skills, particularly the ability to retrieve names and quickly process information, inevitably diminish over time. What normal changes should you expect? Here is a preview:

- ✔ **Recalling information takes longer.** As individuals reach their mid- to late sixties, the brain slows down, but usually just by a matter of milliseconds. As long as they're not rushed, older adults eventually adapt and perform just as well as younger ones.
- ✔ **Distractions become more disruptive.** College students can study and listen to the stereo at the same time. Thirty-something moms can soothe the baby, field questions about homework, and put together a dinner all at once. But as individuals pass age 50, they find it much more difficult to divide their attention or to remember details of a story after having switched their attention to something else.
- ✔ **"Accessing" names gets harder.** The ability to remember names, especially those you don't use frequently, diminishes by as much as 50 percent between ages 25 and 65. Preventive strategies can help, such as repeating a person's name when introduced, writing down the name as soon as possible, and making obvious associations (the Golden Gate for a man named Bridges).
- ✔ **Learning new information is harder.** The quality of memory doesn't change, just the speed at which we receive, absorb, and react to information. That's why strategies like taking notes or outlining material become critical for older students, especially when learning new skills. However, adding to existing knowledge remains as easy as ever.
- ✔ **Wisdom matters.** In any memory test involving knowledge of the world, vocabulary, or judgment, older people outperform their younger counterparts.

## Moving Through Midlife

Although men don't experience the dramatic midlife hormonal changes that women do, their primary sex hormone, testosterone, gradually declines by 30 to 40 percent between ages 48 and 70. This change, sometimes called *andropause,* may cause decreased muscle mass, greater body fat, loss of bone density, flagging energy, lowered fertility, and impaired virility. Some researchers are experimenting with testosterone supplements, but their safety and efficacy are not yet known.

The major changes that occur during a woman's middle years are more evident than those in men. In the next decade, the number of women between the ages of 45 and 54 will increase by half, from 13 million to 19 million. Thus, a large segment of the population will be entering **perimenopause,** the period from a woman's first irregular cycles to her last menstruation.

## Perimenopause

During this time, the egg cells, or oocytes, in a woman's ovaries start to *senesce* or die off at a faster rate. Eventually, the number of egg cells drops to a tiny fraction of the estimated 2 million packed into her ovaries at birth. Trying to coax some of the remaining oocytes to ripen, the pituitary gland churns out extra follicle-stimulating hormone (FSH). This surge is the earliest harbinger of menopause, occurring six to ten years before a woman's final periods. Eventually the other menstrual messenger, luteinizing hormone (LH), also increases, but at a slower rate.

These hormonal shifts can trigger an array of symptoms. The most common are night sweats (a *subdromal hot flash,* in medical terms), which can be just intense enough to disrupt sleep. About 10 to 20 percent of perimenopausal women also experience daytime hot flashes, a symptom that becomes more prevalent with the more drastic and enduring hormonal changes of menopause itself.

## Menopause

**Menopause,** defined as the complete cessation of menstrual periods for 12 consecutive months, generally arrives at age 51 or 52. About 10 to 15 percent of women breeze through this transition with only trivial symptoms. Another 10 to 15 percent are virtually disabled. The majority fall somewhere in between these extremes. Women who undergo surgical or medical menopause (the result of removal of their ovaries or chemotherapy) often experience abrupt symptoms, including flushing, sweating, sleeplessness, early morning awakenings, involuntary urination, changes in libido, mood swings, perception of memory loss, and changes in cognitive function.

Dwindling levels of estrogen subtly affect many aspects of a woman's health, from her mouth (where dryness, unusual tastes, burning, and gum problems can develop) to her skin (which may become drier, itchier, and overly sensitive to touch). The drop in estrogen levels also may cause hot flashes (bursts of perspiration that last from

a few seconds to 15 minutes), which often happen at night, disturbing sleep and causing fatigue. With less estrogen to block them, a woman's androgens, or male hormones, may have a greater impact, causing acne, hair loss, and, according to some anecdotal reports, surges in sexual appetite. (Other women, however, report a drop in sexual desire.)

At the same time, a woman's clitoris, vulva, and vaginal lining begin to shrivel, sometimes resulting in pain or bleeding during intercourse. Since the thinner genital tissues are less effective in keeping out bacteria and other pathogens, urinary tract infections may become more common. Some women develop breast or ovarian cysts, which usually go away on their own. Eventually, a woman's ovaries don't respond at all to her pituitary hormones. After the last ovulatory cycle, progesterone is no longer secreted, and estrogen levels decrease rapidly.

In the United States, the average woman who reaches menopause has a life expectancy of about 30 years. However, she faces risks of various diseases, including a 46 percent risk of heart disease, a 20 percent risk of stroke, and a 10 percent risk of breast cancer.[12] Because estrogen or progestin may play a role in these risks, for many years **hormone replacement therapy (HRT)** was routinely prescribed to ease short-term symptoms of menopause, such as hot flashes, improve a woman's quality of life, and reduce long-term health risks.[13] However, recent research has challenged this practice.[14] (See Savvy Consumer: "Hormone Replacement Therapy.")

Because of the findings of increased risk of heart attack, stroke, and breast cancer, many medical groups have revised their guidelines for HRT. The American College of Obstetricians and Gynecologists and the North American Menopause Society recommend against the use of HRT for preventing heart disease in both healthy women and those who already have heart problems. Although both groups consider HRT an acceptable treatment for menopausal symptoms, they advise caution regarding its prolonged use. The American Heart Association has advised physicians against starting HRT for women with diagnosed heart disease, and suggests physicians base the use of HRT in women without known heart disease on "noncoronary benefits and risks."[15]

There are alternatives, both in terms of medication and lifestyle changes, to HRT. Clonidine, which reduces blood pressure and heart rate, may relieve hot flashes. Testosterone creams, used in the vagina, can help with dryness and irritation. Some women have reported relief from hot flashes, fatigue, depression, and other menopausal symptoms with vitamins and herbal therapies, although there are no scientific studies supporting these benefits. Many postmenopausal women relieve symptoms and lower their risk of future health problems by making lifestyle changes. Exercise lowers the risk of heart disease and strengthens bones; calcium-rich foods and supplements help keep bones strong.

## Savvy Consumer

### Hormone Replacement Therapy

Many people, including physicians, believed that hormone replacement therapy (HRT) would prevent heart disease and strokes and help women live longer. However, this assumption has not lived up to its promise. Several controlled trials have found that rather than protecting women from heart attacks, HRT increased their risk. How could so many people have been so wrong about a therapy used by millions of women? Even though HRT has been around for half a century, rigorous scientific evidence on its benefits and risks emerged only in the last few years.

In 2002 the International Position Paper on Women's Health and Menopause, financed in part by the National Institutes of Health, analyzed existing studies that used "evidence-based medicine"—that is, treatments tested in controlled trials in which patients were assigned at random to either HRT or a placebo. Observational studies, in which women themselves decided to take HRT, had suggested many health benefits from hormone replacement, but these have not held up in evidence-based trials. The reason, researchers say, may be that women who opted for HRT were healthier and had better habits than women who did not choose HRT.

In 2002 the U.S. Preventive Services Task Force reviewed the evidence on the use of HRT and cardiovascular disease, osteoporosis, blood clots, brain function, and cancer (breast, colon, and ovarian). It recommended against the routine use of estrogen and progestin for the prevention of chronic health problems. Despite potential benefits—increased bone mineral density, reduced risk of fractures, and lower risk for colon cancer—the task force concluded that the benefits were outweighed by the dangers, including increased risk of breast cancer, blood clots, heart disease, stroke, and gallbladder disease. HRT's impact on the brain, ovarian cancer, mortality from breast cancer or heart disease, and all-cause mortality was deemed "inconclusive." The task force also concluded that the evidence is insufficient to recommend for or against the use of estrogen alone in women who have had a hysterectomy.

## Sexuality and Aging

Health and sexuality interact in various ways as we age. In a review of sexual function in 1,202 aging men, both the men's health status and their partners' perceived responsiveness were key factors in sexual frequency. When they were in good health and had a willing partner, a substantial number of older men continued to be sexually active.[16] A recent study of a group of physically active men and women over age 50 found that the fittest men and women reported more frequent sexual activity; the fittest men (but not women) also showed the greatest sexual satisfaction.

According to the results of AARP's Maturity Sexual Survey, few of those with self-reported problems took impotence drugs, and those who did said sexual frequency didn't increase, but the sex was better. Among men, 33 percent reported having sex once a week or more after using Viagra or another treatment, compared to 25 percent reporting weekly intercourse before treatment.[17]

Other research has found a relationship between sex and longevity. A Swedish study found that men, but not women, who had discontinued intercourse had higher death rates. A study of the entire male population of a small Welsh town found that the sexually active men had

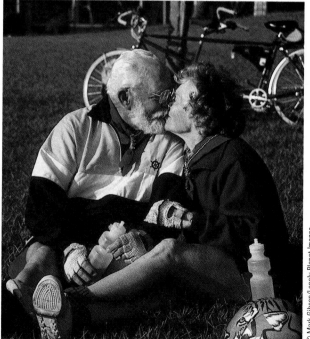

▲ For older couples, sexual desire and pleasure can be enhanced by years of intimacy and affection.

half the mortality of the inactive group. In a Duke University study, longevity in women correlated with enjoyment of sexual intercourse, rather than with its frequency.

Aging does cause some changes in sexual response: Women produce less vaginal lubrication. An older man needs more time to achieve an erection or orgasm and to attain another erection after ejaculating. Both men and women experience fewer contractions during orgasm. However, none of these changes reduces sexual pleasure or desire.

## ???? Do Nutritional Needs Change over Time?

As many as 40 percent of elderly people who live independently do not get adequate amounts of one or more essential nutrients. The reasons are many: limited income, difficulty getting to stores, chronic illness, medications that interfere with the metabolism of nutrients, problems chewing or digesting, poor appetite, inactivity, illness, depression. Among the nutrients often lacking in older Americans are folate, vitamin D, calcium, vitamin E, magnesium, vitamin $B_6$, vitamin C, and zinc.

Nutritionists urge the elderly, like other Americans, to concentrate on eating healthful foods; many also recommend daily nutritional supplements, which may provide the added benefit of improving cognitive function in healthy people over 65. In a study of 86 older people living independently who took either a supplement or a placebo, those taking the supplement showed significant improvements in short-term memory, problem-solving ability, abstract thinking, and attention. Vitamin supplements may help cognitive function by bolstering the immune system, thereby warding off brain changes associated with Alzheimer's disease and other forms of dementia.[18]

The Food Guide Pyramid for Older Americans was designed specifically for adults over age 70, but the USDA urges anyone age 50 or older to heed its recommendations. (See Figure 15-3). The new guidelines advise eight or more 8-ounce glasses of water daily to reduce the risk of dehydration and constipation, which become increasing risks because of decreased thirst sensation in the elderly. The Pyramid also calls for dietary supplements of calcium and vitamins $B_{12}$ and D.[19]

## The Challenges of Age

Aging brains and bodies become vulnerable to diseases like Alzheimer's and osteoporosis. Other common life problems, such as depression, substance misuse, and safe driving, become more challenging as we age.

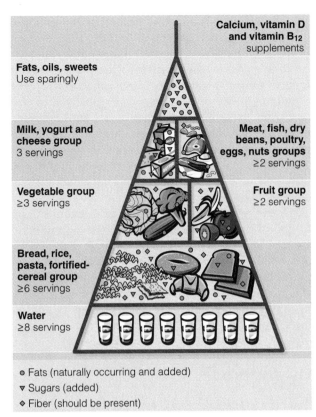

▲ **Figure 15-3** Food Guide Pyramid for Older Adults
The Pyramid shows the USDA-recommended daily servings for adults 70 or older.

## Alzheimer's Disease

About 15 percent of older Americans lose previous mental capabilities, a brain disorder called **dementia.** Sixty percent of these—a total of 4 million men and women over age 65—suffer from the type of dementia called **Alzheimer's disease,** a progressive deterioration of brain cells and mental capacity. Studies using brain imaging indicate that some cognitive deficits associated with age may be reversible. In a study that compared younger and older adults who were asked to memorize a series of words, researchers found that training may help the brains of elderly individuals function more like those of younger people.[20]

 Women are more likely to develop Alzheimer's than men. By age 85, as many as 28 to 30 percent of women suffer from Alzheimer's, and women with this form of dementia perform significantly worse than men in various visual, spatial, and memory tests. African Americans have higher rates of Alzheimer's disease than Africans living in Africa, according to the first study to find differences in the incidence of this illness in an industrial and a nonindustrial country.[21]

The American Academy of Neurology has developed new guidelines, based on a review of 1,000 peer-reviewed papers, for diagnosing Alzheimer's. Based on clinical criteria, these guidelines should allow doctors to diagnose this form of dementia with 90 to 95 percent accuracy.[22] The early signs of dementia—insomnia, irritability, increased sensitivity to alcohol and other drugs, and decreased energy and tolerance of frustration—are usually subtle and insidious. Diagnosis requires a comprehensive assessment of an individual's medical history, physical health, and mental status, often involving brain scans and a variety of other tests.

Even though medical science cannot restore a brain that is in the process of being destroyed by an organic brain disease like Alzheimer's, medications can control difficult behavioral symptoms and enhance or partially restore cognitive ability. Often physicians find other medical or psychiatric problems, such as depression, in these patients; recognizing and treating these conditions can have a dramatic impact.

## Osteoporosis

Another age-related disease is **osteoporosis,** a condition in which losses in bone density become so severe that a bone will break after even slight trauma or injury. (See Figure 15-4.) Among those who live to age 90, 32 percent of women and 19 percent of men will suffer a hip fracture as a result of osteoporosis. Women, who have smaller skeletons, are more vulnerable than men; in extreme cases, their spines may become so fragile that just bending causes severe pain. "Osteoporosis is a terrible crippler and killer," says endocrinologist Joseph Goldzieher, M.D., professor emeritus at Baylor College of Medicine. "The life expectancy for a woman over 70 who breaks her hip is only six months."[23]

 Osteoporosis doesn't begin in old age. In fact, the best time for preventive action is early in life. Increased calcium intake, particularly during childhood and the growth spurt of adolescence, can produce a heavier, denser skeleton and reduce the risk of the complications of bone loss later in life. College-age women also can strengthen their bones and reduce their risk of osteoporosis by increasing their calcium intake and physical activity. Adequate dietary calcium in adulthood can help maintain bone density for years.

Various factors can increase a woman's risk of developing osteoporosis, including family history (a mother, grandmother, or sister with osteoporosis, fractures, height loss, or humped shoulders); petite body structure; white or Asian background; menopause before age 40; smoking; heavy alcohol consumption; loss of ovarian function through chemotherapy, radiation, or hysterectomy; low calcium intake; and a sedentary lifestyle.

In the past, doctors often prescribed hormone replacement therapy to protect aging bones; this is no longer the recommended practice.[24] Alternatives include raloxifene, a SERM (selective estrogen receptor modulator) that prevents bone loss but may cause blood clots in some women; alendronate and risedronate, bisphosphonates that slow the breakdown of bone and may even increase bone density; and calcitonin, a naturally occurring hormone that

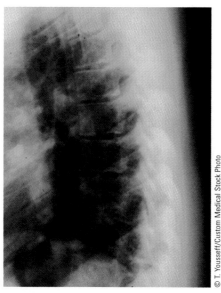

(a)

© T. Youssef/Custom Medical Stock Photo

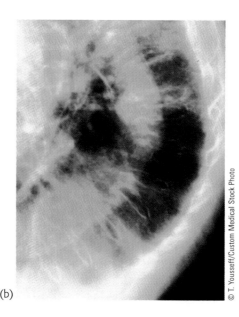

(b)

© T. Youssef/Custom Medical Stock Photo

▲ **Figure 15-4** The Effect of Osteoporosis on the Back (a) A healthy spine: the bony segments (vertebrae) are square with no loss of height. (b) An osteoporotic spine: The curvature is due to compression fractures that occur because the bones are weakened due to loss of mineral density.

## STRATEGIES FOR PREVENTION

### Lowering Your Risk of Osteoporosis

Regardless of your age and gender, you can prevent future bone problems by taking some protective steps now. The most important guidelines are as follows:

▲ Get adequate calcium. Most researchers recommend 500–800 milligrams a day.

▲ Exercise regularly. Both aerobic exercise and weight training can help preserve bone density.

▲ Drink alcohol only moderately. More than two or three alcoholic beverages a day impairs intestinal calcium absorption.

▲ Don't smoke. Smokers tend to be thin (a risk factor for osteoporosis) and enter menopause earlier, thus extending the period of jeopardy from estrogen loss.

▲ Let the sunshine in (but don't forget your sunscreen). Vitamin D, a vitamin produced in the skin in reaction to sunlight, boosts calcium absorption.

increases bone mass in the spine. Other possible therapies are sodium fluoride, parathyroid hormone (PTH), and some forms of vitamin D.

## Substance Misuse and Abuse

Misuse and abuse of prescription and over-the-counter medications occur frequently among the elderly. In part this is because people over age 65 consume one-quarter of all drugs prescribed in the United States. Moreover, many older people have multiple health problems, requiring several medications at the same time. The drugs may interact and cause a confusing array of symptoms and reactions.

The most commonly misused drugs are sleeping pills, tranquilizers, pain medications, and laxatives. Sometimes a person innocently uses more than the prescribed dose or simultaneously takes several prescriptions of the same drug. Some older people are aware of their overreliance on drugs but don't like how they feel when they don't take the pills.

Problems remembering, concentrating, and thinking are the most common psychological side effects of drugs in the elderly. As people age, their bodies take longer to

metabolize drugs, so medications like sleeping pills build up in the body. Almost any amount of alcohol can make mental confusion and memory problems worse. Whenever older people become confused, forgetful, or paranoid, family members should find out which medications they've been taking.

Community surveys suggest that people older than 65 years consume less alcohol and have fewer alcohol-related problems than younger drinkers. In contrast, surveys conducted in health-care settings have found increasing prevalence of alcoholism among older adults. In acute-care hospitals, rates of alcohol-related admissions are similar to rates for heart attacks, and some surveys found the prevalence of problem drinking in nursing homes to be as high as 49 percent. In addition to the direct risks of alcohol, older individuals face related dangers when they drink, including falls, fractures, traffic accidents, medication interactions, depression, and cognitive changes.[25] Brief treatment can be effective in helping the elderly overcome alcohol problems.

## ???? Is It Ever Too Late to Quit Smoking?

The sooner a smoker stops using tobacco, the greater the health benefits, and it is never too late to quit. Quitting at any age, even after age 65, can improve health and extend life—even after thirty or more years of regular smoking. A person who smokes more than 20 cigarettes a day and quits at age 65 increases life expectancy by two or three years.

Despite the well-documented benefits of quitting, an estimated 13 percent of seniors over age 65 smoke. They account for about 70 percent of the smoking-related deaths in the United States. When older people stop tobacco use, their circulation and lung function increase, they suffer less cardiovascular illness, and their quality of life improves.[26]

## Depression

Depression is a serious problem among the elderly. According to the National Institute of Mental Health, 6 percent of Americans aged 65 or older experience some form of depression. Older people face many challenges, including declining health, the loss of loved ones, social isolation, and physical limitations. However, depression is not inevitable, and the elderly are as likely to benefit from psychotherapy and medication as younger individuals.

Older individuals are less likely to seek treatment for depression than younger ones, in part because they may view depression as a weakness rather than a treatable illness. However, the elderly respond just as well to treatment.[27] More than 70 percent of the depressed elderly improve dramatically with treatment. Since loneliness and loss are often important contributing factors, psychiatrists often combine counseling, such as brief psychotherapy, with medication. Because of various physiological differences, the elderly usually respond more slowly to antidepressants than younger people, and the benefits thus may not be apparent for 6 to 12 weeks.

The consequences of not recognizing and treating depression late in life can be tragic. Older Americans have the highest suicide rate in our society, with some 8,500 elderly persons killing themselves every year. The suicide rate is five times higher for those aged 65 than for younger individuals. And depressed older men and women are also more likely to die of other causes.

## Driving Risks

About a third of all drivers are over age 55; their number will increase as the baby-boom generation ages. Driving is very important to seniors, and most want to stay on the road as long as possible. While age alone is not an indicator of impairment, age-related changes can affect driving ability.

The rate of drivers involved in car accidents, including fatal ones, rises after age 70. Drivers aged 70 to 74 are twice as likely to die in an accident than those 30 to 59 years old. The risk for drivers over 80 is five times higher. The most common contributing factors in accidents involving older drivers include pulling out from the side of the road or changing lanes without looking, careless backing, inaccurate turning, failure to yield the right of way, and difficulty reading traffic signs. Unlike younger drivers, older drivers' accidents seldom involve high speeds or alcohol use. Rather, problem driving in older adults involves visual, cognitive, and motor skills, which may decline with aging. The ability of those over 85 to operate a vehicle when they have to divide their attention is half that of people under age 65.

Although half the people over age 85 meet motor vehicle licensing's vision standards, many suffer weaknesses in other critical aspects of vision, such as recovery from glare and depth perception. As various regulatory agencies struggle with better ways to evaluate the safety of older drivers, seniors can lower their risks by limiting night driving, avoiding freeways, driving during less crowded periods of the day, making practice runs of new or difficult routes, and identifying and using alternate means of transportation.

## Death and Dying

The average baby born in 1900 could expect to live 47.3 years. By 1950 life expectancy had climbed to 68.2; by 2000, it had reached a record high of 76.9 years. (See Table 15-1.)

| Table 15-1 Life Expectancy in the United States (Years) | |
| --- | --- |
| **At Birth** | |
| All Americans | 76.9 |
| All males | 74.1 |
| All females | 79.5 |
| **At Age 65** | |
| All Americans | 17.9 |
| All males | 16.3 |
| All females | 19.2 |

Source: *National Vital Statistics Reports*, Vol. 49, No. 12, 2002.

The gaps between blacks and whites and men and women have narrowed over time. While genes may play a role in longevity, lifestyle and healthful behaviors can influence both how long and how well we live.[28] In a landmark study that has tracked the mental and physical health of 724 men as they aged over a 60-year period, seven factors predicted long life and successful aging: moderate alcohol use, no smoking, a stable marriage, exercise, appropriate weight, positive coping mechanisms, and no depressive illness.[29]

More than 2 million people die in the United States each year. Although most are older, death occurs in all age groups. The causes of death vary with both age and gender. Among those under age 35, intentional and nonintentional injury is the primary cause of death. (See Student Snapshot: "Dying Young.") Among older Americans, cancer and heart disease are the top killers. Men typically die at a younger age than women. (See The X&YFiles: "Why Do Women Live Longer Than Men?" on page 386.)

## Defining Death

In our society, death isn't a part of everyday life, as it once was. Because machines can now keep people alive who, in the past, would have died, the definition of death has become more complex. Death has been broken down into the following categories:

✔ **Functional death.** The end of all vital functions, such as heartbeat and respiration.
✔ **Cellular death.** The gradual death of body cells after the heart stops beating. If placed in a tissue culture or, as is the case with various organs, transplanted to another body, some cells can remain alive indefinitely.
✔ **Cardiac death.** The moment when the heart stops beating.

## Student Snapshot ⟩ Dying Young

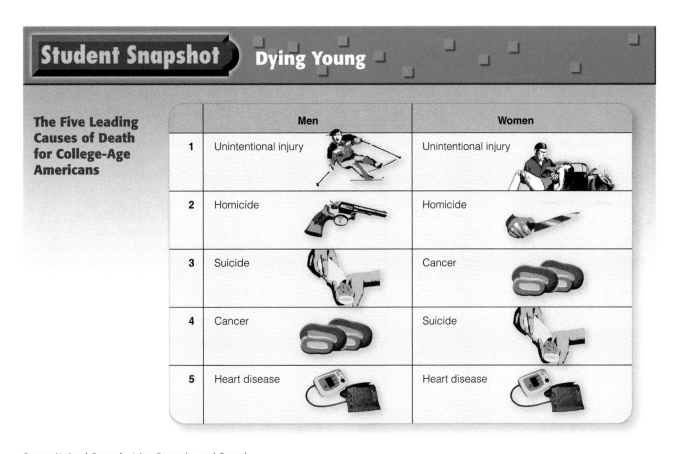

**The Five Leading Causes of Death for College-Age Americans**

| | Men | Women |
|---|---|---|
| 1 | Unintentional injury | Unintentional injury |
| 2 | Homicide | Homicide |
| 3 | Suicide | Cancer |
| 4 | Cancer | Suicide |
| 5 | Heart disease | Heart disease |

Source: National Center for Injury Prevention and Control.

✔ **Brain death.** The end of all brain activity, indicated by an absence of electrical activity (confirmed by an electroencephalogram, or EEG) and a lack of reflexes. The notion of brain death is bound up with what we consider to be the actual person, or self. The destruction of a person's brain means that his or her personality no longer exists; the lower brain centers controlling respiration and circulation no longer function.

✔ **Spiritual death.** The moment when the soul, as defined by many religions, leaves the body.

## Denying Death

Most of us don't quite believe that we're going to die. A reasonable amount of denial helps us focus on the day-to-day realities of living. However, excessive denial can be life-threatening. Some drivers, for instance, refuse to buckle their seat belts because they refuse to acknowledge that a drunk driver might collide with them. Similarly, cigarette smokers deny that lung cancer will ever strike them, and people who eat high-fat meals deny that they'll ever suffer a heart attack.

One important factor in denial is the nature of the threat. It's easy to believe that death is at hand when someone's pointing a gun at you; it's much harder to think that cigarette smoking might cause your death 20 or 30 years down the road. Elisabeth Kübler-Ross, a psychiatrist who has extensively studied the process of dying, describes the downside of denying death in *Death: The Final Stage of Growth.*

> It is the denial of death that is partially responsible for people living empty, purposeless lives; for when you live as if you'll live forever, it becomes too easy to postpone the things you know that you must do. You live your life in preparation for tomorrow or in the remembrance of yesterday—and meanwhile, each today is lost. In contrast, when you fully understand that each day you awaken could be the last you have, you take the time that day to grow, to become more of who you really are, to reach out to other human beings.[30]

## Emotional Responses to Dying

Elisabeth Kübler-Ross has identified five typical stages of reaction that a person goes through when facing death (see Figure 15-5).

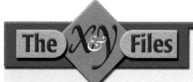

## The X & Y Files          Why Do Women Live Longer Than Men?

The gender gap in longevity has been shrinking since 1990. According to the National Center for Health Statistics, life expectancy for American women now stands at 79.5 years; for men, it is a record high of 74.1 years. Women in other developed nations—Australia, Canada, France, Greece, Italy, Japan, Netherlands, Norway, Spain, Sweden, Switzerland—live up to two years longer than those in the United States and about seven years longer than men. In the former Soviet Union, life expectancy for females is thirteen years longer than for males. By the year 2020, according to current projections for the United States, the average woman's life may increase by ten years, the average man's by six.

The gender difference in mortality rates emerges from the moment of conception. Baby girls are less likely to die in the womb or after delivery than baby boys. Once past age 30, women consistently outnumber and outlive men. By age 85, there are three women for every man.

Why do men die sooner? The female edge may begin at conception with the extra X chromosome, which provides a backup for defects on the X gene and a double dose of the genetic factors that regulate the immune system. In addition, the female hormone estrogen bolsters immunity and protects heart, bone, brain, and blood vessels.

In some cancers, estrogen may somehow protect against distant metastases. In contrast, testosterone may dampen the immune response in males—possibly to prevent attacks on sperm cells that might otherwise be mistaken as alien invaders. When the testes are removed from mice and guinea pigs, their immune systems become more active. In men, lessened immunity may lower resistance to cancer as well as infectious disease. Half of all men—compared with a third of women—develop cancer. Smoking, which for a long time was much more prevalent among men, accounts for some of this difference. However, this is changing; 23 percent of American women smoke, and lung cancer rates in women have doubled since the early 1970s.

Testosterone also has been implicated in men's risk of heat disease and stroke. Originally designed to equip men with an instantaneous burst of power—essential for survival in Stone Age times—this potent male hormone may surge so intensely that it wreaks havoc throughout the cardiovascular system.

Males also die more often as a result of intentional and nonintentional injury. Overall, men are three times more likely than women to die in accidents, mainly in cars and on the job. Men also are four times more likely to die violently. Nine in ten murderers and eight in ten murder victims are men.

---

1. *Denial ("No, not me").* At first knowledge that death is coming, a terminally ill patient rejects the news. The denial overcomes the initial shock and allows the person to begin to gather together his or her resources. Denial, at this point, is a healthy defense mechanism. It can become distressful, however, if it's reinforced by the relatives and friends of the dying patient.

2. *Anger ("Why me?").* In the second stage, the dying person begins to feel resentment and rage regarding imminent death. The anger may be directed at God or at the patient's family and caregivers, who can do little but try to endure any expressions of anger, provide comfort, and help the patient on to the next stage.

3. *Bargaining ("Yes, me, but . . .").* In this stage, a patient may try to bargain, usually with God, for a way to reverse, or at least postpone, dying. The patient may promise, in exchange for recovery, to do good works or to see family members more often. Alternatively, the patient may say, "Let me live long enough to see my grandchild born" or "to see the spring again."

4. *Depression ("Yes, it's me").* In the fourth stage, the patient gradually realizes the full consequences of his or her condition. This may begin as grieving for health that has been lost and then become anticipa-

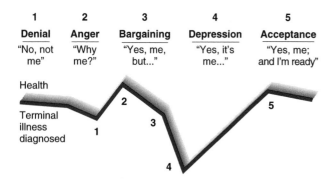

▲ **Figure 15-5** Kübler-Ross's Five Stages of Adjustment to Death

tory grieving for the loss that is to come of friends, loved ones, and life itself. This stage is perhaps the most difficult: The dying person should not be left alone during this period. Neither should loved ones try to cheer up the patient, who must be allowed to grieve.

5. *Acceptance ("Yes, me; and I'm ready").* In this last stage, the person has accepted the reality of death: The moment looms as neither frightening nor painful, neither sad nor happy—only inevitable. The person who waits for the end of life may ask to see fewer visitors, to separate from other people, or perhaps to turn to just one person for support.

Several stages may occur at the same time and some may happen out of sequence. Each stage may take days or only hours or minutes. Throughout, denial may come back to assert itself unexpectedly, and hope for a medical breakthrough or a miraculous recovery is forever present.

Some experts dispute Kübler-Ross's basic five-stage theory as too simplistic and argue that not all people go through such well-defined stages in the dying process. The way a person faces death is often a mirror of the way he or she has faced other major stresses in life: Those who have had the most trouble adjusting to other crises will have the most trouble adjusting to the news of their impending death.

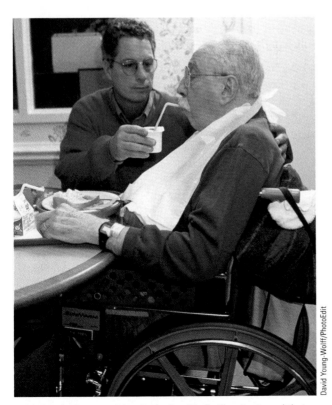

▲ Humanitarian caregiving for both critically ill patients and their loved ones can help to take some of the fear out of death.

An individual's will to live can postpone death for a while. In a study of elderly Chinese women, researchers found that their death rate decreased before and during a holiday during which the senior women in a household play a central role; it increased after the celebration. A similar temporary drop occurs among Jews at the time of Passover. However, different events may have different effects. The prospect of an upcoming birthday postpones death in women but hastens it in men. The will to live typically fluctuates in terminal patients, varying along with depression, anxiety, shortness of breath, and a sense of well-being.[31]

The family of a dying person experiences a spectrum of often wrenching emotions. Family members, too, may deny the verdict of death, rage at the doctors and nurses who can't do more to save their loved one, bargain with God to give up their own health if necessary, sink into helplessness and depression, and finally accept the reality of their anticipated loss.

## Preparing for Death

Throughout this book we have stressed the ways in which you can determine how well and how long you live. You can also make decisions about the end of your life, particularly its impact on other people. To clarify your thinking on this difficult subject, ask yourself the following questions:

✔ Would I prefer to receive or refuse any specific treatments if I were unconscious or incapable of voicing my opinion?
✔ Would I like my bodily systems to be kept functioning by extraordinary life-sustaining measures, even though my natural systems had failed? If I could not survive without mechanical assistance, would I want to be kept alive or resuscitated if my heart were to stop?
✔ Would I like the state to decide how to distribute my property or would I rather name the recipients of my estate?
✔ Would I like to decide how to handle my funeral arrangements?

You can assure that your wishes are heeded by several means, including advance directives, such as a health-care proxy and a living will, and a holographic will.

### ???? What Are Advance Directives?

Every state and the District of Columbia have laws authorizing the use of **advance directives** to specify the kind of medical treatment individuals want in case of a medical crisis. However, few Americans have any type of advance directive. These documents are important because, without clear indications of a person's preferences, hospitals and other institutions often make decisions on an individual's behalf, particularly if family members are not available or disagree. Advance directives also help physicians, who often do not feel comfortable making these kinds of decisions about life-extending treatments for their terminally ill patients.[32]

According to the Patient Self-Determination Act, health-care facilities that receive Medicare or Medicaid reimbursements must advise patients of their right to sign advance directives for health-care decisions, including whether they want to be kept alive by artificial means. These statements allow medical professionals to know and follow an individual's wishes, or the wishes of a person to whom the patient has given authority to make decisions on his or her behalf. Figure 15-6 shows what you can include in an advance directive and the possible limitations on it because of differing state laws. Although the idea of advance directives is popular among patients and physicians, they are rarely discussed. In one study of patients who were either seriously ill or over age 70, only 2 percent had discussed advance directives with their doctors.[33]

A *health-care proxy* is an advance directive that gives someone else the power to make decisions on your behalf. (Figure 15-7 on page 390 shows the Medical Power of Attorney form for Texas.) People typically name a relative or close friend as their agent. Let family and friends know your thoughts about treatments and life support. You also should let your primary physician know about the type of care you would or wouldn't want to receive in various circumstances, such as an accident that results in an irreversible coma, but you should not designate your doctor as your agent. Many states prohibit this. Even when allowed, it is not a good idea because your doctor's primary responsibility is to administer care.

You can also sign an advance directive specifying that you want to be allowed to die naturally—you do not want to be resuscitated in case your heart stops beating. **Do-not-resuscitate (DNR)** orders apply mainly to hospitalized, terminally ill patients. However, in some states, it is possible to complete a *nonhospital DNR* form that specifies an individual's wish not to be resuscitated at home. Patients in the final stages of advanced cancer or AIDS may choose to use such forms to protect their rights in case paramedics are called to their home.

### ???? What Is a Living Will?

A **living will** isn't just for people who don't want to be kept alive by artificial means. Individuals can also use these advance directives to indicate that they want all pos-

sible medical treatments and technology used to prolong their lives. Most states recognize living wills as legally binding, and a growing number of health-care professionals and facilities offer patients help in drafting living wills. You can obtain state-specific forms for living wills and health-care proxies free from Partnership for Caring (www.partnershipforcaring.org, 1-800-989-WILL). Computer software for preparing such documents is also available.

Once the forms are completed, make copies of your living will and other advance directives, and give them to anyone who might have input in decisions on your behalf. Also give copies to your physician or health-care organization, and ask that they be made part of your medical record.

## Holographic Will

Perhaps you think that only wealthy or older people need to write wills. However, if you're married, have children, or own property, you should either hire a lawyer to draw up a will or write a **holographic will** yourself, specifying who you wish to raise your children and who should have your property. If you die *intestate* (without a will), the state will make these decisions for you. Even a modest estate can be tied up in court for a long period of time, depriving family members of money when they need it most.

Many states will recognize a handwritten (not typed) statement by you, through which you can accomplish the following:

✔ Name a family member or friend as the executor, the person who sees that your wishes are carried out.
✔ List the things you own and to whom you want them to go; include addresses and telephone numbers, if possible.
✔ Select a guardian for your children (if any), presumably someone whose ideas about raising children are similar to your own. Be sure that any named guardians are willing and able to accept this responsibility before writing them into your will.
✔ Specify any funeral arrangements.

Be sure to keep the will in a safe place, where your executor, family members, or closest beneficiary can find it quickly and easily; tell them where it is.

## Suicide

Suicide is among the ten leading causes of death in the United States; each year 25,000 to 55,000 people kill themselves. And for every completed suicide, there are 10 to 40

Except in California, where they must be renewed every five years, living wills are effective until they're revoked. Still, it's considered a good idea to initial and date your living will every few years to show that it still expresses your wishes.

"Imminent" is used on many living wills to express the inevitability and timing of death, but it's open to varying interpretations. A recent Virgina court found that it doesn't necessarily mean "immediately, at once, within a few days," and that a comatose person who's within a few months of death falls within the definition.

Except in California, Idaho, and Oregon, living wills have a space to specify treatment you do or don't want. Ask your physician what to include here. You can:

• Ask for or prohibit use of artificial feeding tubes, cardiopulmonary resuscitation, antibiotics, dialysis, and respirators.

• Ask for pain medication to keep you comfortable.

• State whether you would prefer to die in the hospital or at home.

• Designate a proxy—someone to make decisions about your treatment when you're unable.

• Donate organs or other body parts.

If your directions are contrary to state law, they'll be ignored, but the rest of the directive will remain in force.

## DIRECTIVE TO PHYSICIANS

Directive made this _____ day of _____ (month, year). I, _____ being of sound mind, willfully and voluntarily make known my desire that my life shall not be artificially prolonged under the circumstances set forth below, and do hereby declare:

If at any time I should have an incurable condition caused by injury, disease, or illness certified to be a terminal condition by two physicians, and where the application of life-sustaining procedures would serve only to artificially prolong the moment of death and where my attending physician determines that my death is imminent whether or not life-sustaining procedures are utilized, I direct that such procedures be withheld or withdrawn, and that I be permitted to die naturally.

In the absence of my ability to give directions regarding the use of such life-sustaining procedures, it is my intention that this directive shall be honored by my family and physicians as the final expression of my legal right to refuse medical or surgical treatment and accept the consequences from such refusal.

If I have been diagnosed as pregnant and that diagnosis is known to my physician, this directive shall have no force or effect during the course of my pregnancy.

Other directions:
This directive shall be in effect until it is revoked. I understand the full import of this directive, and I am emotionally and mentally competent to make this directive. I understand that I may revoke this directive at any time.

Signed _____

City, County, and State of Residence _____

The declarant has been personally known to me and I believe him/her to be of sound mind. I am not related to the declarant by blood or marriage, nor would I be entitled to any portion of the declarant's estate on his/her decease, nor am I the attending physician of the declarant or an employee of the attending physician or a health facility in which the declarant is a patient, or a patient in the health care facility in which the declarant is a patient, or any person who has a claim against any portion of the estate of the declarant upon his/her decease.

Witness _____ Witness _____

"Life-sustaining procedures" are those that only prolong the process of dying. Most states include feeding and hydration tubes in this definition.

In some states a physician who will not carry out a patient's wishes must make a "good faith effort" to locate a doctor who will. Other states require the physician to actually find someone and specify penalties—in some cases, jail terms—for failure to do so.

In some states the living will is valid for pregnant women. Others exclude women during all or part of their pregnancy, although that has been challenged on the grounds that a woman's right to privacy doesn't end when she becomes pregnant.

You can revoke or amend your living will at any time simply by making a statement to a physician, nurse, or other health-care worker.

Several states provide for the appointment of a proxy. In others decisions may be delegated through a document called a Durable Power of Attorney.

In some states, your signature must be notarized. Elsewhere, the signature of the witnesses is adequate; if you're in a hospital or nursing home in some states you may need as an additional witness the chief of staff or medical director.

▲ **Figure 15-6** Preparing a Physician's Directive

Source: "A Guide to the Living Will," *Hippocrates* (May–June, 1988).

TEXAS MEDICAL POWER OF ATTORNEY — PAGE 1

## TEXAS MEDICAL POWER OF ATTORNEY

**INSTRUCTIONS**

**DESIGNATION OF HEALTH CARE AGENT.**

**PRINT YOUR NAME**
I, _____, appoint:
*(name)*

**PRINT THE NAME, ADDRESS AND HOME AND WORK TELEPHONE NUMBERS OF YOUR AGENT**

_____
*(name of agent)*

_____
*(address)*

_____
*(work telephone number)*     *(home telephone number)*

as my agent to make any and all health care decisions for me, except to the extent I state otherwise in this document. This medical power of attorney takes effect if I become unable to make my own health care decisions and this fact is certified in writing by my physician.

**STATE LIMITATIONS ON YOUR AGENT'S POWER (IF ANY)**

**LIMITATIONS ON THE DECISION MAKING AUTHORITY OF MY AGENT ARE AS FOLLOWS.**

---

TEXAS MEDICAL POWER OF ATTORNEY — PAGE 2

**PRINT THE NAME, ADDRESS AND HOME AND WORK TELEPHONE NUMBERS OF YOUR FIRST AND SECOND ALTERNATE AGENTS**

**DESIGNATION OF ALTERNATE AGENT.**
(You are not required to designate an alternate agent but you may do so. An alternate agent may make the same health care decisions as the designated agent if the designated agent is unable or unwilling to act as your agent. If the agent designated is your spouse, the designation is automatically revoked by law if your marriage is dissolved.)

If the person designated as my agent is unable or unwilling to make health care decisions for me, I designate the following persons to serve as my agent to make health care decisions for me as authorized by this document, who serve in the following order:

**FIRST ALTERNATE**
A. First Alternate Agent

_____
*(name of first alternate agent)*

_____
*(home address)*

_____
*(work telephone number)*     *(home telephone number)*

**SECOND ALTERNATE**
B. Second Alternate Agent

_____
*(name of second alternate agent)*

_____
*(home address)*

_____
*(work telephone number)*     *(home telephone number)*

**LOCATION OF ORIGINAL**
The original of this document is kept at: _____

---

TEXAS MEDICAL POWER OF ATTORNEY — PAGE 3

**LOCATION OF COPIES**
The following individuals or institutions have signed copies:

Name: _____

Address: _____

Name: _____

Address: _____

**DURATION.**
I understand that this power of attorney exists indefinitely from the date I execute this document unless I establish a shorter time or revoke the power of attorney. If I am unable to make health care decisions for myself when this power of attorney expires, the authority I have granted my agent continues to exist until the time I become able to make health care decisions for myself.

**EXPIRATION DATE (IF ANY)**
(IF APPLICABLE) This power of attorney ends on the following date:

_____

**PRIOR DESIGNATIONS REVOKED.**
I revoke any prior medical power of attorney.

**ACKNOWLEDGMENT OF DISCLOSURE STATEMENT.**
I have been provided with a disclosure statement explaining the effect of this document. I have read and understood that information contained in the disclosure statement.

(YOU MUST DATE AND SIGN THIS POWER OF ATTORNEY)

**PRINT THE DATE**
I sign my name to this medical power of attorney on _____
*(date)*

**PRINT YOUR LOCATION**
day of _____, at _____
*(month)*  *(year)*     *(city and state)*

**SIGN THE DOCUMENT**

_____
*(signature)*

**PRINT YOUR NAME**

_____
*(print name)*

© 2000
PARTNERSHIP FOR CARING, INC.

---

TEXAS MEDICAL POWER OF ATTORNEY — PAGE 4

**STATEMENT OF FIRST WITNESS.**
I am not the person appointed as agent by this document. I am not related to the principal by blood or marriage. I would not be entitled to any portion of the principal's estate on the principal's death. I am not the attending physician of the principal or an employee of the attending physician. I have no claim against any portion of the principal's estate on the principal's death. Furthermore, if I am an employee of a health care facility in which the principal is a patient, I am not involved in providing direct patient care to the principal and am not an officer, director, partner or business office employee of the health care facility of any parent organization of the health care facility.

Signature: _____

Print Name: _____ Date: _____

Address: _____

**SIGNATURE OF SECOND WITNESS**

Witness Signature: _____

Print Name: _____ Date: _____

Address: _____

© 2000
PARTNERSHIP FOR CARING, INC.

Courtesy of Partnership for Caring, Inc.      9/99
1620 Eye Street, NW, Suite 202, Washington, DC 20006 800-989-9455

▲ **Figure 15-7** Health-Care Proxy
A medical power of attorney is another advance directive. This example is from the state of Texas.

Source: Reprinted by permission of Partnership for Caring, Inc. Washington, DC 20006. 1-800-989-9455.

unsuccessful attempts. (Chapter 3 presents a detailed discussion of the risk factors and warning signs of suicide.)

One of the main factors leading to suicide is illness, especially terminal illness. A great deal of debate centers on quality of life, yet there is no reliable or consistent way to measure this. Patients who are dying may feel some quality of life, even when others do not recognize it, or their evaluations of the quality of their lives may fluctuate. Dying patients who say their lives are not worth living may be suffering from depression; hopelessness is one of its characteristic symptoms.[34]

Approximately three-fourths of those who commit suicide consult a physician, most with medical complaints, within the six-month period prior to their deaths. Disease, medication, and the fear of pain or of being a burden to one's family can breed depression; treatment can make a difference. Only 10 to 14 percent of those who survive a suicide attempt to take their lives in the next ten years. Fatally ill individuals who talk about suicide should be taken seriously; family physicians can arrange for them to talk with a psychotherapist.

## "Rational" Suicide

An elderly widow suffering from advanced cancer takes a lethal overdose of sleeping pills. A young man with several AIDS-related illnesses shoots himself. A woman in her fifties, diagnosed with Alzheimer's disease, asks a doctor to help her end her life. Are these suicides "rational" because these individuals used logical reasoning in deciding to end their lives?

The question is intensely controversial. Advocates of the right to self-deliverance argue that individuals in great pain or faced with the prospect of a debilitating, hopeless battle against an incurable disease can and should be able to decide to end their lives. As legislatures and the legal system tackle the thorny issue of an individual's right to die, mental health professionals worry that suicidal wishes, even in those with fatal diseases, often stem from undiagnosed depression.

In one classic study of 44 terminally ill individuals, 34 had never been suicidal or wished for death. The remaining ten (seven who did desire early death and three who specifically considered suicide) all had severe depression. Their despair and preoccupation with dying may have contributed to their willingness to consider suicide. Numerous studies have indicated that most patients with painful, progressive, or terminal illnesses do not want to kill themselves. The percentage of those who report thinking about suicide ranges from 5 to 20 percent, and most of these have major depressions. Many mental health professionals argue that what makes patients with severe illnesses suicidal is depression, not their physical condition.

Because depression may indeed warp the ability to make a rational decision about suicide, mental health professionals urge physicians and family members to make sure individuals with chronic or fatal illnesses are evaluated for depression and treated with medication, psychotherapy, or both. It is also important for everyone to allow enough time—an average of three to eight weeks—to see if treatment for depression will make a difference in their desire to keep living.

## Practicalities of Death

At a time of great emotional pain, grieving family members of a deceased loved one must cope with medical, legal, and practical concerns, including obtaining a medical certificate of the cause of death, registering the death, and making funeral arrangements. They may also want to arrange

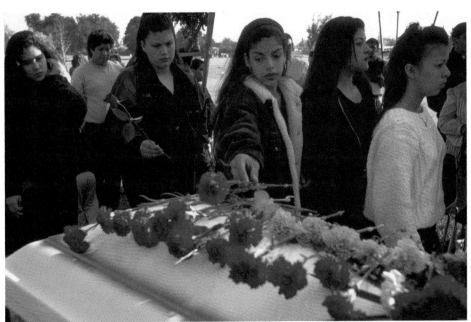

▲ Funerals and memorial services allow those in mourning to honor the deceased and to come to terms with their loss.

for organ donations and, in some circumstances, an autopsy.

A body can be either buried or cremated. Burial requires the purchase of a cemetery plot, which many families do decades before death. A burial is typically the third most expensive purchase of a lifetime, behind the cost of a house and car. The average national costs range as high as $6,000, although they vary considerably. Memorial societies are voluntary groups that help people plan in advance for death. They obtain services at moderate cost, keep the arrangements simple and dignified, and—most important, perhaps—ease the emotional and financial burden on the rest of the family when death finally does come.

If the body is to be cremated, you must comply with some additional formalities, with which the funeral director can help you. After a *cremation* (incineration of the remains), you can either collect the ashes to keep, bury, or scatter yourself, or ask the crematorium to dispose of them.

The tradition of a funeral may help survivors come to terms with the death, enabling them to mourn their loss and to celebrate the dead person's life. Funerals are usually held two to four days after the death. Many have two parts: a religious ceremony at a church or funeral home, and a burial ceremony at the grave site.

Alternatively, the body may be disposed of immediately, through burial, cremation, or bequeathal to a medical school, and a memorial service held later. In a memorial service, the body is not present, which may change the focus of the service from the person's death to his or her life.

## Grief

An estimated 8 million Americans lose a member of their immediate family each year. The death of a loved one may be the single most upsetting and feared event in a person's life.

Losing a parent in childhood can have a lasting impact. A study that followed 100 orphans found that as young adults they suffered significantly higher depressive symptoms.[35] The death of a family member produces a wide range of reactions, including anxiety, guilt, anger, and financial concern. Many may see the death of an old person as less tragic than the death of a child or young person. A sudden death is more of a shock than one following a long illness. A suicide can be particularly devastating, because family members may wonder whether they could have done anything to prevent it. The cause of

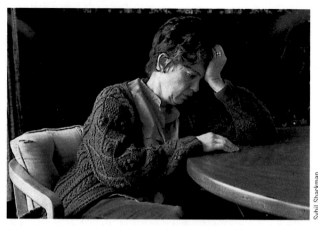

▲ Grief can take an enormous physical and psychological toll on the deceased's family members and loved ones.

death can also affect the reactions of friends and acquaintances. Some people express less sympathy and support when individuals are murdered or take their own lives.

Encountering death can make us feel alone and vulnerable. The most common and one of the most painful experiences is the death of a parent. When both parents die, individuals may feel like orphaned children. They mourn not just for the father and mother who are gone, but also for their lost role of being someone's child.

The death of a child can be even more devastating. Grieving may continue for many years. Eventually parents may be able to resolve their grief and accept the death as "God's will" or as "something that happens." Time erases their pain and they feel a desire to get on with their lives, consciously putting the loss behind them. Others deal with their grief by keeping busy, or by substituting other problems or situations to take their minds off their loss. Yet many parents who lose a child continue to grieve for many years. Although the pain of their loss diminishes with time, they view it as part of themselves and describe an emptiness inside—even though most have rich, meaningful, and happy daily lives.

The loss of a mate can also have a profound impact, although men's and women's responses to the death—and their subsequent health risks—may depend on how their spouses died. Men whose wives die suddenly face a much greater risk of dying themselves than those whose wives die after a long illness. On the other hand, women whose husbands die after a long illness face greater risk of dying than other widows. The reason may be that men whose wives were chronically ill learned how to cope with the loss of their nurturers, while women who spend a long time caring for an ill husband may be at greater risk because of the combined burdens of caregiving and loss of financial support.

Bereavement is not a rare occurrence on college campuses, but it is largely an ignored problem. Counselors have called upon universities to help students who have lost a loved one through initiatives such as training nonbereaved students to provide peer support and raising consciousness about bereavement.[36]

## Grief's Effect on Health

Men and women who lose partners, parents, or children endure so much stress that they're at increased risk of serious physical and mental illness, and even of premature death. Studies of the health effects of grief have found the following:

✔ Grief produces changes in the respiratory, hormonal, and central nervous systems, and may affect functions of the heart, blood, and immune systems.

✔ Grieving adults may experience mood swings between sadness and anger, guilt and anxiety. They may feel physically sick, lose their appetite, sleep poorly, or fear that they're going crazy because they "see" the deceased person in different places.

✔ Friendships and remarriage offer the greatest protection against health problems.

✔ Some widows may have increased rates of depression, suicide, and death from cirrhosis of the liver. The greatest risk factors are poor previous mental and physical health and a lack of social support.

✔ Grieving parents, partners, and adult children are at increased risk of serious physical and mental illness, suicide, and premature death.

## Methods of Mourning

Grief is a psychological necessity, not self-indulgence. Psychotherapists refer to grief as work, and it is—slow, tedious, and painful. Yet only by working through grief—dealing with feelings of anger and despair, and adjusting emotionally and intellectually to the loss—can bereaved individuals make their way back to the living world of hope and love.

Some widows and widowers move through the grieving process without experiencing extreme distress. Others stop somewhere in the midst of normal grieving and continue to pine for the deceased, become overly reliant on others, or show signs of denial, avoidance, or

anxiety. Individuals who lose children or spouses in car accidents are particularly likely to remain depressed and anxious years later. One of the most devastating losses is the death of a child killed by a drunk driver. Many years afterward parents often cannot find any meaning in what happened.

## ???? How Can You Help Survivors of a Loss?

Although we grieve for the dead, the living are the ones who need our help. Bereavement is such an intense state that survivors may be too numb or too stunned to ask for help. Family and friends must take the initiative and spend time with those who are mourning the loss of a loved one, even if that means sitting together silently. Offer empathy and support, and let the grieving person know with verbal and nonverbal expressions that you care and wish to help. Simply being there is enough to let your friend know you care.

You may also wish to write a simple note expressing your sympathy. "I want to let you know I'm thinking of you and praying for you" can mean a great deal. A small gift, such as a book or plant, is also thoughtful. Or you can invite your friend to do something with you. Choose something you know your friend might enjoy—a walk in the country or a concert. And don't just give your help over the first few days or weeks and then withdraw. Grieving people continue to need support for many months. The first anniversary of a death or the first holiday spent alone can be particularly difficult.

Most bereaved people don't need professional psychological counseling. In most instances, sharing their feelings with friends is all that's needed. However, you should urge a friend or relative to seek help if he or she shows no sign of grieving, or exhibits as much distress a year after the loss as during the first months. The family members of a suicide victim are those most likely to need, and benefit from, professional help in sorting out their feelings of failure, anger, and sorrow. Therapy and medication can be enormously helpful—and potentially life-saving.

 What are the stages of emotional response to dying?

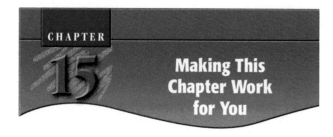

**CHAPTER**

**15**

**Making This Chapter Work for You**

1. Factors that contribute to a long life and successful aging include all of the following except
   a. healthy weight.
   b. moderate smoking.
   c. regular exercise.
   d. social involvement.

2. Physically fit people over age 60
   a. have lower risk of dying from chronic heart disease.
   b. can regain the fitness level of a 25-year-old.
   c. show no difference in levels of anxiety and depression.
   d. have higher body-fat percentages.

3 Which statement about the aging brain is false?
   a. When brain cells die, surrounding cells can fill the gaps to maintain cognitive function.
   b. Remembering names and recalling information may take longer.
   c. "Use it or lose it."
   d. Mental ability and physically ability both decline with age.

4. Which statement about aging is false?
   a. People over age 70 who take vitamin supplements showed improvement in short-term memory and problem-solving ability.
   b. Fitness and frequency of sexual activity are linked.
   c. Hormone replacement therapy reduces the risk of heart disease in menopausal women.
   d. Seniors who take up new hobbies late in life may slow aging within the brain.

5. Which statement about age-related problems is correct?
   a. Osteoporosis affects only women.
   b. Alzheimer's disease is a form of dementia.
   c. Depression is no more prevalent in the older population.
   d. Drug interactions do not occur in the elderly.

6. When should concern change to intervention?
   a. Uncle Charlie is 85 and continues to drive himself to the grocery store and to the Senior Center during the daytime.
   b. Nana takes pills at breakfast, lunch, and dinner, but sometimes mixes them up.
   c. Mom's hot flashes have become a family joke.
   d. Your older brother can never remember where he put his car keys.

7. According to Elisabeth Kübler-Ross, an individual facing death goes through all of the following emotional stages except
   a. bargaining.
   b. acceptance.
   c. denial.
   d. repression.

8. The gender gap related to longevity
   a. is due to deficiencies in the Y chromosome.
   b. results from the presence of a mutant gene.
   c. may be due to the X chromosome and its hormonal influences on the immune system.
   d. is about 13 years in the United States.

9. An advance directive
   a. indicates who should have your property in the event you die.
   b. may authorize which individuals may not participate in your health care if you are unable to care for yourself.
   c. can specify your desires related to the use of medical treatments and technology to prolong your life.
   d. should specify which physician you designate to be your health-care proxy.

10. You can best help a friend who is bereaved by
    a. encouraging him to have a few drinks to forget his pain.
    b. simply spending time with her.
    c. avoiding talking about his loss because it is awkward.
    d. reminding her about all she still has in her life.

Answers to these questions can be found on page 415.

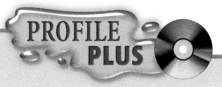

## Critical Thinking

1. How are your parents or other mentors staying fit and alert as they age? Do you think you might use similar strategies?

2. Do you think that coming to terms with mortality allows an individual to live each day to its fullest, rather than putting off what he or she would like to do until tomorrow? How does this concept affect your own life? Explain. Do you believe in a next life? How does this affect your view of life and death?

3. Have your living parents and grandparents written advanced directives or a living will? Have you discussed with them their preferences regarding treatment in the event of a medical crisis? If you haven't had this discussion with your family, how can you

begin the process of helping your parents or grandparents communicate their wishes?

4. As many as 10,000 people in this country are chronically unconscious, kept alive by artificial respirators and feeding tubes. If you were in an accident that left you in a vegetative state, would you want doctors to do everything possible to fight for your life? Would you want to spend months or even years totally unaware of your surroundings? Should health-care professionals have the right to declare that anyone is too old, too ill, or too frail to try to save? Should they have the right to insist that someone live on even if that person isn't experiencing much of a life?

## PROFILE PLUS

Life has only one inevitable conclusion. Explore your responses to death with this activity on

your Profile Plus CD-ROM:

How Do You Feel About Death?

## SITES & BYTES

### National Institute on Aging
**www.nia.nih.gov**

This governmental site features a comprehensive array of resources on aging, including publications on a variety of geriatric health topics, current news events, and a resource directory for older people.

### RealAge Interactive
**www.realage.com**

The RealAge Test on this site is an interactive health assessment survey designed to lead you toward "age-reduction benefits" that will reduce your risk of disease. After answering a series of questions, you will receive a calculated age based on your individual lifestyle as well as suggestions on how you may achieve a younger age score by adopting healthier behaviors. Included here are an encyclopedia of medical conditions and health ailments as well as interactive diet and fitness tools.

### The End of Life
**www.npr.org/programs/death**

This site, sponsored by National Public Radio, focuses on how Americans deal with death and dying. Features include transcripts of personal stories, a place where you can tell your story, and a comprehensive list of organizations that can help families who are copying with death, dying, and the diseases of old age.

Please note that links are subject to change. If you find a broken link, use a search engine such as www.yahoo.com and search for the website by typing in keywords.

### InfoTrac College Edition Activity "Dying and Preparatory Grief." *American Family Physician,* Vol. 65, No. 5, March 1, 2002, p. 897.

1. What is the first phase of the preparatory grief process?

2. During which phase do the bereaved balance the past with the future?
3. What are the signs of depression in terminally ill patients?

You can find additional readings relating to aging and death with InfoTrac College Edition, an online library of more than 900 journals and publications. Follow the instructions for accessing InfoTrac that were packaged with your textbook; then search for articles using a keyword search.

For additional links, resources, and suggested readings on InfoTrac, visit our Health & Wellness Resource Center at http://health.wadsworth.com.

## Key Terms

The terms listed here are used within the chapter on the page indicated. Definitions of the terms are in the Glossary at the end of the book.

advance directives 387
aging 375
Alzheimer's disease 381
dementia 381

do-not-resuscitate (DNR) 388
holographic will 388

hormone replacement therapy (HRT) 379
living will 388

menopause 379
osteoporosis 382
perimenopause 379

## References

1. Gardner, Jon. "Geriatric Provider Shortage Suggests Health Care Needs to Improve with Age." *Health Behavior News Service,* Center for the Advancement of Health, September 5, 2002.
2. National Institute of Aging, www.nia.nih.gov/health.
3. U.S. Census Bureau.
4. Manton, Kenneth, and XiLing, Gu. "Changes in the Prevalence of Chronic Disability in the United States Black and Nonblack Population Above Age 85 from 1982 to 1999." *Proceedings of the National Academy of Sciences of the United States,* Vol. 98, No. 11, May 22, 2001, p. 6354.
5. Roizen, Michael. Personal interview.
6. Kahana, Eva, et al. "Long-Term Impact of Preventive Proactivity on Quality of Life of the Old-Old." *Psychosomatic Medicine,* Vol. 64, May–June, 2002, p. 392.
7. Myers, Jonathan, et al. "Exercise Capacity and Mortality Among Men Referred for Exercise Testing." *New England Journal of Medicine,* Vol. 346, No. 11, March 14, 2002, p. 793.
8. Gibson, Healther. "UF Study: Healthy Aging Depends on Social As Well As Physical Activity." University of Florida News Office, January 29, 2002.
9. Andrews, Gary. "Care of Older People: Promoting Health and Function in an Aging Population." *British Medical Journal,* Vol. 322, No. 7288, March 24, 2001, p. 728.
10. Tabbarah, Melissa, et al. "The Relationship Between Cognitive and Physical Performance." *Journals of Gerontology,* Series A, Vol. 57, No. 4, April 2002, p. 228.
11. Rowe, John. Personal interview.
12. U.S. Preventive Services Task Force. *Hormone Replacement Therapy for Primary Prevention of Chronic Conditions.* Rockville, MD: Agency for Healthcare Research and Quality, 2002.
13. Hlatky, Mark, et al. "Quality-of-Life and Depressive Symptoms in Postmenopausal Women After Receiving Hormone Therapy: Results from the Heart and Estrogen/Progestin Replacement Study (HERS) Trial." *Journal of the American Medical Association,* Vol. 287, No. 5, February 6, 2002, p. 591.
14. Nelson, Heidi, et al. "Postmenopausal Hormone Replacement Therapy Scientific Review." *Journal of the American Medical Association,* Vol. 288, No. 7, August 21, 2002, p. 872.
15. Nelson, Heidi. "Assessing Benefits and Harms of Hormone Replacement Therapy." *Journal of the American Medical Association,* Vol. 288, No. 7, August 21, 2002, p. 882.
16. Bortz, Walter, et al. "Sexual Function in 1,202 Aging Males." *Journal of Gerontology,* Vol. 54, No. 5, May 1999.
17. "AARP's Modern Maturity Reveals Survey Results on Sexual Attitudes, Looks at Top Issues Affecting Relationships. American Association of Retired Persons Press Release, August 3, 1999.
18. Sato, R., et al. "A Prospective Study of Vitamin C and Cognitive Function in Older Adults." *Gerontologist,* October 15, 2000, p. 218.
19. "Modified Food Guide Pyramid for Adults Age 70+." *Geriatrics,* Vol. 56, No. 1, January 2001, p. 16.
20. Logan, Jessica, et al. "Under-Recruitment and Nonselective Recruitment: Dissociable Neural Mechanisms Associated with Aging." *Neuron,* Vol. 33, No. 5, February 28, 2002, p. 827.
21. Josefson, Deborah. "African Americans More At Risk Than Africans from Alzheimer's Disease." *British Medical Journal,* Vol. 322, No. 7286, March 10, 2001, p. 574.
22. Larkin, Marilyn. "New U.S. Guidelines for Alzheimer's Disease Released." *Lancet,* Vol. 357, May 12, 2001, p. 1505. Quality Standards Subcommittee of the American Academy of Neurology. "Early Detection of Dementia: Mild Cognitive Impairment. *Neurology.* 2001, Vol. 56, p. 1133.
23. Goldzieher, Joseph. Personal interview.
24. National Heart, Lung, and Blood Institute, www.nhlbi.nih.gov/whi/hrtupd/ep_facts.htm.

25. Thomas, Vince, and Kenneth Rockwood. "Alcohol Abuse, Cognitive Impairment, and Mortality Among Older People." *Journal of the American Geriatrics Society,* Vol. 49, No. 4, April 2001, p. 415.

26. "Even for Older Adults, It's Not Too Late to Quit." *Facts of Life: Issue Briefing for Health Reporters,* Vol. 6, No. 3, March–April 2001, p. 5.

27. "Treating Depression at Older Ages." *On the Brain,* Spring–Summer 2002, p. 5.

28. "Genetics and Longevity." *On the Brain,* Spring–Summer 2002, p. 7.

29. Vaillant, George, and Kenneth Mukamal. "Successful Aging." *American Journal of Psychiatry,* Vol. 158, No. 6, June 2001, p. 839.

30. Kübler-Ross, Elisabeth. *Death: The Final Stage of Growth.* Englewood Cliffs, NJ: Prentice Hall, 1975.

31. Carpenter, E. "The End of Life Odyssey." *Gerontologist,* October 15, 2001, p. 51.

32. Landers, Susan. "Decisions on End-of-Life Care Shouldn't Be Left to the End." *American Medical News,* September 2, 2002.

33. Tierney, William, et al. "Discussion of Advance Care Directives." *Journal of General Interest Medicine,* January 2001.

34. Farsides, Bobbie, and Robert Dunlop. "Measuring Quality of Life: Is There Such a Thing As a Life Not Worth Living?" *British Medical Journal,* Vol. 322, No. 7300, June 16, 2001, p. 1481.

35. Ifeagwazi, Chuka, et al. "The Influence of Early Parents' Death on Manifestations of Depressive Symptoms Among Young Adults." *Omega—Journal of Death and Dying,* Vol. 42, No. 2, March 2001, p. 151.

36. Balk, David. "College Student Bereavement, Scholarship, and the University." *Death Studies,* Vol. 25, No. 1, January 2001, p. 67.

# Working Toward a Healthy Environment

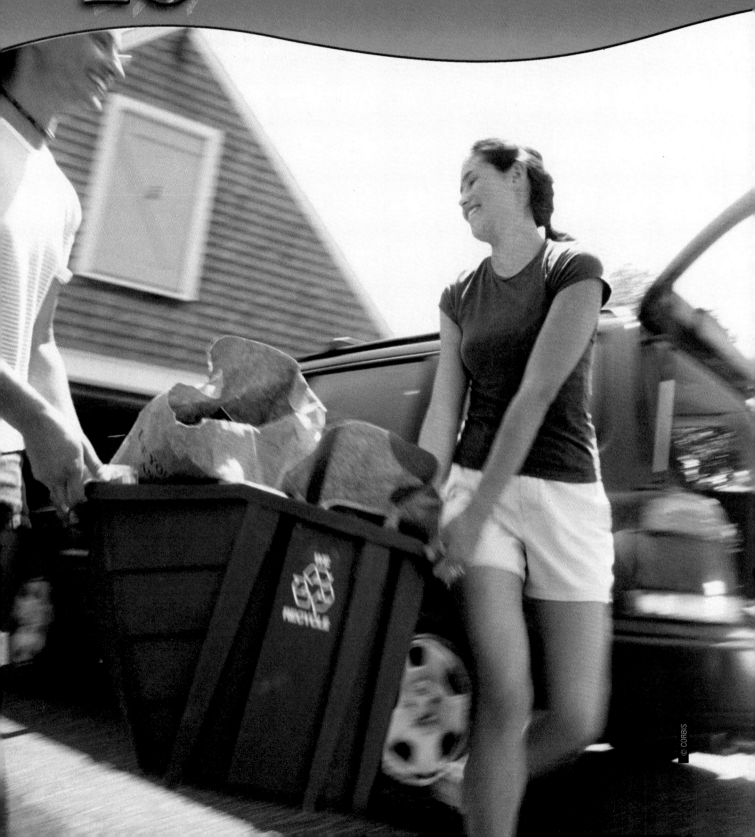

Ours is a planet in peril. A recent report by the United Nations documented increasing dangers to the planet Earth and its inhabitants. Sea levels are rising. Forests are being destroyed. Droughts in Asia and Africa have become more frequent and more intense. Despite some recent improvements, more than 3 million people die every year from the effects of air pollution while 2.2 million people die from contaminated water.[1]

No one has more stake in the future of the planet than the young. Environmental concerns may seem so enormous that nothing any individual can do will have an effect. This is not the case. All of us, as citizens of the world, can help find solutions to the challenges confronting our planet. The first step is realizing that you have a personal responsibility for safeguarding the health of your environment and, thereby, your own well-being.

This chapter explores the complex interrelationships between your world and your well-being. It discusses major threats to the environment—including atmospheric changes; air, water, and noise pollution; chemical risks; and radiation—and provides specific guidance on what you can do about them.

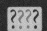

# The State of the Environment

The planet Earth—once taken for granted as a ball of rock and water that existed for our use for all time—now is seen as a single, fragile **ecosystem** (a community of organisms that share a physical and chemical environment). Our environment is a closed ecosystem, powered by the sun. The materials needed for the survival of this planet must be recycled over and over again. Increasingly, we're realizing just how important the health of this ecosystem is to our own well-being and survival. However, as shown in Student Snapshot: "Do Students Care About the Environment?" the majority of undergraduates do not share this concern.

At the beginning of the twenty-first century, environmental experts predicted new dangers to human life and health. These include acts of biological or chemical terrorism, natural disasters, contamination of water supplies, and hazardous waste disposal. One of the greatest challenges is the creation of a shared vision of a global society that is fair and equitable to all people, today and for generations to come. Making this happen will require a different type of health decision-making—one that takes into account both individual and societal risks and that may lead to recommended action, such as bans on potential toxins, before definitive scientific knowledge is available.

## Our Planet, Our Health

Our environment affects our well-being both directly and indirectly. Changes in temperature and rainfall patterns disturb ecological processes in ways that can be hazardous to health. The environment may account for 25 to 40 percent of diseases worldwide. Children are the most vulnerable because of their greater sensitivity to toxic threats.[2] In response to this trend, Congress has approved funding to create a nationwide system to track environmental links to chronic diseases.[3]

No individual is immune to environmental health threats. Depletion of the ozone layer has already been implicated in the increase in skin cancers and cataracts. Global warming, according to some theorists, might lead to changes in one-third to one-half of the world's vegetation types and to the extinction of many plant and animal species. A warmer world is expected to produce more severe flooding in some places and more severe droughts in others, jeopardizing natural resources and the safety of our water supply. Warmer weather—a consequence of changes in atmospheric gases and climate—worsens urban-industrial air pollution and, if the air also is moist, increases concentrations of allergenic pollens and fungal spores. These are truly problems without borders.

For good or for ill, we cannot separate our individual health from that of the environment in which we live. The air we breathe, the water we drink, the chemicals we use all

**Student Snapshot** — Do Students Care About the Environment?

| | |
|---|---|
| All students | 17.0% |
| Men | 17.1% |
| Women | 16.9% |
| Four-year colleges | 16.8% |
| All-black colleges | 22.5% |

*Percentage of freshmen who say that "becoming involved in programs to clean up the environment" is essential or very important.
Source: Sax, Linda, et al. *The American Freshman: National Norms for Fall 2001.* Los Angeles: Higher Education Research Institute, UCLA, 2001.

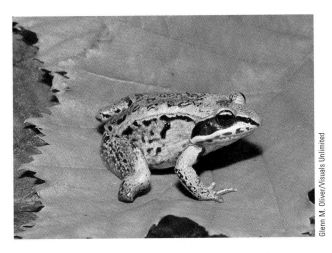

▲ Environmental factors may be to blame for a rise in the number of deformed frogs, toads, and salamanders that have been discovered in recent years.

have an impact on the quality of our lives. At the same time, the lifestyle choices we make, the products we use, the efforts we undertake to clean up a beach or save wetlands affect the quality of our environment.

## Multiple Chemical Sensitivity

The proliferation of chemicals in modern society has led to an entirely new disease, **multiple chemical sensitivity (MCS),** also called environmentally triggered illness, universal allergy, or chemical AIDS. MCS was first described almost a half century ago when a Chicago allergist treated a number of patients who reported becoming ill after being exposed to various petrochemicals. Since that time, many more cases of MCS have been reported, yet there is no agreed-upon definition for the condition, no medical test that can diagnose it, and no proven treatment.

According to medical theory, people become chemically sensitive in a two-step process: First, they experience a major exposure to a chemical, such as a pesticide, a solvent, or a combustion product. The sensitized person then begins to react to low-level chemical exposures from ordinary substances, such as perfumes and tobacco smoke. In other words, these low-level exposures trigger a physiological response. Over time, chemically unrelated substances may induce symptoms such as chest pain, depression, difficulty remembering, dizziness, fatigue, headache, inability to concentrate, nausea, and aches and pains in muscles and joints.

Individuals who may be at risk of MCS include Persian Gulf veterans, industrial workers, occupants of "sick buildings" with high levels of indoor pollutants, and people who live near contaminated sites. Because of the variety of racial, ethnic, and socioeconomic groups affected, medical professionals have become convinced that MCS is a real and serious health problem that requires investigation.[4]

## Pollution

Any change in the air, water, or soil that could reduce its ability to support life is a form of **pollution.** Natural events, such as smoke from fires triggered by lightning, can cause pollution. The effects of pollution depend on the concentration (amount per unit of air, water, or soil) of the **pollutant,** how long it remains in the environment, and its chemical nature. An *acute effect* is a severe immediate reaction, usually after a single, large exposure. For example, pesticide poisoning can cause nausea and dizziness, even death. A *chronic effect* may take years to develop or may be a recurrent or continuous reaction, usually after repeated exposures. The development of cancer after repeated exposure to a pollutant such as asbestos is an example of a chronic effect.

Environmental agents that trigger changes, or **mutations,** in the genetic material (the DNA) of living cells are called **mutagens.** The changes that result can lead to the development of cancer. A substance or agent that causes cancer is a *carcinogen:* All carcinogens are mutagens; most mutagens are carcinogens. Furthermore, when a mutagen affects an egg or a sperm cell, its effects can be passed on to future generations. Mutagens that can cross the placenta of a pregnant woman and cause a spontaneous abortion or birth defects in the fetus are called **teratogens.**

Pollution is a hazard to all who breathe. Deaths caused by air pollution exceed those from motor vehicle injuries, according to research in Austria, France, and Switzerland.[5] Those with respiratory illnesses are at greatest risk during days when smog or allergen counts are high. However, even healthy joggers are affected; carbon monoxide has been shown to impair their exercise performance. The effects of carbon monoxide are much worse in smokers, who already have higher levels of the gas in their blood.

Toxic substances in polluted air can enter the human body in three ways: through the skin, through the digestive system, and through the lungs. The combined interaction of two or more hazards can produce an effect greater than that of either one alone. Pollutants can affect an organ or organ system directly or indirectly.

Among the health problems that have been linked with pollution are the following:

- ✔ Headaches and dizziness.
- ✔ Eye irritation and impaired vision.
- ✔ Nasal discharge.
- ✔ Cough, shortness of breath, and sore throat.
- ✔ Constricted airways.
- ✔ Constriction of blood vessels and increased risk of heart disease.[6]

✔ Chest pains and aggravation of the symptoms of colds, pneumonia, bronchial asthma, emphysema, chronic bronchitis, lung cancer, and other respiratory problems.

✔ Birth defects and reproductive problems.

✔ Nausea, vomiting, and stomach cancer.

## ???? What Is Global Warming?

In the last century Earth's average surface temperature has risen by an estimated 0.6 to 1.2 degrees Fahrenheit.[7] (See Figure 16-1.) More of the warming has occurred over land than over water, more at night than during the day, and more in winter than in summer. No one can predict exactly the effects of a continuing temperature rise, but some experts have predicted severe drought and a rise in ocean levels of 2 to 20 feet—conditions that will affect everyone on Earth. Ways to prevent these consequences include increasing the globe's tree cover (which accelerates carbon dioxide removal) and reducing fossil fuel combustion.[8]

Why is our planet getting warmer? Scientists and policy makers have been heatedly debating this question for years. Global warming may have many causes, including natural processes like volcanic activity, solar radiation, and human activities that have resulted in atmospheric changes. (See Figure 16-2.) Some scientists argue that the mean surface temperatures of the last 100 years are not unusual, but the extremely rapid warming in the last 15 years cannot be explained by natural forces alone.[9]

For the last ten years, world leaders have been focusing on global warming and its potential consequences. In 2001, 165 countries—not including the United States—signed the first international treaty to fight global warming by implementing the rules known as the Kyoto Protocol. The treaty calls on about 40 industrialized nations to limit carbon emissions or reduce them to levels below those of 1990. The United States rejected the accord as harmful to the U.S. economy and unfair because it excused heavily polluting nations, such as India and China, from any obligation.[10]

## ???? What Can I Do to Protect the Planet?

By the choices you make and the actions you take, you can improve the state of the world. (See Savvy Consumer: "Save Energy, Save Money, Save the Planet" on p. 404.) No one expects you to sacrifice every comfort or spend great amounts of money. However, for almost everyone, there's plenty of room for improvement. If enough people make small individual changes, they can have an enormous impact.

One basic environmental action is **precycling:** buying products packaged in recycled materials. According to Earthworks, a consumer group, packaging makes up a third of what people in the United States throw away. When you precycle, you consider how you're going to dispose of a product and the packaging materials before purchasing it. For example, you might choose eggs in recyclable cardboard packages rather than in plastic cartons, and look for juice and milk in refillable bottles.

**Recycling**—collecting, reprocessing, marketing, and using materials once considered trash—has become a necessity for several reasons: We've run out of space for all the garbage we produce; waste sites are often health

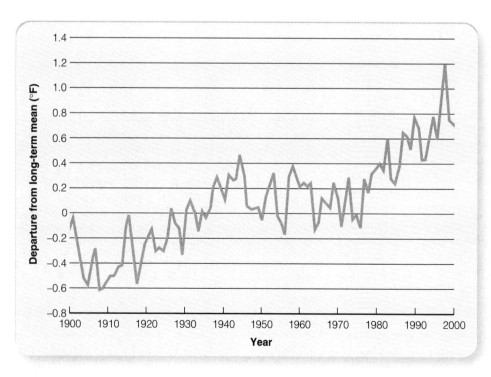

▲ **Figure 16-1** Global Temperature Changes in the Twentieth Century
Source: National Climatic Data Center, 2000 (www.epa.gov/globalwarming/climate/index.html).

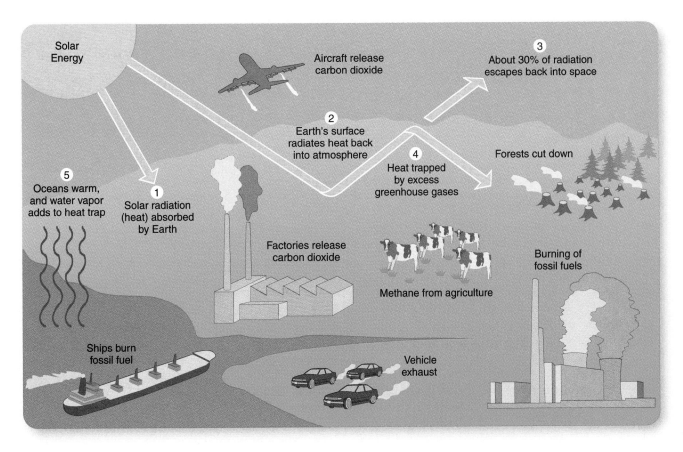

▲ **Figure 16-2** Why the World is Heating Up
The buildup of carbon dioxide and other greenhouse gases in the atmosphere could result in
the greatest climate change in human history. A combination of factors, including the burning of
fossil fuels and deforestation, is causing the atmosphere to retain heat. Scientists estimate that
the world will become hotter within a hundred years—the hottest it's been in 2 million years.

and safety hazards; recycling is cheaper than landfill storage
or incineration (a major source of air pollution); and recycling helps save energy and natural resources. Different
communities take different approaches to recycling. Many
provide regular curbside pickup of recyclables, which is so
convenient that a majority of those eligible for such services
participate. Most programs pick up bottles, cans, and newspapers—either separated or mixed together. Other communities have drop-off centers where consumers can leave
recyclables. Conveniently located and sponsored by community organizations (such as charities or schools), these
centers accept beverage containers, newspapers, cardboard,
metals, and other items.

Buyback centers, usually run by private companies,
pay for recyclables. Many centers specialize in aluminum
cans, which offer the most profit. Some operate in supermarket parking lots; other centers have regular hours and
staff members who carefully weigh and evaluate recyclables. In some places, reverse vending machines accept
returned beverage containers and provide deposit
refunds, in the form of either cash or vouchers. Discarded

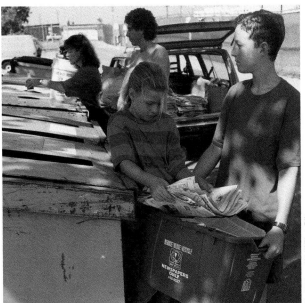

▲ Recycling is an easy way to help save energy and conserve
resources.

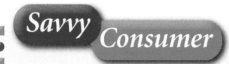

computers and other electronic devices should also be recycled, by donating them to schools or charitable organizations. "Tech trash" buried in landfills is creating a new hazard because trace amounts of potentially hazardous agents, such as lead and mercury, can leak into the ground and water.[11] Enthusiasm and support for recycling has grown, and, thanks to these efforts along with new manufacturing techniques and other technological advances, people in the United States are consuming some natural materials, such as aluminum and steel, at lower rates.

With *composting*—which some people describe as nature's way of recycling—the benefits can be seen as close as your backyard. Organic products, such as leftover food and vegetable peels, are mixed with straw or other dry material and kept damp. Bacteria eat the organic material and turn it into a rich soil. Some people keep a compost pile (which should be stirred every few days) in their backyard; others take their organic garbage (including mowed grass and dead leaves) to community gardens or municipal composting sites.

## Clearing the Air

In most places in the United States, you can breathe easier today than you would have a quarter century ago. Smog has declined by about a third, although there are now 85 percent more vehicles being driven 105 percent more miles a year. Current model automobiles emit an average of 80 percent less pollution per mile than was emitted by new cars in 1970. However, tailpipe emissions from cars and trucks still account for almost a third of the air pollution in the United States.[12]

According to the Harvard School of Public Health, living in a city with even moderately sooty air may shorten your lifespan by about a year. In fact, air pollution can be as harmful to breathing capacity as smoking. Residents of polluted cities are exposed to some of the same toxic gases, such as nitrogen oxide and carbon monoxide, found in cigarettes.

Air pollution of any sort can cause numerous ill effects. As pollutants destroy the hairlike cilia that remove irritants from the lungs, individuals may suffer chronic bronchitis, characterized by excessive mucus flow and continuous coughing. Emphysema may develop or worsen, as pollutants constrict the bronchial tubes and destroy the air sacs in the lungs, making breathing more difficult. In addition to respiratory diseases, air pollution also contributes to heart disease, cancer, and weakened immunity. For the elderly and people with asthma or heart disease, polluted air can be life-threatening. Even healthy individuals can be affected, particularly if they exercise outdoors during high-pollution periods.

## Smog

A combination of smoke and fog, **smog** is made up of chemical vapors from auto exhaust, industrial and commercial pollutants (volatile organic compounds, carbon monoxide, nitrogen oxides, sulfur oxides, particulates), and ozone. The most obvious sources of these pollutants are motor vehicles, industrial factories, electric utility plants, and wood-burning stoves. These chemicals react with sunlight, especially during high-pressure systems and periods of low wind speeds, to form smog.

*Sulfur-dioxide smog* (gray-air smog), often seen in Europe and much of the eastern United States, is produced by burning oil of high sulfur content. Among the cities that must deal with gray-air smog are Chicago, Baltimore, Detroit, and Philadelphia. Like cigarette smoke, gray-air smog affects the cilia in the respiratory passages; the lungs are unable to expel particulates, such as soot, ash, and dust, which remain and irritate the tissues. This condition is hazardous to people with chronic respiratory problems.

*Photochemical smog* (brown-air smog) is found in large traffic centers such as Los Angeles, Salt Lake City, Denver, Mexico City, and Tokyo. This type of smog results principally from nitric oxide in car exhaust reacting with oxygen in the air, forming nitrogen dioxide, which produces a brownish haze and, when exposed to sunlight, other pollutants.

One of these, *ozone,* the most widespread pollutant, can impair the body's immune system and cause long-term lung damage. (Ozone in the upper atmosphere protects us by repelling harmful ultraviolet radiation from the sun, but ozone in the lower atmosphere is a harmful component of air pollution.) Automobiles also produce carbon monoxide, a colorless and odorless gas that diminishes the ability of red blood cells to carry oxygen. The resulting oxygen deficiency can affect breathing, hearing, and vision.

## Indoor Pollutants

Because people in industrialized nations spend more than 90 percent of their time in buildings, the quality of the air they breathe inside can have an even greater impact on their well-being than outdoor pollution. The most haz-

ardous form of indoor air pollution is cigarette smoke. Passive smoking—inhaling others' cigarette smoke—may rank behind active smoking and alcohol use as the third-leading preventable cause of death. Each year secondhand cigarette smoke kills 53,000 nonsmokers.

## Formaldehyde

Unlike outdoor contaminants from exhaust pipes or smokestacks, indoor pollutants come from the very materials the buildings are made of and from the appliances inside them. For instance, formaldehyde, commonly used in building materials, carpet backing, furniture, foam insulation, plywood, and particle board, can cause nausea, dizziness, headaches, heart palpitations, stinging eyes, and burning lungs. Formaldehyde has been shown to cause cancer in animals. Most manufacturers have voluntarily quit using it, but many homes already contain materials made with urea-formaldehyde, which can seep into the air. To avoid formaldehyde exposure, buy solid wood or nonwood products whenever possible, and ask about the formaldehyde content of building products, cabinets, and furniture before purchasing them.

## Asbestos

Asbestos, a mineral widely used for building insulation, has been linked to lung and gastrointestinal cancer among asbestos workers and their families, although it may take 20 to 30 years for such cancer to develop. Fibers from asbestos home insulation or fireproofing that become airborne can cause progressive and deadly lung diseases, including cancer. More than 200,000 lawsuits have been filed for asbestos-related injuries, and as many as 300,000 American workers may have died from asbestos-linked diseases, including lung cancer. The danger may be greatest for those who smoke and are also exposed to asbestos.

If you're concerned about asbestos in your home, don't waste money searching for asbestos in the air. The results of such tests are meaningless. To check a building material for asbestos, put three small pieces in a film canister and send it to a laboratory approved by the U.S. Environmental Protection Agency (EPA). The cost for testing is usually $25 to $75 per sample. If you find asbestos in your house, sealing the source (for example, an old linoleum floor) may be safer than removing it. Contact your state or city health department for advice. If asbestos must be removed, have it done by professionals.

## Lead

A danger both inside and outside our homes is lead, which lurks in some 57 million American homes, most built before 1960, with walls, windows, doors, and banisters

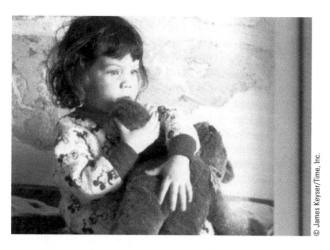

▲ Lead-based paint poses a hazard, especially to children, who can be poisoned even by ingesting small amounts of paint chips.

© James Keyser/Time, Inc.

coated with more than 3 million metric tons of lead-based paint. The Centers for Disease Control and Prevention (CDC) estimates that one of every twenty U.S. children—more than 2 million—suffers from some sort of lead poisoning.[13] Millions more are at risk of poisoning from lead in the air they breathe or the water they drink. "In terms of the number of children affected, the number at risk and the dire effects of exposure, lead is the number-one environmental threat to our youngsters," says pediatrician John Rosen, M.D., chairman of the advisory committee on childhood lead poisoning for the CDC.

Fetuses and children under age 7 are particularly vulnerable to lead because their nervous systems are still developing and because their body mass is so small that they ingest and absorb more lead per pound than adults. Even 10 micrograms (millionths of a gram) of lead per deciliter of blood—the CDC standard for lead poisoning—can kill a child's brain cells and cause poor concentration, reduced short-term memory, slower reaction times, and learning disabilities.

Adults exposed to low levels of lead (which once were thought to be safe) may develop headaches, high blood pressure, irritability, tremors, and insomnia. Health effects increase with exposure to higher levels and include anemia, stomach pain, vomiting, diarrhea, and constipation. Long-term exposure can impair fertility and damage the kidneys. Workers exposed to lead may become sterile or suffer irreversible kidney disease, damage to their central nervous system, stillbirths, or miscarriages.

The CDC and the American Academy of Pediatrics recommend annual testing of blood levels of lead in all children from age 9 months to 6 years, regardless of where they live. High-risk youngsters—those who live or play in older housing (especially if a building is in poor condition or undergoing renovation), those who live with someone who uses lead for a job or hobby, and those who live near a lead smelter, a processing plant, or a heavily traveled road

or highway—should be screened every two or three months until age 3 and every six months until age 6. High levels of ascorbic acid (vitamin C) have been associated with a lower rate of elevated blood lead levels.

## Mercury

While free of lead, some popular, easy-to-use latex paints may contain potentially hazardous mercury, which manufacturers routinely added, until a 1990 ban, to prevent the growth of mold and mildew. The threat of mercury poisoning is greatest during painting and immediately after. Even mercury in medical devices, such as sphygmomanometers that measure blood pressure, can be a hazard. Symptoms of mercury poisoning include a racing heartbeat, sweating, aching limbs, kidney problems, hand tremors, peeling skin, and emotional problems.

## Carbon Monoxide and Nitrogen Dioxide

Carbon monoxide (CO) gas, which is tasteless, odorless, colorless, and nonirritating, can be deadly. Produced by the incomplete combustion of fuel in space heaters, furnaces, water heaters, and engines, it reduces the delivery of oxygen in the blood. Every year an estimated 10,000 Americans seek treatment for CO inhalation; at least 250 die because of this silent killer. Those most at risk are the chronically ill, the elderly, pregnant women, and infants. Typical symptoms of CO poisoning are headache, nausea, vomiting, fatigue, and dizziness. A blood test can measure CO levels; inhaling pure oxygen speeds removal of the gas from the body. Most people who don't lose consciousness as a result of CO poisoning recover completely.

Another dangerous gas, nitrogen dioxide, can reach very high levels if you use a natural gas or propane stove in a poorly ventilated kitchen. This gas may lead to respiratory illnesses. Pilot lights are a steady source of nitrogen dioxide; to reduce exposure, switch to spark ignition.

## Radon

Radioactive radon—which diffuses from rock, brick, concrete building materials, and natural soil deposits under some homes—produces charged decay products that cling to dust particles. Once trapped inside a building, radon can reach levels that may increase the risk of lung cancer. The EPA estimates that the inhalation of indoor radon is responsible for approximately 14,000 lung cancer deaths per year. Radon levels tend to be highest in areas with granite and black shale topped with porous soil.

If you live in a high-radon area, don't panic. Your hypothetical risk of dying from radon-caused lung cancer is about equal to the known risk of dying in a home fire or fall. Check with the geology department at the nearest university or with your state health department to find out if they've performed radon tests in your area. If there may be danger, you can buy a radon detector. In most homes, the readings turn out to be low. If not, your state health department can provide guidelines for bringing them down.

# Protecting Your Hearing

Loud noises cause hearing loss in an estimated 10 million Americans every year.[14] Loudness, or the intensity of a sound, is measured in **decibels (dB).** A whisper is 20 decibels; a conversation in a living room is about 50 decibels. On this scale, 50 isn't two and a half times louder than 20, but 1,000 times louder: Each 10-dB rise in the scale represents a tenfold increase in the intensity of the sound. Very loud but short bursts of sounds (such as gunshots and fireworks) and quieter but longer-lasting sounds (such as power tools) can induce hearing loss.

Sounds under 75 dB don't seem harmful. However, prolonged exposure to any sound over 85 dB (the equivalent of a power mower or food blender) or brief exposure to louder sounds can harm hearing. The noise level at rock concerts can reach 110 to 140 dB, about as loud as an air raid siren. Personal sound systems (boom boxes) can blast sounds of up to 115 dB. Cars with extremely loud music systems, known as boom cars, can produce an earsplitting 145 dB—louder than a jet engine or thunderclap. (See Figure 16-3.)

Most hearing loss occurs on the job. The people at highest risk are firefighters, police, military personnel, construction and factory workers, musicians, farmers, and truck drivers. Other sources of danger include live or recorded high-volume music, recreational vehicles, airplanes, lawn-care equipment, woodworking tools, some appliances, and chain saws.

Common "sound offenders" are nightclubs (with sustained levels of well over 100 decibels), restaurants (with levels of 80 to 96 decibels), and street traffic (80 decibels or more).[15] However, even low-level office noise can undermine well-being and increase health risks.[16]

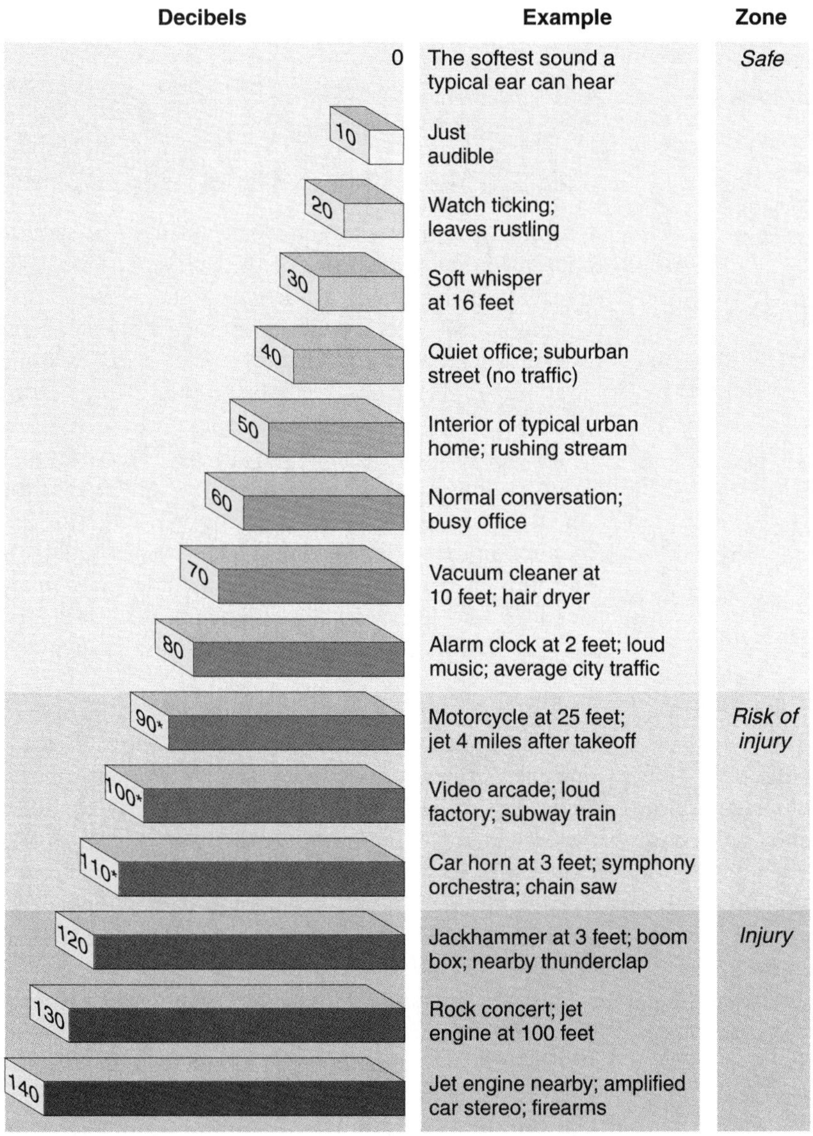

## Effects of Noise

Noise-induced hearing loss is 100 percent preventable—and irreversible. Hearing aids are the only treatment, but they do not correct the problem; they just amplify sound to compensate for hearing loss.

The healthy human ear can hear sounds within a wide range of frequencies (measured in hertz), from the low-frequency rumble of thunder at 50 hertz to the high-frequency overtones of a piccolo at nearly 20,000 hertz. High-frequency noise damages the delicate hair cells that serve as sound receptors in

| Decibels | Example | Zone |
|---|---|---|
| 0 | The softest sound a typical ear can hear | Safe |
| 10 | Just audible | |
| 20 | Watch ticking; leaves rustling | |
| 30 | Soft whisper at 16 feet | |
| 40 | Quiet office; suburban street (no traffic) | |
| 50 | Interior of typical urban home; rushing stream | |
| 60 | Normal conversation; busy office | |
| 70 | Vacuum cleaner at 10 feet; hair dryer | |
| 80 | Alarm clock at 2 feet; loud music; average city traffic | |
| 90* | Motorcycle at 25 feet; jet 4 miles after takeoff | Risk of injury |
| 100* | Video arcade; loud factory; subway train | |
| 110* | Car horn at 3 feet; symphony orchestra; chain saw | |
| 120 | Jackhammer at 3 feet; boom box; nearby thunderclap | Injury |
| 130 | Rock concert; jet engine at 100 feet | |
| 140 | Jet engine nearby; amplified car stereo; firearms | |

*Note: The maximum exposure allowed on the job by federal law, in hours per day: 90 decibels, 8 hours; 100 decibels, 2 hours; 110 decibels, ½ hour.

▲ **Figure 16-3** Loud and Louder
The human ear perceives a 10-decibel increase as a doubling of loudness. Thus, the 100 decibels of a subway train sound much more than twice as loud as the 50 decibels of a rushing stream.

## STRATEGIES FOR CHANGE

### Protecting Your Ears

▲ If you must live or work in a noisy area, wear hearing protectors to prevent exposure to blasts of very loud noise. Don't think cotton or facial tissue stuck in your ears can protect you; foam or soft plastic earplugs are more effective. Wear them when operating lawn mowers, weed trimmers, or power tools.

▲ Soundproof your home by using draperies, carpets, and bulky furniture. Put rubber mats under washing machines, blenders, and other noisy appliances. Seal cracks around windows and doors.

▲ When you hear a sudden loud noise, press your fingers against your ears. Limit your exposure to loud noise. Several brief periods of noise seem less damaging than one long exposure.

▲ Be careful if you wear Walkman-type stereos. The volume is too high if you can feel the vibrations.

▲ Beware of large doses of aspirin. Researchers have found that eight aspirin tablets a day can aggravate the damage caused by loud noise; twelve a day can cause ringing in the ears (tinnitus).

▲ Don't drink in noisy environments. Alcohol intensifies the impact of noise and increases the risk of lifelong hearing damage.

the inner ear. Damage first begins as a diminished sensitivity to frequencies around 4,000 hertz, the highest notes of a piano.

Early symptoms of hearing loss include difficulty understanding speech and *tinnitus* (ringing in the ears). Brief, very loud sounds, such as an explosion or gunfire, can produce immediate, severe, and permanent hearing loss. Longer exposure to less intense but still hazardous sounds, such as those common at work or in public places, can gradually impair hearing, often without the individual's awareness.

Conductive hearing loss, often caused by ear infections, cuts down on perception of low-pitched sounds. Sensorineural loss involves damage or destruction of the sensory cells in the inner ear that convert sound waves to nerve signals.

Noise can harm more than our ears: High-volume sound has been linked to high blood pressure and other stress-related problems that can lead to heart disease, insomnia, anxiety, headaches, colitis, and ulcers. Noise frays the nerves; people tend to be more anxious, irritable, and angry when their ears are constantly barraged with sound.

Chronic airport noise can affect children's physical and mental health.[17] Even unborn babies respond to sounds; some researchers speculate that noise, particularly if it stresses the mother, may be hazardous to the fetus. As a result of exposure to damaging noise levels, 12.5 percent of young Americans, an estimated 5.2 million, between ages 6 and 19 have incurred permanent damage to the hair cells within the ear.[18]

## The Quality of Our Drinking Water

According to a survey by the Water Quality Association, some 86 percent of the people in the United States are concerned about the quality of their tap water, while 32 percent think their water is not as safe as it should be. About two-thirds take steps to drink purer water, either by using filtration and distillation methods or by drinking bottled water.[19] Fears about the public water supply have led many Americans to turn off their taps. However, Consumer Union, a nonprofit advocacy group, maintains that the United States has the safest water supply in the world.[20] The Environmental Protection Agency has set standards for some 80 contaminants. These include many toxic chemicals and heavy metals—including lead, mercury, cadmium, and chromium—that can cause kidney and nervous system damage and birth defects.

Each year the CDC reports an average of 7,400 cases of illness related to the water people drink. The most common culprits include parasites, bacteria, viruses, chemicals, and lead. Health officials suggest having your water tested if you live near a hazardous waste dump or industrial park, if the pipes in your house are made of lead or joined together with lead solder, if your water comes from a well, or if you purchase water from a private company. Check to see if your state health department or local water supplier will provide free testing. If not, use a state-certified laboratory that tests water in accordance with EPA standards.

Is bottled water better than tap water? In the past, the Food and Drug Administration (FDA) simply defined bottled water as "sealed in bottles or other containers and intended for human consumption." Bottled water wasn't required to be "pure" or even to be tested for toxic chemicals. The FDA has now called for federal monitoring of the purity of bottled water. Some states, including California and New York, have their own bottled-water safety standards to ensure that bottled water is at least as safe as public drinking water.

## Fluoride

About half (53 percent) of Americans drink water containing fluoride, an additive to water and toothpaste that helps teeth resist decay. According to the American Dental Association, the incidence of tooth decay is 50 to 70 percent lower in areas with fluoridated water. However, laboratory rats given fluoridated water have shown a high rate of bone cancer. The more fluoride they drank in their water, the more likely they were to develop this cancer. But this type of cancer is extremely rare in humans, and the estimated lifetime risk to any individual from drinking fluoridated water is less than one in 5,000.

Federal health officials have found no evidence that fluoride causes cancer in humans and have concluded that its benefits far outweigh any risks. However, excessive fluoride can increase bone loss and fractures in pre- and postmenopausal women. Health professionals advise consumers to use only small amounts of fluoridated toothpaste, rinse thoroughly after brushing, and use fluoride supplements only when the home water supply is known to be deficient.

## Chlorine

Three-quarters of the population of the United States drinks water treated with chlorine to kill disease-causing bacteria. The Council on Environmental Quality has warned that people drinking chlorinated water have a 53 percent greater risk of getting colon and bladder cancer and a 13 to 93 percent greater risk of getting rectal cancer than those not drinking chlorinated water. There may even be a link between soft water and a higher rate of cardiovascular disease, perhaps because soft water in some areas tends to have more sodium in it.

## Lead

Long recognized as a hazard in paint and dust, lead can also leach into the drinking supply from pipes made of or soldered with lead. The highest risk exists in cities with older housing and with lead pipes or water lines.

## Chemical Risks

According to a 2001 report by the CDC, there have been declines of levels of potentially harmful chemicals, including pesticides and lead, in the country's blood.[21] No relationship has been found between fertility, as measured by time to pregnancy (that is, the time taken for a couple to conceive once they decide they want to), and male exposure to pesticides. Exposure to pesticides may, however, pose a risk to pregnant women and their unborn children. Exposure to toxic chemicals causes about 3 percent of developmental defects.[22]

An estimated 50,000 to 70,000 U.S. workers die each year of chronic diseases related to past exposure to toxic substances, including lung cancer, bladder cancer, leukemia, lymphoma, chronic bronchitis, and disorders of the nervous system. **Endocrine disruptors,** chemicals that act as or interfere with human hormones, particularly estrogen, may pose a different threat. Scientists are investigating their impact on fertility, falling sperm counts, and cancers of the reproductive organs.

## ??? What Health Risks Are Caused by Pesticides?

The FDA estimates that 33 to 39 percent of our food supply contains residues of pesticides that may pose a long-term danger to our health.[23] Scientists have detected traces of pesticides in groundwater in both urban and rural areas.[24]

Various chemicals, including benzene, asbestos, and arsenic, have been shown to cause cancer in humans. Probable carcinogens include DDT and PCB. Risks can be greatly increased with simultaneous exposures to more than one carcinogen, for example, tobacco smoke and asbestos.[25] However, no link to pesticides has been found with clusters of breast cancer.[26]

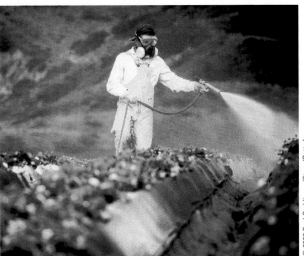

▲ Pesticides protect crops from harmful insects, plants, and fungi but may endanger human health.

**Chlorinated hydrocarbons** include several high-risk substances—such as DDT, kepone, and chlordane—that have been restricted or banned because they may cause cancer, birth defects, neurological disorders, and damage to wildlife and the environment. They are extremely resistant to breakdown.

**Organic phosphates,** including chemicals such as malathion, break down more rapidly than the chlorinated hydrocarbons. Most are highly toxic, causing cramps, confusion, diarrhea, vomiting, headaches, and breathing difficulties. Higher levels in the blood can lead to convulsions, paralysis, coma, and death.

Farmworkers and those in the communities surrounding agricultural land are at greatest risk for pesticide exposure. However, even city dwellers aren't out of range. About half (52 percent) of the nation uses insect repellents, including some made with potent insecticides.

## Invisible Dangers

Among the unseen threats to health are various forms of *radiation,* energy radiated in the form of waves or particles.

## Electromagnetic Fields

Any electrically charged conductor generates two kinds of invisible fields: electric and magnetic. Together they're called **electromagnetic fields (EMFs).** For years, these fields, produced by household appliances, home wiring, lighting fixtures, electric blankets, and overhead power lines, were considered harmless. However, epidemiological studies have revealed a link between exposure to high-voltage lines and cancer (especially leukemia, a blood cancer) in electrical workers and children.

Laboratory studies on animals have shown that alternating current, which changes strength and direction 60 times a second (and electrifies most of North America), emits EMFs that may interfere with the normal functioning of human cell membranes, which have their own electromagnetic fields. The result may be mood disorders, changes in circadian rhythms (our inner sense of time), miscarriage, developmental problems, or cancer. Researchers have documented an increase in breast cancer deaths in women who worked as electrical engineers, electricians, or in other high-exposure jobs, and a link between EMF exposure and an increased risk of leukemia and possibly brain cancer.[27]

After six years of congressionally mandated research, the National Institute of Environmental Health Sciences concluded that the evidence of a risk of cancer and other human disease from the electric and magnetic fields around power lines is "weak." This finding applies to the extremely low frequency electric and magnetic fields surrounding both the big power lines that distribute power and the smaller but closer electric lines in homes and appliances. However, the researchers also noted that EMF exposure "cannot be recognized as entirely safe."

Appliances that are used only briefly, such as hair dryers, are probably less dangerous than electric blankets, which people sleep under for an entire night. Expectant mothers who often use electric blankets or heated water beds during winter have a higher miscarriage rate than nonusers. Babies conceived in the winter by electric blanket-users grow more slowly in the womb and tend to have a lower birthweight than others. Federal officials urge "prudent avoidance" of electric blankets for women who are pregnant or hoping to conceive.

## Video Display Terminals

Chances are there's a **video display terminal (VDT)**—a computer monitor—in your life: at the school library, at the office where you work, in your home. Is it a health hazard? The answer is a definite maybe. Although VDTs have been blamed for increases in reproductive problems, miscarriages, low birthweights, and cataracts, repeated measurements of radiation from VDTs have shown that leakage is well below present standards for safe occupational exposure. However, VDTs emit electromagnetic fields from all sides, not just the screen, and the strongest emissions are from the sides, backs, and tops of monitors. At least in theory, working next to someone using a computer may be more hazardous than using one yourself. Scientists are continuing to investigate possible links between VDT use and health hazards.

## Microwaves

**Microwaves** (extremely high frequency electromagnetic waves) increase the rate at which molecules vibrate; this vibration generates heat. There's no evidence that existing levels of microwave radiation encountered in the environment pose a health risk to people, and all home microwave ovens must meet safety standards for leakage.

Another concern about the safety of microwave ovens stems from the chemicals in plastic wrapping and plastic containers used in microwave ovens. Chemicals may leak into food. In high concentrations, some of the chemicals (such as DEHA, which makes plastic more pliable) can cause cancer in mice. Consumers should be cautious about using clingy plastic wrap when reheating leftovers, and plastic-encased metal "heat susceptors" included in convenience foods such as popcorn and pizza. Although these materials seem safe when tested in conventional ovens at temperatures of 300° to 350° Fahrenheit, microwave ovens can boost temperatures to 500° Fahrenheit.

## ???? Are Cellular Phones Safe to Use?

Since cellular phone service was introduced in the United States in 1984, mobile and handheld phones have become ubiquitous. More than 86 million people use cell phones, and concern has grown about their possible health risks, particularly brain cancer. Because of the close proximity of the antenna to the brain, researchers hypothesized that radio frequency signals might increase the danger. In experimental studies, researchers have documented changes in biological tissues exposed to radio frequency waves.[28]

Researchers have found no link between cell phone use and brain cancer, but further studies are needed to determine whether exposure to radio waves from radio phones might cause slow-growing brain tumors.[29] No studies have continued long enough to rule out any long-term risk of cancer or cardiac and neurological effects.[30]

## Irradiated Foods

The use of radiation on food, from either radioactive substances or devices that produce X rays, is known as **irradiation.** It doesn't make the food radioactive—its primary benefit is to prolong the food's useful life. Like the heat in canning, irradiation can kill all the microorganisms that might grow in food; the sterilized food can then be stored for years in sealed containers at room temperature without spoiling. In addition, low-dose irradiation can inhibit the sprouting of vegetables such as potatoes and onions, and delay the ripening of some fruits, such as bananas, mangoes, tomatoes, pears, and avocados—cost-saving benefits of great appeal to the food industry.

Irradiated foods are believed to be safe to eat, and the federal government has approved their distribution. Most research has focused on low-dose irradiation to delay ripening and destroy insects. Nutritional studies have shown no significant decreases in the quality of the foods, but high-dose treatments may cause vitamin losses similar to those that occur during canning. It's also possible that the ionizing effect of radiation creates new compounds in foods that may be mutagenic or carcinogenic.

 Can the sights and smells of nature improve your health?

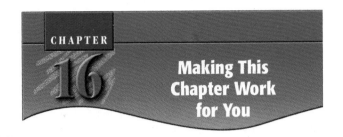

### CHAPTER 16 Making This Chapter Work for You

1. Threats to the environment include
   a. an open ecosystem
   b. depletion of the oxygen layer
   c. ecological processes
   d. global warming

2. Mutagens
   a. are caused by birth defects.
   b. result in changes to the DNA of body cells.
   c. are agents that trigger changes in the DNA of body cells.
   d. are caused by repeated exposure to pollutants.

3. Which of the following statements about global warming is true?
   a. In 2001, the United States signed the first international treaty to fight global warming.
   b. Global warming may result in severe drought and a rise in ocean levels.
   c. Increasing tree cover and agricultural lands will contribute to global warming.
   d. Increasing carbon dioxide production will slow the progress of global warming.

4. One of the most important things you can do to help protect the environment is
   a. recycle paper, bottles, cans, and unwanted food.
   b. use as much water as possible to help lower the ocean water levels.
   c. avoid energy-depleting fluorescent bulbs.
   d. use plastic storage containers and plastic wrap to save trees from being cut down.

5. Which of the following statements about air pollution is false?
   a. Current model automobiles emit much less pollution per mile than new cars in 1970.
   b. The three types of smog include sulfur-dioxide smog, produced by burning oil; photochemical smog, resulting from car exhaust; and carbon-monoxide smog, caused by fossil fuels.
   c. Ozone in the upper atmosphere protects us from harmful ultraviolet radiation from the sun, but in the lower atmosphere, it is a harmful air pollutant.
   d. Air pollution can cause the same types of respiratory health problems as smoking.

6. Indoor pollutants include
   a. lead, which is often found in paint and can result in nervous system damage in adults and impaired fertility and kidney damage in children.
   b. radon, which is found in building materials and can cause heart disease.
   c. asbestos, which may be found in building insulation and can cause lung diseases.
   d. carbon monoxide, which can be produced by furnaces and engines and can result in chronic illnesses such as emphysema.

7. You can protect your hearing by
   a. avoiding prolonged exposure to sounds under 75 decibels.
   b. using foam earplugs when operating noisy tools or attending rock concerts.
   c. limiting noise exposure to short bursts of loud sounds such as fireworks.
   d. drinking alcohol in noisy environments to mute the sounds.

8. Drinking water safety
   a. may be compromised if your water comes from a well.
   b. is high in the United States because of the use of sodium chloride to kill disease-causing bacteria.
   c. can be guaranteed by using bottled water, which is completely free of chemical contaminants.

   d. has been significantly decreased in those communities that add fluoride to the water.

9. Which of the following statements about electromagnetic fields is true?
   a. Overwhelming evidence indicates a strong link between electromagnetic fields around power lines and cancer and other diseases.
   b. The electromagnetic fields emitted by electric blankets are probably less dangerous than those from hair dryers.
   c. The amount of radiation from video display terminals exceeds present standards for safe occupational exposure.
   d. Electrical engineers and electricians who have high exposure to EMFs may be at greater risk for developing leukemia.

10. Which statement about radiation usage is false?
    a. Chemicals in plastic wrap may leak into foods heated in microwave ovens.
    b. Radiofrequency signals from cell phones cause brain cancer.
    c. Irradiation can be used to kill microorganisms in food.
    d. Irradiation can delay the ripening of fruits.

Answers to these questions can be found on page 415.

## Critical Thinking

1. How do you contribute to environmental pollution? How might you change your habits to protect the environment?

2. An excerpt from a recent newspaper article stated, "Children living in a public housing project near a local refinery suffer from a high rate of asthma and allergies, and an environmental group says the plant may be to blame." The refinery has met all the local air quality standards, employs hundreds in the community, and pays substantial city taxes, which support police, fire, and social services. If you were a city council member, how would you balance health and environmental concerns with the need for industry in your community? What actions would you recommend in this particular situation?

3. In one Harris poll, 84 percent of Americans said that, given a choice between a high standard of living (but with hazardous air and water pollution and the depletion of natural resources) and a lower standard of living (but with clean air and drinking water), they would prefer clean air and drinking water and a lower standard of living. What about you? What exactly would you be willing to give up: air conditioning, convenience packaging and products, driving your own car rather than using public transportation? Do you think most people are willing to change their lifestyles to preserve the environment?

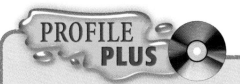

The health of the planet contributes to the health and well being of all its inhabitants. Discover how you can contribute to a healthy environment with this activity on your Profile Plus CD-ROM.

Are You Doing Your Part for the Planet?

## SITES & BYTES

### Environmental Protection Agency
**www.epa.gov**

This comprehensive government site features environmental topics including ecosystems, air and water pollution, compliance and enforcement, pesticides and toxins, accident prevention, and treatment.

### National Center for Environmental Health (NCEH)
**www.cdc.gov/nceh**

This site, sponsored by the U.S. Centers for Disease Control and Prevention, features a searchable database as well as fact sheets and brochures on a variety of environmental topics, from emergency preparedness and public health tracking to environmental hazards and lead poisoning prevention.

### EnviroLink
**www.envirolink.org**

This nonprofit organization maintains a comprehensive database of environmental resources, including current news events as well as information on agriculture, air quality, ecosystems, environmental ethics, environmental legislation, and much more.

### InfoTrac College Edition Activity
Jane K. Dixon and John P. Dixon. "An Integrative Model for Environmental Health Research." *Advances in Nursing Science,* Vol. 24, No. 3, March 2002, p. 43.

1. Describe the four domains and the interrelationships that make up the authors' integrative model of environmental health research.

2. Which four elements of the domain have been most emphasized in environmental health research?

3. What are the most common agents of environmental diseases? What requirements must be met for an agent to pose a health risk to humans?

You can find additional readings relating to safeguarding the environment with InfoTrac College Edition, an online library of more than 900 journals and publications. Follow the instructions for accessing InfoTrac that were packaged with your textbook; then search for articles using a keyword search.

For additional links, resources, and suggested readings on InfoTrac, visit our Health &Wellness Resource Center at http://health.wadsworth.com.

## Key Terms

The terms listed here are used within the chapter on the page indicated. Definitions of terms are in the Glossary at the end of the book.

**chlorinated hydrocarbons** 410
**decibel (dB)** 407
**ecosystem** 400
**electromagnetic fields (EMFs)** 410

**endocrine disruptors** 409
**irradiation** 411
**microwaves** 410
**multiple chemical sensitivity (MCS)** 401
**mutagen** 401

**mutation** 401
**organic phosphates** 410
**pollutant** 401
**pollution** 401
**precycling** 402
**recycling** 402

**smog** 404
**teratogen** 401
**video display terminal (VDT)** 410

# References

1. U.N. Department for Economic and Social Affairs. *Global Outlook 3.* New York: United Nations, 2002.

2. "Children Greatest Victims of Degrading Environment." *Medical Letter on the CDC & FDA,* June 9, 2002, p. 3.

3. "Is Your Environment a Health Hazard?" *Natural Health,* Vol. 32, No. 5, July 2002, p. 19.

4. Sadovsky, Richard. "Assessing Patients with Medically Unknown Symptoms." *American Family Physician,* Vol. 61, No. 11, June 1, 2000, p. 3455.

5. Richter, Elihu, and Tamar Berman. "Speed, Air Pollution, and Health: A Neglected Issue." *Archives of Environmental Health,* Vol. 56, No. 4, July 2001, p. 296.

6. Brook, Robert, et al. "Inhalation of Fine Particulate Air Pollution and Ozone Causes Acute Arterial Vasoconstriction in Healthy Adults." *Circulation,* Vol. 105, No. 10, March 2002, p. 1534.

7. Environmental Protection Agency's website on global warming: www.epa.gov/globalwarming/.

8. Aber, John, et al. "Forest Processes and Global Environmental Change: Predicting the Effects of Individual and Multiple Stressors." *BioScience,* Vol. 51, No. 9, September 2001, p. 735.

9. Weaver, Andrew, et al. "The Causes of 20th Century Warming." *Science,* Vol. 290, No. 5499, December 15, 2000, p. 2081.

10. Staver, A. "The Collapse of the Kyoto Protocol and the Struggle to Slow Global Warming." *Choice,* Vol. 39, No. 2, October 2001, p. 347.

11. "Stemming the Tide of Tech Trash." *Business Week,* October 7, 2002, p. 36A.

12. Environmental Protection Agency, www.epa.gov.

13. "Living with Lead." *Journal of Environmental Health,* Vol. 65, No. 1, July–August 2002, p. 29.

14. "Noise-Induced Hearing Loss: Common Condition Easily Prevented." *Facts of Life: Issue Briefing for Health Reporters,* Vol. 6, No. 5, July–August 2001.

15. "Recent Findings Suggest Urban Setting Means More Noise Exposure and More Hearing Loss." *Facts of Life: Issue Briefing for Health Reporters,* Vol. 6, No. 5, July–August 2001.

16. Lang, Susan. "Even Low-Level Office Noise Can Increase Health Risks." Cornell University News Office, January 22, 2001.

17. "Aircraft Noise and Public Health." *Journal of Environmental Health,* Vol. 63, No. 5, December 2000, p. 46.

18. "Noise-Induced Hearing Loss."

19. "Water, Water, Everywhere." *American Demographics,* October 1, 2001, p. 50.

20. Napoli, Maryann. "Consumer Reports Looks at Bottled Water." *HealthFacts,* August 2000.

21. Revkin, Andrew. "Study of Chemicals in Americans Shows Encouraging Trends." *New York Times,* March 22, 2001.

22. "Advances in Biology Could Help in Assessing the Impact of Chemicals on Children." *Journal of Environmental Health,* Vol. 63, No. 3, October–September 2000, p. 55.

23. Crain, Ellen. "Environmental Threats to Children's Health." *Pediatrics,* Vol. 106, No. 4, October 2000, p. 871.

24. Koplin, Dana, et al. "Pesticides in Ground Water of the United States." *Ground Water,* Vol. 38, No. 6, November 2000.

25. "Environmental Cancer Risks." *Cancer Facts & Figures 2001,* American Cancer Society, 2001.

26. "U.S. Study Shows No Link to Pollution." *Medical Devices & Surgical Technology Week,* September 8, 2002, p. 11.

27. Doube, Clare. "Electromagnetic Exposure: Real Risks or Paranoia?" *New Internationalist,* July 2002, p. 7.

28. Frey, Allan. "Cellular Phones: Are They Safe to Use?" *Scientists,* Vol. 14, No. 23, November 27, 2000.

29. Jones, David. "Phones and the Brain." *Nature,* Vol. 411, No. 6841, June 28, 2001, p. 1012.

30. Doube. "Electromagnetic Exposure."

## Answers: Making This Chapter Work for You

**Chapter 1**
1. b; 2. a; 3. d; 4. c; 5. a; 6. d; 7. b; 8. c; 9. d; 10. a

**Chapter 2**
1. b; 2. d; 3. a; 4. d; 5. a; 6. b; 7. c; 8. a; 9. c; 10. d

**Chapter 3**
1. b; 2. d; 3. a; 4. c; 5. c; 6. d; 7. b; 8. a; 9. d; 10. b

**Chapter 4**
1. c; 2. c; 3. d; 4. b; 5. b; 6. a; 7. d; 8. c; 9. b; 10. d

**Chapter 5**
1. c; 2. a; 3. d; 4. d; 5. b; 6. a; 7. c; 8. a; 9. d; 10. b

**Chapter 6**
1. d; 2. b; 3. b; 4. c; 5. c; 6. a; 7. c; 8. d; 9. a; 10. c

**Chapter 7**
1. d; 2. a; 3. b; 4. a; 5. c; 6. d; 7. c; 8. a; 9. d; 10. b

**Chapter 8**
1. c; 2. d; 3. a; 4. c; 5. c; 6. b; 7. d; 8. a; 9. b; 10. d

**Chapter 9**
1. a; 2. c; 3. d; 4. b; 5. c; 6. a; 7. a; 8. d; 9. b; 10. c

**Chapter 10**
1. b; 2. a; 3. a; 4. b; 5. d; 6. a; 7. d; 8. a; 9. c; 10. b

**Chapter 11**
1. a; 2. c; 3. d; 4. b; 5. c; 6. c; 7. d; 8. a; 9. b; 10. d

**Chapter 12**
1. b; 2. a; 3. b; 4. c; 5. d; 6. c; 7. c; 8. b; 9. b; 10. c

**Chapter 13**
1. b; 2. c; 3. c; 4. d; 5. b; 6. a 7. d; 8. d; 9. c; 10. b

**Chapter 14**
1. d; 2. b; 3. c; 4. b; 5. d; 6. c; 7. b; 8. a; 9. c; 10. b

**Chapter 15**
1. b; 2. a; 3. d; 4. c; 5. b; 6. b; 7. d; 8. c; 9. c; 10. b

**Chapter 16**
1. d; 2. c; 3. b; 4. a; 5. b; 6. c; 7. b; 8. a; 9. d; 10. b

# Glossary

**abscess** A localized accumulation of pus and disintegrating tissue.

**abstinence** Voluntary refrainment from sexual activities that include vaginal, anal, and oral intercourse.

**acquired immune deficiency syndrome (AIDS)** The final stages of human immune deficiency virus (HIV) infection, characterized by a variety of severe illnesses and decreased levels of certain immune cells.

**acupuncture** A Chinese medical practice of puncturing the body with needles inserted at specific points to relieve pain or cure disease.

**acute injuries** Physical injuries, such as sprains, bruises, and pulled muscles, that result from sudden traumas, such as falls or collisions.

**adaptive response** The body's attempt to reestablish homeostasis or stability.

**addiction** A behavioral pattern characterized by compulsion, loss of control, and continued repetition of a behavior or activity in spite of adverse consequences.

**advance directives** Documents that specify an individual's preferences regarding treatment in a medical crisis.

**aerobic exercise** Physical activity in which sufficient or excess oxygen is continually supplied to the body.

**aging** The characteristic pattern of normal life changes that occur as humans grow older.

**alcohol abuse** Continued use of alcohol despite awareness of social, occupational, psychological, or physical problems related to its use, or use of alcohol in dangerous ways or situations, such as before driving.

**alcohol dependence** Development of a strong craving for alcohol due to the pleasurable feelings or relief of stress and anxiety produced by drinking.

**alcoholism** A chronic, progressive, potentially fatal disease characterized by an inability to control drinking, a preoccupation with alcohol, continued use of alcohol despite adverse consequences, and distorted thinking, most notably denial.

**altruism** Acts of helping or giving to others without thought of self-benefit.

**Alzheimer's disease** A progressive deterioration of intellectual powers due to physiological changes within the brain; symptoms include diminishing ability to concentrate, disorientation, depression, apathy, and paranoia.

**amenorrhea** The absence or suppression of menstruation.

**amino acids** Organic compounds containing nitrogen, carbon, hydrogen, and oxygen; the essential building blocks of proteins.

**amnion** The innermost membrane of the sac enclosing the embryo or fetus.

**amphetamine** A stimulant that triggers the release of epinephrine, which stimulates the central nervous system; users experience a state of hyper-alertness and high energy, followed by a crash as the drug wears off.

**anaerobic exercise** Physical activity in which the body develops an oxygen deficit.

**angioplasty** Surgical repair of an obstructed artery by passing a balloon catheter through the blood vessel to the area of obstruction and then inflating the catheter to compress the plaque against the vessel wall.

**anorexia nervosa** A psychological disorder in which refusal to eat and/or an extreme loss of appetite leads to malnutrition, severe weight loss, and possibly death.

**antibiotics** Substances produced by microorganisms or synthetic agents that are toxic to other types of microorganisms; in dilute solutions, used to treat infectious diseases.

**antidepressant** A drug used primarily to treat symptoms of depression.

**antioxidants** Substances that prevent the damaging effects of oxidation in cells.

**antiviral drug** A substance that decreases the severity and duration of a viral infection if taken prior to or soon after onset of the infection.

**anxiety** A feeling of apprehension and dread, with or without a known cause; may range from mild to severe and may be accompanied by physical symptoms.

**anxiety disorders** A group of psychological disorders involving episodes of apprehension, tension, or uneasiness, stemming from the anticipation of danger and sometimes accompanied by physical symptoms; causes significant distress and impairment to an individual.

**aorta** The main artery of the body, arising from the left ventricle of the heart.

**appetite** A desire for food, stimulated by anticipated hunger, physiological changes within the brain and body, the availability of food, and other environmental and psychological factors.

**arteriosclerosis** Any of a number of chronic diseases characterized by degeneration of the arteries and hardening and thickening of arterial walls.

**artificial insemination** The introduction of viable sperm into the vagina by artificial means for the purpose of inducing conception.

**assertive** Behaving in a nonhostile, confident manner to make your needs and desires clear to others.

**atherosclerosis** A form of arteriosclerosis in which fatty substances (plaque) are deposited on the inner walls of arteries.

**atrium** (plural, **atria**) Either of the two upper chambers of the heart, which receive blood from the veins.

**attention deficit/hyperactivity disorder (ADHD)** A spectrum of difficulties in controlling motion and sustaining attention, including hyperactivity, impulsivity, and distractibility.

**autonomy** The ability to draw on internal resources; independence from familial and societal influences.

**aversion therapy** A treatment that attempts to help a person overcome a dependence or bad habit by making the person feel disgusted or repulsed by that habit.

**416**

**ayurveda** A traditional Indian medical treatment involving meditation, exercise, herbal medication, and nutrition.

**bacteria** (singular, **bacterium**) One-celled microscopic organisms; the most plentiful pathogens.

**bacterial vaginosis** A vaginal infection caused by overgrowth and depletion of various microorganisms living in the vagina, resulting in a malodorous white or gray vaginal discharge.

**barbiturates** Antianxiety drugs that depress the central nervous system, reduce activity, and induce relaxation, drowsiness, or sleep; often prescribed to relieve tension, treat epileptic seizures, or as a general anesthetic.

**barrier contraceptives** Birth-control devices that block the meeting of egg and sperm, by physical barriers (such as condoms, diaphragms, or cervical caps) or by chemical barriers (such as spermicide), or both.

**basal body temperature** The body temperature upon waking, before any activity.

**basal metabolic rate (BMR)** The number of calories required to sustain the body at rest.

**behavior therapy** Psychotherapy that emphasizes application of the principles of learning to substitute desirable responses and behavior patterns for undesirable ones.

**benzodiazepines** Antianxiety drugs that depress the central nervous system, reduce activity, and induce relaxation, drowsiness, or sleep; often prescribed to relieve tension, muscular strain, sleep problems, anxiety, or panic attacks; also used as an anesthetic and in the treatment of alcohol withdrawal.

**bidis** Skinny, sweet-flavored cigarettes.

**binge drinking** For a man, having five or more alcoholic drinks at a single sitting; for a woman, having four drinks or more at a single sitting.

**binge eating** The rapid consumption of an abnormally large amount of food in a relatively short time.

**biofeedback** A technique of becoming aware, with the aid of external monitoring devices, of internal physiological activities in order to develop the capability of altering them.

**bipolar disorder** Severe depression alternating with periods of manic activity and elation.

**bisexual** Sexually oriented toward both men and women.

**blended family** A family formed when one or both of the partners bring children from a previous union to the new marriage.

**blood-alcohol concentration (BAC)** The amount of alcohol in the blood, expressed as a percentage.

**body composition** The relative amounts of fat and lean tissue (bone, muscle, organs, water) in the body.

**body mass index (BMI)** A mathematical formula that correlates height and weight with body fat; a better predictor of disease than weight alone.

**botulism** Possibly fatal food poisoning, caused by a type of bacterium that produces a toxin in the absence of air; found in improperly canned food.

**breech birth** A birth in which the infant's buttocks or feet pass through the birth canal first.

**bulimia nervosa** Episodic binge eating, often followed by forced vomiting or laxative abuse, and accompanied by a persistent preoccupation with body shape and weight.

**caesarean delivery** The surgical procedure in which an infant is delivered through an incision made in the abdominal wall and uterus.

**calorie** The amount of energy required to raise the temperature of 1 gram of water by 1 degree Celsius. In everyday usage related to the energy content of foods and the energy expended in activities, a calorie is actually the equivalent of a thousand such calories, or a kilocalorie.

**candidiasis** An infection of the yeast *Candida albicans,* commonly occurring in the vagina, vulva, penis, or mouth, and causing burning, itching, and a whitish discharge.

**capillary** A minute blood vessel that connects an artery to a vein.

**carbohydrates** Organic compounds, such as starches, sugars, and glycogen, that are composed of carbon, hydrogen, and oxygen; sources of bodily energy.

**carbon monoxide** A colorless, odorless gas produced by the burning of gasoline or tobacco; displaces oxygen in the hemoglobin molecules of red blood cells.

**carcinogen** A substance that produces cancerous cells or enhances their development and growth.

**cardiorespiratory fitness** The ability of the heart and blood vessels to efficiently circulate blood through the body.

**celibacy** Abstention from sexual activity; can be partial or complete, permanent or temporary.

**cell-mediated immunity** The portion of the immune response that protects against parasites, fungi, cancer cells, and foreign tissue, primarily by means of T cells, or lymphocytes.

**certified social worker** A person who has completed a two-year graduate program in counseling people with mental problems.

**cervical cap** A thimble-sized rubber or plastic cap that is inserted into the vagina to fit over the cervix and prevent the passage of sperm into the uterus during sexual intercourse; used with a spermicidal foam or jelly, it serves as both a chemical and a physical barrier to sperm.

**cervix** The narrow, lower end of the uterus that opens into the vagina.

**chanchroid** A soft, painful sore or localized infection usually acquired through sexual contact.

**chiropractic** A method of treating disease, primarily through manipulating the bones and joints to restore normal nerve function.

**chlamydia** A sexually transmitted disease caused by the bacterium *Chlamydia trachomatis,* often asymptomatic in women but sometimes characterized by urinary pain; if undetected and untreated, may result in pelvic inflammatory disease (PID).

**chlorinated hydrocarbons** Highly toxic pesticides, such as DDT and chlordane, that are extremely resistant to breakdown; may cause cancer, birth defects, neurological disorders, and damage to wildlife and the environment.

**cholesterol** An organic substance found in animal fats; linked to cardiovascular disease, particularly atherosclerosis.

**circumcision** The surgical removal of the foreskin of the penis.

**clitoris** A small erectile structure on the female, corresponding to the penis on the male.

**club drugs** Illegally manufactured psychoactive drugs (including ecstasy, Special

K, and Rohypnol) that have dangerous physical and psychological effects; often used at all-night rave or trance events.

**cocaine** A white crystalline powder extracted from the leaves of the coca plant that stimulates the central nervous system and produces a brief period of euphoria followed by a depression.

**cognitive therapy** A technique used to identify an individual's beliefs and attitudes, recognize negative thought patterns, and educate in alternative ways of thinking.

**cohabitation** Two people living together as a couple, without official ties such as marriage.

**coitus interruptus** The removal of the penis from the vagina before ejaculation.

**colpotomy** Surgical sterilization by cutting or blocking the fallopian tubes through an incision made in the wall of the vagina.

**complementary and alternative medicine (CAM)** A term used to apply to all health-care approaches, practices, and treatments not widely taught in medical schools, not generally used in hospitals, and not usually reimbursed by medical insurance companies.

**complementary proteins** Incomplete proteins that, when combined, provide all the amino acids essential for protein synthesis.

**complete proteins** Proteins that contain all the amino acids needed by the body for growth and maintenance.

**complex carbohydrates** Starches, including cereals, fruits, and vegetables.

**conception** The merging of a sperm and an ovum.

**conditioning** The gradual building up of the body to enhance one or more of the three main components of physical fitness: flexibility, cardiorespiratory fitness, and muscular strength and endurance.

**condom** A latex sheath worn over the penis during sexual acts to prevent conception and/or the transmission of disease; some condoms contain a spermicidal lubricant.

**constant-dose combination pill** An oral contraceptive that releases synthetic estrogen and progestin at constant levels throughout the menstrual cycle.

**contraception** The prevention of conception; birth control.

**corpus luteum** A yellowish mass of tissue that is formed immediately after ovulation from the remaining cells of the follicle; it secretes estrogen and progesterone for the remainder of the menstrual cycle.

**Cowper's glands** Two small glands that discharge into the male urethra.

**crucifers** Plants, including broccoli, cabbage, and cauliflower, that contain large amounts of fiber, proteins, and indoles.

**culture** The set of shared attitudes, values, goals, and practices of a group that are internalized by an individual within the group.

**cunnilingus** Sexual stimulation of a woman's genitals by means of oral manipulation.

**cystitis** Inflammation of the urinary bladder.

**daily values (DV)** Reference values developed by the U.S. Food and Drug Administration specifically for use on food labels.

**decibel (dB)** A unit for measuring the intensity of sounds.

**defense mechanism** A psychological process that alleviates anxiety and eliminates mental conflict; includes denial, displacement, projection, rationalization, reaction formation, and repression.

**deleriants** Chemicals, such as solvents, aerosols, glue, cleaning fluids, petroleum products, and some anesthetics, that produce vapors with psychoactive effects when inhaled.

**dementia** Deterioration of mental capability.

**dendrites** Branching fibers of a neuron that receive impulses from axon terminals of other neurons and conduct these impulses toward the nucleus.

**depression** In general, feelings of unhappiness and despair; as a mental illness, also characterized by an inability to function normally.

**depressive disorders** A group of psychological disorders involving pervasive and sustained depression.

**diabetes mellitus** A disease in which the inadequate production of insulin leads to failure of the body tissues to break down carbohydrates at a normal rate.

**diaphragm** A bowl-like rubber cup with a flexible rim that is inserted into the

vagina to cover the cervix and prevent the passage of sperm into the uterus during sexual intercourse; used with a spermicidal foam or jelly, it serves as both a chemical and a physical barrier to sperm.

**diastole** The period between contractions in the cardiac cycle, during which the heart relaxes and dilates as it fills with blood.

**dietary fiber** The nondigestible form of carbohydrates found in plant foods, such as leaves, stems, skins, seeds, and hulls.

**dietary reference intakes (DRI)** A set of values for the dietary nutrient intakes of healthy people (Estimated Average Requirements, Recommended Dietary Allowances, Adequate Intakes, and Tolerable Upper Intake levels); used for planning and assessing diets.

**dilation and evacuation (D and E)** A medical procedure in which the contents of the uterus are removed through the use of instruments.

**distress** A negative stress that may result in illness.

**do-not-resuscitate (DNR)** An advance directive expressing an individual's preference that resuscitation efforts not be made during a medical crisis.

**drug** Any substance, other than food, that affects bodily functions and structures when taken into the body.

**drug abuse** The excessive use of a drug in a manner inconsistent with accepted medical practice.

**drug misuse** The use of a drug for a purpose (or person) other than that for which it was medically intended.

**dynamic flexibility** The ability to move a joint quickly and fluidly through its entire range of motion with little resistance.

**dysfunctional** Characterized by negative and destructive patterns of behavior between partners or between parents and children.

**dysmenorrhea** Painful menstruation.

**dyspareunia** A sexual difficulty in which a woman experiences pain during sexual intercourse.

**dysthymia** Frequent, prolonged mild depression.

**eating disorders** Bizarre, often dangerous patterns of food consumption, including anorexia nervosa and bulimia nervosa.

**ecosystem** A community of organisms sharing a physical and chemical environment and interacting with each other.

**ecstasy (MDMA)** A synthetic compound, also known as methylenedioxymethamphetamine, that is similar in structure to methamphetamine and has both stimulant and hallucinogenic effects.

**ectopic pregnancy** A pregnancy in which the fertilized egg has implanted itself outside the uterine cavity, usually in the fallopian tube.

**ejaculatory duct** The canal connecting the seminal vesicles and vas deferens.

**electromagnetic fields (EMFs)** The invisible electric and magnetic fields generated by an electrically charged conductor.

**embryo** An organism in its early stage of development; in humans, the embryonic period lasts from the second to the eighth week of pregnancy.

**emergency contraception (EC)** Types of oral contraceptive pills usually taken within 72 hours after intercourse that can prevent pregnancy.

**emotional health** The ability to express and acknowledge one's feelings and moods.

**emotional intelligence** A term used by some psychologists to evaluate the capacity of people to understand themselves and relate well with others.

**endocrine disruptors** Synthetic chemicals that interfere with the ways hormones work in humans and wildlife.

**endometrium** The mucous membrane lining the uterus.

**endorphins** Mood-elevating, pain-killing chemicals produced by the brain.

**endurance** The ability to withstand the stress of continued physical exertion.

**environmental tobacco smoke** Secondhand cigarette smoke; the third leading preventable cause of death.

**epididymis** That portion of the male duct system in which sperm mature.

**epidural block** An injection of anesthesia into the membrane surrounding the spinal cord to numb the lower body during labor and childbirth.

**essential nutrients** Nutrients that the body cannot manufacture for itself and must obtain from food: water, carbohydrates, fats, vitamins, and minerals.

**estrogen** The female sex hormone that stimulates female secondary sex characteristics.

**ethyl alcohol** The intoxicating agent in alcoholic beverages; also called ethanol.

**eustress** A positive stress, which stimulates a person to function properly.

**failure rate** The number of pregnancies that occur per year for every 100 women using a particular method of birth control.

**fallopian tubes** The pair of channels that transports ova from the ovaries to the uterus; the usual site of fertilization.

**family** A group of people united by marriage, blood, or adoption, residing in the same household, maintaining a common culture, and interacting with one another on the basis of their roles within the group.

**fellatio** Sexual stimulation of a man's genitals by means of oral manipulation.

**fertilization** The fusion of the sperm and egg nuclei.

**fetal alcohol effects (FAE)** Milder form of fetal alcohol syndrome, including low birthweight, irritability as newborns, and permanent mental impairment; caused by the mother's alcohol consumption during pregnancy.

**fetal alcohol syndrome (FAS)** A cluster of physical and mental defects in the newborn, including low birthweight, smaller-than-normal head circumference, intrauterine growth retardation, and permanent mental impairment; caused by the mother's alcohol consumption during pregnancy.

**fetus** The human organism developing in the uterus from the ninth week until birth.

**fiber** Indigestible materials in food that lower blood cholesterol and facilitate digestion and elimination.

**FIT** A formula that describes the frequency, intensity, and length of time for physical activity.

**flexibility** The range of motion allowed by one's joints; determined by the length of muscles, tendons, and ligaments attached to the joints.

**food toxicologists** Specialists who detect toxins in food and treat the conditions toxins produce.

**frostbite** The freezing or partial freezing of skin and tissue just below the skin, or even muscle and bone; more severe than frostnip.

**frostnip** Sudden blanching or lightening of the skin on hands, feet, and face, resulting from exposure to high wind speeds and low temperatures.

**functional fiber** Isolated, nondigestible carbohydrates with beneficial effects in humans.

**fungi** (singular, **fungus**) Organisms that reproduce by means of spores.

**gamma globulin** The antibody-containing portion of the blood fluid (plasma).

**gamma hydroxybutyrate (GHB)** A brain messenger chemical (also known as *blue nitro* or the *date rape drug*) that stimulates the release of the human growth hormone; commonly abused for its high and its alleged ability to trim fat and build muscles.

**general adaptation syndrome (GAS)** The sequenced physiological response to a stressful situation; consists of three stages: alarm, resistance, and exhaustion.

**generalized anxiety disorder (GAD)** An anxiety disorder characterized as chronic distress.

**gonorrhea** A sexually transmitted disease caused by the bacterium *Neisseria gonorrhoeae;* male symptoms include discharge from the penis, women are generally asymptomatic.

**guided imagery** An approach to stress control, self-healing, or the motivation of life changes by means of visualizing oneself in the state of calmness, wellness, or change.

**hallucinogen** A drug that causes hallucinations.

**hashish** A concentrated form of cannabis containing the psychoactive ingredient TCH; causes a sense of euphoria when inhaled or eaten.

**health** A state of complete well-being, including physical, psychological, spiritual, social, intellectual, and environmental components.

**health maintenance organization (HMO)** An organization that provides health services on a fixed-contract basis.

**health promotion** An educational and informational process in which people are helped to change attitudes and behaviors in an effort to improve their health.

**heat cramps** Painful muscle spasms caused by vigorous exercise and heavy sweating in the heat.

**heat exhaustion** Faintness, rapid heart beat, low blood pressure, an ashen appearance, cold and clammy skin, and nausea, resulting from prolonged sweating with inadequate fluid replacement.

**heat stress** Physical response to prolonged exposure to high temperature; occurs simultaneously with or after heat cramps.

**heat stroke** A medical emergency consisting of a fever of at least 105° Fahrenheit, hot dry skin, rapid heartbeat, rapid and shallow breathing, and elevated or lowered blood pressure, caused by the breakdown of the body's cooling mechanism.

**helminth** A parasitic roundworm or flatworm.

**hepatitis** An inflammation and/or infection of the liver caused by a virus, often accompanied by jaundice.

**herbal medicine** An ancient form of medical treatment using substances derived from trees, flowers, ferns, seaweeds, and lichens to treat disease.

**herpes simplex** A condition caused by one of the herpes viruses and characterized by lesions of the skin or mucous membranes; herpes virus type 2 is sexually transmitted and causes genital blisters or sores.

**heterosexual** Primary sexual orientation toward members of the opposite sex.

**holistic** An approach to medicine that takes into account body, mind, emotions, and spirit.

**holographic will** A will wholly in the handwriting of its author.

**homeopathy** A system of medical practice that treats a disease by administering dosages of substances that would produce symptoms in healthy people similar to those of the disease.

**homeostasis** The body's natural state of balance or stability.

**homosexual** Primary sexual orientation toward members of the same sex.

**hormone replacement therapy (HRT)** The use of supplemental hormones during and after menopause.

**host** A person or population that contracts one or more pathogenic agents in an environment.

**human immune deficiency virus (HIV)** A type of virus that causes a spectrum of health problems, ranging from a symptomless infection to the development of life-threatening diseases because of impaired immunity.

**human papilloma virus (HPV)** A pathogen that causes genital warts and increases the risk of cervical cancer.

**humoral immunity** A portion of the immune response that provides lifelong protection against bacterial or viral infections, such as mumps, by means of antibodies whose production is triggered by the release of antigens upon first exposure to the infectious agent.

**hunger** The physiological drive to consume food.

**hypertension** High blood pressure occurring when the blood exerts excessive pressure against the arterial walls.

**hypothermia** An abnormally low body temperature; if not treated appropriately, coma or death could result.

**hysterectomy** The surgical removal of the uterus.

**hysterotomy** A procedure in which the uterus is surgically opened and the fetus inside it removed.

**immunity** Protection from infectious diseases.

**implantation** The embedding of the fertilized ovum in the uterine lining.

**incomplete proteins** Proteins that lack one or more of the amino acids essential for protein synthesis.

**incubation period** The time between a pathogen's entrance into the body and the first symptom.

**indoles** Naturally occurring chemicals found in foods such as winter squash, carrots, and crucifers; may help lower cancer risk.

**infertility** The inability to conceive a child.

**infiltration** A gradual penetration or invasion.

**inflammation** A localized response by the body to tissue injury, characterized by swelling and the dilation of the blood vessels.

**influenza** Illness caused by one of the highly contagious influenza viruses; symptoms include stuffy nose, headache, body aches, fever, and cough.

**informed consent** Permission (to undergo or receive a medical procedure or treatment) given voluntarily, with full knowledge and understanding of the procedure or treatment and its possible consequences.

**inhalants** Substances that produce vapors having psychoactive effects when inhaled.

**integrative medicine** An approach that combines traditional medicine with alternative and/or complementary therapies.

**intercourse** Sexual stimulation by means of entry of the penis into the vagina; coitus.

**interpersonal therapy (IPT)** A technique used to develop communication skills and relationships.

**intimacy** A state of closeness between two people, characterized by the desire and ability to share one's innermost thoughts and feelings with each other, both verbally and nonverbally.

**intoxication** Maladaptive behavioral, psychological, and physiologic changes that occur as a result of substance abuse.

**intramuscular** Into or within a muscle.

**intrauterine device (IUD)** A device inserted into the uterus through the cervix to prevent pregnancy by interfering with implantation.

**intravenous** Into a vein.

**irradiation** Exposure to or treatment by some form of radiation.

**isokinetic** Having the same force; exercise with specialized equipment that provides resistance equal to the force applied by the user throughout the entire range of motion.

**isometric** Of the same length; exercise in which muscles increase their tension without shortening in length, such as when pushing an immovable object.

**isotonic** Having the same tension or tone; exercise requiring the repetition of an action that creates tension, such as weight lifting or calisthenics.

**labia majora** The fleshy outer folds that border the female genital area.

**labia minora** The fleshy inner folds that border the female genital area.

**labor** The process leading up to birth: effacement and dilation of the cervix; the movement of the baby into and through the birth canal, accompanied by strong contractions; and contraction of the uterus and expulsion of the placenta after the birth.

**lacto-vegetarians** People who eat dairy products as well as fruits and vegetables (but not meat, poultry, or fish).

**Lamaze method** A method of childbirth preparation taught to expectant parents to help the woman cope with the discomfort of labor; combines breathing and psychological techniques.

**laparoscopy** A surgical sterilization procedure in which the fallopian tubes are observed with a laparoscope inserted through a small incision, and then cut or blocked.

**laparotomy** A surgical sterilization procedure in which the fallopian tubes are cut or blocked through an incision made in the abdomen.

**licensed clinical social worker (LCSW).** *See* certified social worker.

**lipoproteins** Compounds in blood that are made up of proteins and fat; a high-density lipoprotein (HDL) picks up excess cholesterol in the blood; a low-density lipoprotein (LDL) carries more cholesterol and deposits it on the walls of arteries.

**listeria** A bacterium commonly found in deli meats, hot dogs, and soft cheeses that can cause an infection called listeriosis.

**living will** A written statement providing instructions for the use of life-sustaining procedures in the event of terminal illness or injury.

**lochia** The vaginal discharge of blood, mucus, and uterine tissue that occurs after birth.

**locus of control** An individual's belief about the source of power and influence over his or her life.

**lumpectomy** The surgical removal of a breast tumor and its surrounding tissue.

**lymph nodes** Small tissue masses in which some immune cells are stored.

**macronutrients** Nutrients required by the human body in the greatest amounts, including water, carbohydrates, proteins, and fats.

**mainstream smoke** The smoke inhaled directly by smoking a cigarette.

**major depression** Sadness that does not end.

**male pattern baldness** The loss of hair at the vertex, or top, of the head.

**mammography** A diagnostic X-ray exam used to detect breast cancer.

**managed care** Health-care services and reimbursement predetermined by third-party insurers.

**marijuana** The drug derived from the cannabis plant, containing the psychoactive ingredient THC, which causes a mild sense of euphoria when inhaled or eaten.

**marriage and family therapist** A psychiatrist, psychologist, or social worker who specializes in marriage and family counseling.

**massage therapy** A therapeutic method of using the hands to rub, stroke, or knead the body to produce positive effects on an individual's health and well-being.

**mastectomy** The surgical removal of an entire breast.

**masturbation** Self-stimulation of the genitals, often resulting in orgasm.

**medical abortion** Method of ending a pregnancy within 9 weeks of conception using hormonal medications that cause expulsion of the fertilized egg.

**meditation** The use of quiet sitting, breathing techniques, and/or chanting to relax, improve concentration, and become attuned to one's inner self.

**meningitis** An extremely serious, potentially fatal illness in which the bacterium *Neisseria meningitis* attacks the membranes around the brain and spinal cord.

**menopause** The complete cessation of ovulation and menstruation for 12 consecutive months.

**menstruation** Discharge of blood from the vagina as a result of the shedding of the uterine lining at the end of the menstrual cycle.

**mental disorder** Behavioral or psychological syndrome associated with distress or a significantly increased risk of suffering pain, disability, loss of freedom, or death.

**mental health** The ability to perceive reality as it is, to respond to its challenges, and to develop rational strategies for living.

**metabolic syndrome** A cluster of symptoms that increases the risk of heart disease and diabetes.

**metastasize** To spread to other parts of the body via the bloodstream or the lymphatic system.

**micronutrients** Vitamins and minerals needed by the body in very small amounts.

**microwaves** Extremely high frequency electromagnetic waves that increase the rate at which molecules vibrate, thereby generating heat.

**mindfulness** A method of stress reduction that involves experiencing the physical and mental sensations of the present moment.

**minerals** Naturally occurring inorganic substances; small amounts of some minerals are essential in metabolism and nutrition.

**minilaparotomy** A surgical sterilization procedure in which the fallopian tubes are cut or sealed by electrical coagulation through a small incision just above the pubic hairline.

**minipill** An oral contraceptive containing a small amount of progestin and no estrogen; prevents contraception by making the mucus in the cervix so thick that sperm cannot enter the uterus.

**miscarriage** A pregnancy that terminates before the 20th week of gestation; also called *spontaneous abortion.*

**mononucleosis** An infectious viral disease characterized by an excess of white blood cells in the blood, fever, fatigue, bodily discomfort, a sore throat, and kidney and liver complications.

**monophasic pill** *See* constant-dose combination pill.

**mons pubis** The rounded, fleshy area over the junction of the female pubic bones.

**mood** A sustained emotional state that colors one's view of the world for hours or days.

**multiphasic pill** An oral contraceptive that releases different levels of estrogen and progestin to mimic the hormonal fluctuations of the natural menstrual cycle.

**multiple chemical sensitivity (MCS)** A sensitivity to low-level chemical exposure from ordinary substances, such as perfumes and tobacco smoke, that results in physiological responses such as chest pain, depression, dizziness, fatigue, and nausea. Also known as *environmentally triggered illness.*

**muscular fitness** The amount of strength and level of endurance in the body's muscles.

**mutagen** An agent that causes alterations in the genetic material of living cells.

**mutation** A change in the genetic material of a cell or cells that is brought about by radiation, chemicals, or natural causes.

**myocardial infarction (MI)** A condition characterized by the dying of tissue areas in the myocardium, caused by interruption of the blood supply to those areas; the medical name for a heart attack.

**naturopathy** An alternative system of treatment of disease that emphasizes the use of natural remedies such as sun, water, heat, and air. Therapies may include dietary changes, steam baths, and exercise.

**neoplasm** Any tumor, whether benign or malignant.

**nicotine** The addictive substance in tobacco; one of the most toxic of all poisons.

**non-exercise activity thermogenesis (NEAT)** The process of burning calories through nonvolitional activities such as walking and gardening.

**nongonococcal urethritis (NGU)** Inflammation of the urethra caused by organisms other than the gonococcus bacterium.

**nonopioids** Chemically synthesized drugs that have sleep-inducing and pain-relieving properties similar to those of opium and its derivatives.

**norms** The unwritten rules regarding behavior and conduct expected or accepted by a group.

**nutrition** The science devoted to the study of dietary needs for food and the effects of food on organisms.

**obesity** The excessive accumulation of fat in the body; a condition of having a body mass index (BMI) of 30 or above.

**obsessive-compulsive disorder (OCD)** An anxiety disorder characterized by obsessions and/or compulsions that impair one's ability to function and form relationships.

**opioids** Drugs that have sleep-inducing and pain-relieving properties, including opium (and its derivatives) and nonopioid, synthetic drugs.

**optimism** The tendency to seek out, remember, and expect pleasurable experiences.

**oral contraceptives** Preparations of synthetic hormones that inhibit ovulation; also referred to as *birth control pills* or simply *the pill.*

**organic** Term designating food produced with, or production based on the use of, fertilizer originating from plants or animals, without the use of pesticides or chemically formulated fertilizers.

**organic phosphates** Toxic pesticides that may cause cancer, birth defects, neurological disorders, and damage to wildlife and the environment.

**osteoporosis** A condition common in older people in which the bones become increasingly soft and porous, making them susceptible to injury.

**ovaries** The paired female sex organs that produce egg cells, estrogen, and progesterone.

**overload principle** Providing a greater stress or demand on the body than it is normally accustomed to handling.

**overloading** Method of physical training in which the number of repetitions or the amount of resistance is gradually increased to work the muscle to temporary fatigue.

**over-the-counter (OTC) drugs** Medications that can be obtained without a prescription from a medical professional (i.e., over the counter at a retail outlet).

**overtrain** Working muscles too intensely or too frequently, resulting in persistent muscle soreness, injuries, unintended weight loss, nervousness, and an inability to relax.

**overuse injuries** Physical injuries to joints or muscles, such as strains, fractures, and tendinitis, which result from overdoing a repetitive activity.

**overweight** A condition of having a body mass index (BMI) between 25.0 and 29.9.

**ovo-lacto-vegetarians** People who eat eggs, dairy products, and fruits and vegetables (but not meat, poultry, or fish).

**ovulation** The release of a mature ovum from an ovary approximately 14 days prior to the onset of menstruation.

**ovulation method** A method of birth control based on the observation of changes in the consistency of the mucus in the vagina to predict ovulation.

**ovum** (plural, **ova**) The female egg cell.

**panic attack** A short episode characterized by physical sensations of light-headedness, dizziness, hyperventilation, and numbness of extremities, accompanied by an inexplicable terror, usually of a physical disaster such as death.

**panic disorder** An anxiety disorder in which the apprehension or experience of recurring panic attacks is so intense that normal functioning is impaired.

**pathogen** A microorganism that produces disease.

**PCP (phencyclidine)** A synthetic psychoactive substance that produces effects similar to other psychoactive drugs when swallowed, smoked, sniffed, or injected, but may also trigger unpredictable behavioral changes.

**pelvic inflammatory disease (PID)** An inflammation of the internal female genital tract, characterized by abdominal pain, fever, and tenderness of the cervix.

**penis** The male organ of sex and urination.

**perimenopause** The period from a woman's first irregular cycles to her last menstruation.

**perinatology** The medical specialty concerned with the diagnosis and treatment of pregnant women with high-risk conditions and their fetuses.

**perineum** The area between the anus and vagina in the female and between the anus and scrotum in the male.

**phobia** An anxiety disorder marked by an inordinate fear of an object, a class of objects, or a situation, resulting in extreme avoidance behaviors.

**physical dependence** The physiological attachment to, and need for, a drug.

**physical fitness** The ability to respond to routine physical demands, with enough reserve energy to cope with a sudden challenge.

**phytochemicals** Chemicals that exist naturally in plants and have disease-fighting properties.

**placenta** An organ that develops after implantation and to which the embryo attaches, via the umbilical cord, for nourishment and waste removal.

**plaque** Deposits of fat, fibrin, cholesterol, calcium, and other cell parts on the lining of the arteries.

**pollutant** A substance or agent in the environment, usually the by-product of human industry or activity, that is injurious to human, animal, or plant life.

**pollution** The presence of pollutants in the environment.

**polyabuse** The misuse or abuse of more than one drug.

**postpartum depression** The emotional down-swing that occurs after having a baby due to hormonal changes, physical exhaustion, and psychological pressures.

**posttraumatic stress disorder (PTSD)** The repeated reliving of a trauma through nightmares or recollection.

**preconception care** Health care to prepare for pregnancy.

**precycling** The use of products that are packaged in recycled or recyclable material.

**preferred provider organization (PPO)** A group of physicians contracted to provide health care to members at a discounted price.

**premature labor** Labor that occurs after the 20th week but before the 37th week of pregnancy.

**premenstrual dysphoric disorder (PMDD)** A disorder that causes symptoms of psychological depression during the last week of a woman's menstrual cycle.

**premenstrual syndrome (PMS)** A disorder that causes physical discomfort and psychological distress prior to a woman's menstrual period.

**prevention** Information and support offered to help healthy people identify their health risks, reduce stressors, prevent potential medical problems, and enhance their well-being.

**progesterone** The female sex hormone that stimulates the uterus, preparing it for the arrival of a fertilized egg.

**progestin-only pill** *See* minipill.

**progressive overloading** Gradually increasing physical challenges once the body adapts to the stress placed upon it to produce maximum benefits.

**progressive relaxation** A method of reducing muscle tension by contracting, then relaxing certain areas of the body.

**proof** The alcoholic strength of a distilled spirit, expressed as twice the percentage of alcohol present.

**prostate gland** A structure surrounding the male urethra that produces a secretion that helps liquefy the semen from the testes.

**protection** Measures that an individual can take when participating in risky behavior to prevent injury or unwanted risks.

**protein** A substance that is basically a compound of amino acids; one of the essential nutrients.

**protozoa** Microscopic animals made up of one cell or a group of similar cells; their enzymes and toxins can harm or destroy healthy cells.

**psychiatric drugs** Medications that regulate a person's mental, emotional, and physical functions to facilitate normal functioning.

**psychiatric nurse** A nurse with special training and experience in mental health care.

**psychiatrist** Licensed medical doctor with additional training in psychotherapy, psychopharmacology, and treatment of mental disorders.

**psychoactive** Mood-altering.

**psychodynamic** Interpreting behaviors in terms of early experiences and unconscious influences.

**psychological dependence** The emotional or mental attachment to the use of a drug.

**psychologist** Mental health professional who has completed a doctoral or graduate program in psychology and is trained in a variety of psychotherapeutic techniques, but who is not medically trained and does not prescribe medications.

**psychoprophylaxis** *See* Lamaze method.

**psychotherapy** Treatment designed to produce a response by psychological rather than physical means, such as suggestion, persuasion, reassurance, and support.

**psychotropic** Mind-affecting.

**pyelonephritis** Inflammation of the kidney.

**quackery** Medical fakery; unproven practices claiming to cure diseases or solve health problems.

**rape** Sexual penetration of a female or a male by means of intimidation, force, or fraud.

**recycling** The processing or reuse of manufactured materials to reduce consumption of raw materials.

**reflexology** A treatment based on the theory that massaging certain points on the foot or hand relieves stress or pain in corresponding parts of the body.

**reinforcement** Reward or punishment for a behavior that will increase or decrease one's likelihood of repeating the behavior.

**relapse prevention** An alcohol recovery treatment method that focuses on social skills training to develop ways of preventing or minimizing a relapse.

**relative risk** The risk of developing cancer in persons with a certain exposure or trait compared to the risk in persons who do not have the same exposure or trait.

**resting heart rate** The number of heartbeats per minute during inactivity.

**reuptake** Reabsorption by the originating cell of neurotransmitters that have not connected with receptors and have been left in synapses.

**reversibility principle** The physical benefits of exercise are lost through disuse or inactivity.

**rhythm method** A birth-control method in which sexual intercourse is avoided during those days of the menstrual cycle in which fertilization is most likely to occur.

**rubella** An infectious disease that may cause birth defects if contracted by a pregnant woman; also called *German measles.*

**satiety** A feeling of fullness after eating.

**saturated fat** A chemical term indicating that a fat molecule contains as many hydrogen atoms as its carbon skeleton can hold. These fats are normally solid at room temperature.

**schizophrenia** A general term for a group of mental disorders with characteristic psychotic symptoms, such as delusions, hallucinations, and disordered thought patterns during the active phase of the illness, and a duration of at least six months.

**scrotum** The external sac or pouch that holds the testes.

**sedative-hypnotics** A drug that depresses the central nervous system, reduces activity, and induces relaxation and sleep; includes the benzodiazepines and the barbiturates.

**self-actualization** A state of wellness and fulfillment that can be achieved once certain human needs are satisfied; living to one's full potential.

**self-efficacy** Belief in one's ability to accomplish a goal or change a behavior.

**self-esteem** Confidence and satisfaction in oneself.

**self-talk** Repetition of positive messages about one's self-worth to learn more optimistic patterns of thought, feeling, and behavior.

**semen** The viscous whitish fluid that is the complete male ejaculate; a combination of sperm and secretions from the prostate gland, seminal vesicles, and other glands.

**seminal vesicles** Glands in the male reproductive system that produce the major portion of the fluid of semen.

**set** A person's expectations or preconceptions about a situation or experience; mind-set.

**set-point theory** The proposition that every person has an unconscious control system for keeping body fat (and therefore weight) at a predetermined level, or set point.

**sexual coercion** Sexual activity forced upon a person by the exertion of psychological pressure by another person.

**sexual orientation** The physiological, psychological, and social factors that attract a person to members of the same sex or members of the opposite sex.

**sexually transmitted diseases (STDs)** Any of a number of diseases that are acquired through sexual contact.

**sidestream smoke** The smoke emitted by a burning cigarette and breathed by everyone in a closed room, including the smoker; contains more tar and nicotine than mainstream smoke.

**simple carbohydrates** Sugars; like all carbohydrates, they provide the body with glucose.

**smog** A grayish or brownish haze caused by the presence of smoke and/or chemical pollutants in the air.

**social isolation** A feeling of unconnectedness with others caused by and reinforced by infrequency of social contacts.

**social phobia** A severe form of social anxiety marked by extreme fears and avoidance of social situations.

**specificity principle** Each part of the body adapts to a particular type and amount of stress placed upon it.

**sperm** The male reproductive cell produced by the testes and transported outside the body through ejaculation.

**spermatogenesis** The process by which sperm cells are produced.

**spinal block** An injection of anesthesia directly into the spinal cord to numb the lower body during labor and childbirth.

**spiritual health** The ability to identify one's basic purpose in life and to achieve one's full potential; the sense of connectedness to a greater power.

**spiritual intelligence** The capacity to sense, understand, and tap into ourselves, others, and the world around us.

**static flexibility** The ability to assume and maintain an extended position at one end point in a joint's range of motion.

**sterilization** A surgical procedure to end a person's reproductive capability.

**stimulant** An agent, such as a drug, that temporarily relieves drowsiness, helps in the performance of repetitive tasks, and improves capacity for work.

**strength** Physical power; the maximum weight one can lift, push, or press in one effort.

**stress** The nonspecific response of the body to any demands made upon it; may be characterized by muscle tension and acute anxiety, or may be a positive force for action.

**stressor** Specific or nonspecific agents or situations that cause the stress response in a body.

**stroke** A cerebrovascular event in which the blood supply to a portion of the brain is blocked.

**subcutaneous** Under the skin.

**suction curettage** A procedure in which the contents of the uterus are removed by means of suction and scraping.

**syphilis** A sexually transmitted disease caused by the bacterium *Treponema pallidum;* characterized by early sores, a latent period, and a final period of life-threatening symptoms including brain damage and heart failure.

**systemic disease** A pathologic condition that spreads throughout the body.

**systole** The contraction phase of the cardiac cycle.

**tar** A thick, sticky dark fluid produced by the burning of tobacco, made up of several hundred different chemicals, many of them poisonous, some of them carcinogenic.

**target heart rate** The heart rate at which one derives maximum cardiovascular benefit from aerobic exercise; 60 to 85 percent of the maximum heart rate.

**teratogen** Any agent that causes spontaneous abortion or defects or malformations in a fetus.

**testes** (singular, **testis**) The paired male sex organs that produce sperm and testosterone.

**testosterone** The male sex hormone that stimulates male secondary sex characteristics.

**toxicity** The dosage level at which a drug becomes poisonous to the body, causing either temporary or permanent damage.

**trans-fatty acids** Fats formed when liquid vegetable oils are processed to make table spreads or cooking fats, and also found in dairy and beef products; considered to be especially dangerous dietary fats.

**trichomoniasis** An infection of the protozoan *Trichomonas vaginalis;* females experience vaginal burning, itching, and discharge, but male carriers may be asymptomatic.

**triglycerides** Fats that flow through the blood after meals and that are linked to increased risk of coronary artery disease.

**tubal ligation** The suturing or tying shut of the fallopian tubes to prevent pregnancy.

**tubal occlusion** The blocking of the fallopian tubes to prevent pregnancy.

**12-step program** Self-help group program based on the principles of Alcoholics Anonymous.

**unsaturated fat** A fat molecule that contains fewer hydrogen atoms than its carbon skeleton can hold. These fats are normally liquid at room temperature.

**urethra** The canal through which urine from the bladder leaves the body; in the male, also serves as the channel for seminal fluid.

**urethral opening** The outer opening of the thin tube that carries urine from the bladder.

**urethritis** Infection of the urethra.

**uterus** The female organ that houses the developing fetus until birth.

**vagina** The canal leading from the exterior opening in the female genital area to the uterus.

**vaginal contraceptive film (VCF)** A small dissolvable sheet saturated with spermicide that can be inserted into the vagina and placed over the cervix.

**vaginal spermicide** A substance that kills or neutralizes sperm, inserted into the vagina as a foam, cream, jelly, or suppository.

**values** The criteria by which one makes choices about one's thoughts, actions, goals, and ideals.

**vas deferens** Two tubes that carry sperm from the epididymis into the urethra.

**vasectomy** A surgical sterilization procedure in which each vas deferens is cut and tied shut to stop the passage of sperm to the urethra for ejaculation.

**vector** A biological or physical vehicle that carries the agent of infection to the host.

**vegans** People who eat only plant foods.

**ventricles** The two lower chambers of the heart that pump blood out of the heart and into the arteries.

**video display terminal (VDT)** A screen or monitor that emits electromagnetic fields from all sides; these fields may lead to increased reproductive problems, miscarriages, low birthweights, and cataracts.

**virus** A submicroscopic infectious agent; the most primitive form of life.

**visualization** An approach to stress control, self-healing, or motivating life changes by means of guided imagery.

**vital signs** Measurements of physiological functioning: temperature, blood pressure, pulse rate, and respiration rate.

**vitamins** Organic substances that are needed in very small amounts by the body and that carry out a variety of functions in metabolism and nutrition.

**waist-to-hip ratio** The proportion of waist circumference to hip circumference; an indicator of cardiovascular disease risk.

**wellness** A state of optimal health.

**withdrawal** Development of symptoms that cause significant psychological and physical distress when an individual reduces or stops drug use.

**zygote** A fertilized egg.

# Photo Credits

**Chapter 1**

**p. 2,** © Lori Adamski Peek/Stone/Getty Images; **p. 4,** © David H. Wells/CORBIS; © Walter Hodges/CORBIS; © Kelly Harriger/CORBIS; **p. 6,** © AFP/CORBIS; **p. 7,** © Lorenzo Ciniglio/Corbis Sygma; **p. 20,** © Neil Rabinowitz/CORBIS

**Chapter 2**

**p. 26,** © Laurence Monneret/Stone/Getty Images; **p. 28,** © CORBIS; © 2000 PhotoDisc; **p. 34,** © Ulrike Welsch; **p. 36,** © Will and Deni McIntyre/Photo Researchers, Inc.; **p. 37,** AP/Wide World Photos; **p. 39,** © Richard T. Nowitz/Photo Researchers, Inc.; © CORBIS; **p. 41,** © CORBIS

**Chapter 3**

**p. 46,** © LWA-Dann Tardif/CORBIS; **p. 48,** © Susan Van Etten/Photo Edit; **p. 49,** David Young-Wolff/PhotoEdit; © Phil Schermeisater/CORBIS; **p. 52,** © Robert W. Ginn/PhotoEdit; **p. 54,** © Mark Richards/PhotoEdit; **p. 58,** © 2000 PhotoDisc, Inc.; **p. 59,** © David Young-Wolff/PhotoEdit; **p. 61,** Paul Avis/Getty Image; **p. 64,** Mary Kate Denny/PhotoEdit; **p. 65,** "My Head Is Going Round and Round" from *Art As Healing* by Edward Adamson/Coventure, Limited; **p. 67,** Michael Newman/PhotoEdit

**Chapter 4**

**p. 72,** © Warren Morgan/CORBIS; **p. 76,** © 2001 Lori Adamski Peek/Stone/Getty Images; © Jurgen Reisch/Stone/Getty Images; © Paul Almasy/CORBIS; © 2000 PhotoDisc, Inc.; **p. 81,** © 2001 PhotoDisc; © David Hanover; © David Hanover; **p. 83,** Left to Right, © Digital Vision/PictureQuest; © RubberBall Productions/PictureQuest; © RubberBall Productions/PictureQuest; © Duomo/CORBIS; **p. 86,** ©Jim Cummins/Taxi/Getty Images; **p. 87,** © 2000 PhotoDisc, Inc.; **p. 91,** © David Madison, all

**Chapter 5**

**p. 96,** © LWA-Stephen Welstead/CORBIS; **p. 99,** © Polara Studios, Inc.; **p. 114,** (left) Canada's Food Guide to Healthy Eating, http://www.hc-sc.gc.ca/hpfb-dgpsa/onppbppn/food_guide_rainbow_e.html, Health Canada, 1992 Reproduced with the permission of the Minister of Public Works and Government Services Canada, 2003 (right) Reproduced by kind permission of the Food Standards Agency; **p. 116,** © Marc Alcarez/Index Stock Imagery

**Chapter 6**

**p. 122,** © Bruce Dale/National Geographic/Getty Images; **p. 124,** © Christie's Images, London/SuperStock, Inc.;

**p. 132,** © Richard T. Nowitz/CORBIS; **p. 134,** © 2000 Bruce Ayres/Stone/Getty Images; **p. 139,** © Michael Newman/PhotoEdit

**Chapter 7**

**p. 144,** © M. J. Cardenas Productions/The Image Bank/Getty Images; **p. 146,** © 2000 David Roth/Stone/Getty Images; **p. 149,** © David Hanover/Stone/Getty Images; **p. 153,** © 2000 PhotoDisc, Inc.; Photo used with permission of Sylvia Chaney; **p. 161,** © 2000 Marc Dolphin/Stone/Getty Images; **p. 164,** © Deborah Davis/PhotoEdit; **p. 168,** © 2001 Carol Ford/Stone/Getty Images

**Chapter 8**

**p. 172,** © Stewart Cohen/Stone/Getty Images; **p. 179,** © Joel Gordon Photography; **p. 181,** Organon USA; Ortho-McNeil Pharmaceutical; **p. 182–190,** © Joel Gordon Photography; **p. 197,** AP/Wide World Photos; **p. 199,** © Petit Format/Nestle/ScienceSource/Photo Researchers, Inc.; **p. 201,** © SIU/Peter Arnold, Inc.; **p. 203,** © Dana Fineman/CORBIS-Sygma

**Chapter 9**

**p. 208,** © Andrew Brookes/CORBIS; **p. 213,** Boehringer Ingelheim International GmbH Photo Lennart Nilsson Bonnier Alba AB (both); **p. 214,** © F. Hoffman/The Image Works; **p. 216,** © Myrleen Ferguson Cate/PhotoEdit; **p. 226,** © LWA/CORBIS; **p. 228,** © Science VU/Visuals Unlimited; **p. 229,** St. Bartholomew's Hospital/Science Photo Library/Photo Researchers, Inc.; Biophoto Associates/Photo Researchers, Inc.; **p. 231,** © Marazzi/Photo Researchers, Inc.; © E. Gray/Photo Researchers, Inc.

**Chapter 10**

**p. 240,** © Bruce Ayres/Stone/Getty Images; **p. 243,** © Charles Gupton/Stock, Boston; **p. 253,** © Cabisco/Visuals Unlimited; © Sloop-Ober/Visuals Unlimited; **p. 254,** © 2000 Bruce Ayres/Stone/Getty Images; **p. 259,** © 2000 PhotoDisc, Inc.; **p. 260,** © Corbis Images; © Bill Crump/Brand X Pictures/PictureQuest; © 2001 PhotoDisc, Inc.; © Corbis Images; © 2001 PhotoDisc, Inc.; **p. 261,** © 2001 PhotoDisc, Inc.; **p. 262,** Courtesy of Skin Cancer Foundation; **p. 263,** © Will and Deni McIntyre/Photo Researchers, Inc.; **p. 266,** © Damien Lovegrove/Science Photo Library/Photo Researchers, Inc.

**Chapter 11**

**p. 272,** © Barbara Peacock/Taxi/Getty Images; **p. 278,** © CORBIS; **p. 290,** © TekImage/SPL/Photo Researchers, Inc.; **p. 293,** © Roy Morsch/CORBIS; **p. 295,** Mimi Forsyth

Photography; **p. 296,** © Oscar Burriel/Latin Stock/Photo Researchers, Inc.; **p. 297,** Hank Morgan/Science Source/ Photo Researchers, Inc.

### Chapter 12

**p. 302,** © Jim Bastardo/The Image Bank/Getty Images; **p. 309,** © 2000 PhotoDisc, Inc.; **p. 312,** © Evan Schneider Photography; **p. 314,** © Mark Richards/PhotoEdit; **p. 315,** © Michael Weisbrot/Stock, Boston; **p. 316,** © K. L. Jones/LLRResearch; **p. 317,** © Tony Freeman/ PhotoEdit; **p. 318,** © SuperStock, Inc.; **p. 319,** Mark Nielsen (both); **p. 326,** © Lawrence Migdale; **p. 329,** AP/Wide World Photos; **p. 329,** Leonard Morse/Medical Images; **p. 330,** Felicia Martinez/PhotoEdit; **p. 331,** Michael Newman/PhotoEdit; © David M. Grossman/ Photo Researchers, Inc.; © A. Ramey/PhotoEdit; **p. 333,** © Michael Newman/PhotoEdit; © Billy E. Barnes/Stock, Boston

### Chapter 13

**p. 338,** © Bruce Ayres/Stone/Getty Images; **p. 342,** © Michael Newman/PhotoEdit; © 2000 PhotoDisc, Inc.; **p. 346,** © 2000 PhotoDisc, Inc.; **p. 348,** © Kevin R. Morris/CORBIS; **p. 350,** © Tim Maloy/Paul Biddle/SPL/ Photo Researchers, Inc.

### Chapter 14

**p. 356,** © Zoom Agence/Allsport Concepts/Getty Images; **p. 360,** © 2000 PhotoDisc, Inc.; **p. 361,** © Tony Freeman/ PhotoEdit; **p. 362,** © Lewis Merrim/Photo Researchers, Inc.; **p. 367,** © Yvonne Hemsey/Gamma Liaison/Getty Images; **p. 368,** © 2000 PhotoDisc, Inc.; **p. 369,** © Rhoda Sidney/PhotoEdit; **p. 370,** © B. Mahoney/The Image Works

### Chapter 15

**p. 374,** © EyeWire Collection/Getty Images; **p. 377,** © 2000 PhotoDisc, Inc.; **p. 380,** © Mark Gibson/Lonely Planet Images; **p. 382,** © T. Yousseff/Custom Medical Stock Photo (both); **p. 387,** David Young-Wolff/PhotoEdit; **p. 391,** A. Ramey/PhotoEdit; **p. 392,** Sybil Shackman

### Chapter 16

**p. 398,** © Tom Stewart/CORBIS; **p. 401,** Glenn M. Oliver/Visuals Unlimited; **p. 403,** David Young-Wolff/ PhotoEdit; **p. 406,** © James Keyser/Time, Inc.; **p. 409,** © 2000 Paul Grebliunas/Stone/Getty Images

# Index